Steve,

May all of your canals be straight,
May all of your exposures be planned,
May all your instruments have
clean white filings and,
May you never hear the word perforate.

Thanks for everything and please keep in touch.

Bill

6/16/76

To Steve;

With my very best regards.
I hope you find it useful in your career.

Don Morse

CLINICAL ENDODONTOLOGY

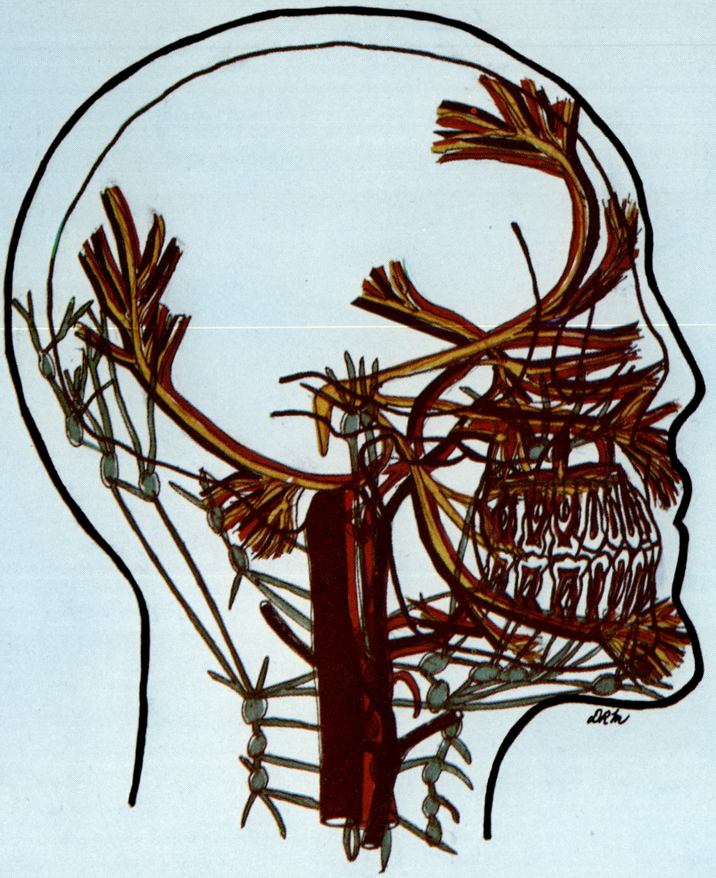

NERVE, BLOOD, AND LYMPH SUPPLY TO TEETH AND ASSOCIATED REGIONS

Frontispiece

CLINICAL ENDODONTOLOGY

A Comprehensive Guide to Diagnosis,
Treatment and Prevention

Text and Illustrations by

DONALD R. MORSE, B.S., D.D.S., M.A.

Associate Professor and Former Director
Advanced Education Division
Acting Chairman and Director
Predoctoral Division
Department of Endodontology
Temple University School of Dentistry
Diplomate American Board of Endodontics
Active Member American Academy of Implant Dentistry
Member American Society for Microbiology
Member American Analgesia Society

With a Foreword by

Samuel Seltzer, B.S., D.D.S.

Professor, Former Chairman,
Director Advanced Education Division
Department of Endodontology
Temple University School of Dentistry
Diplomate and President
American Board of Endodontics

CHARLES C THOMAS · PUBLISHER
Springfield · Illinois · U. S. A.

Published and Distributed Throughout the World by

CHARLES C THOMAS • PUBLISHER
Bannerstone House
301-327 East Lawrence Avenue, Springfield, Illinois, U. S. A.

ISBN 0-398-03121-5

Library of Congress Catalog Card Number: 74-718

With THOMAS BOOKS careful attention is given to all details of manufacturing and design. It is the Publisher's desire to present books that are satisfactory as to their physical qualities and artistic possibilities and appropriate for their particular use. THOMAS BOOKS will be true to those laws of quality that assure a good name and good will.

Printed in the United States of America
C-1

Library of Congress Cataloging in Publication Data

Morse, Donald R.
Clinical endodontology: a comprehensive guide to diagnosis, treatment, and prevention.

1. Endodontics. I. Title. [DNLM: 1. Endodontics. WU230 M884c 1974]
RK351.M67 617.6'34 74-718
ISBN 0-398-03121-5

To

Dr. Samuel Seltzer, without whose inspiration and assistance it never would have been written, and to Diane, my lovely wife, and Andy, Brian and Caryn, my wonderful children, for their considerable patience and understanding.

FOREWORD

DENTISTRY IS FINALLY EMERGING from its cocoon. The art and mechanics have always been necessary. Dentists are practitioners of a healing branch of medicine. As such, they have always needed to be craftsmen—gentle in touch and delicate in manipulation. Knowing "how to" has always been important. Now, a new breed is emerging. Being an excellent craftsman is no longer adequate. Knowing "why to" is assuming its rightful significance. It is axiomatic that correct diagnosis dictates correct treatment. The days of needless and ruthless extraction of teeth are over. People need their teeth, want their teeth and are psychologically upset at the thought of losing their teeth. And rightly so! Patients have every right to expect their dentists to advise them on methods of prevention of all types of dental disease. They have the right to expect their dentists to know how to prevent pulp and periapical disease. They have the right to expect their dentists to differentiate between pain of dental and non-dental origin. They have the right to expect their dentists to know the effects of dental disease on systemic health. They have the right to expect their dentists to know the interactions of drugs prescribed. Finally, they have the right to expect their dentists to plan and perform optimum treatment. All of these expectations can be accomplished by a profession which is dedicated to educating dentists who are inquisitive, knowledgable and trained in the scientific method. Furthermore, the dentist should be stimulated to keep abreast of the literature and to remain a continuing student.

In my view, this book, "Clinical Endodontology," takes a giant step toward accomplishing the objectives of progressive dental education. It is a book that serves the needs of the present-day curriculum and points the way toward the future. I am proud to have been responsible, in a small way, for providing some of the stimulus needed for its preparation. However, Donald Morse deserves tremendous credit for his devotion and dedication in the preparation of this book. How well I know the toil and turmoil needed to write a book of such tremendous breadth and scope. I congratulate him for this outstanding achievement. A dentist who knows and understands the material in this book will have gone a long way toward becoming the kind of dentist that every patient deserves.

SAMUEL SELTZER, D.D.S.

PREFACE

PATIENTS WHO COME to the dental office in extreme pain and/or swelling desire one thing; relief. Heretofore, many patients with similar symptoms obtained relief only after removal of the involved teeth. However, in recent years, many dentists and patients have become aware of the effectiveness of endodontic therapy, to allow for the retention of previously infected teeth. It is now known that extreme pain and swelling by themselves, are not contraindications to endodontic therapy.

There has also been a renewed interest in prevention in dentistry and as a result many patients who were formerly seen by general practitioners and oral surgeons for extractions are now being seen by general practitioners and endodontists for endodontic therapy. Endodontic therapy, along with proper periodontal and restorative procedures, provides a basis for saving teeth. The maintenance of natural teeth can have important psychic rewards for many patients. The loss of teeth may create tremendous psychologic trauma, that may be conscious or unconscious. There is also ample proof that natural teeth function much better than artificial replacements.

General practitioners and endodontists are now engaged in treating patients with severe oral pain, swelling, and periapical lesions. Therefore it becomes imperative that these practitioners have the facility to correctly evaluate the cause of these clinical manifestations. It is extremely important that these dental practitioners are aware of all aspects of differential diagnosis. Especially relevant is the differential diagnosis of head and neck pain, swelling, and bony lesions. A complete medical history is essential, because in the age bracket of many endodontic patients, chronic and degenerative diseases may be present. The presence of these disease conditions can affect the decision for or against treatment, the type of treatment rendered, and the outcome of treatment. Also, patients may be taking a wide variety of drugs, some of the most damaging of which may be self-prescribed. Interactions can take place between the drugs patients are taking, drugs the dentist prescribes, natural metabolites, foods the patients are taking, and external irritants. The dentist must be aware of the consequences of these potential interactions.

New findings have been discovered relative to the etiology of pulpal and periapical disease. Prevention of pulpal and periapical damage must be an important consideration for general dentists as well as endodontists. There are also new and improved methods of diagnosis and treatment of endodontically-involved teeth. It is therefore imperative that dental practitioners have the facility to diagnose, treat, and prevent pulpal and periapical conditions, as well as the ability to refer non-endodontic cases to the appropriate specialist.

As a result of these various considerations, this book was written. Rather than just adding another clinical book to the already expanding list of endodontic texts, it was felt that a book that stressed diagnosis, treatment planning, and prevention was needed. Therefore, although treatment is considered, a complete discussion of this aspect of clinical endodontology is not included. However, all treatment methodologies are covered. It is hoped that this book will prove useful to the student, the general practitioner, and the endodontist. Oral surgeons, periodontists, oral pathologists, pedodontists, oral radiologists, and physicians may also find certain sections to be of interest.

The book is written in the form of a step-by-step guide through diagnostic procedures, treatment planning considerations, methods of prevention, and methods of treatment. The basic sciences: anatomy, biochemistry, histology, microbiology, pathology, pharmacology, and physiology are considered only as they relate to the clinical concepts covered.

The book is composed of four divisions. The first division is involved with diagnosis. Chapter 1 is concerned with diagnostic factors, with the endodontic relevance of all aspects of the medical and dental history discussed. Examination procedures and diagnostic tests are detailed. Chapter 2 is devoted to the differential diagnosis of endodontic lesions from non-endodontic lesions and normal anatomic landmarks and physiological conditions.

The second division is concerned with treatment planning. For each condition presented, one or more alternative treatments are discussed.

In the third division, an account of all treatment procedures in the discipline of endodontology is presented. There are chapters on drug therapy, analgesia and anesthesia, pulp conservation treatments, acute situation treatments, nonsurgical endodontic therapy, periapical surgery, root amputation and hemisection, plantation procedures, bleaching, restorations, sterilization procedures, endodontic aids, and medical emergencies.

The fourth division is devoted to prevention in endodontic practice. Among the subjects discussed are techniques and methods to prevent endodontic diseases, caries control methods, prevention of extraction, prevention of treatment complications, and prevention of retreatments. The appendix is limited to medical tests, giving both normal values and abnormal ranges of endodontically-relevant diseases and conditions, calcification and eruption times of teeth and a table of drug interactions.

ACKNOWLEDGEMENTS

THE CREATION OF A TEXTBOOK is never an individual undertaking; many people have helped me in my efforts. I hope that these acknowledgements can in some way let all my friends know that I appreciate everything that was done on my behalf.

To

DR. JOEL WEISS, clinical assistant professor, department of endodontology, Temple University School of Dentistry, for proofreading the entire text. The suggestions were appreciated.

MR. ALEX V. MUCHA, director of visual education, Temple University School of Dentistry, for the excellence of the photographic reproductions of both my illustrations and of the many pathologic cases. If the illustrations are favorably received, much of the credit must go to Mr. Mucha.

DR. LES MULDORF, second year graduate student, department of endodontology, Temple University School of Dentistry, for the many excellent clinical photographs and for his clinical cases.

DR. MARVIN GROSS, clinical associate professor and director graduate clinic, department of endodontology, Temple University School of Dentistry, for his contribution to the chapter on periapical surgery and for his clinical cases.

DR. GEORGE BIRON, clinical assistant professor and director undergraduate clinic, department of endodontology, Temple University School of Dentistry, for his contribution to the chapter on nonsurgical endodontics therapy.

DR. HAROLD NAZIMOFF, formerly clinical assistant professor, department of endodontology, Temple University School of Dentistry, for his contribution to the chapter on endodontic aids.

DR. KURT BOMZE, diplomate, American Board of Pedodontics, for his contribution to the pedodontic-endodontics section and for his clinical cases.

DR. NORMAN SIEGEL, diplomate, American Board of Internal Medicine and Hematology, for his contribution to the section on hemorrhagic disorders.

DR. THEODORE SIMPSON, professor and chairman, department of oral diagnosis, Temple University School of Dentistry, for the outstanding collection of pathological cases that he allowed me to use. Without these cases, the diagnosis division would have been incomplete. Thanks also to the other members of the department who have helped in the collection.

DR. WILLIAM UPDEGRAVE, professor and chairman, department of radiology, Temple University School of Dentistry, for the many interesting radiographs that he allowed me to reproduce.

DR. I. B. BENDER, formerly president, American Association of Endodontists, for the use of his radiographs of bony diseases and for the use of pictures from *The Dental Pulp*.

DR. SAMUEL SELTZER, professor and chairman, department of endodontology, Temple University School of Dentistry, for the use of his histologic pictures and for the use of pictures from *The Dental Pulp* and *Endodontology*.

DR. DAVID LITWACK, associate professor, departments of periodontology and pathology, Temple University School of Dentistry, for the use of his pathologic cases.

DR. ALAN SCHLOSSBERG, assistant professor, department of periodontology, Temple University School of Dentistry, for the use of his clinical cases and for his advice.

DR. ROBERT LOEB, endodontist in Babylon, New York, for the use of cases of his polycarboxylate obturation technique.

DR. WALTER SOLTANOFF, DR. HERBERT SPASSER, DR. NOAH CHIVIAN, DR. JAN LEVY, DR. RON WOLLARD, DR. CALVIN LEIFER, DR. ELIE WOLFSON and DR. SEYMOUR GOLDMAN, for the use of their clinical cases.

DR. ROBERT THOMPSON, assistant professor of pharmacology, Temple University School of Pharmacy, for his help in the sections on drugs.

MS. MARY GARDNER, medical illustrator, Temple University School of Dentistry, for her advice on medical illustrations.

ALL MY GRADUATE STUDENTS, for their thoughtful suggestions.

MS. ANN CARNEY, ALBERTA O'HARGAN, MARY FLYNN, JUNE BIRNBAUM, GILDA SEGAL, and LAURIE FURMAN, for their help in the typing of the manuscript and finally to MR. PETER FINLEY and MR. PAYNE THOMAS of Charles C Thomas, Publisher, for their sincere cooperation in the publication of this text.

CONTENTS

CLINICAL ENDODONTOLOGY

DIVISION ONE

DIAGNOSIS

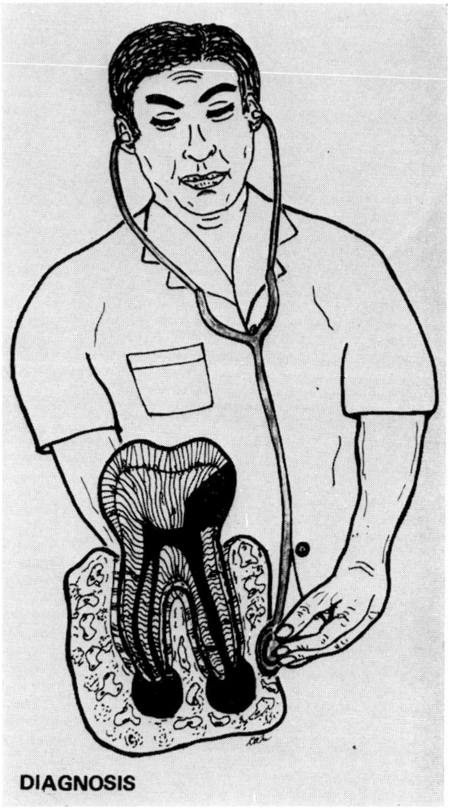

CHAPTER 1

DIAGNOSTIC FACTORS

The personal information, medical history, and oral history are determined by having the patient fill out and sign a detailed history form, followed by the patient answering leading questions. The diseases and questions involved in the questionnaire and their relevance to endodontics are discussed below. After the history is completed, a visual examination is made. This is followed by diagnostic tests, such as radiographs, pulp testing, palpation, mobility, and percussion. Any medical tests that are deemed appropriate are taken or ordered. Any necessary medical and dental consultations are made. Upon completion of the history, visual examination, objective tests, and consultations, the dentist is ready to make a differential diagnosis.

PERSONAL INFORMATION

The patient's name, address, telephone number, age, sex, race, nationality, religion, height, weight, occupation, family physician, family dentist (if an endodontist is treating the patient), and family pharmacy are obtained. All of these factors are necessary. There are certain diseases more prevalent among particular races, religions, age groups, sexes and occupations. Also, drug dosages may have to be altered for some of these factors.

Name

The patient's surname may give you some clue to his nationality.

Address

The neighborhood that the patient lives in may also give some clue to the patient's race, nationality and religion. Certain diseases are more prevalent among people living in crowded neighborhoods. An example is tuberculosis. Water is fluoridated in some locations and not in others. Some of the former residents may have enamel fluorosis (mottled enamel) (Fig. 1). Polluted city air contains carbon monoxide, hydrocarbons, sulfur, nitrogen and phosphorus compounds and many other chemicals. Some of these agents may interfere with drugs the dentist prescribes (See section on drug interactions).

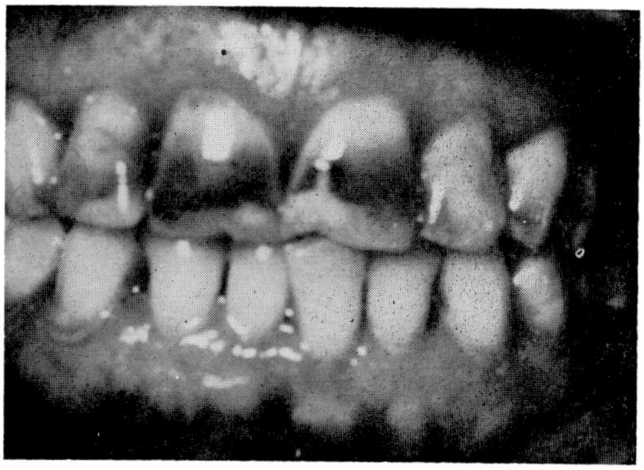

Figure 1. Enamel fluorosis. ("Mottled enamel," Courtesy of Dr. T. Simpson, Philadelphia, Pa.)

Age

Some women patients are reluctant to reveal their age, and the dentist may have to make a calculated guess. Most infectious diseases are more severe in the very young and the very old. The infant possesses a lesser reserve of dietary material and has fewer antibodies to infectious organisms than does an older individual. In the aged, arteriosclerotic changes occur in blood vessels with consequent reduction in blood flow. Increased viscosity of ground substance, increased fibrosis of connective tissue, and less lymphatic tissue (source of antibodies), makes repair more difficult in the aged. Certain diseases, such as cherubism are seen primarily in the young. Prognosis for endodontic therapy is poorer in older people. In the very young and the very old, drug dose has to be decreased relative to the average adult. A useful formula for the compilation of a child's dose is the surface area rule. The formula is $0.7 \times$ wgt in lbs $+ 10 =$ % of adult dose.

Sex

Infectious and cardiovascular diseases are more severe in males than females. This is probably related to the female hormones. The estrogens are important in aiding repair, and they appear to deter atherosclerotic changes in blood vessels. Postmenopausal women (with markedly decreased estrogens) have difficulties in healing. This can be observed in the occasional retention of periapical areas following endodontic therapy. Postmenopausal patients also have an increased incidence of cardiovascular disease.

Race

Sickle Cell Anemia is a genetic disease with possible oral manifestations that occurs predominantly in blacks. Oriental patients may have genetically-determined extra roots and root canals.

Nationality

Cooley's Anemia is another genetic disease that can show oral changes. It occurs primarily in Mediterranean types such as Italians and Greeks.

Religion

Certain diseases are found principally in individuals of a particular religion. Examples are diabetes mellitus and Gaucher's disease which are found predominately in Jews.

Occupation

There are diseases more prevalent among workers in certain industries. The following are examples of diseases with oral manifestations:

(1) Radiation workers have a higher incidence of leukemia.

(2) Workers in industrial chemical plants often have stained teeth and gingiva. Some of the chemicals that may be involved are arsenic, mercury, bismuth, phosphorus, copper, iron, chromium, silver, and lead.

(3) Citrus workers may have extensive dental erosion (Fig. 2).

(4) Occupational dental abrasion can occur with the following classes of workers: seamstresses, upholsterers (Fig. 3), carpenters, shoemakers, glass blowers, musi-

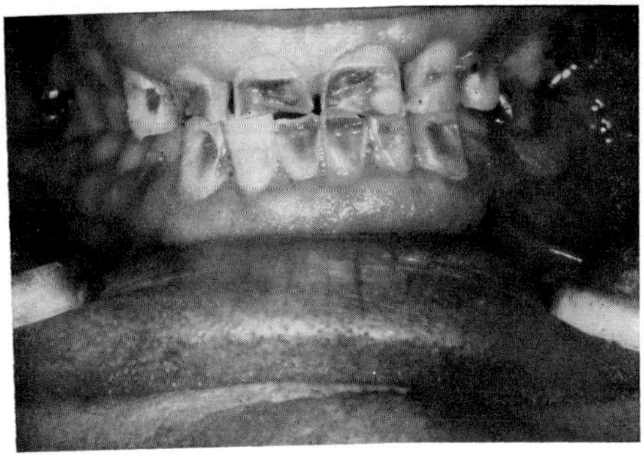

Figure 2. Extensive erosion of anterior teeth. (Courtesy of Dr. T. Simpson, Philadelphia, Pa.)

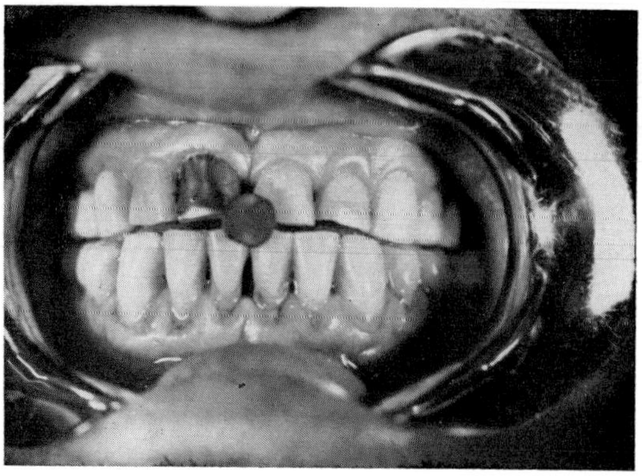

Figure 3. Upholsterer with a tack between the central incisors; a cause of abrasion. (Courtesy of Dr. T. Simpson, Philadelphia, Pa.)

cians, hairdressers, and policemen (whistle blowing).

(5) Granulomatous disease (e.g. silicosis) can occur among workers in coal and other mines, factories where excessive dust is produced (such workers as rock drillers, sand blasters and foundrymen), and dental lab technicians.

(6) Osteosclerotic bone changes can be seen in workers in phosphorus mines.

Height and Weight

Obese individuals have greater tendencies toward certain diseases such as diabetes and cardiac diseases. Very thin patients are predisposed toward anemias and tuberculosis. Drug dosages may have to be modified for these individuals, with obese patients requiring more of the particular drug (because of greater surface area to affect, poorer circulation and sluggish metabolism). Thin individuals would require less (because of lesser surface area, presumably better circulation and faster metabolism).

Family Physician

This is essential to know as medical consultation is frequently necessary. The dentist should also have recorded the name of specialists (such as cardiologists or internists) by whom the patient is currently being treated.

Family Dentist

If an endodontist is treating the patient, it is important for him or her to know the name of the general practitioner involved in the case. There are often discussions between the general practitioner and the endodontist. Also if there are other specialists involved in the case, such as periodontists, this should be noted on the patient's record.

Family Pharmacy

This is important to know as the dentist may have to telephone a prescription (which must be followed by a written prescription sent to the pharmacy). Also, the dentist may want to call the pharmacist to verify that the patient had received a particular prescription. The dentist may also want to check whether the patient has received too much of a particular drug. Some patients are addicted to drugs and go from one practitioner to the next to fulfill their need. The dentist may also want to know what other drugs the patient is taking because of possible drug interactions.

SUBJECTIVE

This section includes the systemic history, the oral history, and the visual examination.

Systemic History

This covers past history, current manifestations, habits, and drug, nutritional supplement, and food intake.

Miscellaneous Cardiac Diseases

These include rheumatic fever, heart murmur (functional or not), congenital heart disease, and bacterial endocarditis. Symptoms and signs of rheumatic fever include previous acute hemolytic streptococcal infection (several days to several weeks before), fever, carditis, joint pain, chorea, erythema, subcutaneous nodules, epistasis, abdominal pain, anorexia, sore throat, weight loss, fatigability, and weakness. Carditis manifestations include palpitations, precordial pain, heart murmurs, possible heart enlargement, and electrocardiograph changes. Patients with subacute bacterial endocarditis usually have had a previous history of rheumatic heart disease or congenital heart disease. The clinical manifestations are insidious and slow to occur. They include weakness, low grade fever, anorexia, malaise, chills, sweating, painful joints, finger and toe nodules (Osler nodes), petechiae, significant heart murmurs, and signs and symptoms attributable to emboli in various organs. In approximately 5 to 10 per cent of the cases, a history is given of extraction or a manipulative dental procedure 2 to 3 weeks prior to the onset of manifestations.

The dentist must premedicate patients with heart murmurs with antibiotics before performing manipulative endodontic procedures.* This is because of the possibility of oral microbes being disseminated into the blood stream and becoming fixed to damaged heart valves. The resultant disease, subacute bacterial endocarditis, is very serious and difficult to treat. The dentist should premedicate these patients with penicillin before each visit. If a patient is allergic to this drug, then erythromycin should be used. The treatment schedule as recommended by the American Heart Association is the following: procaine penicillin G, 600,000 units plus crystalline penicillin G, 200,000 units intramuscularly one hour before the procedure. The same dose is given for the following two days. In cooperative patients, oral penicillin can be substituted. The dosage schedule is 500 mg of penicillin V (V-cillin-K®, Pen-V-K®, Compocillin V-K®) or potassium phenethicillin (Darcil®, Maxpen®, Syncillin®) one hour before the procedure. A 250 mg dose every six hours is given for the remainder of that day and for the following two days. Penicillin G (Pentids 400®) can be substituted if the patient takes the pills at least one hour before eating or two hours after

* Recent findings have shown that chronic drug abusers may have heart valve damage and should also be premedicated with antibiotics.

eating (to prevent gastric inactivation). The dose schedule is 1,200,000 units one hour before the procedure; then 600,000 units every 6 hours for the remainder of that day and for the following two days. For patients who are allergic to penicillin or who are being maintained on continuous oral penicillin to prevent recurrences of rheumatic fever, erythromycin (e.g. Erythrocin® stearate, Ilosone®) should be used. The dose is 500 mg one and one-half to two hours prior to the procedure and then 250 mg every six hours for the following two days.

The dentist should ask the patient before the visit whether he (or she) has taken the medication. The case should be performed in as few visits as possible in order to decrease the number of possible bacteremias.

Cardiovascular Diseases

These include coronary insufficiency, angina pectoris, coronary thrombosis, coronary occlusion, myocardial infarction, arteriosclerosis, atherosclerosis, circulatory diseases, hypertension, congestive heart failure, cardiac arrythmias, and cerebral stroke. The dentist must check with the family physician or cardiologist about the use of the following classes of drugs: antibiotics, sedatives, anticoagulants, vasoconstrictors, antihypertensives, analgesics, diuretics, antiarrhythmics, digitalis-type drugs, and vasodilators. Also to be discussed is whether the patient can have complete therapy including surgery or only palliative treatment.

General manifestations of cardiac diseases are dyspnea (difficulty in breathing), chest pains after exercise that may radiate down the left arm (angina pectoris symptom), bluish coloration of lips or fingernails, and ankle edema. Manifestations and treatment of cardiac emergencies are discussed in chapter 16. It has been reported that in patients with edema, who only take their medications at particular periods, flare-ups can occur during endodontic therapy. These flare-ups occur during the period when the patient is not on their anti-diuretic therapy (for the treatment of edema) and may be related to periapical fluid accumulation.

It has been shown that administration of a local anesthetic and the start of surgery causes considerable anxiety in angina patients. A good preventative procedure is to administer one tablet of nitroglycerine (0.4-0.6 mg) two minutes before the start of therapy. For severe reactions, a physician should be called immediately and emergency treatment should be instituted (See Chapter 16).

In treating cardiac patients, there are certain considerations to be taken. Patients should be relaxed. Premedication with sedatives is often necessary. The use of nitrous oxide analgesia, along with adequate local anesthesia is helpful. According to the American Heart Association, the endogenous production of epinephrine is much greater when a local anesthetic without a vasoconstrictor is used (Procaine HCl® 2%, Lidocaine HCl® 2%, Xylocaine HCl® 2%) than the amount of epinephrine from a local anesthetic (concentration of 1:100,000 epinephrine) that could get into the general circulation. However, if the cardiac patients are taking one of the antihypertensive drugs such as the veratrum alkaloids, the organic nitrates, the organic nitrites, the rauwolfia alkaloids, or the ganglionic blocking agents, then epinephrine should not be used. The interaction of epinephrine with any of these antihypertensive drugs could cause the development of a severe hypotensive episode. A local anesthetic without epinephrine should be used for these patients. Examples of drugs that result in good local anesthesia without an added vasoconstrictor are mepivacaine HCl (Carbocaine HCl® 3%), and prilocaine HCl (Citanest HCl® 4%).

Generally, antibiotics should be used only when there are dental indications, such as cellulitis. Cardiac patients usually take narcotic analgesics during their treatment; therefore narcotics can be used during endodontic therapy. Caution must be exercised as addiction to these drugs is a possibility. Many patients who have had *heart attacks* are taking anticoagulants such as bishydroxycoumarin (Dicumarol®), warfarin sodium (Coumadin®), phenindione (Denilone®, Hedulin®), and heparin. Surgical procedures in these individuals might be complicated by serious hemorrhage. Dose adjustments may be necessary. Consultation with the patient's physician is imperative. However, vital pulp extirpation causes very little hemorrhage and is preferable to extraction. Recently, surgical procedures have been performed successfully without modification of the anticoagulant regimen. Use of adequate sutures, firm pressure, hemostatic aids such as thrombin, and careful handling of the tissues have been employed. Nevertheless, it is preferable to perform nonsurgical endodontics for these patients.

Cardiac patients can be taking one of the aforementioned antihypertensive drugs. These drugs can cause patients to develop postural hypotension or syncope. Sudden changes in position can cause temporary loss of consciousness.

Patients with congestive heart failure and cardiac arrhythmias can be taking several drugs that can have oral implications.

Digitalis and Related Drugs. These drugs can cause nausea and vomiting. Therefore the dentist should try not to stimulate the vomiting reflex. The tetracyclines and lincomycin should not be used for these patients as diarrhea can result. The diarrhea results in potassium loss, and this effect increases the toxicity of digitalis.

Antiarrhythmics, Such as Quinidine and Procainamide HCl. Procainamide can cause agranulocytosis to occur, with the oral manifestation of necrotizing gingivitis.

Diuretics. Mercurial diuretics may cause an acute stomatitis to occur. Acetazolamide can cause facial paresthesia. Diuretics can also cause xerostomia to occur.

Patients who have pacemakers present should not have their teeth pulp tested with an electric pulp tester, as there is a possibility that the latter can interfere with the action of the pacemaker. The use of electrocautery on these patients should also be avoided because of possible interference with pacemaker action.

Sinusitis

Sinusitis manifestations can simulate endodontic conditions. Signs and symptoms of nasal or sinus disturbances are fluid discharge from the nose, post-nasal drip into the throat, clogging of nasal passages, sneezing, nasal bleeding, and feeling of fullness in the sinuses. Pain may be referred to the upper anterior teeth for nasal and frontal sinus conditions. For maxillary sinus conditions, pain can be referred to upper posterior teeth. When the roots of infected upper anterior teeth are in close apposition to the nasal fossae, nasal infection may result. Infected posterior teeth may occasionally cause a maxillary sinusitis.

Respiratory Diseases

These conditions include frequent colds, a deviated septum, bronchitis, influenza, and pneumonia. Past or present history of these conditions indicate that the patients' general resistance is poor. If the patient currently has one of these disease states, the use of nitrous oxide analgesia is contraindicated. This is because dissemination of microbes could occur or nasal breathing could be impaired. It is possible, but not probable, that lung infections can be intensified if virulent or large numbers of avirulent oral microbes are aspirated. Pentazocine HCl (Talwin®) and strong narcotics should not be used if the lungs are compromised, as these drugs can cause respiratory depression. The sedative paraldehyde is contraindicated in patients with lung complications, as it is partially metabolized in the lungs. It has been reported that during influenza epidemics, a small proportion of patients develop toothaches. This may be related to the pan-sinusitis that can occur during an influenza attack.

Recurrent Sore Throats, Laryngitis and Inflamed Tonsils

These conditions are also indicative of lowered general resistance. The inflamed tissues could be a site for dissemination of microbes into the blood stream. Whether or not the microbes can become fixed to necrotic pulps or periapical *areas* (anachoresis) is debatable. Tonsillitis can cause a regional lymphadenopathy which may be confused with a pulpally-induced lymphadenopathy.

Allergic Conditions

These conditions include asthma, emphysema, hay fever, hives, and allergies to food or drugs. These allergic individuals must be carefully checked. Patients with asthma, emphysema, hay fever, and hives may also be allergic to drugs the dentist may prescribe. They may also be more prone to hypersensitivity-type cellulitis reactions. Consultation with the patients' physician (or allergist) is mandatory. For patients who are allergic to drugs, the dentist should ascertain the type of reaction, e.g. rash, swelling, shock, or fever, and what particular drug incited the reaction. Regarding local anesthetics, many patients think that they had an allergic reaction, when they actually had a psychogenic reaction. Psychogenic reactions include accelerated heart beat and syncope (fainting). Other possible nonallergic reactions that patients may have to local anesthetic injections are a toxic reaction to the anesthetic resulting in first stimulation and then depression of the central nervous system, and a systemic reaction to the vasoconstrictor resulting in an accelerated heart beat and a rise in blood pressure. Even if a patient has a history of allergic reactions to a local anesthetic such as a rash, swelling, or bronchial constriction, it is possible that the reaction was not due to the local anesthetic per se, but rather to one of the preservatives used in the local anesthetic mixture. Some of the preservatives that can be allergenic are methylparaben and propylparaben. The preservative sodium bisulfite is much less allergenic than either of the other two mentioned. Also, allergy to procaine-type local anesthetics is much more prevalent than allergy to lidocaine-type derivatives. If a patient is truly allergic to a local anesthetic, then there are certain alternative treatments.

(1) If the local anesthetic that the patient is allergic to is an amine-type (e.g. procaine), then an amide-type of local anesthetic (e.g. lidocaine) can be used.

(2) If no local anesthetic can be used, then an antihistamine (e.g. Benadryl®, Pyribenzamine®) may be tried as the latter type drugs do have local anesthetic properties (See Chapter 5).

(3) If none of these drugs can be used, a mummification procedure can be attempted to devitalize the pulp (See Chapter 5).

(4) Other possible methods that can be used are hypnosis, chemical or inhalation analgesia, and general anesthesia (See Chapter 5).

Other drugs used in endodontics that patients might be allergic to include antibiotics, sulfonamides, analgesics, resins, sedatives, zinc oxide and eugenol compounds, and mercury (from amalgam fillings). Skin testing can be used as an aid in determining hypersensitivity to drugs, although allergists find that it is not always reliable.

Patients with asthma often do well under nitrous oxide analgesia, as there is a large volume of oxygen used. The dentist should not use potent narcotic analgesics, mefenamic acid (Pontsel®) and the nonnarcotic analgesic, Talwin, as they all are respiratory depressants. Aspirin should be used with caution, as it can potentiate asthmatic attacks. Other drugs that may induce asthma should be used with care. These include cephaloridine, erythromycin, penicillin, and tetracycline. The practitioner should avoid stressful situations for these patients. Premedication with sedatives would help. The dentist should have anti-asthmatic drugs available such as epinephrine 1:1000 and isoproterenol oral inhalant (See Chapter 16). For patients with emphysema, the dentist should check with the physician to determine if the patient's physical state will allow for more than palliative therapy.

Epilepsy

An epileptic patient should take his medication prior to the appointment and should be handled gently and reassuringly. Knowledge that the patient has the disease helps in the diagnosis of gingival hyperplasia due to diphenyldantoin sodium (Dilantin®) therapy. Care must be exercised while using a local anesthetic in these patients to prevent injection into a blood vessel. The central nervous system stimulatory effect may be enhanced for epileptics.

Patients on oxazolidone derivatives should have blood and urine analysis prior to endodontic surgery, as the use of these drugs can lead to bleeding problems. These patients are usually taking barbiturates and do not require further sedation. Narcolepsy is a form of epilepsy in which the patients' nervous system is depressed rather than stimulated. These patients can be taking stimulants, such as amphetamines. A medical consultation is necessary before any sedatives are prescribed by the dentist. Treatment for an epileptic seizure is discussed in Chapter 16.

Fainting Spells (Syncope) or Dizziness

Repeated spells of syncope may be indicative of cerebral disease and this requires medical consultations and tests. Syncope usually is a sign of an extremely nervous patient who would be helped by nitrous oxide analgesia. During nitrous oxide-oxygen administration, the patient is receiving a high concentration of oxygen, which may prevent cerebral anoxia (the cause of fainting). For treatment, see Chapter 16.

Diabetes Mellitus

Patients with latent diabetes may have no overt clinical manifestations. The disease can only be detected by an abnormal glucose tolerance test or an elevated fasting blood glucose in a patient not under stress.

Signs and symptoms of the overt disease are polyphagia (increased hunger), polydipsia (excessive thirst), polyuria (excessive urination), weight loss, fatigability, repeated infections of skin and urinary tract, pruritis, and in later stages, dyspnea, anorexia, nausea and vomiting, atherosclerotic changes, peripheral nerve changes, acetone breath, and finally mental depression, shock and coma. Diabetic patients can have a toothache that simulates a pulpalgia. The cause is unknown, but it may be related to pulpal blood vessel atherosclerosis or a pulpal arteritis. There is also an increased caries incidence in uncontrolled diabetes which may be related to the decreased salivation present. Before any treatment is begun, a determination must be made of whether or not the patient is under control. The type of control must also be ascertained (drugs or diet). A consultation with the patient's physician is necessary as further control measures may be indicated to prevent the development of insulin shock or diabetic coma. Emergency treatment of the latter conditions is discussed in Chapter 16. Endodontic treatment for uncontrolled diabetics is dangerous. Aside from the possibilities of shock and coma, infection spreads rapidly and healing is poor in these patients. Even with good endodontic therapy, periapical lesions may increase in size. In controlled diabetes, the use of antibiotics during treatment is controversial. Should signs of infection occur, such as swelling, fever and malaise, then antibiotics are indicated. Other treatment precautions should be taken. The patient should not be treated until he (or she) is controlled, either by insulin, oral medication or diet. The patient should be seen in the morning, after he (or she) has eaten and taken insulin (or oral medication). The patient is more likely to have a controlled blood sugar level at that time. The dentist should try to avoid stress, as stress causes a rise in blood sugar. Premedication with a sedative is helpful. The dentist may want to use nitrous oxide analgesia as well as adequate local anesthesia, to keep the patient relaxed. The use of a local anesthetic without epinephrine is desirable, as epinephrine stimulates the breakdown of glycogen to glucose. Alternative local anesthetics that can be used have been described in the section on cardiovascular diseases. As general anesthetics can cause a rise in blood sugar, they should only be used after medical clearance. During surgery, the tissues should be handled as atraumatically as possible. The dentist should not prescribe aspirin or aspirin-containing compounds. Aspirin decreases the blood sugar level and could lead to a dangerous hypoglycemia. Finally, it is important that after surgery the patient has an adequate diet. This includes proteins, carbohydrates, and a vitamin-mineral supplement. The patient's physician should be consulted for the determination of an adequate sugar-free supplement. Adequate nutritional intake is necessary to allow for repair.

Hepatitis and Other Liver Diseases

Clinical manifestations of acute viral hepatitis include fever, chill, anorexia, headache, myalgia, malaise, nausea, jaundice, weakness, and gastrointestinal disturbances. Patients with chronic hepatitis and other liver diseases may have extensive liver damage. Therefore drugs metabolized in the liver should be used with extreme caution, as they may not be detoxified and serious complications can result. Drugs that the dentist should not use unless medical clearance is given include phenacetin (in Empirin compound, Phenaphen®, Sal-Fayne®), acetaminaphen (in Tylenol®, Tempra®, Nebs®, Trigesic®), mefenamic acid (Ponstel), barbiturates, chloral hydrate, paraldehyde, chlordiazepoxide (Librium®), diazepam (Valium®), tetracyclines, sulfonamides, erythromycin estolate (Ilosone), cephalosporins, and ampicillin (Penbritin®, Omnipen®, Polycillin®). Before using any analgesic, antibiotic, or sedative, the dentist should ascertain whether it is metabolized by the liver. A medical consultation is necessary for the determination of the proper drug and dose.

Another possible problem with patients with liver disease is excessive hemorrhage. Hemorrhage may be difficult to control because of the lack of clotting factors such as vitamin K and prothrombin.

In patients with a previous history of hepatitis, viruses may remain viable in the blood stream for a considerable time (weeks to months). To prevent cross contamination, instruments used on these patients should be discarded.

To prevent the transmission of serum hepatitis virus, it is essential that any instrument or needle that contacts the blood stream be sterile.

In patients with liver diseases, protein synthesis is adversely affected. Mineralization and other aspects of internal metabolism are also affected. Therefore, periapical healing can be delayed for these individuals.

Arthritis

It is possible but not proven that microbes found in infected root canals may produce antigens which can cause a secondary response in joint tissues. This auto-immune type response, which may be considered a type of focal infection, can be manifested as arthritis. Patients with arthritis of the neck region can have pain referred to the jaws.

Thyroid Condition and Goiter

Patients with hypothyroidism have a diminished resistance to infection and an inability to withstand prolonged stress. Antibiotic therapy should be used during treatment. These patients may be exceptionally sensitive to barbiturates, narcotics, and related drugs. Dental appointments should be as brief and as atraumatic as possible as these patients are subject to adrenocortical insufficiency. Hypothyroid patients can have facial edema which might simulate swelling due to periapical disease. However, the edema is bilateral, which should differentiate it from the local condition. There have also been reports of abnormal root resorption being associated with hypothyroidism as well as an increased caries incidence.

Clinical manifestations of hyperthyroidism include weakness, increased fatigue, rapid pulse, intolerance to heat, increased sweating, insomnia, weight loss, tremulousness, exopthalmia (Fig. 4) and goitrous enlargement of the thyroid. Women on weight reducing diets may be taking thyroid preparations, and can react as if they were hyperthyroid. Hyperthyroid patients can go into a thyroid crisis (storm) following an epinephrine-containing local anesthetic injection. This is because epinephrine potentiates the action of the thyroid

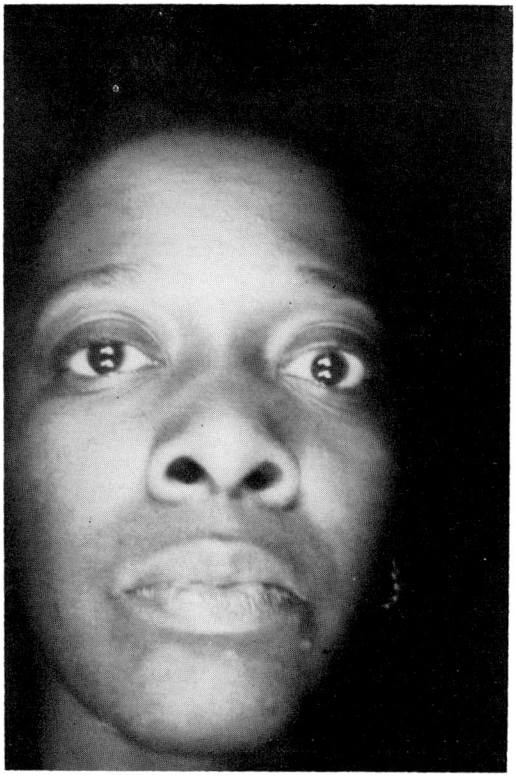

Figure 4. Exophthalmia in a patient with hyperthyroidism. (Courtesy of Dr. T. Simpson, Philadelphia, Pa.)

gland. A local anesthetic without epinephrine (Carbocaine 3%, Citanest 4%) should be used for these patients. Premedication with sedatives is helpful. However, barbiturates should not be used as they can cause a paradoxical stimulatory reaction which can be dangerous. Nonbarbiturate sedatives can be used. If profound anesthesia with local anesthetics is not possible, then a mummification-type procedure should be employed to devitalize the pulp (see Chapter 5). Treatment of thyroid crisis is discussed in Chapter 16.

If hyperthyroid patients are being treated with propylthiouracil, they should have a blood count prior to endodontic surgery, as there is the possibility of a leukopenia developing postsurgically. There have also been reports of an increased caries and erosion incidence in hyperthyroid patients.

Pain can be referred to the teeth from a thyroid tumor or from an acute thyroiditis.

Peptic Ulcers

Clinical manifestations of peptic ulcers are anorexia, stomach pain, nausea, vomiting, belching, and vague epigastric burning sensations. These patients generally are hyperactive, high-strung, emotional individuals and may require sedatives and/or sedation techniques. Tetracyclines should not be administered to ulcer patients taking aluminum containing antacids (see drug section). As ulcer patients generally have gastric hyperacidity, they should only be given drugs that resist gastric acid inactivation. An example would be the use of penicillin V rather than penicillin G. Ulcer patients cannot take aspirin, aspirin containing compounds, and Ponstel because of the possibility of these compounds inducing bleeding in the gastrointestinal tract and complicating the ulcer condition. Vomiting occurs frequently in these patients. After a number of years, extensive erosion of the teeth can occur. This results from the acid content of the vomitus (Figs. 2, 492).

Kidney Diseases

General manifestations of kidney diseases are decreased urination, color changes in the urine, foul smelling urine, painful urination, edema, hypertension, pain in the small of the back, and blood in the urine. However, these manifestations can vary with the particular disease. Patients with nephritis may have a burning sensation in the mouth. Along with some kidney diseases, secondary hyperparathyroidism with associated jaw lesions can occur (Fig. 16). With uremia, patients may have an ulcerative stomatitis. Patients with nephrosis are usually on high corticosteroid therapy. For discussion of patients on these drugs see section on adrenal cortex diseases.

Patients with kidney diseases may have difficulties with breakdown and excretion of the drugs that the dentist prescribes. The patient should receive smaller and less frequent dosages of drugs that are normally eliminated by the kidney. Analgesic drug combinations containing aspirin, Ponstel, phenacetin, and possibly acetaminophen have been implicated in the causation of kidney damage and should be avoided. Other drugs that the dentist should avoid because of possible exacerbation of kidney disease are corticosteroids, narcotics, and vasoconstrictors (epinephrine, nor-epinephrine, levarterenol, etc.). If premedication is used, short acting barbiturates (pentobarbital, Nembutal®; secobarbital, Seconal®) should be given rather than long acting barbiturates (phenobarbital, Luminal®). The former are metabolized in the liver, while the latter are metabolized in the kidney. Chloral hydrate can also cause kidney damage and should be avoided.

Patients with kidney diseases may have an increased susceptibility to infection and retarded healing. Use of antibiotics is generally indicated. As erythromycin is metabolized in the liver, it is advantageous to use this drug in preference to penicillin, the tetracyclines, cephaloridine, and sulfonamides, which are broken down in the kidney.

Patients with severe kidney disorders can have hemorrhagic diatheses and they should be treated with proper methods to establish hemostasis (e.g. use of adequate sutures, firm pressure, etc.).

Patients on renal dialysis (in cases of failing kidneys) receive frequent blood transfusions. There is the possibility of the serum hepatitis virus being present in their blood. Therefore special precautions must be used in handling these patients. Sterilized disposable needles must be available; all materials must be autoclaved; and root canal instruments should be discarded after use on these patients. Sterile disposable rubber gloves and masks should be used.

There have been cases reported of kidney symptoms related to abscessed teeth. However, these reports have not been scientifically documented.

Tuberculosis and Other Debilitating Lung Infections

General manifestations of chronic lung conditions are persistent coughs, hemoptysis (bloody sputum), chest pain, fatigability, weakness, loss of weight, and anorexia. The dentist should not render any treatment, other than palliative care, until the disease is brought under control. The resistance of these patients is poor and repair is usually delayed. The blood is not sufficiently aerated due to the excessive lung destruction. With the insufficient aeration, nutrition is impaired and fibroplasia is retarded. Therefore, periapical repair may be delayed. Another reason for caution by the dentist is the fact that these diseases are contagious. Oral lesions of tuberculosis and other granulomatous diseases can appear as individual ulcers that may simulate paruli (gum boils).

Nervous Breakdown, Mental and Psychiatric Conditions

These patients are difficult to treat and must be handled cautiously. The use of tranquilizers and antidepressants may be necessary. These should only be prescribed after medical consultation. Occasionally, these patients may have

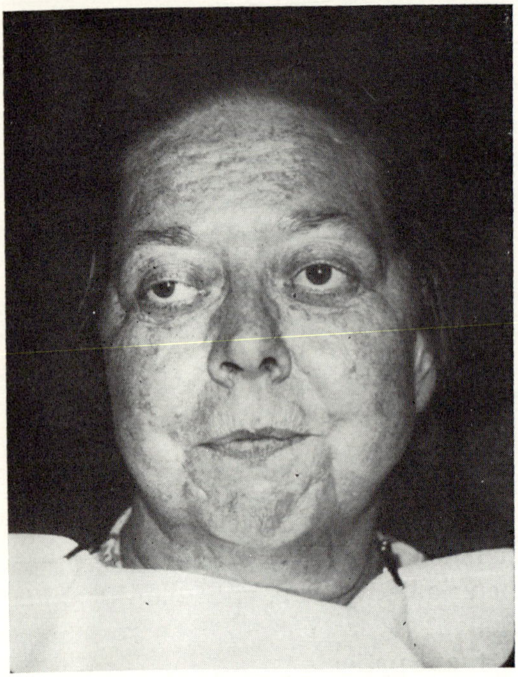

Figure 5. Patient with Cushing's disease showing the typical *moon-face* appearance. (Courtesy of Dr. T. Simpson, Philadelphia, Pa.)

pain of psychogenic origin that can be referred to the teeth.

Adrenal Cortex Diseases and Conditions in Which the Patients Are Receiving Corticosteroids

The adrenal cortex diseases are Addison's disease and Cushing's disease. Certain diseases in which patients receive corticosteroid therapy are lupus erythematosus, rheumatoid arthritis, scleroderma, pemphigus and nephrosis.

Before beginning endodontic therapy, it is important to determine the corticosteroid blood level for these patients. Medical consultation is essential.

Clinical manifestations of Addison's disease (low level of circulating corticosteroids) are easy fatigability, languor, pigmentation of the skin and mucous membranes, weight loss, anorexia, nausea, vomiting, diarrhea, abdominal pain, and nervousness. These patients have poor ability to cope with stressful situations, including infection and surgery. No treatment should be performed until control has been established.

Patients with Cushing's disease (high level of circulating corticosteroids) or patients who are on prolonged corticosteroid therapy, often have osteoporotic bone changes (including the jaws). Clinical manifestations include obesity of face (Fig. 5), neck, and trunk, muscle weakness, ruddy appearance of face and neck, susceptibility to bruises, hypertension, and mood changes. There is usually an impairment of tissue healing for these patients. Adjustments may have to be made in the corticosteroid level prior to surgery. Therefore, a medical consultation is essential. Treatment of shock reaction in these individuals is discussed in Chapter 16. As a consequence of the delayed healing potential, antibiotics should be used during endodontic therapy. The antibiotics will prevent multiplication and dissemination of microbes.

Malnutrition

These individuals have difficulties in repair because of insufficient nutrients (vitamins, minerals and proteins).

Venereal Diseases

It is important to ascertain whether the patient or patient's mother had syphilis. Enamel hypoplasia and Hutchinson's incisors can occur with congenital syphilis (Fig. 6). Syphilis is a contagious disease and can be transmitted

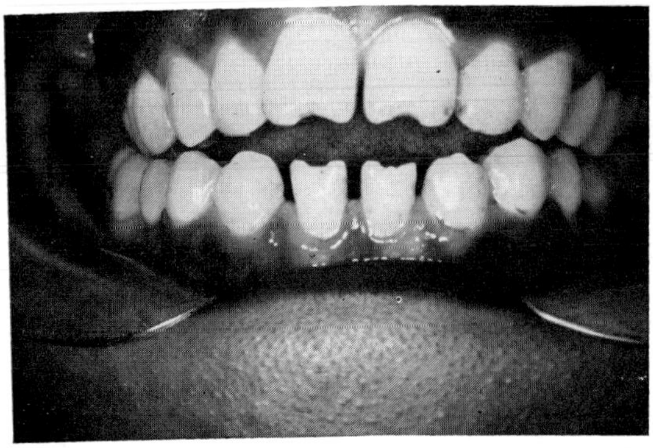

Figure 6. Patient with congenital syphilis showing Hutchinson's incisors and slight hypoplasia. (Courtesy of Dr. T. Simpson, Philadelphia, Pa.)

orally. The dentist has to be careful with any suspicious lesion and use of rubber gloves is essential. Lesions in certain stages of syphilis can be isolated to the alveolar mucosa and may simulate a parulis. In tabes dorsalis, a rarely seen late stage of syphilis, it has been reported that patients have pulpal paresthesia and neuralgic pains of the face. Also in advanced stages, an osteomyelitis of the jaws may occur (Fig. 7). In lymphogranuloma inguinale, there may occur ulcerative oral lesions and a regional lymphadenopathy. In gonorrhea, occasionally oral lesions may be present.

Surgery including Valvular and Transplant Procedures

The dentist should inquire about the reasons for the surgery and consult with the physician as to the disease process that was involved. Especially important are cardiac valvular prostheses, and vascular grafts and transplant (heart, kidney, etc.) procedures. Certain medical authorities believe that these patients should have all their teeth extracted prior to surgery, while others believe endodontic therapy is preferable. These patients can have serious life-endangering infections from normal oral microorganisms, because of the immunosuppressive drugs they are taking. Therefore, large doses of predetermined antibiotics must be used during treatment. These patients are usually treated in hospitals. Before any treatment is attempted, medical consultation is essential regarding the antibiotic of choice and dosage.

Temporal Arteritis

Patients with temporal arteritis can have pain referred to the upper teeth and the zygoma region. The painful symptoms apparently result from an arteritis that involves the maxillary arteries as well as the temporals.

Blood Disorders

These patients require medical consultation and tests prior to endodontic therapy. Problems are related to healing (anemias and blood dyscrasias), bleeding (hemorrhagic disorders), and survival (blocd dyscrasias such as leukemi-

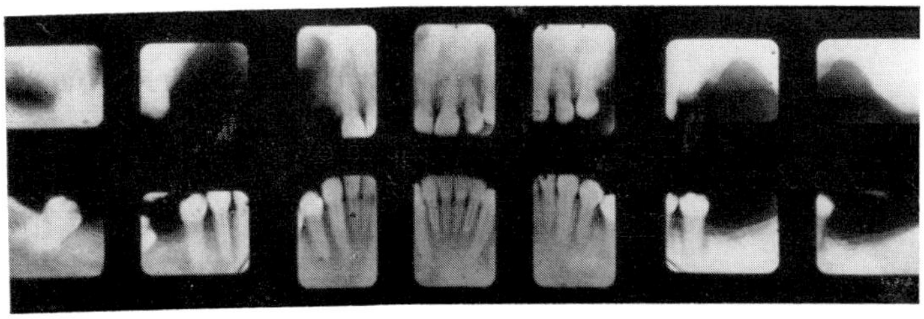

Figure 7. Syphilitic osteomyelitis, predominantly of the maxilla. (Courtesy of Dr. T. Simpson, Philadelphia, Pa.)

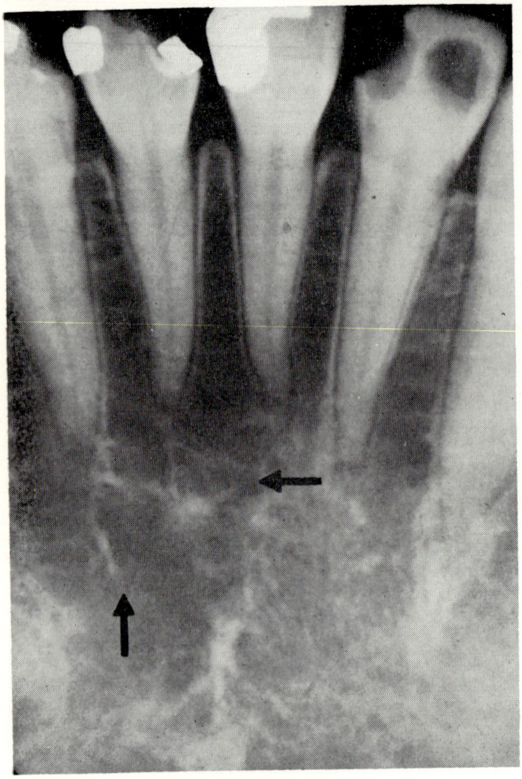

Figure 8. Osteolytic rarefactions seen in sickle cell anemia. (Courtesy of Dr. T. Simpson, Philadelphia, Pa.)

as and polycythemia vera). Patients with anemias have delayed healing because of the poor oxygenation of their tissues. These patients should receive local rather than general anesthesia, because of the already relatively insufficient oxygenation of the cerebral tissues. Sulfonamides, barbiturates, tetracyclines, streptomycin, aspirin, chloramphenicol, and chlorpromazine (Thorazine®) have the capacity to cause aplastic anemia and/or agranulocytosis. These drugs certainly shouldn't be prescribed for patients who already have an anemia or a granulocyte deficiency. Phenacetin and possible acetaminophen can cause acute hemolytic anemia if taken in sufficiently large doses. However, this is rarely a problem in dental usage. A defect found in approximately 15 per cent of American blacks is glucose-6-phosphate-dehydrogenase deficiency. The erythrocytes have an abbreviated life cycle, which is only a problem under conditions of stress or administration of potentially oxidant drugs. Phenacetin is converted *in vivo* to an oxidant compound and hence shouldn't be given to these patients.

In sickle cell anemia and Cooley's anemia, individuals may have periapical osteolytic rarefactions, which may be confused with endodontic lesions (Figs. 8, 9). Patients with Cooley's anemia have a typical facial appearance (Fig. 10). Patients with sickle cell anemia can have toothaches or jaw pain during

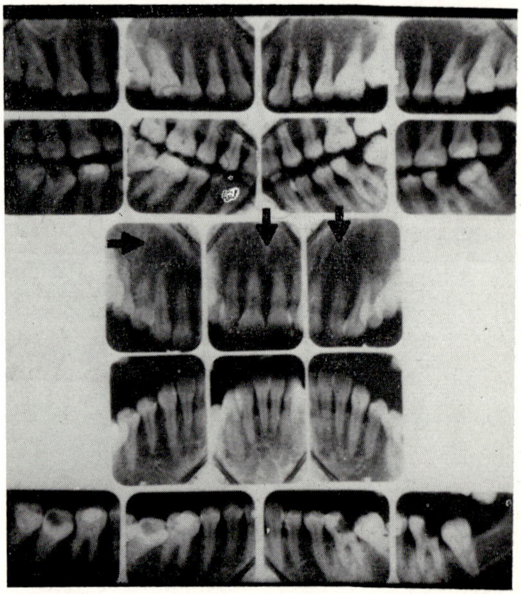

Figure 9. Osteolytic rarefactions seen in Cooley's anemia. (Courtesy of Dr. T. Simpson, Philadelphia, Pa.)

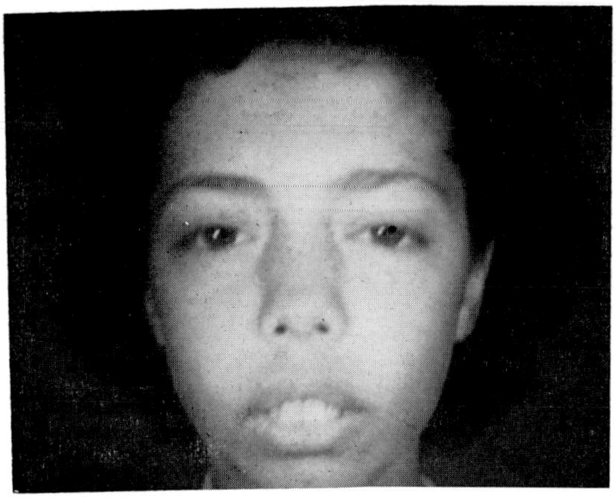

Figure 10. Typical facial appearance in Cooley's anemia; round face (related to hyperplasia of bone marrow) and protruding anterior teeth. (Courtesy of Dr. T. Simpson, Philadelphia, Pa.)

sickling crises, and may have pigmented teeth. Medical consultation is necessary before treating patients with sickle cell anemia because of the problems related to anoxia, pain, and infection. In erythroblastosis fetalis, in which anemia occurs, tooth pigmentation is found.

Leukemic patients may have a gingivitis (Fig. 11), and osteolytic bony rarefactions (Fig. 12). They also can develop toothaches that are unrelated to endodontic lesions. The pulps become infiltrated with leukemic cells. Extractions for leukemic patients have been thought to hasten their deaths; hence endodontic therapy is preferable. This is probably related to the platelet deficiency in these patients and to the possibility of dissemination of leukemic cells throughout the blood stream resulting from the extraction. Medical consultation is necessary to ascertain whether complete therapy should be performed or only palliative treatment. As functional polymorph leucocytes are lacking in these patients, combatting of infection becomes a problem and repair is delayed or impeded.

Polycythemic patients are very susceptible to hemorrhage, thrombosis and infection. This is related to the large increase in erythrocytes and thrombocytes and the presence of immature

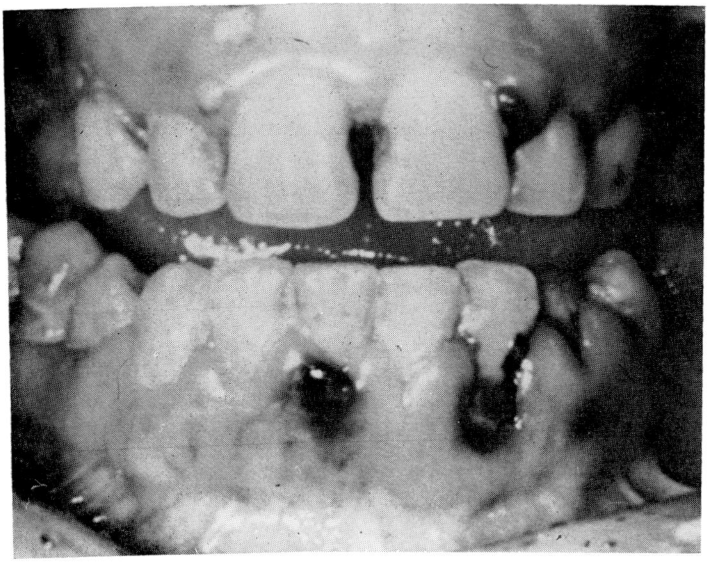

Figure 11. Patient with chronic myelocytic leukemia showing localized gingivitis with bleeding. (Courtesy of Dr. M. Gross, Philadelphia, Pa.)

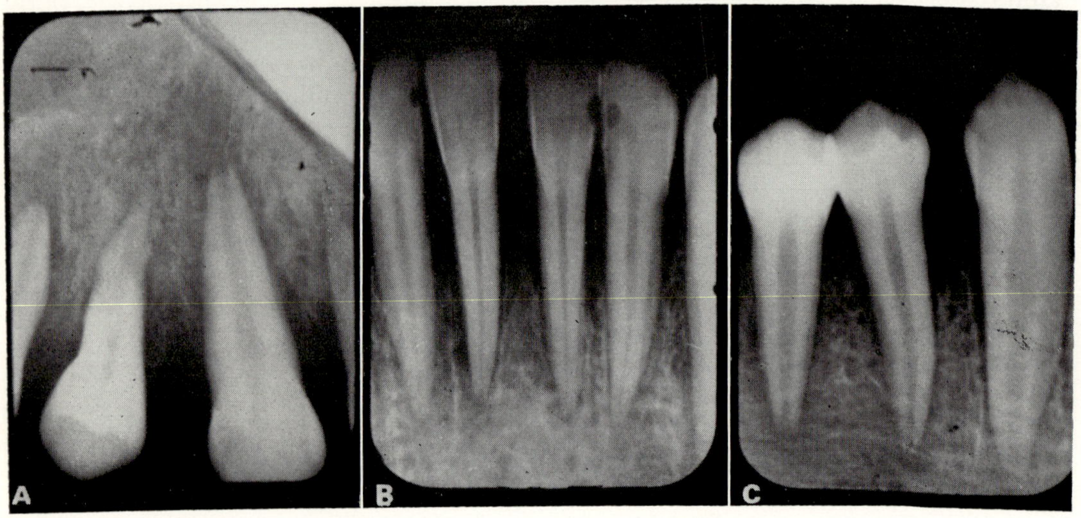

Figure 12. Osteolytic rarefactions seen in a patient with monocytic leukemia. (Courtesy of Dr. I. B. Bender, Philadelphia, Pa.)

polymorph leucocytes (in many cases). Treatment for these patients should be delayed until their blood picture is relatively normal. Antibiotics should be used, and good hemorrhage control should be practiced.

To evaluate hemorrhagic disorders, the patient should be asked whether he (or she) is on anticoagulant or antibiotic therapy, whether high doses of aspirin are being taken, and about previous bleeding problems after dental extractions, pulp extirpations, periodontal treatments, other oral surgical procedures, general surgical procedures, menstruation, and childbirth. It is important to determine whether the bleeding problem was purely a local solitary occurrence (such as a *dry socket*) or whether it had recurred several times. If there is a suspicion of a hemorrhagic disease, medical consultation and blood tests are necessary. Aspirin should not be given to patients with hemorrhagic diatheses as it can intensify the hemorrhage.

There are three general groups of hemorrhagic disorders: vascular defects, platelet disorders, and coagulation defects.*

Vascular Defects. These disorders result from vascular abnormalities. Bleeding of the skin and mucous membranes after minor trauma is common. Ecchymoses and petechiae may be evident. Generally, the bleeding is not as serious as is the case with the other hemorrhagic disorders. Usual screening tests for vascular defects are bleeding time and the tourniquet test, both of which may be abnormally prolonged. The vascular abnormalities include idiopathic simple purpura, allergic purpura

* Preparation of this section was aided by Dr. Norman Siegel, a Diplomate of the American Boards of Internal Medicine and Hematology, Dept. of Medicine. The Cooper Hospital, Camden, N. J.

(Henoch-Schloenlein), drug purpura (e.g. resulting from iodides, chlorthiazides, belladonna alkaloids), senile purpura, steroid purpura, infection (e.g. streptococcal septicemia, rheumatic fever, scarlet fever, rocky mountain spotted fever), vitamin C deficiency, chronic diseases (e.g. obstructive jaundice, kidney failure, macroglobulinemia, amyloidosis, polycythemia vera), and genetic (e.g. Ehlers-Danlos syndrome, hemorrhagic telangiectasia).

Vascular Purpuras. In the vascular purpuras, bleeding is not serious and tends to subside after about one week. However, recurrences are common.

Infection. Increase in capillary fragility is associated with certain infections (see "infection" above). Bleeding episodes are generally mild with no definite treatment required.

Vitamin C Deficiency. This includes scurvy and subclinical vitamin C deficiency. Scurvy as a clinical entity is practically absent in the United States, but subclinical cases of vitamin C deficiency have been reported. These patients may have a painful gingivitis with a tendency toward bleeding episodes, probably resulting from increased capillary permeability. Osteoporotic jaw lesions may occur in more advanced stages. In patients with vitamin C deficiency, periapical healing may be delayed after endodontic therapy. Supplemental vitamin C (approximately 500 mg daily) should be given for at least one week before and after surgery. Crystalluria and gout may occur following high doses of vitamin C tablets. It has been reported that this does not occur with sustained release tablets (Cevi-Bid® capsules, All-Day C-500® tablets).

PLATELET DISORDERS. These defects are of two types: quantitative deficiencies (the thrombocytopenias), and qualitative deficiencies (thrombocytopathia, etc.).

Thrombocytopenias. These disorders are much more common than the qualitative defects. The clinical picture shows easy bruising and extensive bleeding from minor cuts or spontaneously. Usual laboratory test findings in severe cases are platelet count of 70,000 cu/mm or less (examination of stained blood smear), prolonged bleeding time, poor clot retraction, and increased capillary fragility (tourniquet test). Thrombocytopenia has many etiologies, some of which are unknown. Frequently it is induced by certain drugs. Management includes treatment of the underlying disease or in the case of serious bleeding, transfusion with fresh whole blood or platelet concentrates.

Qualitative Platelet Deficiencies. The clinical manifestations of the qualitative platelet disorders are minor skin and mucous membrane bleeding. In these disorders, there are abnormalities detectable by the following tests: bleeding time, tourniquet test, clot retraction, ADP-induced platelet aggregation and tests for platelet adhesiveness. Examples of platelet function disorders include Von Willebrand's disease, the platelet defect associated with aspirin ingestion, and thrombocytopathy. With aspirin ingestion, there is usually no overt bleeding with normal doses. However, in susceptible individuals bleeding can occur with as little as one 300 mg aspirin tablet. Treatment of qualitative platelet deficiencies is dependent upon control of the causative factors. In the case of serious bleeding, management is generally similar to that given for the thrombocytopenias.

COAGULATION DEFECTS. The coagulation disorders are of two types, genetic and acquired. The genetic types (e.g. hemophilia) are more well known, but they are rarer than the acquired defects. With the severe diseases (e.g. classical hemophilia), bleeding can occur spontaneously or after minor trauma.

Screening tests used are observation of the whole blood clot, partial thromboplastin time (PTT), prothrombin time (PT), and thrombin time (TT). Whole blood clotting time (glass, Lee-White method) is a test that gives a gross evaluation of the early clotting *stages*. Formation of a clot in ten minutes or more indicates a coagulation defect. Tests to evaluate the specific deficiencies are the individual factor assays. Thrombin time is a useful test for the determination of quantitative and qualitative fibrinogen abnormalities. Fibrin degradation products (split products) are used in the diagnosis of certain acquired fibrinogen disorders (disseminated intravascular coagulation).

Acquired Coagulation Disorders. The acquired coagulation deficiencies involve more than one coagulation factor, whereas the usual case with the genetic disorders is one deficient coagulation factor.

The acquired coagulation disorders include those that are secondary to vitamin K deficiency, related to circulating anticoagulant (as seen in systemic lupus erythematosus), related to fibrinogen deficiencies or abnormalities, and secondary to heparin therapy.

Vitamin K deficiency. With the deficiency of vitamin K, there are associated deficiencies of Factors II (prothrombin), VII, IX (Christmas factor) and X (Stuart factor). Vitamin K deficiency has the following possible causes: prolonged antibiotic therapy causing suppression of the intestinal bacteria (which normally synthesize most of the vitamin K), administration of coumarin-type anticoagulants (inhibitors of vitamin K), malabsorption of fat-soluble substances, related to biliary obstruction or a primary bowel disorder, and severe liver disease resulting in a reduction of synthesis of vitamin K-related proteins. If these patients are not controlled, hemorrhage can be a serious problem. Vitamin K deficiency can be corrected by vitamin K analogues. Patients on anticoagulants can be corrected only by administration of vitamin K_1 (for other considerations, see Cardiovascular Diseases in this chapter). Patients with severe liver disease cannot be corrected by any vitamin K preparation and serious bleeding may require transfusions of plasma.

Circulating Anticoagulant. With this syndrome, there is moderate hemorrhage. Diagnostic tests used are anticoagulant assays. Results are positive against Factors II, V, VII, or X. Management is based on treatment of the underlying cause (e.g. systemic lupus erythematosus).

Fibrinogen Disorders. The fibrinogen disorders include intravascular coagulation syndrome (disseminated intravascular coagulation), acute fibrinolysis, and liver disease.

With disseminated intravascular coagulation, there are deficiencies in Factors I (Fibrinogen), II (Prothrombin), V, and VIII (AHG). Hemorrhage is severe in these cases. Diagnostic test results usually show a thrombocytopenia, an increased prothrombin time, a small retracted clot that appears to lyse (red cell fall out), presence of fibrin split products, a prolonged thrombin time, and a rapid euglobulin lysis time, if fibrinolysis is present. The syndrome can be related to many disorders including obstetrical complications, acute leukemia, disseminated carcinoma, septicemia, following hemolytic transfusion reactions, accompanying shock, following heat stroke, after lung surgery, and with purpura fulminans. Successful treatment depends upon management of the underlying disease and if bleeding is severe, the use of heparin.

Fibrinolysis is a secondary manifestation of the intravascular coagulation syndrome. Acute fibrinolysis (primary fibrinolysis) is very rare and detection is aided with the use of euglobulin lysis time test. Treatment is the use of specific drugs to counteract the fibrinolysis. With liver disease, treatment of the underlying disease is necessary along with replacement therapy.

Heparin Therapy. In patients on heparin therapy, thrombin is inhibited. Minor bleeding can be controlled by the withdrawal of the drug. Severe bleeding necessitates the administration of protamine, which is a heparin antagonist (also see section on Cardiovascular Diseases, in this chapter).

Genetic Coagulation Disorders. These defects include classical hemophilia (Factor VIII [AHG] deficiency) Von Willebrand's disease, Factor IX deficiency (Christmas disease), Factor V deficiency (parahemophilia), Factor II deficiency (Hypoprothrombinemia), Factor I deficiency (congenital afibrinogenemia, congenital hypofibrinogenemia, congenital dysfibrinogenemia), Factor XI deficiency (PTA deficiency), Factor X deficiency (Stuart disease), Factor VII deficiency (hypoproconvertinemia), Factor XIII deficiency (fibrin-stabilizing factor deficiency), and Factor XII deficiency (Hageman factor deficiency). With all of these disorders, endodontics is preferable to surgery as there is much less bleeding involved. Periapical surgery should be performed only when the clinical entities are under control. Even with maintained cases, good hemorrhage control is essential (See under Classical Hemophilia). All of these deficiencies are rare, but the most common is classical hemophilia.

Classical Hemophilia. This disease primarily affects males. Hemorrhage is severe in uncontrolled cases with cardinal signs being spontaneous bleeding and bleeding after minor trauma. Uncontrolled patients can die from simple procedures. Patients under control receive transfusions of the deficient Factor VIII (AHG). However, even under controlled conditions, fewer complications occur with endodontic therapy than with extractions. Injections of local anesthetics may cause submucosal hemorrhages in these patients. Mummification procedures should be used to devitalize pulp tissue (See Chapter 5). If periapical surgery is performed in maintained cases, it is still essential to have good hemorrhage control. There should be well adapted margins, gentle handling of tissues, an adequate number of sutures, use of hemostatic aids such as thrombin, and firm pressure. Blood tests usually show deficiency of Factor VIII, prolonged clotting time in glass, impaired thromboplastin generation, and prolonged partial thromboplastin time.

Von Willebrand's Disease (Vascular Hemophilia). This genetic disorder occurs in both sexes. The bleeding is not as severe as in hemophilia. There is an abnormality of a vascular factor as well as a reduction of Factor VIII. Blood tests show a reduction in Factor VIII, a prolonged bleeding time, and a decreased platelet adhesiveness.

Factor IX Deficiency (Christmas Disease). In this disease, bleeding can occur into joints and after minor trauma, including dental procedures. The best laboratory test is a specific assay of the patient's plasma for Factor IX. There is also an abnormal partial thromboplastin time and a normal prothrombin time.

Factor V Deficiency (Parahemophilia). This genetic disorder may be found in both sexes. Bleeding can occur into joints, and after minor trauma, including dental procedures. Blood tests show prothombin time significantly prolonged, partial thromboplastin time prolonged, and low levels of Factor V.

Factor II Deficiency (Congenital Hypoprothrombinemia). This very rare genetic disorder can occur in either sex. Bleeding can occur into joints, and after minor trauma, including dental procedures. Diagnosis is aided by an abnormal 2-stage prothrombin time.

Factor I Deficiency (Congenital Afibrinogenemia, Hypofibrinogenemia, or Dysfibrinogenemia). In these diseases, there is an absence, deficiency, or qualitative abnormality in fibrinogen, which is detected by a direct assay. Prolonged bleeding can occur following minor trauma.

Factor XI Deficiency (P.T.A. Deficiency). In this genetic disorder, excessive bleeding can occur following trauma. Diagnosis depends on direct assay for Factor XI. Poor consumption of prothrombin (measured by one-stage prothrombin method) is a usual finding.

Miscellaneous Factor Disorders. The other genetic disorders are very rare and are determined by specific assay of the patient's plasma for the deficient factor. Most of the disorders are not too serious. In fact, with Factor XII deficiency (Hageman factor deficiency) there are no symptoms and there is either no, or a minimal bleeding problem.

Radiation Treatments

If patients have had radiation treatment in the head and neck area, then osteoradionecrosis can occur (Fig. 13). These patients can also have numbness (paresthesia) of the jaws and toothaches can occur. Toothaches may result from radiation damage to the pulpal blood supply with subsequent infection. If the teeth are left in the mouth, sau-

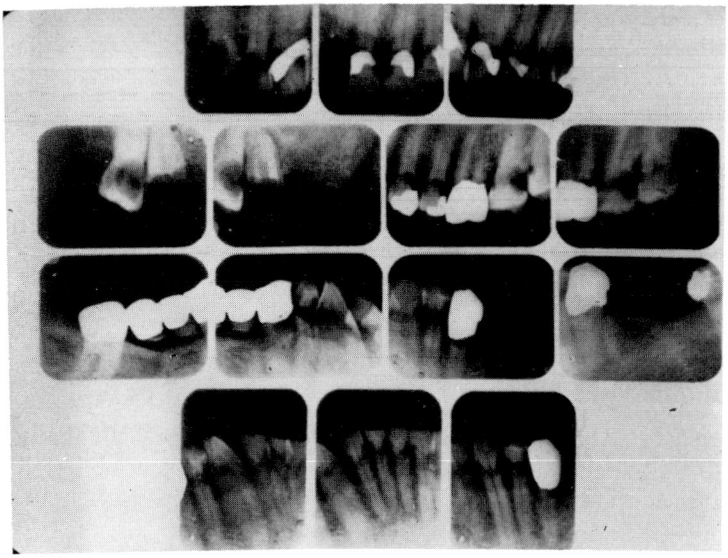

Figure 13. Osteoradionecrosis and rapid root caries secondary to radiation treatment in the head and neck area. (Courtesy of Dr. T. Simpson, Philadelphia, Pa.)

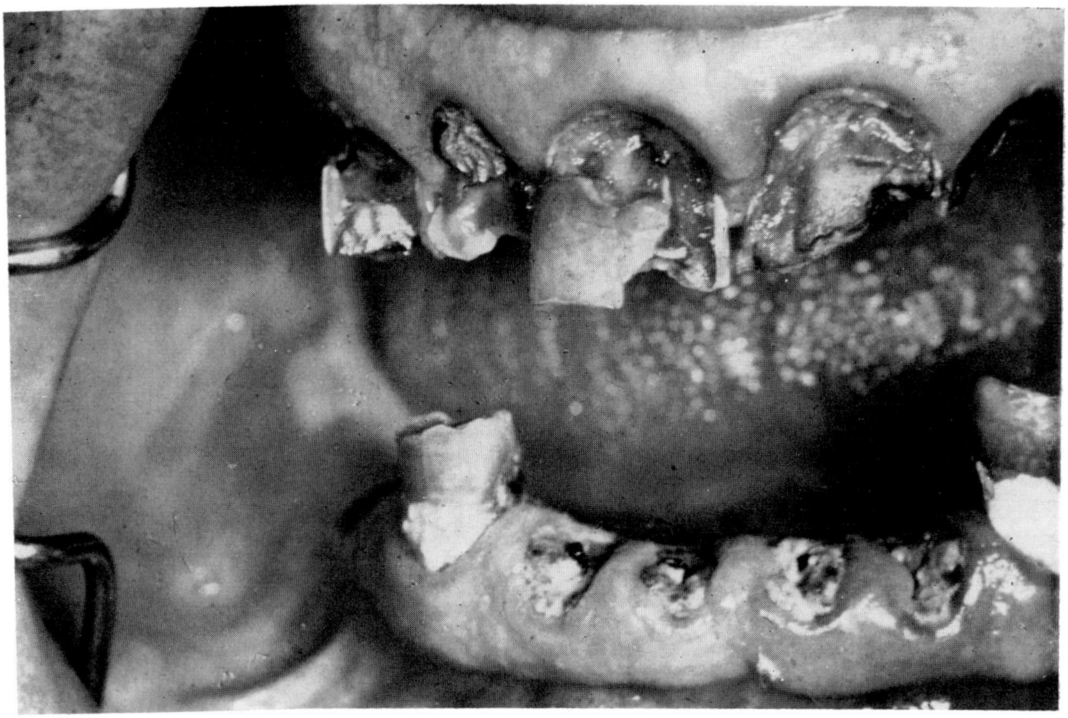

Figure 14. Saucer-shaped coronal destruction and brown-black destruction secondary to radiation treatment of the neck. (From S. Seltzer and I. B. Bender, *The Dental Pulp,* J. P. Lippincott Co., 1965. Used with permission of J. P. Lippincott Company.)

cer-shaped coronal destruction (which may be a form of rapid root caries) and brown-black discoloration often occurs (Fig. 14). Pulpal necrosis is a possible sequlae to the radiation therapy.

There is a difference of opinion among authorities about whether teeth should be extracted prior to radiation therapy of the head and neck. If the teeth are not removed, performing endodontic therapy would not necessarily prevent the onset of osteoradionecrosis. Microbes from the gingival sulcus (or periodontal pocket) can invade the bone that has impaired circulation. If a patient has had previous radiation therapy in the oral region and pulpal involvement occurs, then endodontics is definitely preferred to extraction.

Menstruation Irregularities

During the period, women can have oral herpetic lesions, gingivitis, and toothaches. The toothaches appear to be related to the capillary dilation that can occur. Postoperative hemorrhage occurs more frequently during menstruation then at other times. The latter has been shown for pulpal extirpations. It has also been observed that there is a higher incidence of flare-ups during menstruation. All of these results are apparently related to hormonal changes.

Pregnancy

The dentist should use as few radiographs as possible. To protect the fetus, the patient should be draped with a lead apron. Medical consultation may be necessary concerning the use of drugs and the time of treatment. As the time of greatest vulnerability for the fetus is during the first trimester, it is best to avoid giving or prescribing drugs for the pregnant patient during that period and only to perform symptomatic treatment. If drug use is essential the drugs should be used sparingly and in minimal doses because of the unknown effect on the fetus. Most physicians prefer treatment to be carried out in the second trimester. During pregnancy, women can have signs and symptoms as described under menstruation irregularities. There is a reported clinical study showing that in pregnant women with periapical *infection* present, there is a much higher incidence of pregnancy complications (abortion and pyelitis) than in controls without periapical disease. However, this was not a well-controlled study, and it is not known how infection was determined.

Menopause

Women in the post-menopausal state can have osteoporotic jaw lesions that appear to result from the depletion of estrogen. They also may develop atypical facial neuralgia that can simulate pulpalgia. In these patients, after apparently sound endodontic therapy, periapical areas of rarefaction may not heal. This again seems to be related to the depletion of estrogen. Therefore, as long as there are no clinical symptoms or signs, no further treatment should be attempted. If areas enlarge visibly, and/or the patient has clinical manifestations, then periapical surgery should be attempted. However, there is no documented evidence that periapical surgery will be more successful than extraction. Medical consultation is necessary concerning the possibility of replacement estrogen therapy.

Diseases That "Run" in the Family (Genetic Diseases)

This information gives the dentist clues about possible genetic diseases that can have oral manifestations (such diseases are described in Chapter 2).

Exanthematous Diseases (High Fever Diseases)

These include measles, chicken pox, scarlet fever, and pertussis (whooping cough). If the patient had one or more of these diseases as a child, depending upon the age, his (or her) permanent teeth may show varying degrees of enamel hypoplasia (Fig. 15).

Fever of Unknown Origin

This may result from a bacteremia, viremia or septicemia, among other possibilities.

The presence of fever of unknown origin would alert the dentist to the possibility of some systemic microbial disease being present and calls for a medical consultation prior to treatment.

Occasionally, patients have infected, pulpless teeth with no history of caries, erosion, attrition, abrasion, or periodontal disease. The teeth may have suffered trauma with the pulps becoming necrotic. It is possible that microbes could have been attracted to these teeth (anachoresis) from a blood stream infection (bacteremia or septicemia).

Cerebral Palsy, Parkinson's Disease or Tremors of Unknown Origin

These patients have difficulty in remaining stationary for dental procedures. It may be necessary to use general anesthesia. It has been reported that patients with cerebral palsy have marked tooth abrasion, even up to the point of pulpal exposures.

Muscle and Nerve Diseases

This group encompasses myasthenia gravis, muscular dystrophy, myositis ossificans, multiple sclerosis, lateral sclerosis, poliomyelitis, and other diseases of

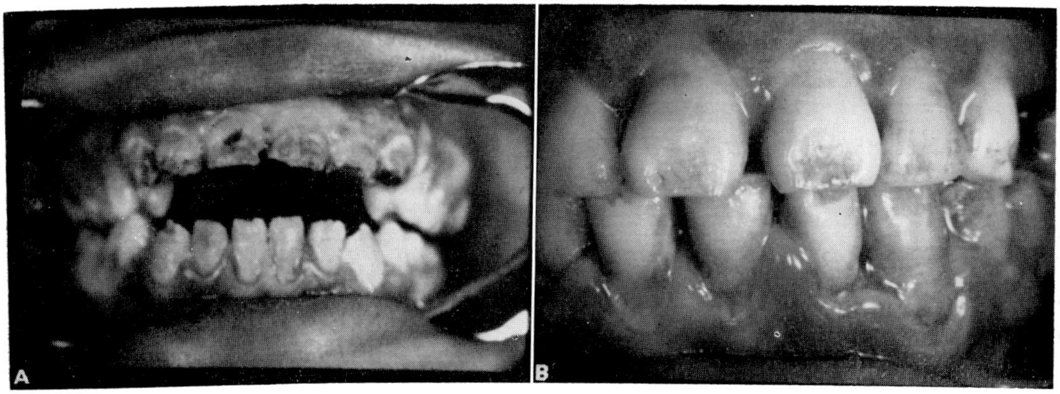

Figure 15. Enamel Hypoplasia—A. Severe case probably resulting from an exanthematous disease during childhood. B. Mild case probably related to a mild *bout* of an exanthematous disease during childhood. (Courtesy of Dr. T. Simpson, Philadelphia, Pa.)

muscles and nerves. Because of these patients' extreme weakness, medical consultation is necessary to determine whether complete therapy or just emergency care should be performed. General anesthesia and hospitalization may be necessary. Myositis ossificans can occur in the temporalis muscle, producing a facial swelling and fan shaped calcifications which may be seen as irregular radiopacities on periapical posterior radiographs.

Cases of myositis have been reported as resulting from abscessed teeth. This focal infection concept is very difficult to prove, but as stated previously, one cannot rule out the possibility of a microbially-incited auto-immune disease. Patients with multiple sclerosis may have paresthesia of the teeth and/or symptoms of trigeminal neuralgia.

Miscellaneous Osteolytic and Osteosclerotic Bone Diseases

Patients with these diseases can have osteoporotic and osteosclerotic jaw lesions that can simulate endodontically-induced lesions. The most endodontically-relevant diseases in this group are Paget's disease and hyperparathyroidism.

Patients with hyperparathyroidism (primary or secondary) may have loss of the lamina dura surrounding their teeth (Fig. 16). Patients with Paget's disease may also show loss of the lamina dura, tooth mobility, hypercementosis and/or root resorption (Fig. 17). As a result of the extensive circulation present within the bone, osteomyelitis can develop rapidly from pulpally-induced periapical pathoses. Patients with Gaucher's disease may have excessive hemorrhage following surgery, especially if splenectomy has not been performed. Therefore, endodontics is preferred. A medical consultation is necessary before performing periapical surgery.

For a description of the various bone diseases that can have jaw manifestations, see Chapter 2.

Eye Disorders and Diseases

Patients with these conditions can have pain referred to the upper teeth. There have been many reported cases of eye diseases, such as retinitis, iritis, optic neuritis, choroiditis, keratitis, and uveitis, resulting from abscessed teeth. Nevertheless, there is much doubt about whether focal infection occurs in these type cases. An auto-immune response cannot be ruled out completely.

Ear Diseases

Patients with ear diseases can have pain that is referred to posterior teeth. As with the eye diseases, cases of otitis media and mastoiditis have been ascribed to infections originating in abscessed teeth. Documentation is lacking, but the possibility of an auto-immune response exists.

Oral Facial-Cranial Neuralgias and Neuritises

Clinical manifestations are discussed in Chapter 2.

These disorders can be a source of referred pain to the teeth and jaws.

Cranial Lesions, Diseases and Injuries

Recurrent headaches, together with facial paresthesia, and other sensory

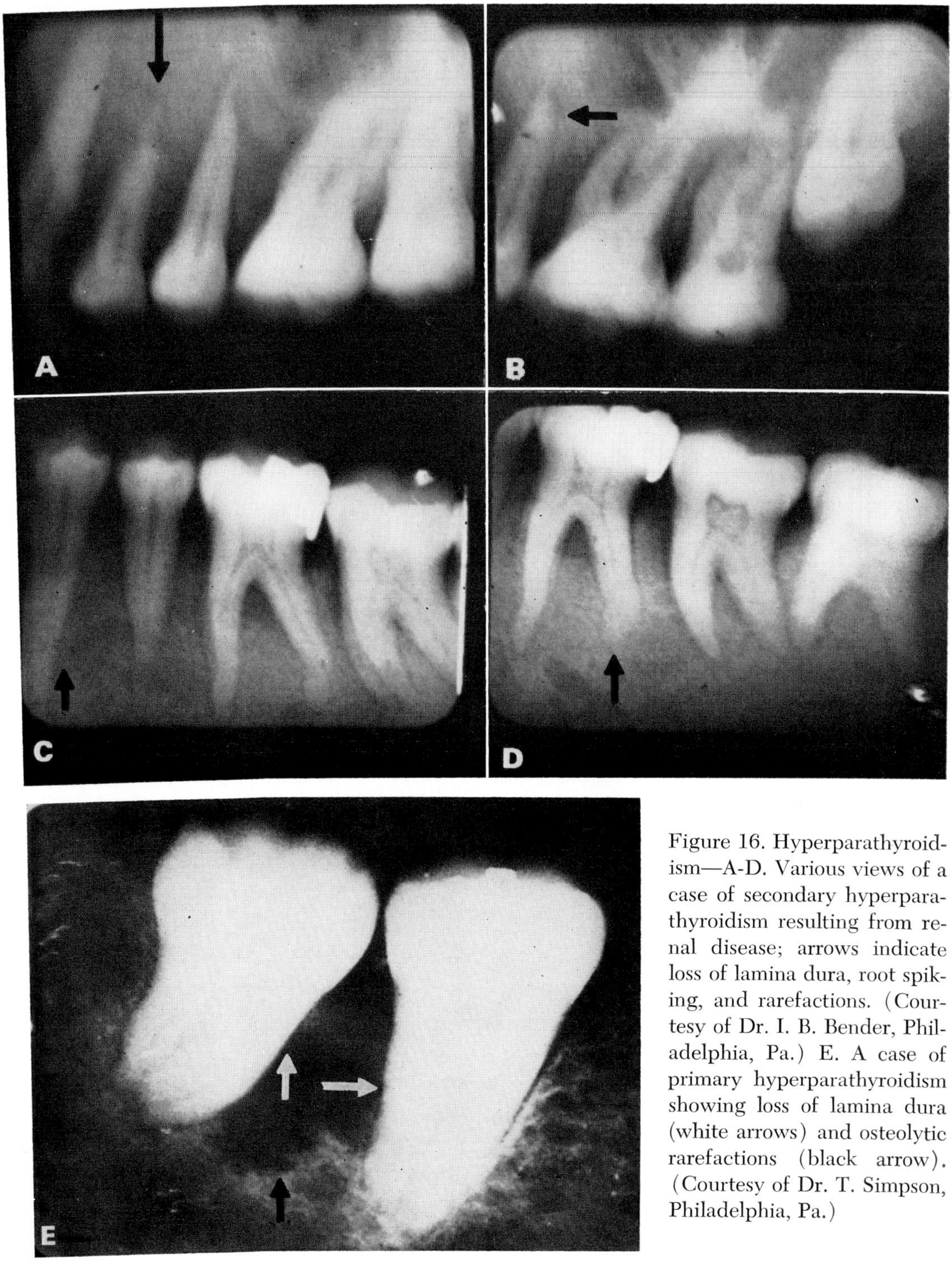

Figure 16. Hyperparathyroidism—A-D. Various views of a case of secondary hyperparathyroidism resulting from renal disease; arrows indicate loss of lamina dura, root spiking, and rarefactions. (Courtesy of Dr. I. B. Bender, Philadelphia, Pa.) E. A case of primary hyperparathyroidism showing loss of lamina dura (white arrows) and osteolytic rarefactions (black arrow). (Courtesy of Dr. T. Simpson, Philadelphia, Pa.)

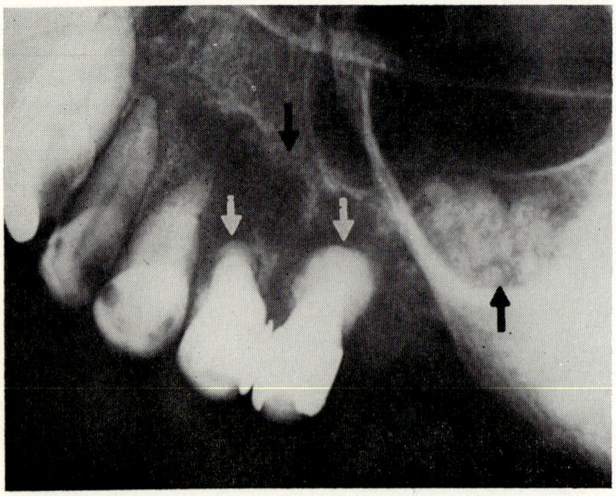

Figure 17. A case of Paget's disease showing root resorption (left white arrow), hypercementosis (right white arrow), osteolytic region (left black arrow) and radiopaque region (right black arrow). (Courtesy of Dr. T. Simpson, Philadelphia, Pa.)

and motor disturbances should make the dentist suspicious of a cranial involvement. Occasionally, oral pain and paresthesia can occur. All drugs, and especially strong narcotics should be prescribed with caution for these patients, as the depressant action can be very dangerous. Before initiating any treatment, a medical consultation is necessary.

Gastrointestinal Diseases, Other than Malnutrition and Peptic Ulcers

General manifestations of gastrointestinal diseases are nausea, vomiting, flatulence, abdominal pain, belching, anorexia, diarrhea, constipation, and blood in the stool.

In these diseases, oral odors may be present that can simulate odors from suppurative pulps. Patients with chronic ulcerative colitis have interference with absorption of nutrients from the gastrointestinal tract. This often results in vitamin deficiencies. Healing may be delayed and this can occur after endodontic therapy. Patients with pyloric obstruction can get dehydration with an interference in water and electrolyte balance. Repair in these individuals is impeded. Cases of exacerbation of gastrointestinal diseases following the swallowing of large numbers of oral microbes have been reported. As with focal infection, evidence for this type of contiguous disease is lacking. It seems probable that the acidic environment of the stomach would destroy most of the swallowed microbes. Patients do ask the dentist if there is danger in swallowing *pus* and the practitioner should explain that any mal-effects are unlikely.

Malignancies

It is important to consult with the patient's physician to determine the present status of the disease. If life expectancy is brief, then pallative treatment may be less traumatic to the patient.

Infectious Mononucleosis

Clinical symptoms include malaise, sore throat, moderate fever from five days to several weeks, slight splenomegaly, headache, general soreness, and anorexia.

Patients with this disease have poor resistance. It is possible to have oral manifestations such as gingival hyperplasia, regional lymphadenopathy, and palatal petechial hemorrhages. Definite treatment for these patients during the active phase of the disease is contraindicated because of their lowered resistance to infection. Palliative treatment should be performed, and then completion of therapy should await the patient's return to normalcy.

Hypoparathyroidism

The most prominent manifestation is tetany which often shows symptoms of tingling and numbness of the fingers, toes and lips.

This is a rare disease, but it has been reported that pain in the bones and teeth can occur. Root resorptions may also be present. These patients have difficulties in healing, including periapical repair.

Rickets, Osteomalacia (Adult Rickets) or Hypovitaminosis D

These patients have generalized bony deformities and may have hypoplastic teeth and osteolytic jaw lesions. Difficulties occur in healing. Vitamin D supplements are necessary but these should be prescribed by the physician treating the condition.

Hypovitaminosis A

This condition is very rare in the United States. The most prominent manifestation is night blindness. These patients may have hypoplastic teeth and an increased susceptibility to infection.

Cystic Fibrosis

This is a childhood pancreatic disease. The patients have malnutrition and are prone to chronic respiratory diseases. Patients with this disease may have osteoporotic jaw lesions and gingivitis. As many of these patients are treated with tetracyclines, tooth discolorations are frequent (Fig. 18).

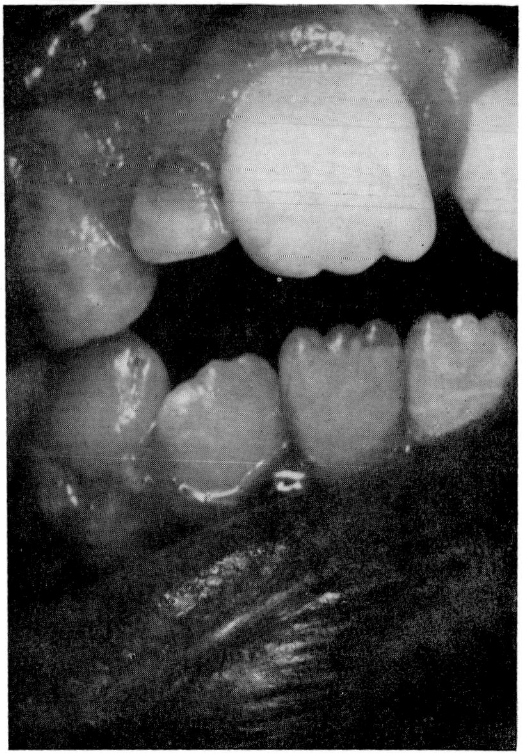

Figure 18. Tooth discoloration in a patient with cystic fibrosis. (Courtesy of Dr. T. Simpson, Philadelphia, Pa.)

Gout

A typical attack is manifested by pain in the big toe or more rarely, in the ankle, knee, elbow, wrist, or a finger. Bones in the various parts of the body, including very rarely the jaws, may show punched out radiolucent areas on radiographs. Patients with gout are usually taking uricosuric drugs for treatment, and shouldn't receive aspirin or aspirin containing-drugs. These preparations antagonize the action of uricosuric drugs.

Skin Diseases (Dermatoses)

In many of these diseases, such as

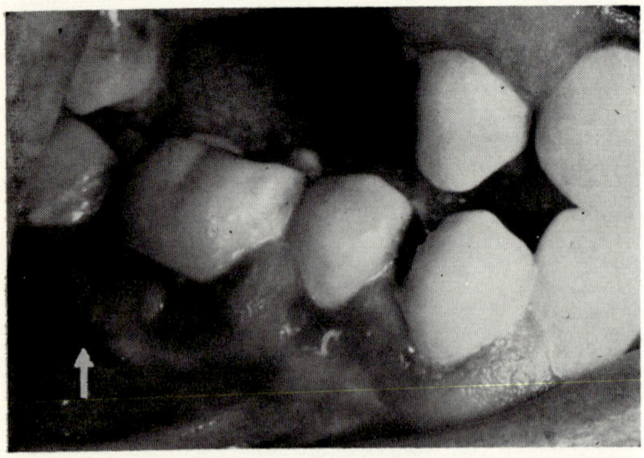

Figure 19. Patient with benign pemphigus showing a lesion in the gingiva-alveolar mucosa area of the lower right first molar. (Courtesy of Dr. T. Simpson, Philadelphia, Pa.)

lupus erythematosus, pemphigus, lichen planus, erythema multiforme and scleroderma, oral ulcerative lesions are present. The lesions are rarely isolated to the alveolar mucosa where they can simulate a parulis (gum boil) (Fig. 19). In scleroderma, the jaws may show radiolucent rarefactions and widening of the periodontal ligament space (Fig. 20). As discussed in the section on adrenal cortex diseases, these patients usually are taking corticosteroids and should be treated accordingly.

Typhoid Fever

This disease is now rare in the United States because of good sanitation procedures. Typical clinical manifestations are gradual onset (10 to 12 days), malaise, fever, headache, nonproductive cough, anorexia, lethargy, nausea, vomiting, constipation, generalized aches, rash, and enlarged spleen. Patients with this disease have been reported to have had the following oral manifestations: oral mucosal ulcerations, pulpal abscesses, periapical abscesses, osteomyelitis, and submaxillary lymphadenopathy. It is not clear whether these dental responses were due to the typhoid microbes per se or to poor patient resistance. In these reported cases, it is probable that caries became rampant, with resultant pulpal exposures, leading to the various oral manifestations.

Prostatitis and Seminal Vesiculitis

These are two genital tract diseases that have been reported to be related to oral foci of infection. The same possibilities exist as has been discussed previously.

Porphyria

There are several types of porphyria but typical clinical manifestations include bullae or vesicles on hands or face upon exposure to sunlight, skin lesions, abdominal pain, and nervous system symptomatology (neuritis, palsy, paralysis). Patients with congenital porphyria

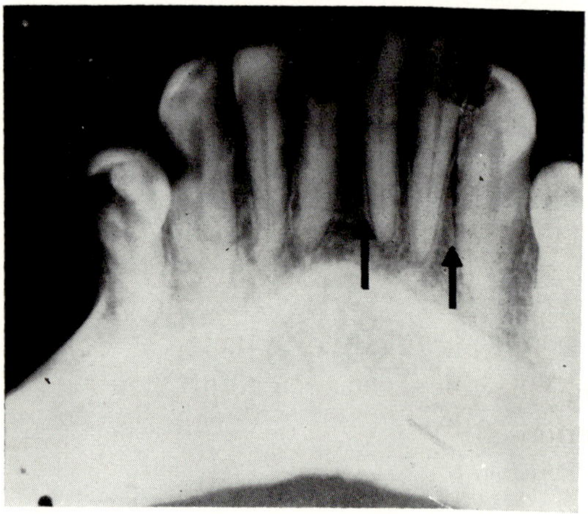

Figure 20. A case of scleroderma in which there is moderate widening of the periodontal ligament space (black arrows) and rarefaction in the lower anterior region. (Courtesy of Dr. T. Simpson, Philadelphia, Pa.)

(a very rare disease) characteristically have brownish-red coloration of their teeth. Tetracyclines, barbiturates, sulfonamides, and alcohol should not be prescribed for these patients. Severe life-threatening reactions can occur as the result of the interactions of these drugs with the porphyrin compounds.

Hemangiomas and Encephalofacial Angiomatosis (Sturge-Weber Syndrome)

In the latter syndrome, hemangiomas are present. Surgery should not be performed on patients with oral-facial hemangiomas as uncontrollable hemorrhage can occur.

Smoking Habits

Smoking can cause the oral manifestations of bad breath, tooth staining, leukoplakia, and oral carcinoma. There also have been reports that smoking causes a depletion in vitamin C levels, which then could cause an interference with repair. Smoking also inhibits certain drugs (see drug section).

Usual Blood Pressure and Pulse Rate

This is noted on the patient's chart so that deviations from normal can readily be determined.

Present and Past Hospitalization

The patient should be asked if he (or she) has ever been hospitalized for any serious disease. This should be entered on the patient's record. If hospitalization was for any of the previously described conditions, then the appropriate section should be consulted. If the patient is currently under medical treatment, this should also be recorded. If any conditions are found that could conceivably affect endodontic therapy, it is essential that the dentist have a medical consultation prior to the start of therapy.

Drug and Nutritional Supplement Intake

Drug, food, and vitamin-mineral supplement intake are important for two basic reasons. These are (1) foods and nutritional supplements that a patient takes or is lacking have a great influence on the patient's resistance. The patient's resistance can affect the outcome of endodontic therapy, and (2) drug interaction can take place between drugs that the dentist prescribes and drugs that the patient has taken, foods that the patient has ingested, nutritional supplements that the patient has taken, external irritants (e.g. air pollutants), and normal tissue metabolites.

The dentist should inquire about drug intake before each visit. It is a good idea to ask the dental assistant, especially if she is young, to question patients about drug intake. Especially important are the drug abuse preparations, such as marijuana, LSD, heroin, amphetamines, barbiturates, Quaalude®, etc. As the young assistant is in the age group of many drug abusers, the patients may be more willing to respond to her than to the doctor. A thorough summary of drug interactions is given in the appendix. Important drug and nutritional supplement interactions are discussed below.

FOODS. It is becoming apparent that not only do drugs interact with other drugs, but foods can also interact with drugs. Certain foods contain drugs naturally, other foods have chemical agents added that may act *in vivo* as drugs. Not only foods, but water also may have excesses of toxic substances. Early in 1973, high levels of chromium were found in the drinking water in a southern New Jersey city. Foods may naturally contain any of these products: vitamins, minerals, hormones, various enzymes, pressor amines, toxins which can act as CNS stimulants, CNS depressants, and hallucinogenic agents, potentially carcinogenic agents, cholesterol, etc. Additives are intentional and nonintentional and they may be used as flavoring agents, preservatives, coloring agents, pesticides, lubricants, plasticizers, stabilizers, sweetening agents, growth promotors (hormones, vitamins, minerals, antibiotics), etc.

Some specific examples are pressor amines which are found in cheeses, yogurt, pickled herring, figs, raisins, wines, etc.; egg yolk which is a prolific source of cholesterol; tannic acid which is in tea; caffeine and other CNS stimulants which are in tea, coffee, cocoa, and cola drinks; mono-sodium glutamate, which can cause a severe throbbing headache, chest pressure, burning pain, and nausea, is found in Chinese foods, baby foods, and in a proprietary seasoner (Accent®); and minerals such as copper, zinc, manganese, mercury, and cadmium may be found in foods. Cadmium is found in tea, coffee, peanuts, and sea foods; various foods have different levels of sodium and potassium; sodium nitrites and nitrates found in frankfurters may interact with amines *in vivo* to form dimethylnitrosamine which can cause migraine-like headaches. The latter compound has also been shown to be carcinogenic in certain animals. Cabbage is high in vitamin K (important in patients on anticoagulants), bread and cereals are high in phenylalanine (a problem for patients with phenylketonuria), DDT, other pesticides, growth hormones, and antibiotics may be found in milk and certain foods, many potential allergins can be found in foods, excessive ingestion of licorice (contains glycyrrhizic acid) can cause pseudoaldosteronism, a serious syndrome that can lead to congestive heart failure, and this is only a small sample of drugs in foods.

As far as drug intake and foods is concerned, generally most drugs are absorbed better on an empty stomach, but there are certain exceptions. Drug manufacturers usually supply this information. If fat is in the stomach, gastric emptying time is increased. This can prolong the action of an ingested drug.

A very interesting recent finding concerns the effects of foods on drug excretion. Certain drugs are only excreted in an acid urine, while others require an alkaline urine. If the pH is not correct for the particular drug, instead of being broken down and excreted, the drug may be reabsorbed. This can lead to a prolonged and dangerous effect. Wheat, cranberry juice, fowl, and fish tend to make the urine acid. Milk and coffee lead to an alkaline urine (a more complete list is in the Appendix).

Generally foods taken within an hour of drug ingestion have the potentiality of interacting with the drug. Some examples of known interactions are calcium carbonate and milk leading to an acute alkalosis and hypercalcemia; MAO inhibitors (anti-depressants) given with any of these foods: cheese, yeast, pickled herring, figs, raisins, broad beans, yogurt, wines, and beer, can lead to a severe hypertensive crisis; cabbage interferes with the action of anticoagulants; crackers have a high starch content and the starch may complex with the particular drug given and interfere with its action.

Many other examples could be given. As it is very difficult to evaluate all the foods a patient may be eating, it is important that the dentist obtains a general survey of the patient's dietary intake. This would help in determining the overall resistance of the patient. Generally the dentist should insist that drugs should not be taken if food has been ingested within two hours.

Amphetamines and Other CNS Stimulants. These patients would require a higher dose of a sedative for the required action. These patients may also appear to be *jumpy* when they come to the dental office. Commonly used drugs are amphetamine (Benzedrine®, Raphetamine®), methamphetamine (Desoxyn®, Amphedroxyn®, Desyphed®, Desoxyephedrine®, Doxyfed®, Dexoval®, Norodin®, Efroxine®, Semoxydrine®, Syndrox®), and dextro amphetamine (Dexedrine®, d-Amfetasul®). Patients should also be questioned about their beverage habits as several cups of coffee, tea, or other caffeinated beverages can cause excitability.

There are also patients that regularly use nasal decongestants. These drugs can cause elevation of blood pressure and increased excitability. Such drugs are phenylephrine nose drops (Neo-Synephrine®), cyclopentamine (Clopane®), naphazoline (Privine®), hydroxyamphetamine (Paredrine®), and phenylpropanolamine (Propadrine®).

Alcohol. Alcohol is the most widely used drug in the United States. Responses of other drugs with alcohol depend upon whether its use is chronic or acute. Acute administration of alcohol inhibits the action of liver microsomal enzymes that normally break down other drugs. This would tend to prolong the action of those other drugs. Therefore, patients who have taken alcoholic beverages prior to the visit should not receive barbiturates, other sedatives, anti-anxiety agents, or antihistamines for sedation. The interaction between these drugs and alcohol can produce a profound depression of the central nervous system. Morphine in therapeutic doses may be lethal in the presence of high blood alcohol levels.

Chronic use of alcohol causes an increased action of microsomal enzymes that break down alcohol itself and other drugs. Hence, alcoholics tend to be tolerant to sedatives and would require higher doses for effective sedation. This would also be true for nitrous oxide analgesia and general anesthetics. In chronic alcoholism, cirrhotic livers are often present, which may lead to a hemorrhagic tendency. Chronic alcoholics may also tend to suffer from malnutrition, with its attendant problems in repair.

Meprobamate (Miltown®, Equanil®), a tranquilizer, increases the tendency to consume alcohol, hence this tranquilizer should not be prescribed for heavy drinkers.

ANTI-DEPRESSANT AND ANTI-HYPERTENSIVE DRUGS. Many patients are taking monoamine oxidase inhibitor drugs (MAOI'S) for the control of depression. It is imperative that the dentist does not use a vasoconstrictor, such as epinephrine for these patients. The interaction of the sympathomimetic amines with the MAOI'S can cause a *MAOI crisis* in which the patient develops a severe headache and a substantial rise in blood pressure. This may lead to a cerebral hemorrhage or an acute cardiovascular collapse. Some MAOI drugs are furazolidone (Furoxone®), iproniazid, isocarboxazid (Marplan®), mebanazine, procarbazine (Matulane®), nialamide (Niamid®), phenelzine sulfate (Nardil®), pivaloyl hydrazine, tranylcypromine sulfate (Parnate® sulfate) and pargyline (Eutonyl®). These patients should also not receive narcotic analgesics, barbiturates, tranquilizers and general anesthetics. The interaction of these drugs with MAOI drugs can cause bizarre reactions including extreme hypotension with coma, an increased anti-depressant action, and an increased hypoglycemic action. Patients taking anti-hypertensives such as mecamylamine (Inversine®), chlorpromazine (Thorazine®), hydralizine (Apresoline®), pempidine, quanethidine (Ismelin®), bethamidine, alphamethyldopa (Aldomet®), and reserpine should not receive general anesthetics or sedatives unless the latter drugs are given under controlled hospital conditions. The interaction of those drugs with anti-hypertensives can cause a dangerous hypotension. In the dental office, patients taking any of the anti-hypertensives can develop a severe hypotension from a sudden change in position.

ASPIRIN AND ASPIRIN-CONTAINING COMPOUNDS. If a cardiac patient is taking one of the coumarin-type anticoagulant drugs (Dicumarol, Coumadin, Denilone, Hedulin), and he (or she) also receives aspirin, this can lead to an increased anticoagulant effect. The aspirin releases the anticoagulant from its binding sites on plasma proteins. This leads to an increased effect from the anticoagulant. The same type of reaction occurs between aspirin and the corticosteroids resulting in an increased steroid effect. Hence, these patients should receive non-aspirin containing analgesics such as acetaminophen (Tylenol, Nebs). In diabetics taking insulin or the sulfonylureas (Orinase®, Diabinase®, Dymelor®), the interaction of aspirin with these compounds can cause an increased insulin effect. A more pronounced hypoglycemia results. Unless high doses of aspirin are used, this does not become a clinical problem. Ulcer patients should not take aspirin or aspirin-containing compounds, as gastrointestinal bleeding can occur. This is a result of the direct action of the aspirin on the lining of the gastrointestinal tract. Also patients who have had kidney transplants should not have aspirin because of its ulcerogenic potential. Aspirin potentiates the action of penicillin and the sulfonamides by displacing the anti-microbial from its site on plasma proteins. Therefore, this has to be considered if these drug combinations are prescribed. Aspirin produces antagonism of uricosuric drugs used in the treatment of gout. Aspirin should be used with extreme caution in patients with asthma, as the principal allergic manifestation of aspirin is an asthmatic attack. It should also be avoided in patients with hemorrhagic disorders. It has been reported that newborn infants can have bleeding problems as a result of aspirin ingestion by the mother. Therefore, aspirin should not be prescribed during the last month of pregnancy. Patients on high aspirin therapy (such as patients with rheumatoid arthritis) have an increased tendency toward hemorrhagic problems. This may be related to the fact that aspirin impairs platelet function. Also vitamin C is normally found in high levels in platelets. Clinical studies have shown that high doses of aspirin significantly decreases vitamin C levels, both in plasma and platelets. As vitamin C is important for repair, it would appear to be important to give rheumatoid patients supplementary vitamin C before performing surgery. Prior consultation should be obtained with the patient's physician, because of the possibility of exacerbation of the rheumatoid condition by too high a dose of vitamin C.

Giving a compound containing aspirin, phenacetin and caffeine (a typical analgesic preparation) to a patient who has an intake of large amounts of sucrose may lead to growth inhibition. Studies have shown that ingestion of large amounts of sucrose tends to decrease sexual activity. This result is compounded if analgesics such as aspirin, paracetamol, and phenacetin, are taken.

ANTI-ANXIETY AGENTS. The anti-anxiety agents such as chlordiazepoxide (Librium) and diazepam (Valium) should not be given to patients on anti-thyroid drugs, as the interaction of the two groups of drugs causes an increased anti-thyroid effect. The anti-anxiety drugs interfere with the uptake of iodine into the thyroid gland. Patients who are taking anti-anxiety drugs such as the phenothiazine drugs, Thorazine, promazine (Sparine®) and prochlorperazine (Compazine®) require a smaller dose of barbiturates for sedation. They would also require a smaller dosage of nitrous oxide for analgesia.

BARBITURATES, OTHER SEDATIVES AND ANTIHISTAMINE DRUGS. Patients taking these drugs would also require a smaller dosage of nitrous oxide for analgesia. Barbiturates, glutethimide (Doriden®), and ethchorvynol (Placidyl®) antagonize the action of anticoagulants, so that more of the anticoagulant would be necessary. If patients are on anticoagulants and a barbiturate is being used, the barbiturate should not be removed rapidly as bleeding can occur. Dentists should not prescribe barbiturates to patients taking griseofulvin (an antifungal antibiotic) because the barbiturates interfere with the action of griseofulvin. Barbiturates should not be prescribed for epileptic patients taking diphenylhydantoin (Dilantin), as the barbiturates interfere with the action of Dilantin. Barbiturates and anti-histamines should not be prescribed for patients taking steroids, as the former drugs interfere with the action of the steroids. Barbiturates cause the release of posterior pituitary hormones. If the patient is receiving a local anesthetic with felypressin (as in some non U.S. formulations of Citanest), the patient should not also receive a barbiturate. The felypressin plus the released posterior pituitary hormones causes an enhanced effect which can lead to cardiovascular collapse. Barbiturates are contraindicated for patients with porphyria. Barbiturates can be used as a premedicant to counteract the convulsive effect of local anesthetics. However, local anesthetics also have a delayed depressive effect and the barbiturate would not help in counteracting the depression. This is especially true for the amide-type local anesthetics (e.g. lidocaine).

Patients who are taking antihistamines, such as thonzylamine HCl (Anahist®), tripelennamine HCl (Pyribenzamine®), diphenhydramine HCl (Benadryl) and chlorpheniramine maleate (Chlor-Trimeton®), require a smaller dose of barbiturates and other sedatives. The reason is that the antihistamines have sedative action of their own. The sedatives also antagonize the antihistaminic action. It has been reported that antihistamines can also interfere with the action of local anesthetics. If a patient is on an antihistamine, it may take a larger dose and a longer time interval for local anesthesia to occur.

ANTIBIOTICS. If patients are on tetracyclines, the dentist should not prescribe penicillin simultaneously as an antagonistic effect can occur between the two groups of drugs. Antagonism has also been reported between penicillin and erythromycin. Most oral organisms are sensitive to penicillin and this is the drug of choice, provided no hypersensitivity exists and the microbes are not penicillinase producers. Patients taking antibiotics (especially tetracyclines) can have diarrhea. Many intestinal bacteria are destroyed and vitamin K can be lost in excessive amounts. Blood clotting may be impaired. For patients taking anti-coagulants the anticoagulant effect would be enhanced. The dentist should not prescribe antidiarrhea drugs such as Kaopectate®, as these drugs interfere with the gastrointestinal absorption of the antibiotics. Tetracyclines should not be prescribed for patients with congenital porphyria. The interaction of the tetracycline with the heme compounds can cause a severe reaction. Tetracyclines and lincomycin are contraindicated for cardiac patients taking digitalis. The diarrhea that could result from the ingestion of the antibiotic results in an increased toxic effect by the digitalis. Iron, even in small quantities, inhibits the effects of tetracyclines. Iron is in many vitamin-mineral supplements and is often prescribed for women during pregnancy and for patients with iron deficiency anemia.

Patients who are on antacid compounds containing aluminum salts (usually taken by ulcer patients) should not receive tetracyclines within at least an hour of the antacid ingestion. The reason is that most of the tetracycline is bound by the antacids.

The interaction of tetracyclines and ultra-violet rays from sunlight can cause bronzing of the skin. It also has been reported that an aspirin and tetracycline combination leads to increased bleeding.

Patients on immunosuppressive drugs have inhibition of gamma globulins. As tetracyclines inhibit protein synthesis, the interaction of the immunosuppressives and the tetracyclines can cause further inhibition of gamma globulins.

SULFONAMIDES. The dentist should not prescribe sulfonamides to patients taking anticoagulants as these anti-microbial drugs potentiate the action of anticoagulants. Sulfonamides should also not be prescribed for diabetic patients taking insulin or the sulfonylurea compounds. The sulfa drugs cause an increased hypoglycemic effect. Sulfonamides should not be given to patients taking procaine local anesthetics or procaine penicillin, as the sulfa drugs are antagonistic to the latter drugs. Sulfonamides are also contraindicated for patients with liver and kidney diseases.

ANTI-PARKINSONISM PREPARATIONS. Dentists should not prescribe propoxyphene (Darvon®) compounds to Parkinson's disease patients who are taking orphenadrine (Disipal®, Norflex®). The resultant interactions of the two drugs may cause central nervous system stimulation including tremors, mental confusion and anxiety. Dentists should not prescribe multiple vitamin preparations containing pyridoxine for Parkinson's disease patients taking L-Dopa®, as the pyridoxine antagonizes the L-Dopa.

ORAL CONTRACEPTIVES. Women taking birth control pills appear to have a higher incidence of flare-ups during endodontic therapy. This may be related to hormonal changes or depletion of vitamin C by the oral contraceptives.

A recent study has shown that women taking oral contraceptives have a significantly lower level of vitamin C (in leukocytes and platelets) than in women not taking the pills. To aid in repair, women taking oral contraceptives should receive supplementary vitamin C before undergoing surgical procedures.

CORTICOSTEROIDS. Some aspects of corticosteroid therapy have been discussed under the adrenal cortex disease section.

Dentists should not prescribe corticosteroids for patients with viral infections, tuberculosis, peptic ulcers, diabetes, and hypertension. Corticosteroids can cause exacerbation of infection, increase in gastric acidity, development of hyperglycemia and glycosuria, and an increase in blood pressure. They also interfere with inflammation and repair, increase fat at the expense of protein, and lead to the development of osteoporosis. Interaction of aspirin and corticosteroids causes an increased steroid effect. Patients taking corticosteroids with oral infections present must have antibiotic coverage during treatment.

IMMUNOSUPPRESSIVE DRUGS. Patients who are on immunosuppressive drugs (usually recipients of transplants) must have the concomitant administration of antibiotics during therapy. Medical consultation is essential before any treatment is begun. The principal immunosuppressive agents used (aside from the corticosteroids) are azathioprine (Imuran®) and anti-lymphocyte serum.

STIMULATORY DRUG ABUSE PREPARATIONS. Patients who are taking LSD, other hallucinogens, heroin, cocaine and other dangerous addictive drugs are very hyperreactive. Sedation may be difficult. They may also have bizarre reactions in the dental office. Cocaine and epinephrine taken systemically can cause cardiac arrythmias, convulsions, and vasomotor collapse. No definite deleterious effect is known from marijuana, except that the patients' reflexes are slowed. If patients are addicted to narcotics, obtaining analgesia is difficult. Use of nonnarcotic analgesics is not often effective.

Iodine Preparations. There have been cases of thyrotoxicosis that have developed from nontoxic goiters as the result of the use of iodoform pastes in endodontic treatment.

Vitamin, Mineral and Protein Supplements. Although such supplements may be helpful for repair, it is necessary to ascertain the reason the patient is taking them. Are the supplements being prescribed by a physician for a known deficiency or are the supplements self-prescribed? Is the patient taking an overdose of potentially damaging vitamins such as A and D? Also, ingestion of vitamins A, D, E and K can cause erroneous values to be given for some common laboratory tests.

Nicotine. A recent study has shown that chronic smokers gave a poorer response to Librium and Valium (antianxiety agents) than did nonsmokers. This may be related to the interaction of nicotine with these drugs.

Cathartics. The use of mineral oil as a laxative may be taken regularly by some patients. It interferes with vitamin K absorption, which could lead to a hypoprothrombinemia and bleeding complications during dental procedures.

Oral History

This covers past history, current manifestations, habits and chief complaints.

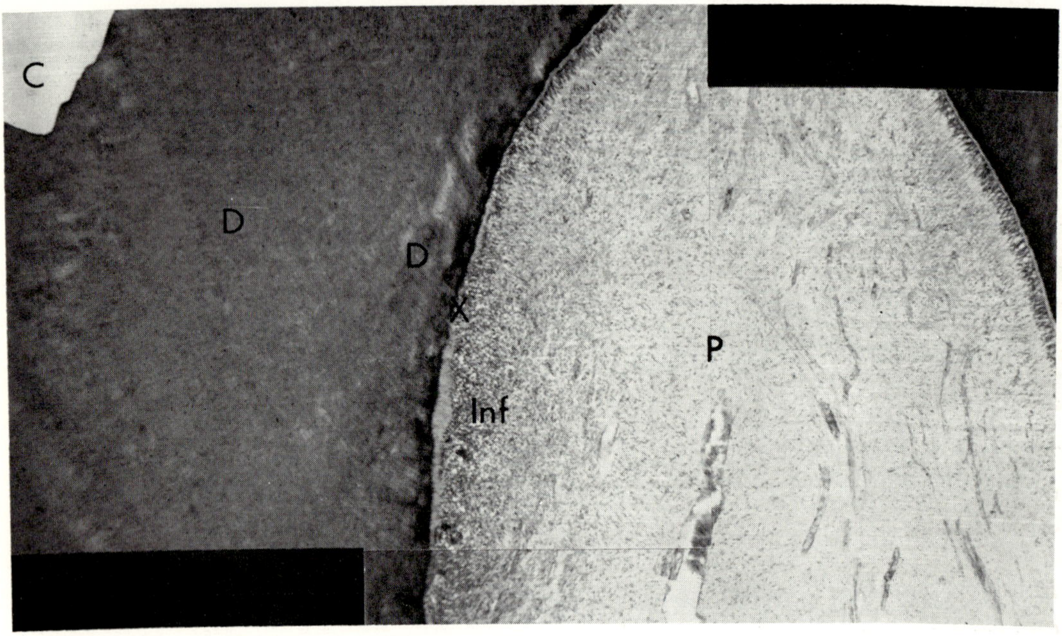

Figure 21. Pulpal inflammation beneath a silicate restoration; P = pulp, Inf = inflammation, D = dentin, C = space where silicate was placed; predentin is missing at region X (×54). (From S. Seltzer and I. B. Bender, *The Dental Pulp*, J. P. Lippincott Co., 1965. Used with permission of J. P. Lippincott Company.)

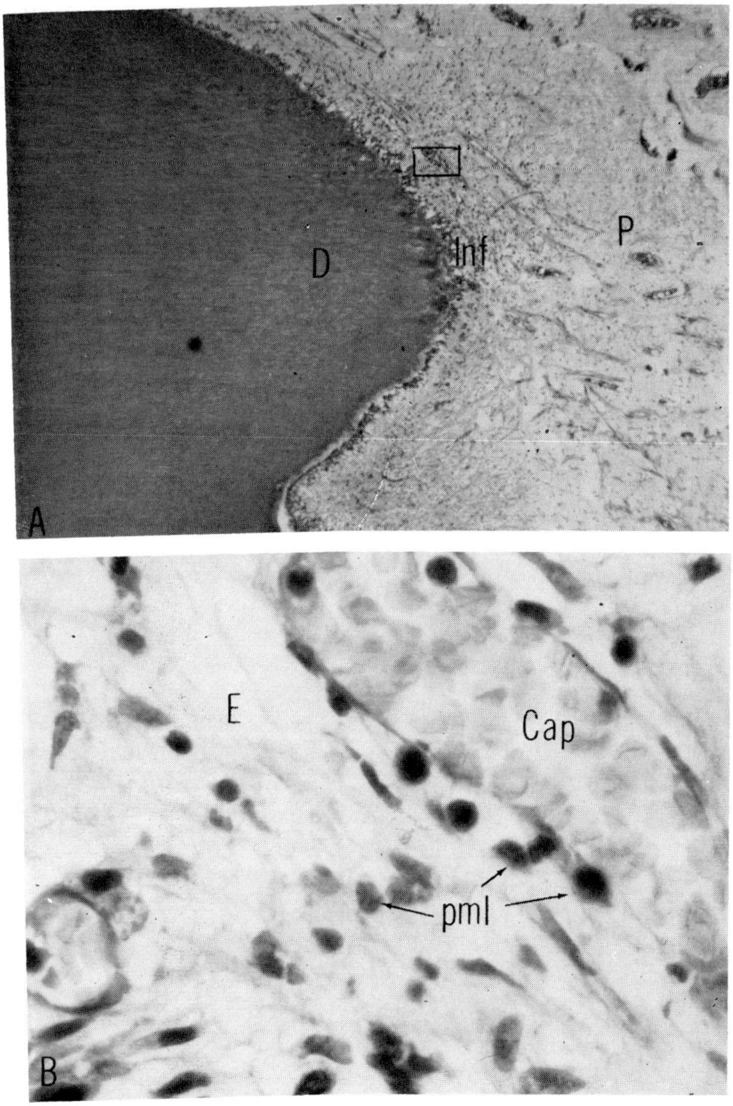

Figure 22. Acute pulpitis beneath a gold foil restoration that had been applied one week previously; the cavity preparation was shallow. A. P = pulp, Inf = inflammation, D = dentin (×54). B. Higher magnification of section indicated by rectangle; Pml = polymorph leucocytes, Cap = dilated capillaries, E = edematous tissue spaces (×960). (From S. Seltzer and I. B. Bender, *The Dental Pulp*, J. P. Lippincott Co., 1965. Used with permission of J. P. Lippincott Company.)

The first section is devoted to history, manifestations, and habits. The next section covers chief complaints.

Extensive Dental Restorations and Caries

Patients that have had extensive caries and restorations are likely candidates for at least some pulpal exposures. Often dental restorations inserted years previously can cause pulps to become chronically inflamed. Then some recent incident can cause an acute flare-up. In some individuals, the presence of gold and amalgam restorations in adjoining or opposing teeth can set up an electrolytic reaction. This could in turn cause an electrical shock that could conceivably result in pulpal damage.

Silicate and Plastic Restorations. The phosphoric acid of silicates and the monomer of acrylic restorations are very damaging to pulps, especially in unlined cavities. Even a shallow unlined cavity restored with a silicate can lead to pulpal necrosis (Fig. 21).

Restorations in General. Regarding synthetic, gold, and amalgam restorations, the dentist should question the patient.

(1) Was automatic malleting performed (Fig. 22)?

(2) Was zinc phosphate used as a cement base or to cement in the restoration?

(3) Were you told that the cavity was close to the *nerve*?

(4) Was a chemical such as silver nitrate or phenol used in the base of the cavity (Figs. 23, 24)?

(5) Was air blown into the cavity?

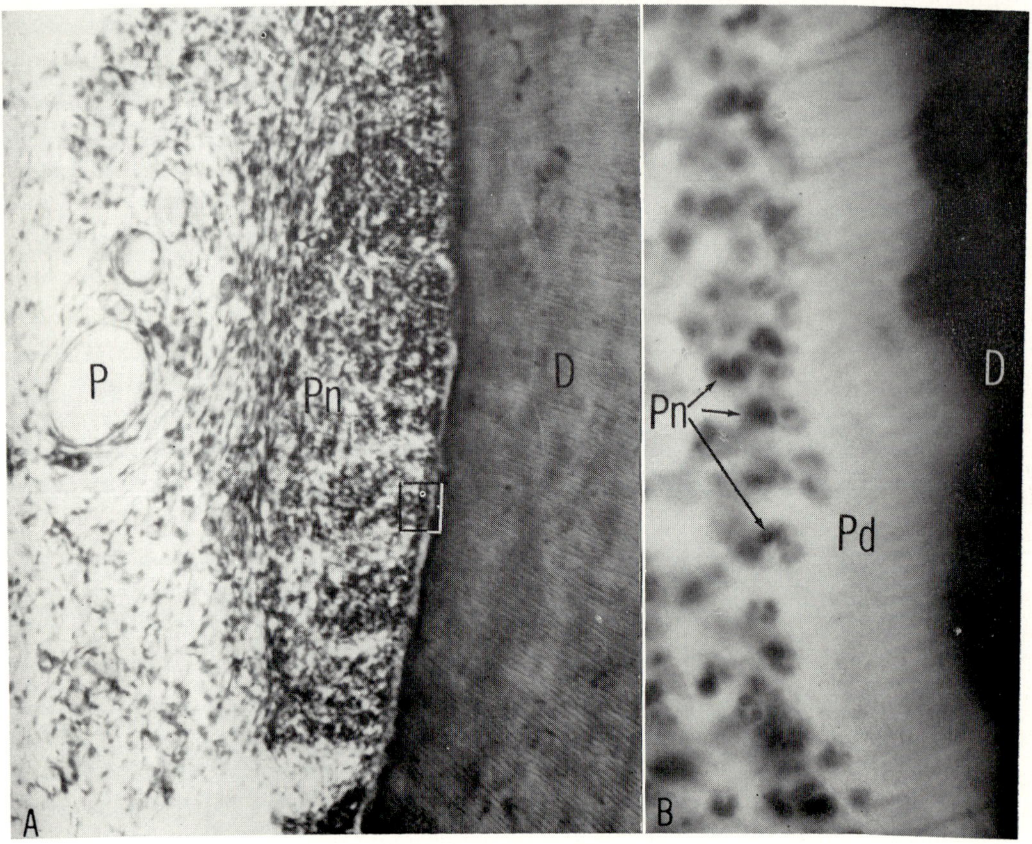

Figure 23. Pulpal inflammation following use of silver nitrate. A. P = pulp, Pn = polymorph leucocytes, D = dentin (×96). B. Higher magnification of section indicated by rectangle; Pn = polymorph leucocytes, Pd = periodontal ligament, D = dentin (×960). (From S. Seltzer and I. B. Bender, *The Dental Pulp*, J. P. Lippincott Co., 1965. Used with permission of J. P. Lippincott Company.)

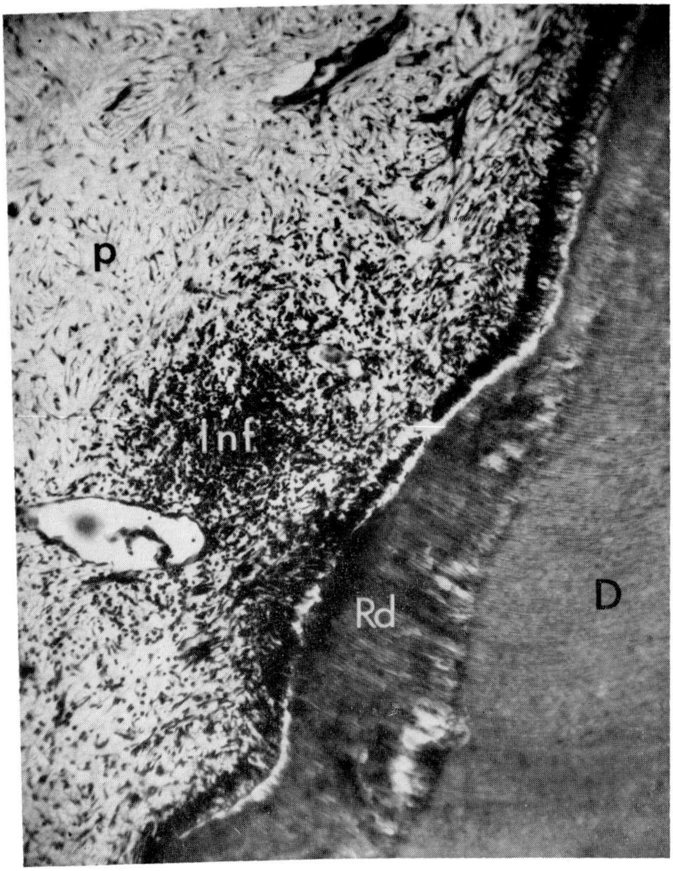

Figure 24. Pulpal inflammation following use of phenol; three months following application of phenol to deep cavity in dentin; P = pulp, Inf = inflammation, Rd = reparative dentin, D = primary dentin (×100). (From S. Seltzer et al, "Histologic Changes in Dental Pulps of Dogs and Monkeys Following Application of Pressure, Drugs, and Microorganisms on Prepared Cavities," *Oral Surg*, 14: 856, 1961.)

(6) Was alcohol or chloroform wiped on the cavity?
(7) Was the tooth drilled on without water?
(8) Was slow speed used? Did you feel vibrations?
(9) Were large burs or stones used?
(10) Was a hot impression taken? Was it taken more than once (Fig. 25)?
(11) Were pins used to reinforce the restoration? Insertion of pins can cause stresses to develop, which may result in pulpal damage or fractures into the pulp.
(12) Were the restorations polished in the mouth? All of these aforementioned procedures or chemicals can cause pulpal damage.
(13) Were there *nerve* exposures (Fig. 26)? If there were, was either pulp capping or pulpotomy performed? Internal resorption (Fig. 27) and calcification (Fig. 28) can result from these procedures.
(14) Did the filling feel *high* during biting or eating? *High* fillings may initiate an acute apical per-

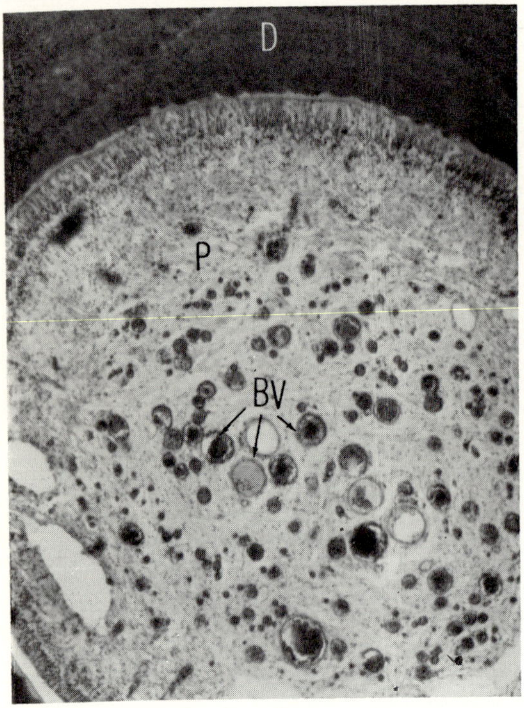

Figure 25. Effect of heat and pressure on the pulp; P = pulp, D = dentin, BV = engorged blood vessels; filled with polymorph leucocytes (×54). (From S. Seltzer and I. B. Bender, *The Dental Pulp*, J. P. Lippincott Co., 1965. Used with permission of J. P. Lippincott Company.)

iodontitis and may cause pulpal damage over a long period of time.

Trauma from Dental and Non-Dental Diseases

The patient should be asked the following questions:

(1) Was there any known blow or fall involving the teeth? Trauma can cause pulpal necrosis, even years after the incident.

(2) Was there any known blow to the primary predecessor? Trauma to a primary tooth can cause damage to the permanent successor. The resulting conditions are hypocalcification, hypoplasia, and dilaceration. Dilacerated teeth often become pulpless.

(3) Was an extraction performed on an adjacent tooth? The pulp of a tooth next to an extracted tooth can become injured from the luxation or extraction procedure. This may be true even if the extraction occurred years previously.

(4) Has the tooth ever been luxated

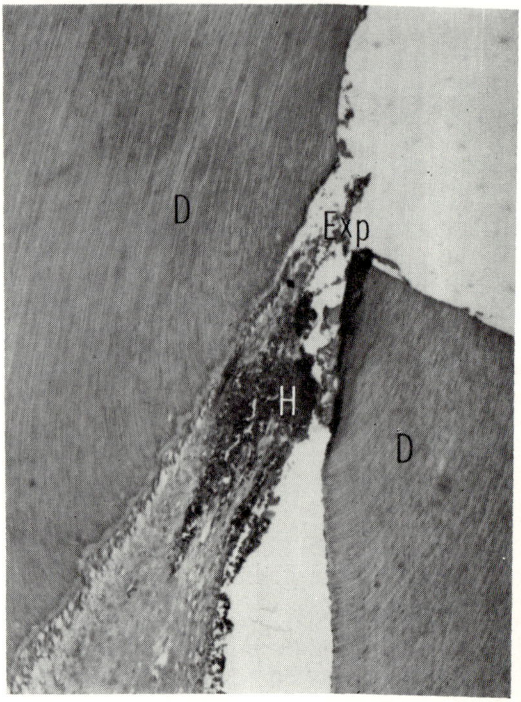

Figure 26. The effect on the pulp of a small mechanical exposure; D = dentin, Exp = exposure, H = hemorrhage (×96). (From S. Seltzer and I. B. Bender, *The Dental Pulp*, J. P. Lippincott Co., 1965. Used with permission of J. P. Lippincott Company).

(pushed up into the socket, displaced partially out of the socket, displaced labially or displaced lingually)? Pulps can become inflamed or necrotic as a result of luxation.

(5) Has the tooth ever been avulsed (knocked out) and then replanted? Certain dentists in particular situations replant teeth without performing endodontics.

(6) Was the tooth transplanted from another site in the same mouth? from another individual? Again, at times endodontics is not performed initially on transplanted teeth.

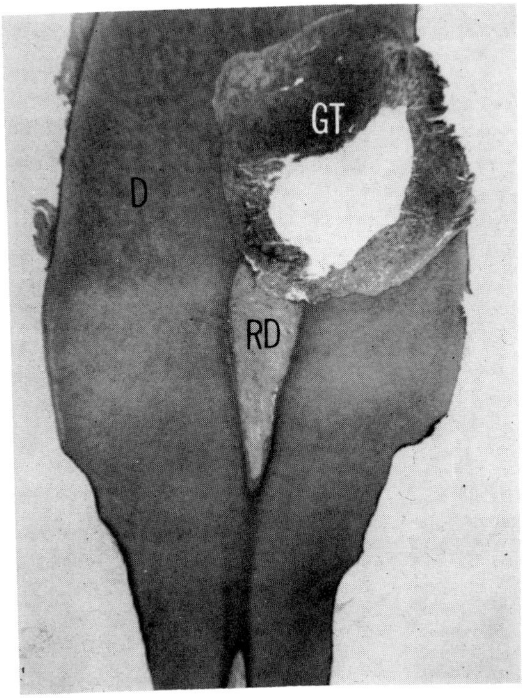

Figure 27. Internal resorption; D = dentin, RD = reparative dentin, GT = granulomatous tissue (×8.6). (From S. Seltzer, *Endodontology*, McGraw-Hill, Inc., 1971. Used with permission of McGraw-Hill Book Company.)

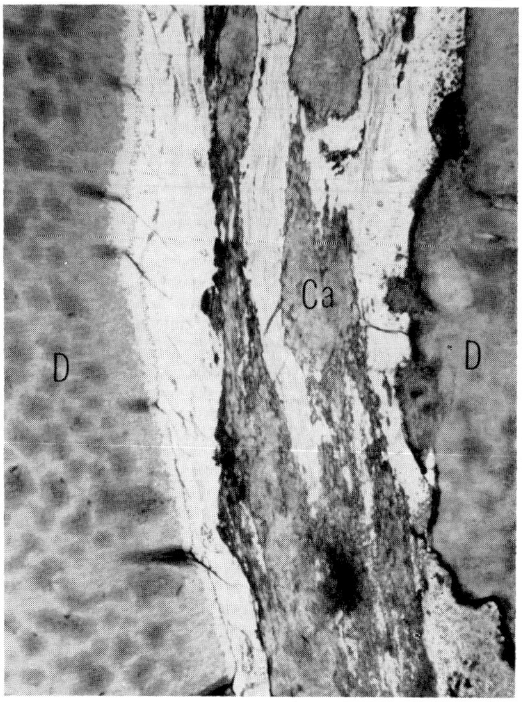

Figure 28. Dystrophic calcification of the pulp; D = dentin, CA = diffuse calcification, P = pulp (×54). (From S. Seltzer and I. B. Bender, *The Dental Pulp*, J. P. Lippincott Co., 1965. Used with permission of J. P. Lippincott Company.)

(7) Have the teeth ever been separated?
   (a) by separating devices during dental treatment?
   (b) by personal objects such as toothpicks, and wedges? These procedures can cause pulpal damage.

(8) Has any form of surgery been performed in the oral-facial area? Was general anesthesia used? Pulpal death can occur in upper anterior teeth following rhinoplasty procedures. Injury to upper posterior teeth can follow

maxillary sinus surgery. Luxation and/or other traumatic injuries can occur to incisors during oral intubation procedures for general anesthesia (Fig. 29).

Previous Endodontic Therapy on any Tooth

The dentist should inquire about the patients' reactions (good or bad) to the previous therapy, so that he (or she) can be better prepared to treat the patient for the current condition, if endodontics is required. If endodontic therapy has been completed on a tooth previously and now needs retreatment, there are certain clinical manifestations:

Persistent Pain Since Therapy. The dentist should suspect an accessory canal, a root fracture, excessive filling material in the alveolar mucosa (possibly due to apical fenestration), a poorly filled canal, an inadequate retrograde seal, an adjacent pulpally-involved tooth, or a perforation during treatment.

Pain on Mastication or Biting. The dentist should suspect a root fracture, a restoration in supraocclusion, an over-

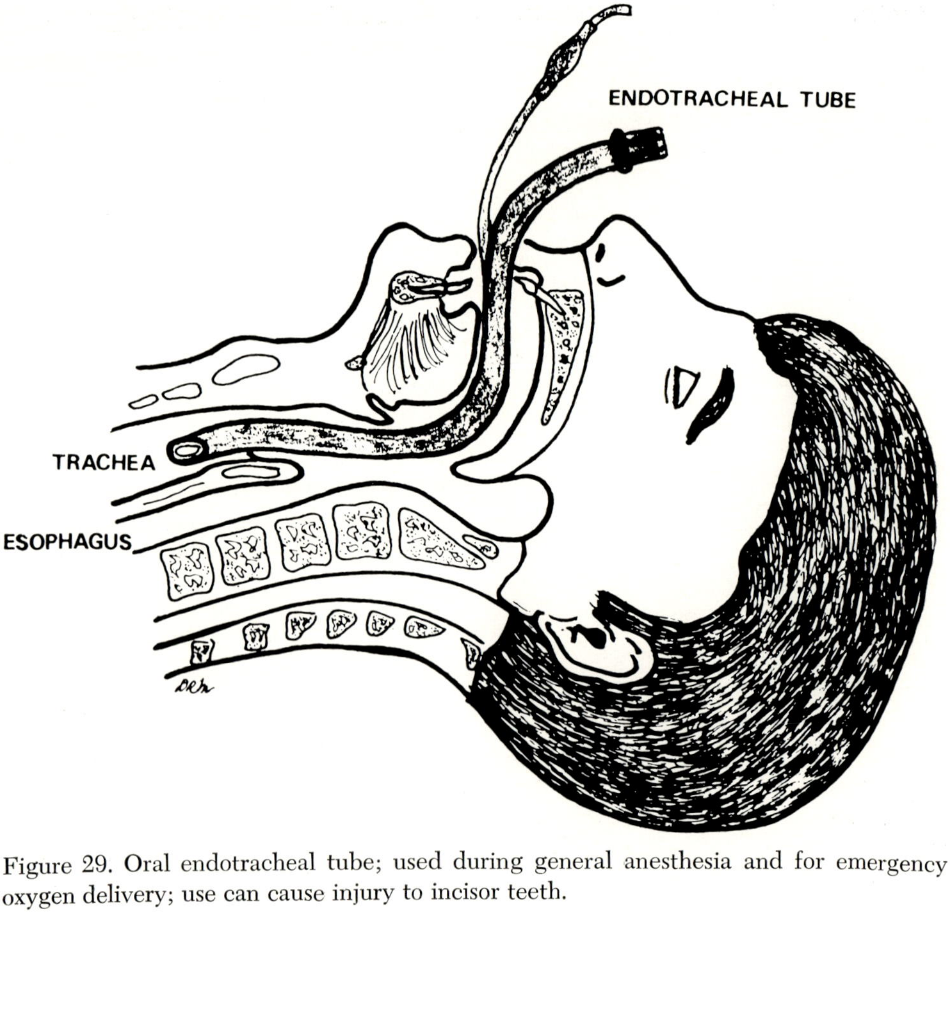

Figure 29. Oral endotracheal tube; used during general anesthesia and for emergency oxygen delivery; use can cause injury to incisor teeth.

filled silver cone, or a perforation (if a post had been placed).

PERSISTENT SWELLING. The dentist should suspect a root fracture, a poorly sealed root canal, excessive filling material in the alveolar mucosa, or a perforation during treatment.

A DRAINING SINUS TRACT. The dentist should suspect a root fracture, a poorly sealed root canal, a perforation during treatment (or from a post), or an endodontic-periodontic lesion.

HISTORY OF A BLOW TO THE TOOTH OR A FALL ON THE TOOTH AFTER THERAPY HAS BEEN COMPLETED. The dentist should suspect a root fracture, or displacement of a root canal filling, especially if an apical amalgam was inserted.

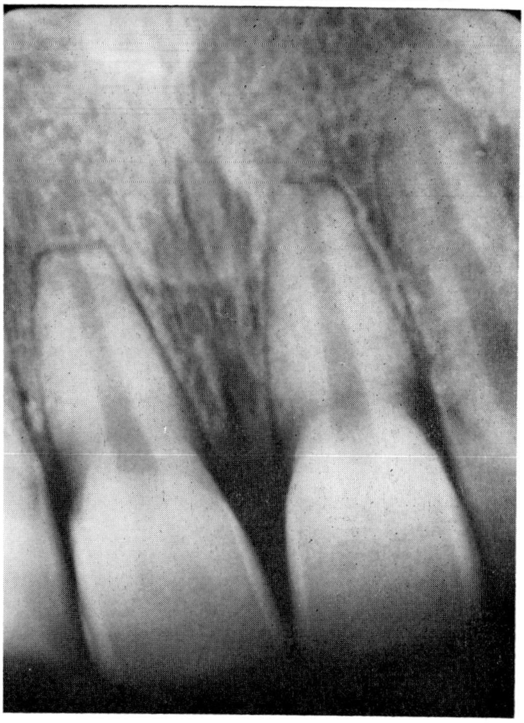

Figure 30. Root resorption on orthodontically treated upper incisors. (Courtesy of Dr. T. Simpson, Philadelphia, Pa.)

Periodontal Diseases

The patient should be asked about previous or present periodontal disease. Symptoms and signs of periodontal disease can simulate endodontic conditions. These manifestations include pain, swelling (local, as well as regional lymphadenopathy), and bleeding. Periodontal conditions can cause pulpal disease and vice versa. Sometimes the periodontal pocket does not regress or stop suppurating after periodontal treatment. The reason may be a vertical fracture that is difficult to detect either clinically or radiographically.

Periodontal Treatment

This includes curettage and/or surgery. The dentist should inquire whether any of these procedures were performed on the tooth in question or on adjacent teeth. Periodontal treatment, especially when cementum is removed can expose lateral canals and open dentinal tubules. This may lead to pulpal damage.

Orthodontic Therapy

The patient should be asked about previous orthodontic therapy. Teeth moved orthodontically can show extensive root resorption, calcifications, and even pulpal necrosis (Fig. 30). Patients can also develop toothaches. Extensive caries may also be found under bands and attachments. Occasionally, orthodontically-moved upper anterior teeth can have bone loss on the palatal bone with a periodontal pocket extending to the apex.

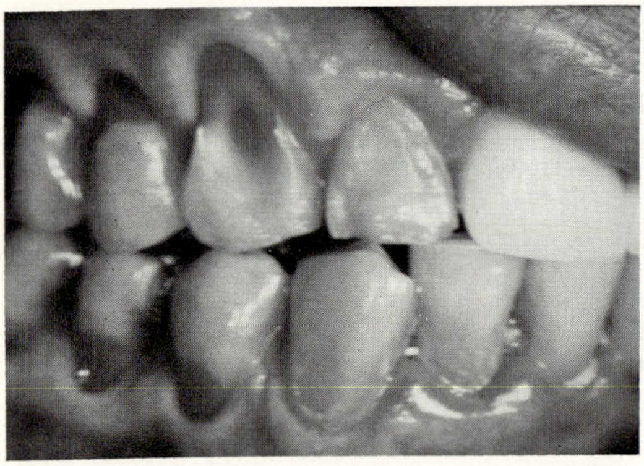

Figure 31. Severe erosion in a patient who often sucked lemons. (Courtesy of Dr. T. Simpson, Philadelphia, Pa.)

Removable Partial Prostheses

The patient should be asked if he (or she) has a removable denture in the mouth. Extensive caries can also develop beneath clasp attachments of partial dentures.

Hypersensitive Dentin Treatments

The patient should be asked if there was any treatment for hypersensitive dentin (or cementum). Caustic chemicals such as silver nitrate as well as electrocautery may induce pulpal damage.

Recent Extractions

The dentist should inquire about recent extractions in the vicinity where the patient has symptoms. Pain from a *dry socket* can be referred to adjacent teeth. There may be a residual root, cyst, or granuloma, that is causing the symptoms. Also, pain may arise from a *phantom* tooth at the site of a former extraction.

Habits

The dentist should ask the patient if he (or she) has any habits that might cause erosion, attrition, abrasion, or trauma. These habits can lead to pulpal damage, pulpal exposure, and periodontal disease.

PINS. Women who often use hair pins or bobby pins may have teeth with characteristic attrition patterns. Periodontal pockets may also develop on the involved teeth.

PIPES. Pipe smokers develop notable abrasions and attritions and can also develop periodontal pockets.

CITRUS FRUITS. Citrus fruit consumers can have severe erosion (Fig. 31).

BRUXISM. Bruxism (clenching or grinding) can cause attrition as well as trauma to the involved teeth (Fig. 32).

HABITS THAT PUT UNUSUAL STRESS ON TEETH. Examples are strong men who pull heavy objects with their teeth, and people who put nails and tacks in and out of their teeth while they are doing carpentry work (Fig. 3). Thumb suck-

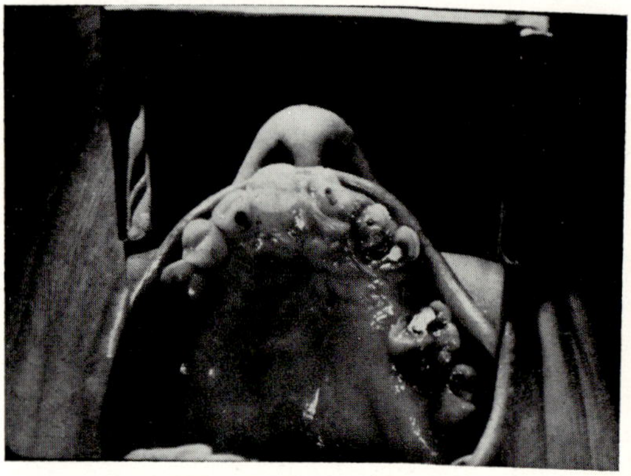

Figure 32. Extensive attrition leading to pulpal exposures; resulting from bruxism. (Courtesy of Dr. T. Simpson, Philadelphia, Pa.)

ing and tongue thrusting may cause pulpal and periodontal disease.

Sialorrhea

The patient should be asked whether he (or she) salivates excessively. This may result from nervousness. The dentist may have to prescribe antisialagogues to combat this condition.

Xerostomia

If the patient has an exceedingly dry mouth, this may be the result of intake of antisialogogues such as atropine and scopolamine. The intake of these drugs can lead to an increased caries incidence.

Temporo-mandibular Joint Pain—Dysfunction Syndrome (Myo-fascial Pain —Dysfunction Syndrome)

These entities are probably the same, although occlusal problems are emphasized in the designation TMJPDS, and muscular imbalances are stressed in the designation, MFPDS. Oral pain may be an important symptom in these conditions. The patient should be asked the following questions if a previous history of a TMJ problem is given or if the condition is suspected:

(1) Is there continuous pain or discomfort?
(2) Is there an earache on the involved side?
(3) Do the teeth seem to meet first on the involved side?
(4) Is the pain intensified upon biting or eating?
(5) Do the jaw muscles feel tense?
(6) Is it difficult to keep your mouth open wide?
(7) Do subluxations or dislocations of the jaw occur?

A yes answer to these questions may be indicative of TMJ dysfunction.

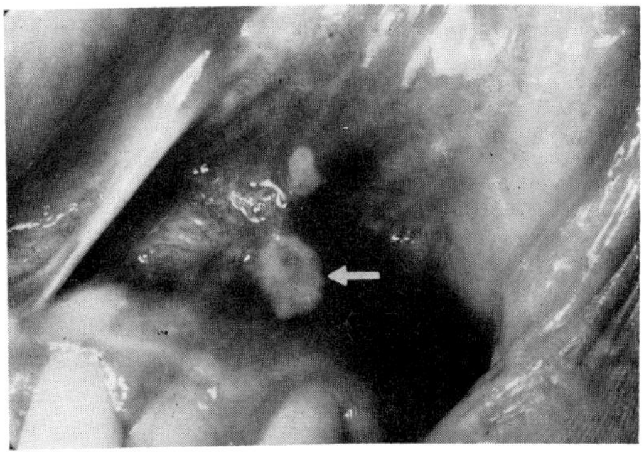

Figure 33. Apthous ulcer located at the mucobuccal fold. (Courtesy of Dr. T. Simpson, Philadelphia, Pa.)

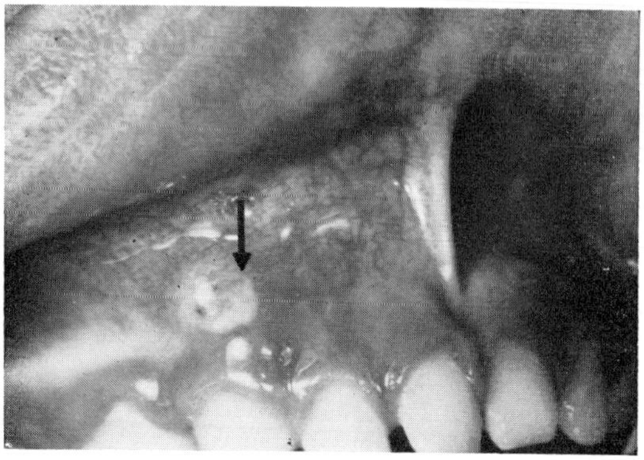

Figure 34. Ulcer on alveolar mucosa related to trauma. (Courtesy of Dr. T. Simpson, Philadelphia, Pa.)

Osteomyelitis

The patient should be asked about any previous history of extensive bone disease in the jaws, such as osteomyelitis. Osteomyelitis may become chronic instead of being completely cured. Acute

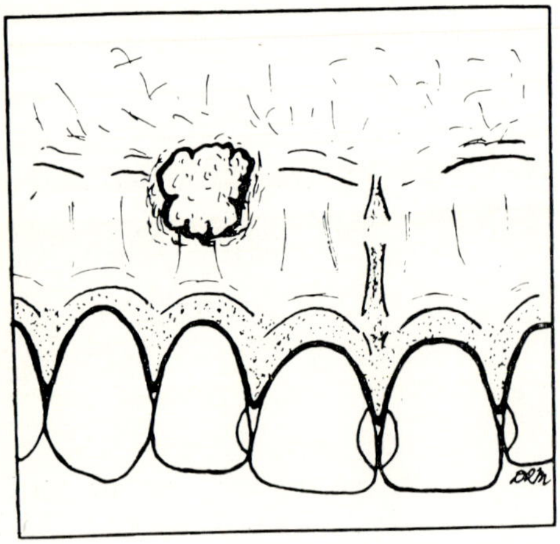

Figure 35. Leukoplakia-type lesion.

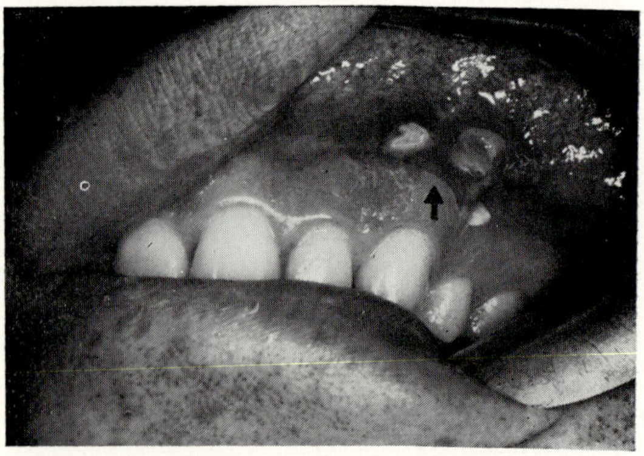

Figure 36. Silver nitrate burn resulting from dental use of silver nitrate. (Courtesy of Dr. T. Simpson, Philadelphia, Pa.)

exacerbations may occur later causing severe pain. The pain may simulate pulpal or periapically-induced pain.

Minor Oral Lesions

Lesions such as herpetic stomatitis, apthous stomatitis (Fig. 33), traumatic ulcers (Fig. 34), herpes zoster, herpangina, leukoplakia (Fig. 35), and thrush may occasionally be isolated to the oral mucosa and simulate paruli (gum boils). The patient should be asked the following questions:

(1) Have you eaten or done anything that could have burned or irritated the mucosa and thus caused this lesion (Figs. 36-38)?

(2) Has the lesion changed in appearance? Paruli (gum boils) increase in size and after they discharge, they decrease in size (Fig. 39). They may then enlarge

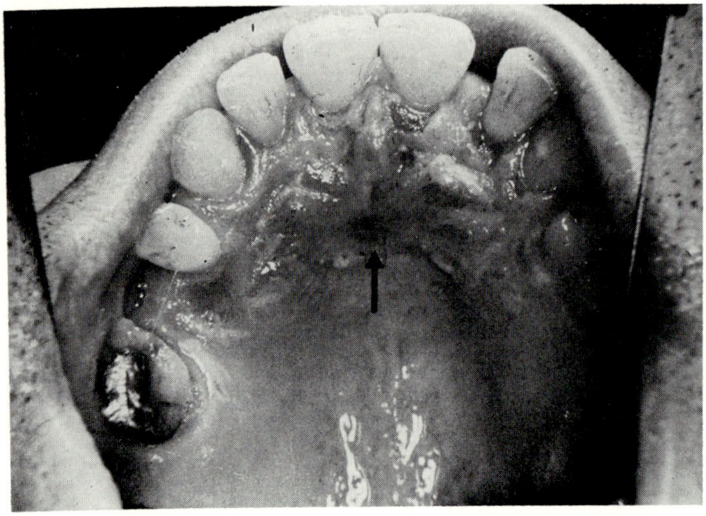

Figure 37. Pizza burn on anterior palate. (Courtesy of Dr. M. Gross, Philadelphia, Pa.)

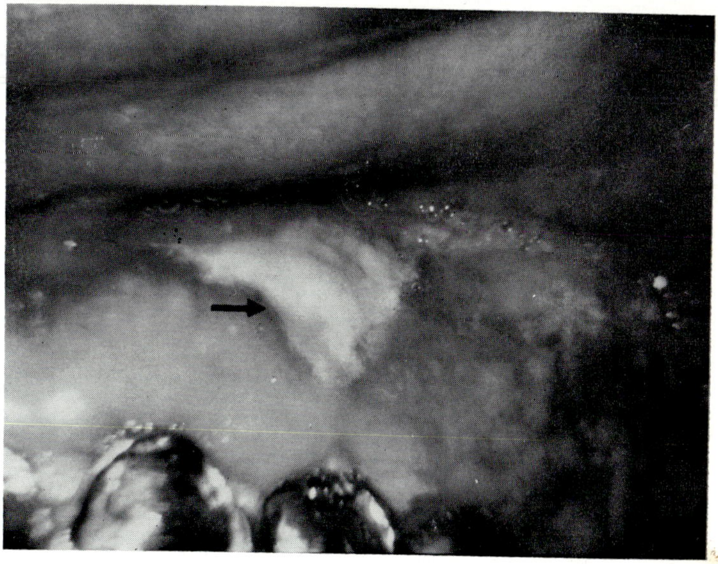

Figure 38. Aspirin burn caused by placement of aspirin in the muco-buccal fold in attempt to relieve a toothache. (Courtesy of Dr. L. Muldorf, Philadelphia, Pa.)

again. Salivary gland swellings follow the same type of pattern according to food ingestion. Tumors may enlarge slowly or rapidly, depending upon the type.

Salivary Gland Diseases

Present occurrence or past history of salivary gland diseases should be elicited from the patient. Salivary gland diseases include mumps, acute sialadenitis, and chronic sialadenitis. Oral lesions from these diseases may rarely be isolated to the alveolar mucosa, thereby simulating paruli. Regional lymphadenopathy can occur which may be misdiagnosed as an endodontically originated lymphadenopathy. On occasion, pain may be referred to teeth from the salivary gland disease.

Tumors and Cysts

Benign tumors and cysts may also simulate paruli. Primary and metastatic lesions can be found in the jaws that may be confused with pulpally-induced periapical pathoses. These malignancies can cause teeth to loosen, roots to resorb, the lamina dura to be lost, and pain and paresthesia to occur. Isolated lesions can occur in the region of the alveolar mucosa, and regional lymphadenopathy can develop.

Chief Complaints

These include pain, swelling, odor, taste, bleeding, mobility, tooth discoloration, cracked tooth, paresthesia, oral lesions, and a discharging sinus tract.

PAIN. Categories covered in this section are location, pathways of referred pain, duration, frequency, type, previous episodes, relieved by, increased by, unchanged by, and initiated by. A chart listing possible etiologies of odontalgia is shown in Table I.

Location: Is it unilateral or bilateral?

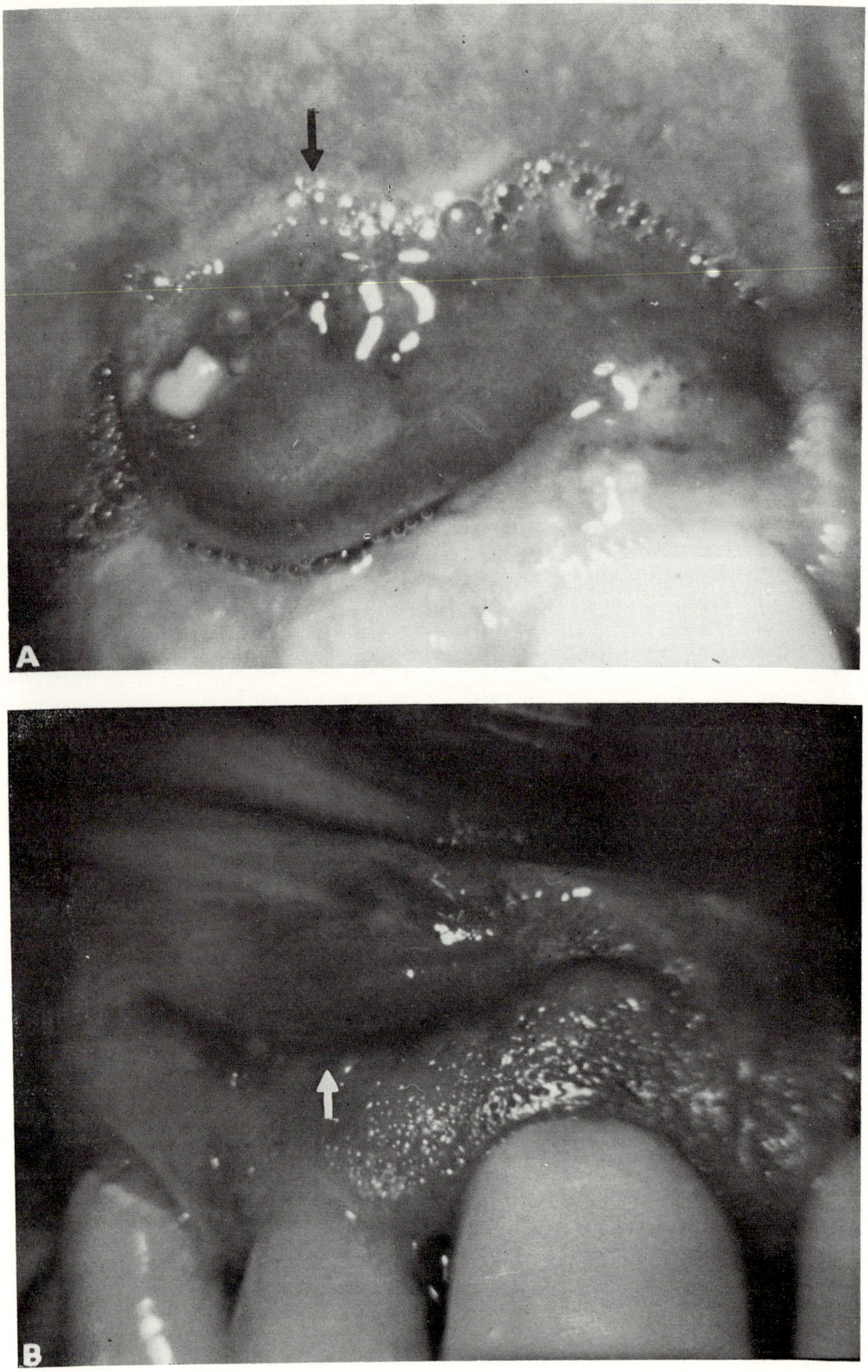

Figure 39. Large parulis (stoma, *gum boil*). A. Before discharging. B. After discharging. (Courtesy of Dr. L. Muldorf, Philadelphia, Pa.)

TABLE I

ODONTALGIA*

The possible etiologies of odontalgia are listed in order of decreasing frequency. This order is an approximation based on clinical experience and a review of the literature.

Condition	*Usual Type of Pain*	*Primary or Referred*	*Causative Factors*
Hypersensitive dentin or cementum	Dentinal; sharp; sudden; stops when stimulus is removed	Primary	Periodontal disease, periodontal treatment, abrasion, erosion, attrition, fracture, caries, operative dentistry procedures
Acute pulpitis	Mild pulpalgia of short duration	Primary	Operative dentistry procedures, direct pulp capping, pulpotomy, periodontal disease, periodontal treatment, rapid orthodontic movement, galvanism, sudden trauma (e.g. extraction of adjoining tooth, nasal and sinus operations, oral intubation procedures)
Chronic pulpitis	Mild to severe pulpalgia; increases with severity of pulpitis; pain is worst when acute exacerbation occurs	Primary	Caries, attrition, erosion, abrasion, periodontal disease, secondary to operative dentistry procedures (may occur years later), secondary to periodontal treatment and rapid or excessive orthodontic tooth movement; exacerbations can occur as a result of trauma (cracked tooth syndrome), operative dentistry, periodontal treatment, and atmospheric pressure (aerodontalgia)
Acute apical periodontitis (acute pericementitis)	Mild odontalgia, intensified by biting	Primary	Occlusal traumatism (usually from a "high" restoration), incipient periapical disease, result of endodontic treatment procedures (instrumentation, irrigation, intracanal medication, "high" temporary restoration, obturation)
Periapical granuloma and radicular cyst	Mild to severe odontalgia; severe pain can occur with acute exacerbation	Primary	Sequel to pulpal disease; original etiology is the same as listed for chronic pulpitis; may also occur after a root canal failure (root fracture, root perforation, foreign body beyond the apex, incomplete obturation)
Acute apical abscess	Moderate to severe odontalgia	Primary	Sequel to pulpal disease; original etiology is the same as listed for chronic pulpitis
Cellulitis (e.g. buccal space, canine space, submaxillary space, sublingual space)	Moderate to severe odontalgia; pain subsides when localization and drainage occurs	Usually primary; may occasionally have a facial cellulitis from a non-dental cause and then dental pain would be of referred type	Usually a sequel to periapical disease; original etiology is the same as listed for chronic pulpitis; may occasionally result from facial trauma, eye diseases (e.g. canine space), etc.

TABLE 1 *(Continued)*

Condition	*Usual Type of Pain*	*Primary or Referred*	*Causative Factors*
Myofascial pain-dysfunction syndrome	Moderate odontalgia	Referred; temporal m. to upper posteriors; masseter m. to lower posteriors	Muscular imbalance; occlusal imbalance; psychological factors; joint discrepancies
Neuralgias	Severe odontalgia	Referred	Unknown
Periodontal diseases	Mild to severe odontalgia; mild with gingivitis, periodontitis more severe with periodontal abscess, acute papillitis, ANUG (Vincent's disease), acute herpes, and acute pericoronitis	Usually primary; can be referred in acute pericoronitis	Calculus, occlusal traumatism, habits, malocclusion, poor dentistry (e.g. overhanging margins, lack of proximal contact), mouth breathing, vitamin deficiencies, blood dyscrasias, various systemic diseases, and Dilantin therapy
Sinusitis (maxillary [more common] and frontal) and sinus lesions	Mild to moderate odontalgia	Referred from sinus to upper teeth (maxillary sinusitis to posteriors, frontal sinusitis to anteriors)	Common cold, allergies, other nasal and sinus diseases and lesions
Eye diseases, inflammations, and lesions	Mild to moderate odontalgia	Referred	Viral diseases, microbial infections, eye lesions, accidents and operations
Ear diseases, inflammations, and lesions	Mild to moderate odontalgia	Referred	Viral diseases, microbial diseases, ear lesions, accidents, and operations
Salivary gland diseases, inflammations, and lesions	Mild to moderate odontalgia	Referred	Viral diseases, microbial diseases, salivary gland lesions, operations, and accidents
Coronary artery diseases	Moderate to severe odontalgia	Referred	Heart diseases related to microbial infections, diet, hereditary, physical activity, habits (smoking, etc.), drug intake
Cranial tumors, diseases and conditions	Moderate to severe odontalgia	Referred	Viral and microbial diseases, cranial accidents, drugs, lesions, emboli, hereditary factors
Diabetes mellitis	Moderate odontalgia	Primary	Hereditary, diet, pain is related to pulpal arteritis or atherosclerosis of pulpal or periapical blood vessels
Menstruation and pregnancy	Mild to moderate odontalgia	Primary	Pain is related to hyperemia and capillary dilatation of pulpal and periapical blood vessels, that results from hormonal changes
Throat diseases, inflammations and lesions	Mild to moderate odontalgia	Referred	Virus infection, microbial disease, and lesions, operations and accidents

Osteomyelitis	Mild to severe odontalgia; severe pain in acute conditions	Referred	As a sequel to periapical disease, radiation therapy, chemicals, and as a late stage in diseases such as syphilis, tuberculosis, and Paget's
Leukemias	Mild to severe odontalgia; severe pain in acute conditions	Primary	Pain may result from accumulation of leukemic cells in pulpal and periapical blood vessels; disease related to hereditary and environmental factors
Sickle cell anemia	Moderate to severe odontalgia	Primary	During "sickling crisis," toothache can occur that may be related to presence of sickle cells in pulpal and periapical blood vessels; disease is of hereditary type
Thyroid diseases, inflammation, and lesions	Mild to moderate odontalgia	Referred	Microbial diseases, lesions, accidents, and operations
Miscellaneous bony lesions, either primary or secondary	Mild to severe odontalgia	Referred	Hereditary and environmental factors
Acute suppurative myositis	Moderate to severe odontalgia	Referred	Secondary to cellulitis or result of facial accident or operation; unsterile injection into muscle
Arthritis of neck	Moderate odontalgia	Referred	Hereditary and environmental factors
Whiplash injury of neck	Moderate odontalgia	Referred	Accident involving the neck region
Miscellaneous systemic diseases including: malaria, aspergillus, gastrointestinal disturbances, urogenital disturbances, gout, influenza, and hypoparathyroidism	Mild to moderate odontalgia	Referred	This group of diseases has been reported to cause odontalgia probably resulting from sympathetic nervous system interconnections with the fifth nerve; results are based solely on case reports
Neuritis	Mild to moderate odontalgia	Referred	The inflammation can result from facial trauma, dental extractions, or severe bites
Temporal arteritis	Moderate to severe odontalgia	Referred	This disease may be a form of periarteritis nodosa (a possible autoimmune disease)
Cavernous sinus, thrombosis (cavernous sinus thrombophlebitis)	Moderate to severe odontalgia	Referred	May follow periapical disease in a debilitated individual; secondary to severe cranial-facial diseases
Various oral soft tissue tumors	Moderate to severe odontalgia	Referred	Pressure on nerve trunk can cause referred pain
Jaw fractures	Moderate to severe odontalgia	Referred	Pressure on nerve trunk can cause referred pain

* Odontalgia refers to pain coming from a tooth. It may be primary or referred from another site. The primary pain may be of dentinal, pulpal, periapical, or periodontal origin. Pulpalgia refers to pain of pulpal origin.

If bilateral, systemic disease should be suspected.

(1) *One tooth only.* The dentist should consider pulpal-periapical disease, periodontal abscess, and occlusal traumatism.

(2) *Several teeth involved.* Possibly etiologies are maxillary sinusitis and periodontal diseases. It is rare for odontalgia to occur simultaneously in two or more teeth.

(3) *No tooth involved.* Consideration should be given to *phantom* tooth pain, an acute alveolitis *(dry socket)* from a recent extraction, a residual root (or tip), or a residual granuloma or cyst.

(4) *Submaxillary lymph nodes.* Here there is a wide range of possibilities including endodontic diseases, salivary gland diseases, periodontal diseases, many oral lesions, and oral manifestations of systemic diseases.

(5) *Facial area.* The possibilities are neuralgias, neuritises, temporal arteritis, buccal space infection, temporal or infratemporal space infection, sinusitis, cranial diseases, oral-facial manifestations of systemic diseases, and myofascial pain-dysfunction syndrome (masseter m.).

(6) *Sinuses.* The practitioner should suspect maxillary or frontal sinusitis or neoplasms of the sinuses.

(7) *Occipital, frontal, and temporal areas.* The patient has a headache. Possible etiology is cranial diseases, migraine, neuralgias, neuritises, systemic diseases, referred pain from teeth, and myo-fascial pain-dysfunction syndrome (temporal m.).

*Pathways of referred pain:**

(1) *Referred from teeth to other teeth and/or from teeth to areas in head and neck.* Referred pain occurs primarily with teeth affected by chronic partial pulpitis. Occasionally, cracked teeth can cause referred pain. Once the apical periodontal ligament becomes involved, the pain becomes localized. These pathways of referred pain are only general guidelines, and may vary in individual cases. Pain may be referred anywhere along the distribution of the fifth cranial nerve, and can occasionally be referred to other areas. This is because of the close anatomic association of the fifth nerve with the third, fourth, sixth, seventh, ninth, and tenth cranial nerves, the cervical nerves, and the sympathetic nervous system (Fig. 40). Referral patterns are depicted in Figure 41. Pathways are the following:

(a) From the upper centrals and laterals to the frontal area, posterior maxilla, lower molar area, and rarely to upper premolars, upper molars, lower premolars, mental area, angle of the mandible, the ear, and temporal area

* Referral pathways are based on findings by Dr. D. H. Glick, Beverly Hills, Ca.; Dr. S. Seltzer, Philadelphia, Pa.; and Dr. N. Chivian, W. Orange, N. J., and Dr. D. R. Morse, Philadelphia, Pa.

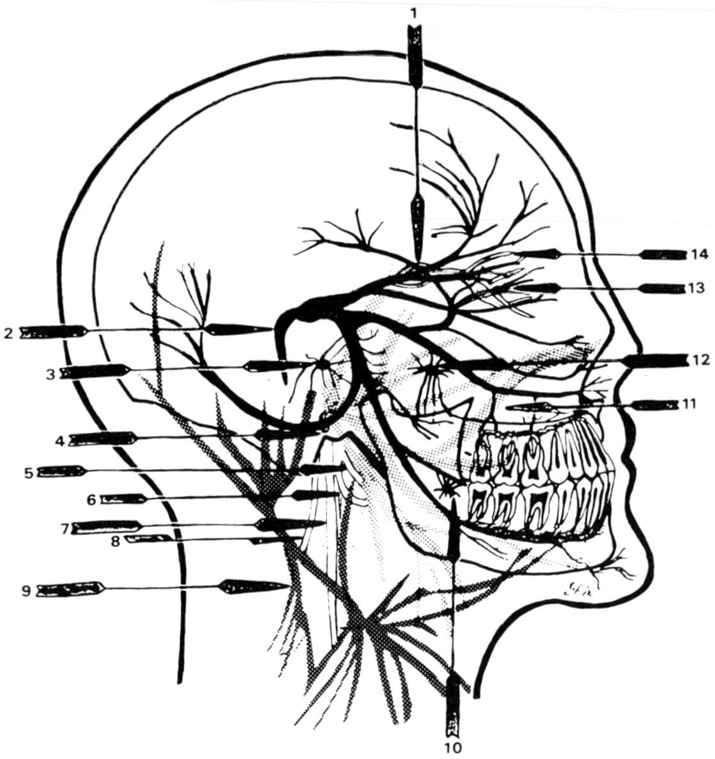

1—4th & 6th nerves
2—5th nerve & trigeminal ganglion
3—Otic ganglion
4—8th nerve
5—9th nerve
6—12th nerve & sympathetic chain
7—10th nerve
8—11th nerve
9—Cervical nerves
10—Submaxillary ganglion
11—7th nerve
12—Sphenopalatine ganglion
13—Ciliary ganglion
14—3rd nerve

Figure 40. Nerve connections of the fifth nerve.

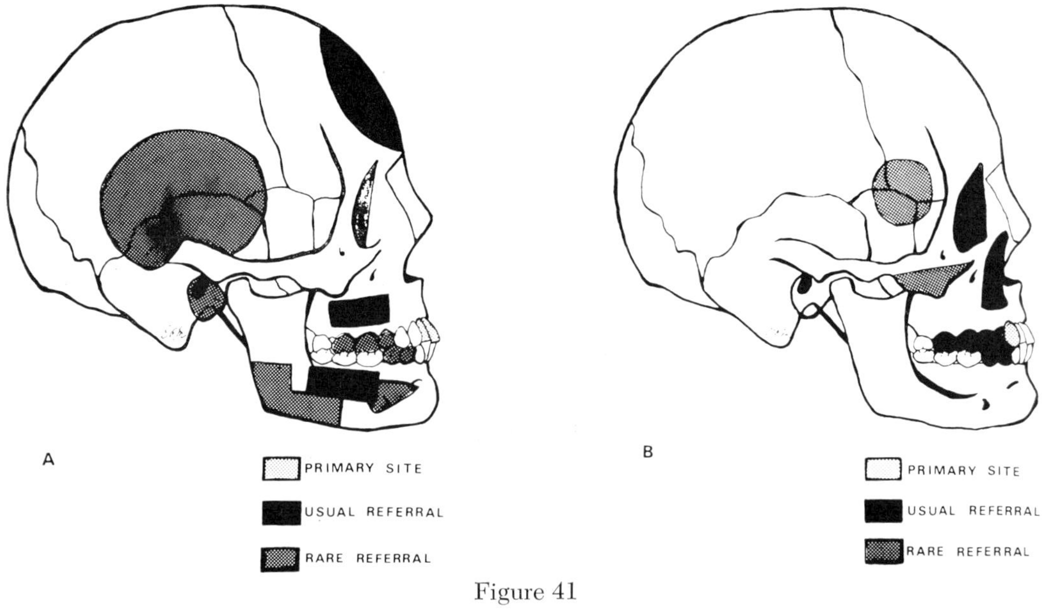

Figure 41

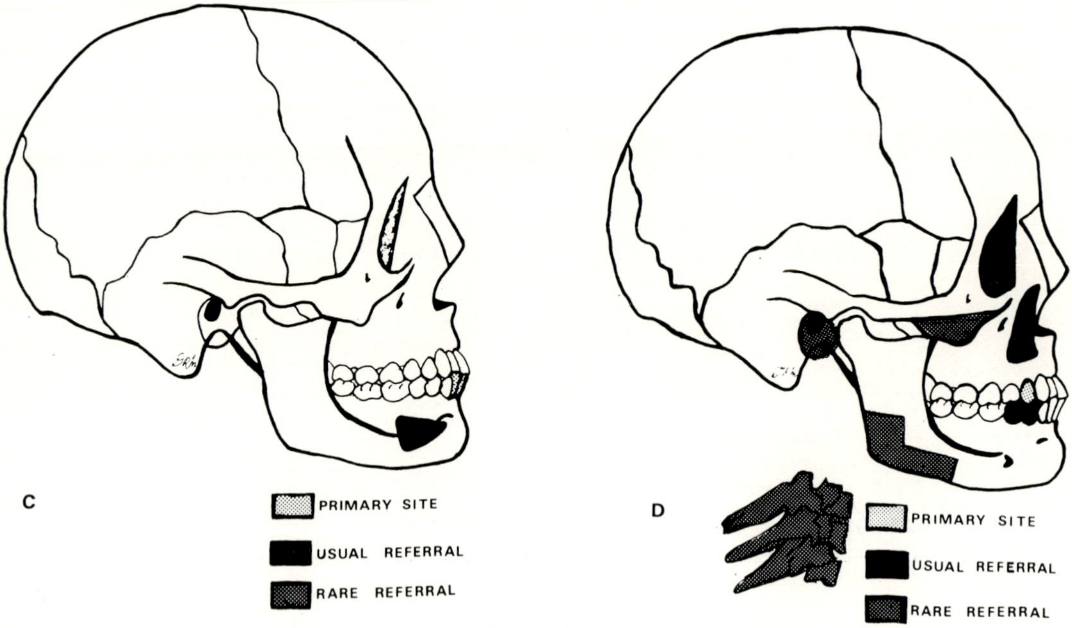

Figure 41

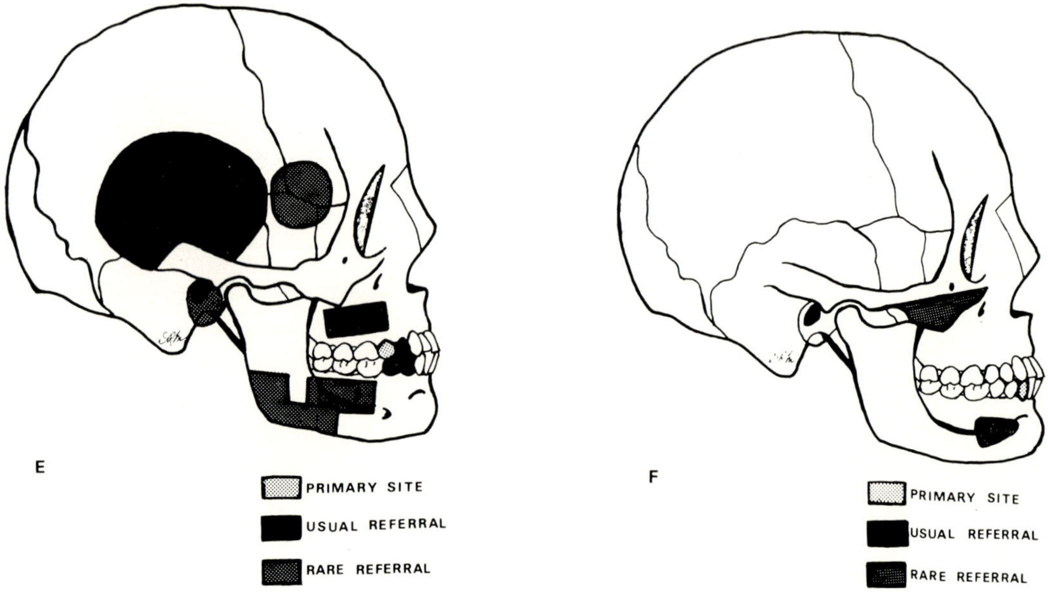

Figure 41

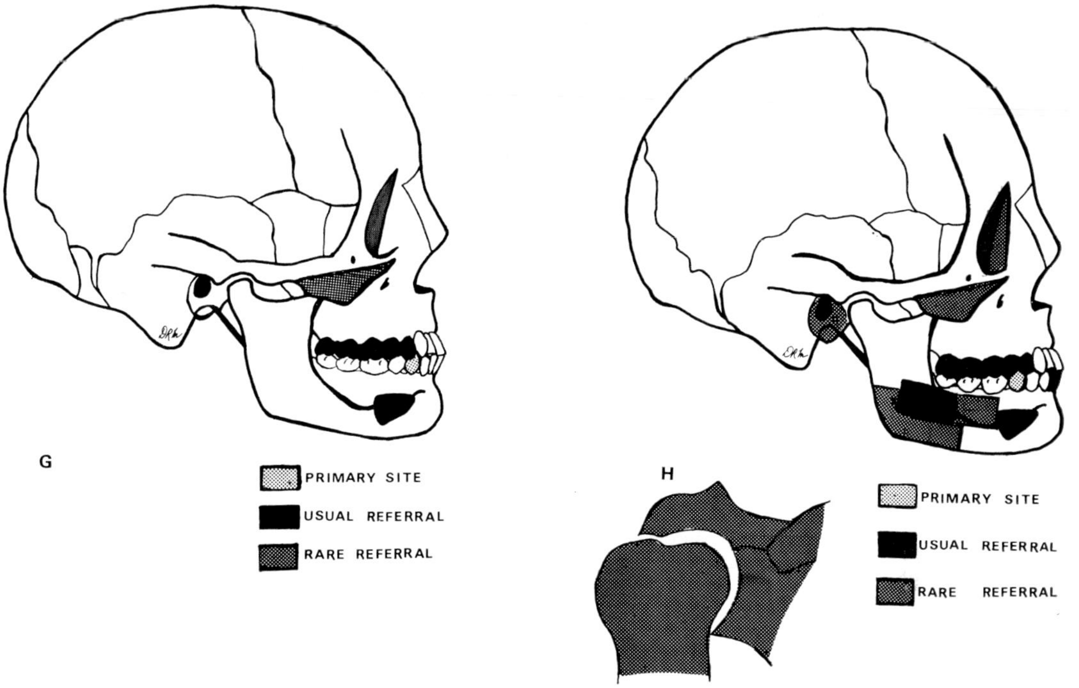

Figure 41

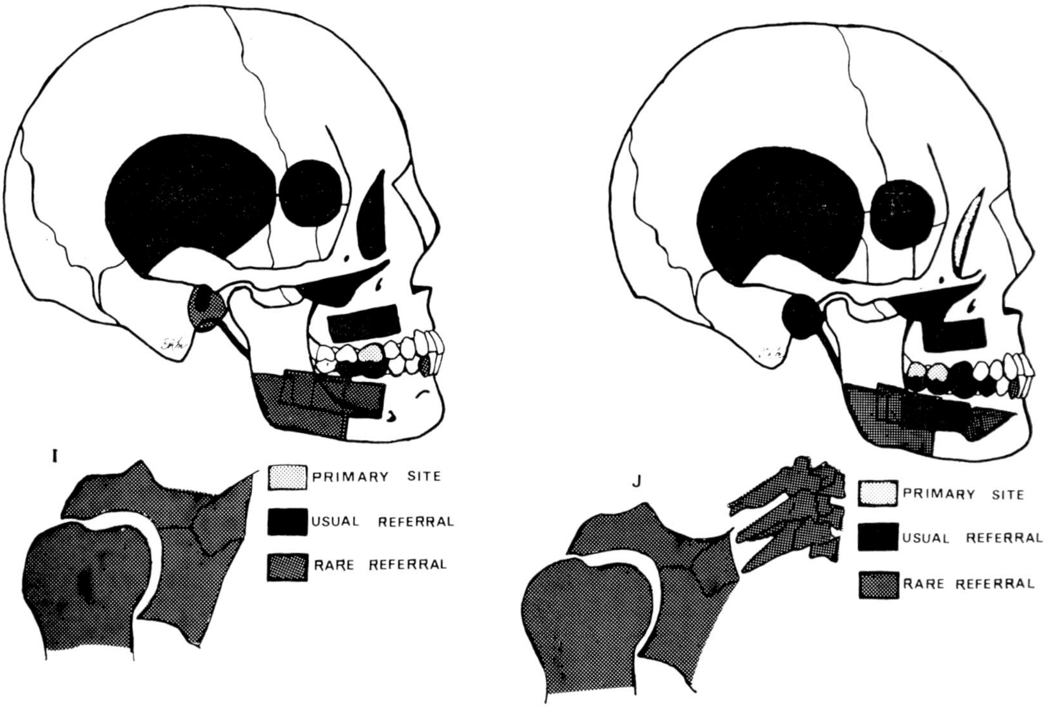

Figure 41

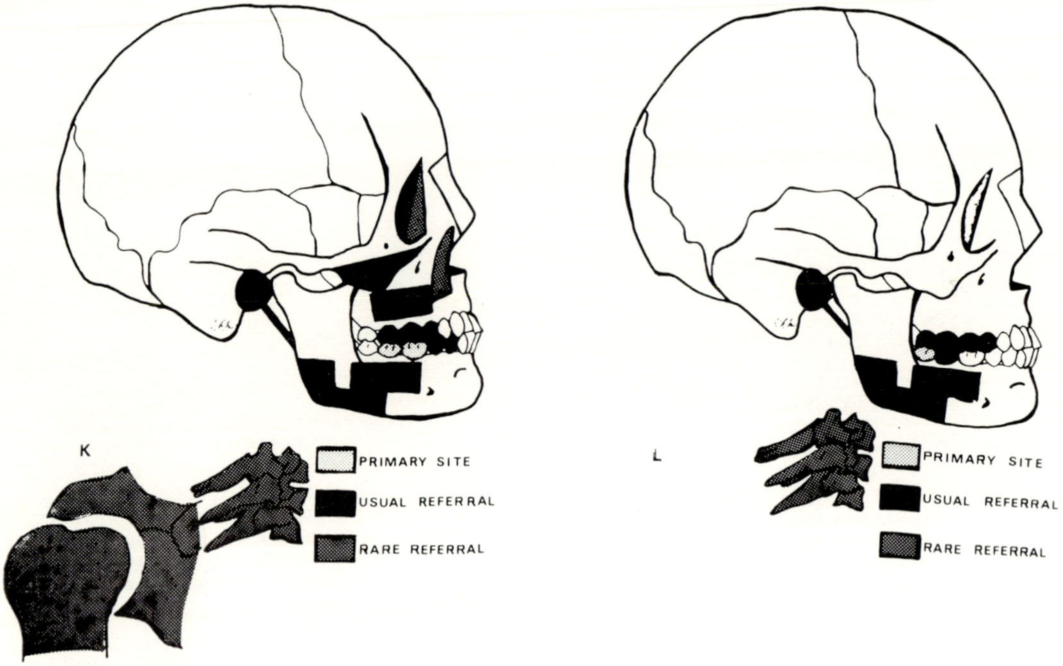

Figure 41 A-L. Referred pathways from the teeth. See text for explanation.

on the same side (Fig. 41A).

(b) From the upper canine to the upper premolars, first and second molars, lower premolars, nasolabial area, orbit, and rarely to the zygoma, and sphenoid area on the same side (Fig. 41B).

(c) From the lower incisors to the mental area on the same side (Fig. 41C).

(d) From the upper first premolar to the nasolabial area, orbit, lower premolars, and rarely to the zygoma, angle of the mandible, ear, and neck on the same side (Fig. 41D).

(e) From the upper second premolar to the upper first premolar, lower premolars, posterior maxilla, temporal region, and rarely to the ear, sphenoid area, lower molar area, and angle of the mandible on the same side (Fig. 41E).

(f) From the lower canine to the mental area, and rarely to the zygoma on the same side (Fig. 41F).

(g) From the lower first premolar to the upper premolars, upper molars, mental area, and rarely to the zygoma on the same side (Fig. 41G).

(h) From the lower second premolar to the upper premolars, upper molars, lower incisors, mental area, mid-ramus area, and rarely to the lower molar area, angle of the mandible, ear, orbit, zygoma, and arm on the same side (Fig. 41H).

(i) From the upper first molar to the posterior maxilla, zygoma, orbit, sphenoid area, temporal region, lower molars, and rarely to the ear, lower molar area, lower canine, mid-ramus area, angle of the mandible, and arm on the same side (Fig. 41I).

(j) From the upper second and third molars to the posterior maxilla, zygoma, sphenoid area, temporal area, lower second premolar, lower molars, lower molar area, ear, and rarely to the lower canine, mid-ramus area, angle of the mandible, mental area, neck, and arm on the same side. An erupting third molar can refer pain to teeth anterior to it (Fig. 41J).

(k) From the lower first and second molars to the lower premolars, upper second premolar, upper first and second molar, angle of the mandible, ear, lower molar area, posterior maxilla, zygoma, and rarely to the orbit, nasolabial area, neck, and shoulder (Fig. 41K).

(l) From the lower third molar to the upper second premolar, upper molars, lower molar area, angle of the mandible, ear, and rarely to the neck on the same side. An erupting third molar and a third molar with an acute pericoronitis can refer pain to teeth anterior to it (Fig. 41L).

(2) *Referred from other areas to the teeth.* The fifth nerve (trigeminal) and the seventh nerve (facial) are in close connection with each other. They also connect with the third, fourth, sixth, eighth, ninth, and tenth cranial nerves, and the sympathetic nervous system. The fifth nerve is closely associated with four sympathetic ganglia: the ciliary, the sphenopalatine, the otic, and the submaxillary. There are also close associations with the cervical nerves. These interconnections (both potential and actual) are shown in Figure 40. Disturbances can occur in different organs and pain can be referred to the teeth as a result of these various nerve associations. Referral patterns are:

(a) From the heart to lower teeth and rarely upper teeth; in coronary artery diseases.

(b) From the neck to lower teeth; in arthritis of the neck.

(c) From the nose to upper anteriors, in nasal diseases, accidents to the nose, and nasal operations.

(d) From the sinuses to the upper anteriors for frontal sinusitis, and upper posteriors for maxillary sinusitis.

(e) From the eyes to upper anteriors and premolars in eye diseases, accidents to the eyes, and eye operations.

(f) From the angle of the mandible to posterior teeth. This can take place with the temporo-mandibular joint pain-dysfunction syndrome.

(g) From the ears to posterior teeth in ear diseases, accidents to the ears, and ear operations.

(h) From the muscles of mastication to posterior teeth; in the myo-fascial pain-dysfunction syndrome (temporal muscle to upper teeth; masseter muscle to lower teeth).

(i) From the temporal area to upper posterior teeth; in temporal arteritis.

(j) From the occipital area to posterior teeth; in cranial diseases, lesions, and neuralgias.

(k) From the palate to upper teeth; in palatal lesions.

(l) From the floor of the mouth to lower teeth; in salivary gland diseases, and lesions in the floor of the mouth.

(m) From the throat to posterior teeth; in throat lesions, diseases, operation and glossopharyngeal neu ralgia.

(n) From the tongue to lowe teeth; in tongue lesions an glossopharyngeal neuralgia

(o) From the mandible or max illa to teeth in the area; i bony lesions, *dry socket* and retained roots (granu lomas or cysts).

(p) There have been reports o reflex pain to the teet from conditions such a constipation, hunger, distended bladder, stomachache, uterine disturbances; gout, malaria, syphilis, the exanthematous diseases (measles, chickenpox, scarlet fever, etc.), anemias, influenza, menstruation, and pregnancy. The pathways may be via the vagus nerve and/or glossopharyngeal nerves via interconnections of the trigeminal nerve. However, these reports have not been scientifically documented.

(q) From diseases along the course of the fifth nerve to various teeth. This has been reported in cases of neuritis, pressure of tumors, and jaw fractures.

(3) *Referred across the midline of either upper or lower jaws.* This is very rare, but may occur in certain cases:

(a) Anterior teeth; in pulpal or periapical conditions when

because of an aberration, the nerve fibers cross the mid-line.

(b) Any teeth; in neuroses, psychoses, and atypical facial neuralgia. No anatomic pathways are involved, as this is related to psychogenic causes. Any bizarre type of referral pathway is possible.

Duration. The duration of the pain helps in differentiating pain from various endodontic diseases as well as pain resulting from other causes. Pain of long duration is arbitrarily considered to be continuous pain of one half-hour or more. Pulpalgia of long duration indicates that the pulp is irreversibly damaged. Sinus pain of long duration is indicative of a possible cyst or tumor.

Frequency. In general, the greater the frequency, the more intense is the pulpal damage.

Type. This aids in differentiating pulpal, periapical and non-endodontic diseases. The various types of pain are sharp, dull, lancinating, boring, deep-seated, and throbbing. An example of differentiation by type of pain is that sharp, short-lived pain may be related to hypersensitive dentin, and the pulp is treatable. A deep-seated, boring type of pain indicates irreversible pulpal disease or periapical disease. Although certain patients may be able to differentiate pain characteristics with great precision, others cannot. Therefore, specific pain characteristics are not considered pathognomonic for any specific pulpal condition.

Previous Episodes. Teeth that may have had a history of previous painful episodes usually have irreversible pulpal disease or failure of previous endodontic therapy.

The pain may be relieved by one of several methods:

(1) *Hot.* This indicates pulp disease, without actually determining the severity.

(2) *Cold.* This usually indicated irreversible pulp disease.

(3) *Mild analgesics.* This may indicate reversible pulp disease.

(4) *Strong analgesics.* This usually indicates irreversible pulp disease.

(5) *Alcohol injections.* This treatment is used for trigeminal neuralgia.

(6) *Vitamin injections.* This treatment has also been used in trigeminal neuralgia.

(7) *Biting.* This usually indicates periodontal involvement, but not necessarily pulp involvement.

(8) *Chewing.* Same as 7.

The pain may be increased by several methods:

(1) *Hot.* This indicates irreversible pulp disease.

(2) *Cold.* Same as (1). If the patient has pain only during the cold application, this indicates hypersensitive dentin or cementum.

(3) *Toothbrushing.* The dentist should consider hypersensitive dentin and/or cementum. In these cases, when no external irritants are applied, the patients do not experience pain.

(4) *Use of dental floss.* Same as 3.

(5) *Use of interdental stimulators and/or toothpicks.* Same as 3. Periodontal disease may also be involved.

(6) *Sweet foods.* Same as 3. Carious involvement may also be involved.

(7) *Sour foods.* Same as 6.

(8) *Tension.* The dentist should consider myo-fascial pain-dysfunction syndrome, as well as a nervous individual.

(9) *Head colds.* The dentist should consider sinusitis.

(10) *Chewing.* The dentist should consider temporomandibular joint pain-dysfunction syndrome, myo-fascial pain-dysfunction syndrome, periodontal disease, periapical pathosis, and maxillary sinusitis. It is also possible for pain of a sharp, transient nature to occur as the result of food packing into a carious lesion. If there is pain only during eating, this condition is most probably hypersensitive dentin.

(11) *Biting.* Same as 10.

(12) *Lying down.* This indicates irreversible pulp disease.

(13) *Bending forward or jumping.* This is indicative of sinusitis.

(14) *Physical exertion.* This is indicative of coronary artery disease.

(15) *High altitudes.* This is a symptom of aerodontalgia.

If the pain is unchanged by all previously listed factors, it is indicative of irreversible pulpal disease.

Pain may be initiated by one of two factors:

(1) *Trigger zones.* This occurs in neuralgias.

(2) *Cold.* This occurs in Bell's palsy.

SWELLING. The categories covered are location, duration, and what the swelling is related to.

Location. Is it unilateral or bilateral? If bilateral, systemic diseases should be suspected.

(1) Intraoral

  (a) *Mucobuccal fold.* The dentist should suspect periapical pathosis, hematoma from an injection (Fig. 42), and an expanding jaw tumor or cyst.

  (b) *Gingiva.* The dentist should suspect a lateral (periodontal) abscess or cyst, a gingival cyst, a pregnancy tumor, a pyogenic granuloma

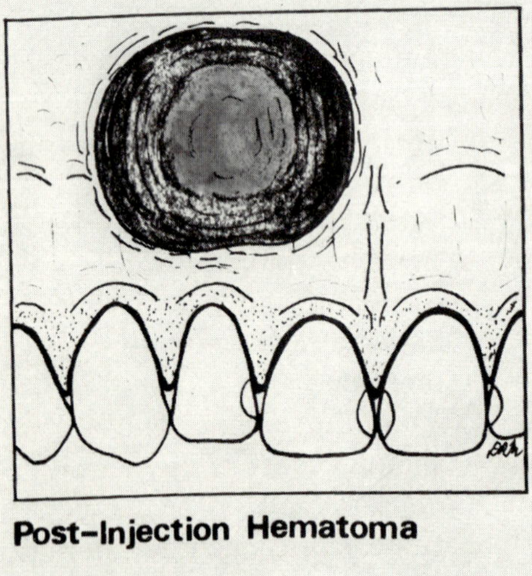

Figure 42. Post-injection hematoma.

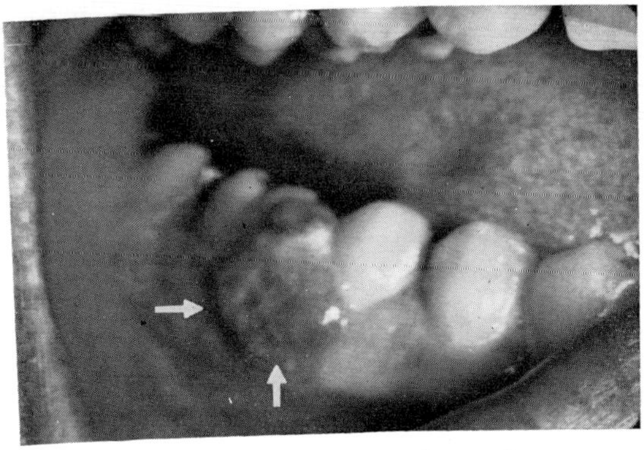

Figure 43. Pregnancy tumor located on interdental papilla. (Courtesy of Dr. T. Simpson, Philadelphia, Pa.)

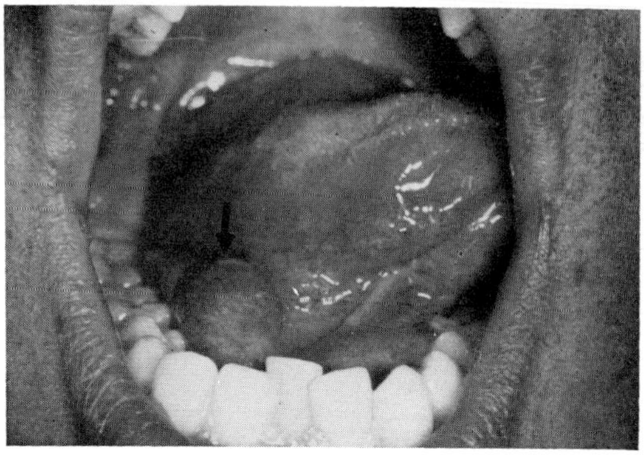

Figure 45. Ranula (Courtesy of Dr. T. Simpson, Philadelphia, Pa.)

or another soft tissue tumor (Figs. 43, 44).

(c) *Palate.* The dentist should consider periapical pathosis related to the root of an upper lateral incisor or a palatal root of an upper posterior tooth and a salivary gland lesion.

(d) *Floor of the mouth.* The practitioner should consider periapical pathosis related to a lower molar, a salivary gland lesion, a ranula (Fig. 45) or mucocoele, and a tumor.

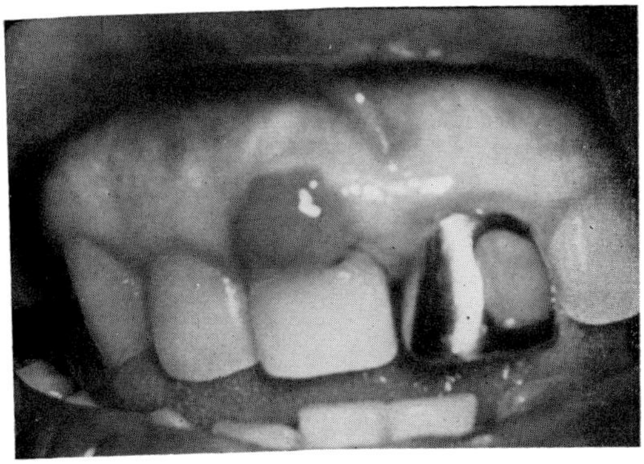

Figure 44. Pyogenic granuloma located on attached gingiva. (Courtesy of Dr. T. Simpson, Philadelphia, Pa.)

(e) *Oral pharynx.* Consideration should be given to sublingual space or deep space infections related to lower molar teeth, throat infections and lesions, and Ludwig's angina.

(2) Extraoral

(a) *Nose.* Possibilities are periapical pathosis related to an upper anterior tooth, nasal diseases, and frontal sinusitis.

(b) *Eye.* The dentist should consider canine space involvement, eye diseases, and angioneurotic edema.

(c) *Cheek.* Possible causes are buccal space involvements (upper or lower molars) (Fig. 46), swelling in buccal fat pad, maxillary sinusitis, facial boils, carbuncles, and insect stings, oral lesions in cheek area, masseteric hypertrophy, myositis, trauma, jaw tumors, and systemic diseases such as Cushing's disease (Fig. 5), hypothyroidism, Cooley's anemia (Fig. 10), and myositis ossificans.

(d) *Submaxillary area.* Consideration should be given to regional lymphadenopathy related to periapical pathosis, submaxillary space infection related to lower molars

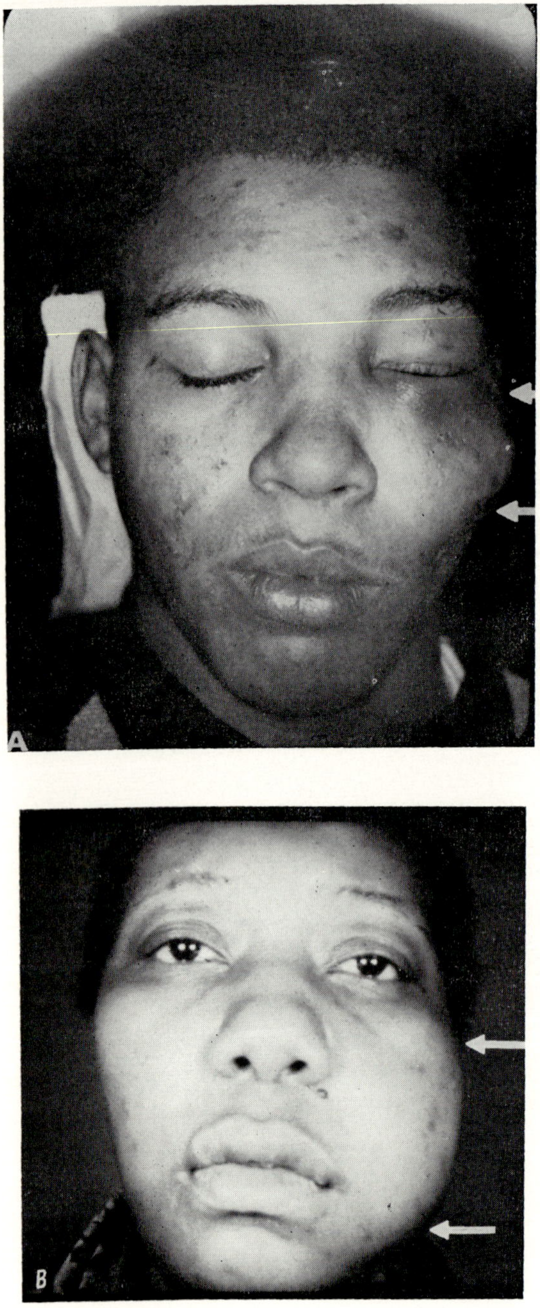

Figure 46. Buccal space involvement. A. Early stage; cheek swollen, eye closed. B. Later stage; cheek swelling has dropped, eye open. (Courtesy of Dr. T. Simpson, Philadelphia, Pa.)

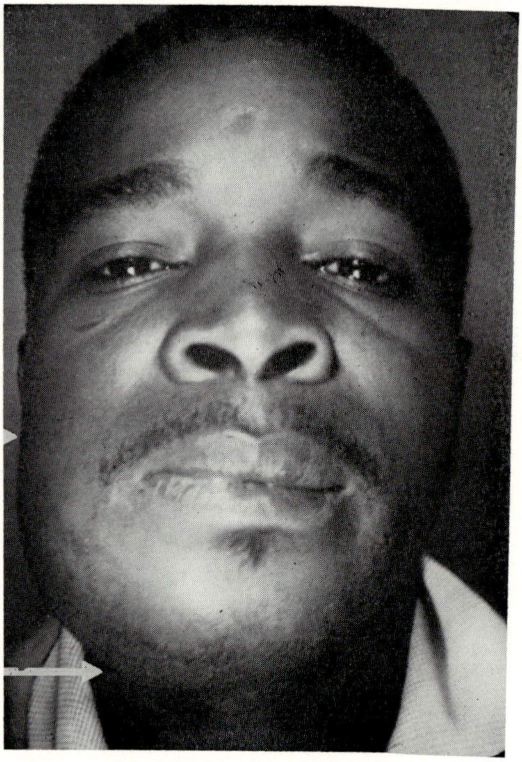

Figure 47. Submaxillary space involvement related to lower molar infectious disease. (Courtesy of Dr. T. Simpson, Philadelphia, Pa.)

TABLE II

SUBMAXILLARY LYMPHADENOPATHY*

The possible etiologies of submaxillary lymphadenopathy are listed in order of decreasing frequency. This order is an approximation based on clinical experience and a review of the literature.

Condition	*Causative Factors*	*Local or Systemic in Origin*
Periapical pathosis from upper and lower posterior teeth (no cellulitis involved)	Pulpal disease, microbes	Local
Submaxillary space involvement from lower posterior teeth with periapical pathosis (contiguous involvement)	Periapical disease; microbes	Local
Various other cellulitises (non-contiguous involvement)	Periapical disease; microbes	Local
Salivary gland diseases, inflammations, and lesions	Viruses, microbes, lesions, operations, and accidents	Local
Throat diseases, inflammations and lesions (e.g. acute follicular tonsillitis; streptococcal sore throat)	Viruses, microbes, lesions, operations, and accidents	Local
Exanthematous diseases (e.g. measles, chickenpox, diphtheria, scarlet fever)	Viruses, microbes	Systemic
Acute necrotizing ulcerative gingivitis (ANUG, Vincent's infection)	Microbes, calculus, poor dentistry	Local
Acute herpetic gingivostomatitis	Herpes virus	Local
Acute pericoronitis	Microbes, food debris, foreign bodies, operculum	Local
Granulomatous diseases (e.g. syphilis, tuberculosis, actinomycosis, lymphogranuloma venerum, infectious mononucleosis, sarcoidosis, histoplasmosis)	Viruses, microbes	Local and/or systemic
Oral surgical procedures, with resultant ecchymosis	Tissue break-down products act as irritants	Local
Nasal diseases, inflammations, and lesions	Viruses, microbes, lesions, operations, and accidents	Local
Eye diseases, inflammations, and lesions	Viruses, microbes, lesions, operations, and accidents	Local
Ear diseases, inflammations, and lesions	Viruses, microbes, lesions, operations, and accidents	Local
Malignant tumors (e.g. carcinomas, sarcomas, lymphomas, etc.)	Hereditary and environmental factors	Local
Metastatic tumors	Hereditary and environmental factors	Local
Leukemias	Hereditary and environmental factors	Local
Multiple myeloma	Hereditary and environmental factors	Local
Hodgkin's disease	Hereditary and environmental factors	Systemic
Typhoid fever	Salmonella typhosa microbe	Systemic
Emphysema	A complication of surgery (air and microbes in the circulation)	Local
Erysipelas	Hemolytic streptococci or staphylococci (microbes)	Local
Osteomyelitis	Extension of periapical disease (microbes); radiation therapy; a late stage in diseases such as syphilis; tuberculosis, and Paget's disease	Local or late complication of systemic disease
Iodism	Chronic iodine poisoning	Systemic
Tangier disease (familial high-density lipoprotein deficiency)	Genetic	Systemic
Cavernous sinus thrombosis (cavernous sinus thrombophlebitis)	Microbes, sequel to periapical disease and other debilitating infections of head and face area	Local

* Lymphadenopathy is found in the submaxillary nodes, but may be present in other nodes, such as the submental, parotid, and cervical.

(Figs. 47, 130), regional lymphadenopathy related to oral and throat lesions, and diseases, and oral manifestations of systemic diseases, surgical emphysema, and jaw tumors (see Table II).

(e) *Parotid area.* The practitioner should suspect mumps or other salivary gland diseases. Mumps can occasionally be unilateral (Fig. 48).

(f) *Chin.* Swelling here indicates mental space infection (chin area) or submental space infection (below chin).

(g) *Neck.* Consideration should be given to Ludwig's angina (Fig. 49), dermoid cysts, goiter, and other neck lesions, and surgical emphysema.

(h) *Frontal area.* One should think of frontal sinusitis.

Duration. The patient should be asked about the length of time the swelling has been present.

Expansion characteristics. Is it a slowly or rapidly expanding swelling? A rap-

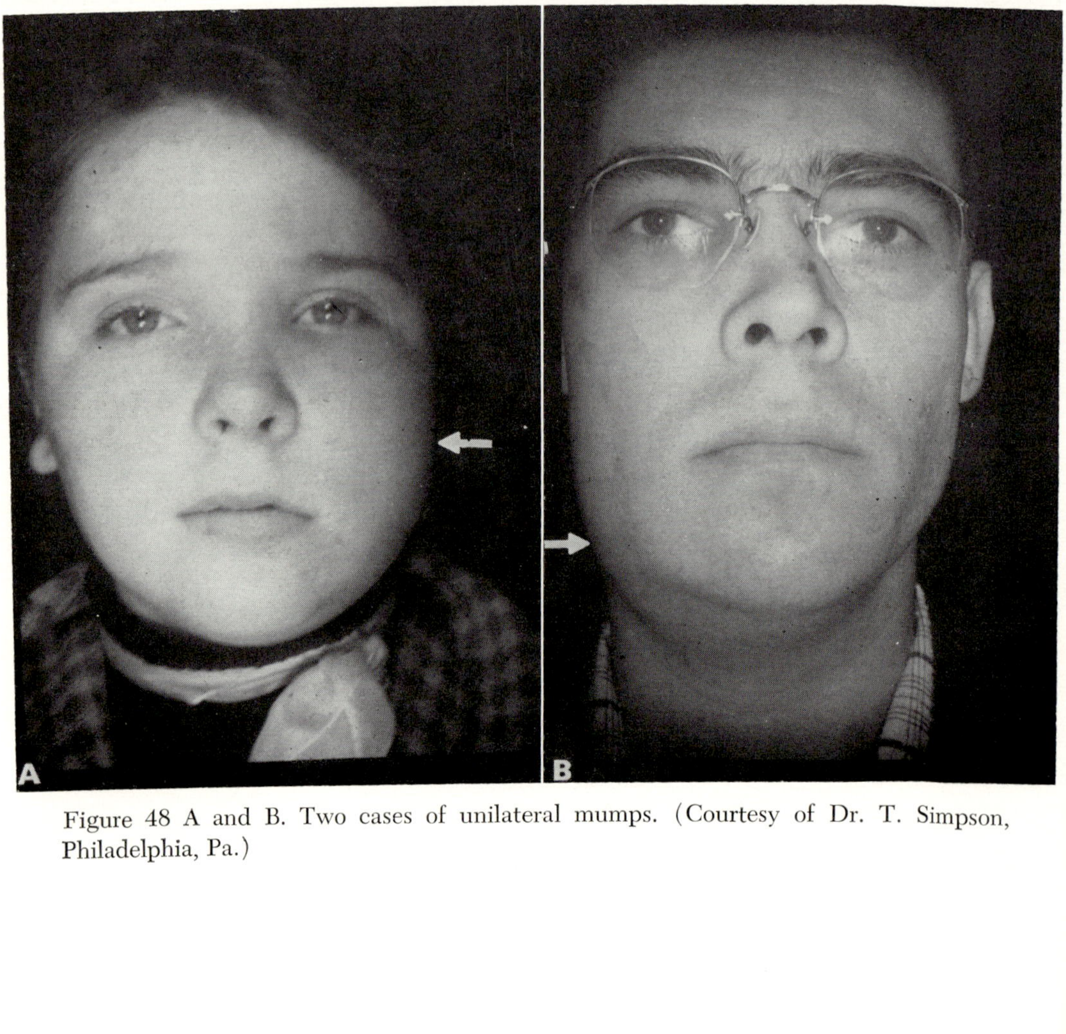

Figure 48 A and B. Two cases of unilateral mumps. (Courtesy of Dr. T. Simpson, Philadelphia, Pa.)

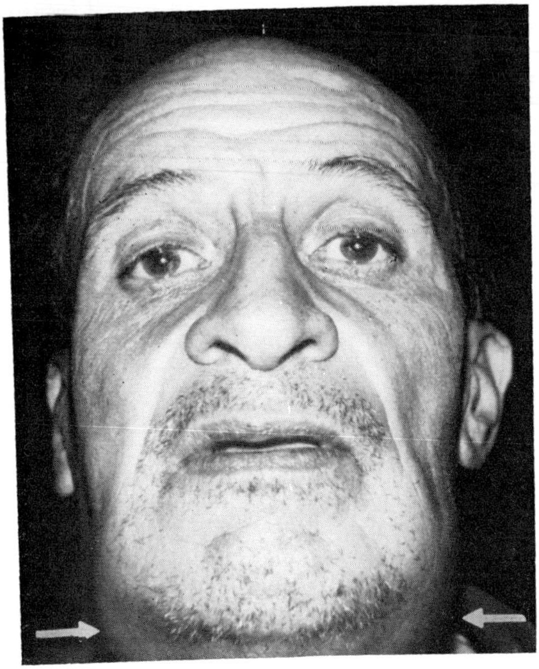

Figure 49. Ludwig's angina resulting from lower molar infectious disease in a debilitated individual. (Courtesy of Dr. T. Simpson, Philadelphia, Pa.)

idly expanding swelling is more likely to be of infectious origin, a slowly expanding swelling is more likely to be a neoplasm.

Type. If it is indurated, except for Ludwig's angina, it is likely to be a tumor. If it is fluctuant, it is likely to be an abscess. If it is discharging, it is also likely to be an abscess.

The swelling may be related to one of the following:

(1) *Pulpalgia.* If there is a history of a toothache prior to the onset of the swelling, the swelling is likely to be derived from an infected pulpless tooth.

(2) *Mastication.* This is pathognomonic of a sialolithiasis (stone in the salivary gland or duct).

(3) *Surgical procedure or trauma.* Facial swelling is normal following trauma to the facial area or after an oral or facial surgical procedure.

Odor and Taste: This can occur as a result of local factors, such as a carious lesion, a discharging sinus tract or gingival sulcus, or from systemic factors such as gases and fluids emanating from the respiratory and gastrointestinal tracts. The location of the odor and taste may be from any of a number of sources:

(1) *Derived from a tooth.* This indicates a pulpal or periapical inflammation.

(2) *Derived from many teeth.* This can result from food debris and carious lesions.

(3) *Derived from the gingival sulcus.* This indicates a gingivitis or an endodontic-periodontic lesion, with drainage through the sulcus.

(4) *Derived from the oral mucous membrane.* This can occur in various types of stomatitises and other oral diseases such as acute necrotizing ulcerative gingivitis and acute herpetic stomatitis.

(5) *Derived from a sinus tract.* This indicates pulpally-induced periapical pathosis.

(6) *Derived from the throat.* This indicates infected tonsils or other throat diseases or lesions.

(7) *Derived from the salivary glands.* This can occur in mumps and

other salivary gland diseases and lesions.

(8) *Derived from the respiratory system.* This indicates lung, bronchial or upper respiratory tract disease.

(9) *Derived from the gastrointestinal tract.* This indicates gastrointestinal diseases, metabolic diseases such as diabetes mellitus (acetone breath), kidney disease such as uremia (ammoniacal odor), eating certain foods (e.g. garlic), which cause bad oral odor, or alcoholism (a foul odor). Pregnant or menstruating women often have a characteristic breath odor during the involved periods (this may be due to gingivitis). Coffee drinkers and cigarette smokers both have characteristic odors.

BLEEDING. The patient should be asked about the origin of the bleeding. Is it the gingiva? the tooth? an extraction socket? the oral mucous membrane? coughed up? The patient's answers will help in the differential diagnosis. Oral bleeding can result from various causes including gingivitis, sanguinous exudate from a pulp, intraoral laceration, throat disease, lung disease, gastrointestinal disease, recent extraction, a hemorrhagic disorder (see discussion in this chapter), facial injury, a hematoma, hemangioma, Sturge-Weber disease, leukemias, and polycythemia.

MOBILITY. Mobility can result from periodontal disease, acute periapical involvement, cellulitis, a traumatic blow or fall involving the tooth, root fracture, crown fracture, bone or soft tissue lesions, a tongue habit, and rapid orthodontic movement. The patient should be asked if he (or she) has a history of a fall, a blow, gum disease, or toothache.

CRACKED RESTORATION, LOST RESTORATION, FRACTURED TOOTH OR CAVITY. The patient's complaints in these instances is based on the sensation mediated by the tongue's probing of a large *hole* in the tooth. Many times the patient is fearful of having lost the entire tooth, as the gap feels enormous. Examination by the practitioner usually reassures the patient that he has not lost his tooth, and that it can be saved by endodontic therapy. A slight crack can cause the cracked tooth syndrome, in which pain can occur on infrequent occasions when the patient bites in a certain way (See Chapter 2).

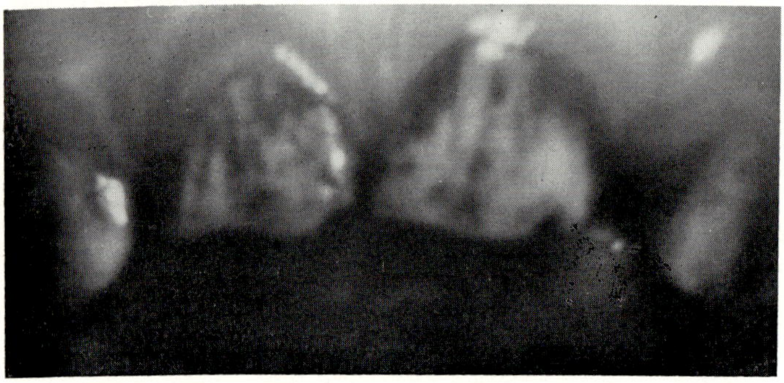

Figure 50. Upper incisors with extrinsic stains probably derived from food products and/or microorganisms. (Courtesy of Dr. K. Bomze, Cherry Hill, N. J.)

DISCOLORED TOOTH. Tooth discoloration can result from a pulpless tooth, smoking, microbial products and food products (Fig. 50), systemic disorders such as congenital porphyria and erythroblastosis fetalis, tetracycline ingestion (Fig. 51), and metallic stains. Generally, only in pulpal necrosis is the discoloration localized to one tooth (Fig. 52).

PARESTHESIA. Paresthesia (numbness) may involve the teeth, the jaws, the oral mucous membrane, the lips or the tongue. The patient should be questioned about previous jaw infection, root canal therapy, periapical surgery, any other oral surgical procedure, history of a jaw fracture, and osteomyelitis. Any of these factors can cause the development of paresthesia. Such diseases as multiple sclerosis, syphilis (tabes dorsalis) and oral malignancies (either primary or metastatic) can also lead to the development of paresthesia.

ORAL LESIONS IN ALVEOLAR MUCOSA. Oral lesions can result from a parulis (gum boil), soft tissue tumors or cysts, periodontal diseases, oral manifestations of systemic diseases, trauma, apthous ulcers, foreign bodies, other oral and pharyngeal diseases, and allergic reactions to drugs. The patient should be asked about the history of the lesion. Specific questions include, does it discharge fluid? does it tend to recur? is it related to a toothache? All of these manifestations are indicative of a parulis.

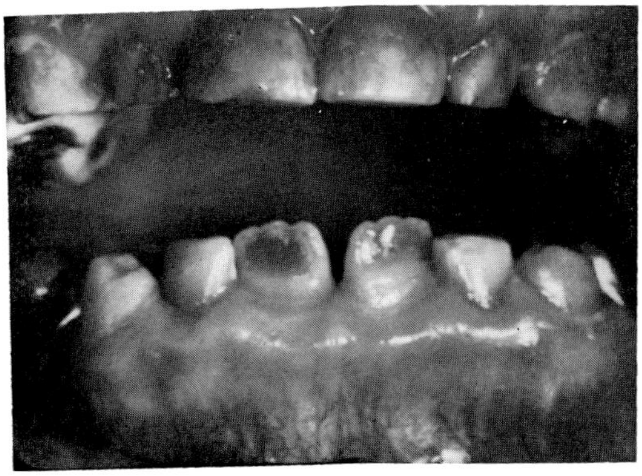

Figure 51. Tooth discoloration resulting from tetracycline ingestion. (Courtesy of Dr. T. Simpson, Philadelphia, Pa.)

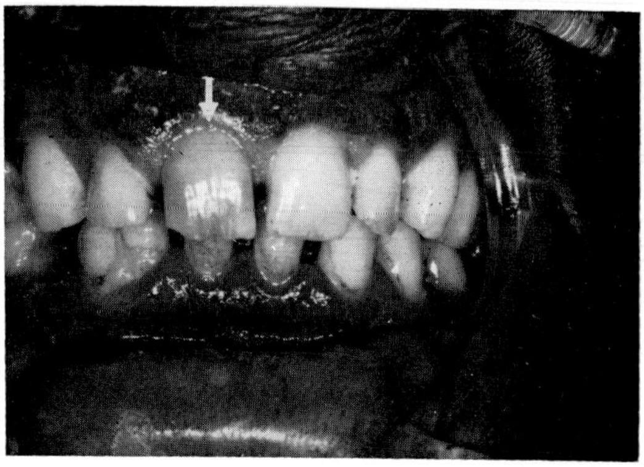

Figure 52. Tooth discoloration localized to one tooth in a case of pulpal necrosis. (Courtesy of Dr. T. Simpson, Philadelphia, Pa.)

DISCHARGING SINUS TRACT. The patient should be asked the same questions discussed under oral lesions. Aside from endodontic involvements, sinus tracts can be related to root fracture, periodontal disease, infected retained roots, infected residual granulomas or cysts, osteomyelitis, infected dentigerous cyst, and unerupted teeth that communicate with the oral cavity. A skin sinus tract can be related to endodontic involvement (Fig. 53). Multiple skin sinus tracts can occur in actinomycosis and branchial neck fistulae (Figs. 54, 55). Lesions simulating skin sinus tracts include tubercular nodules, basal cell carcinoma ulcers, salivary gland fistulae, in-

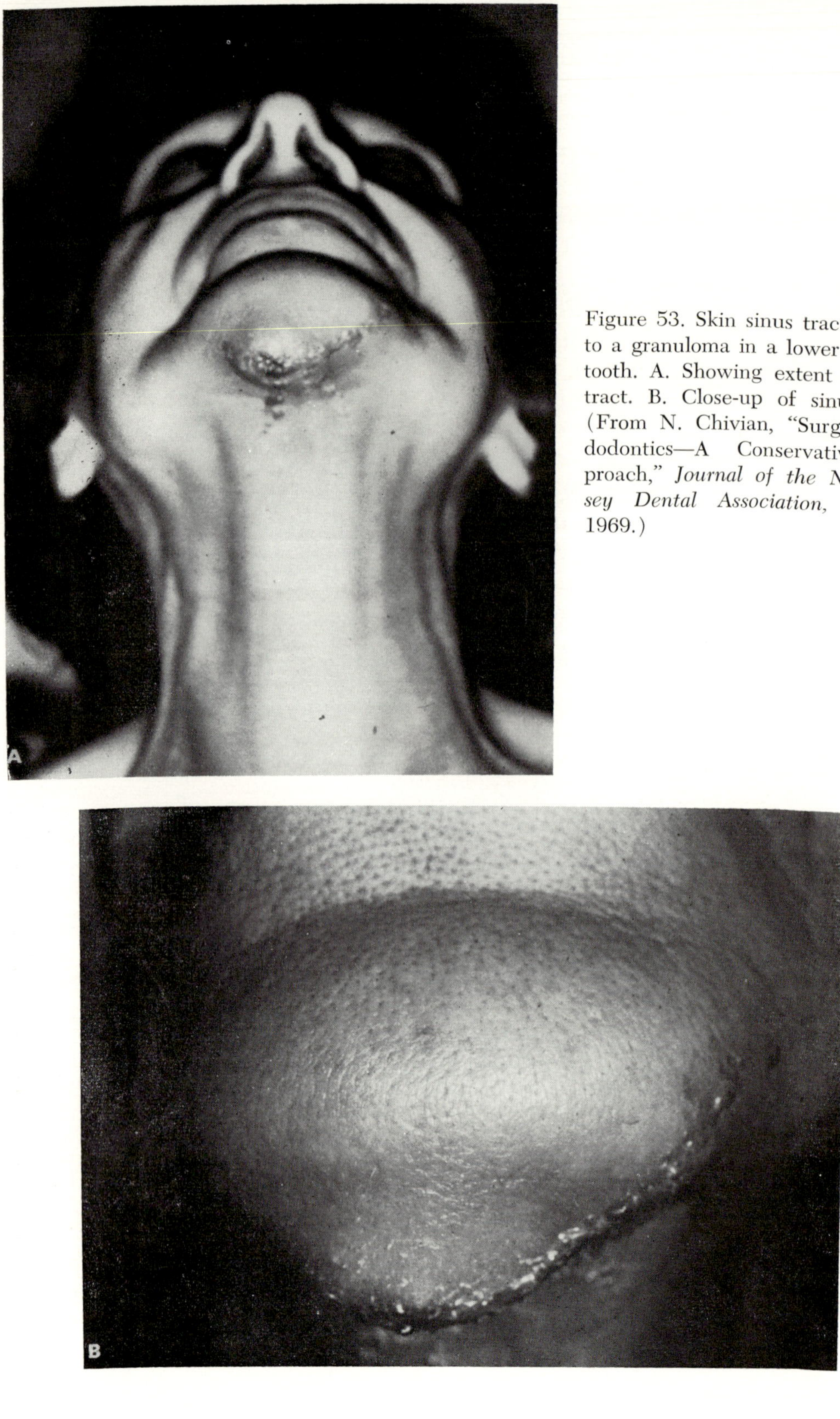

Figure 53. Skin sinus tract related to a granuloma in a lower anterior tooth. A. Showing extent of sinus tract. B. Close-up of sinus tract. (From N. Chivian, "Surgical Endodontics—A Conservative Approach," *Journal of the New Jersey Dental Association*, 40:234, 1969.)

fected sebaceous cysts, carbuncles, and pyogenic granulomas.

General Considerations. If there are any questions about previous or current dental conditions that could conceivably affect endodontic therapy, it is essential that the endodontist (if he is handling the case) or general practitioner have a consultation with the referring (or previous) dentist. This should be done prior to the start of the endodontic therapy.

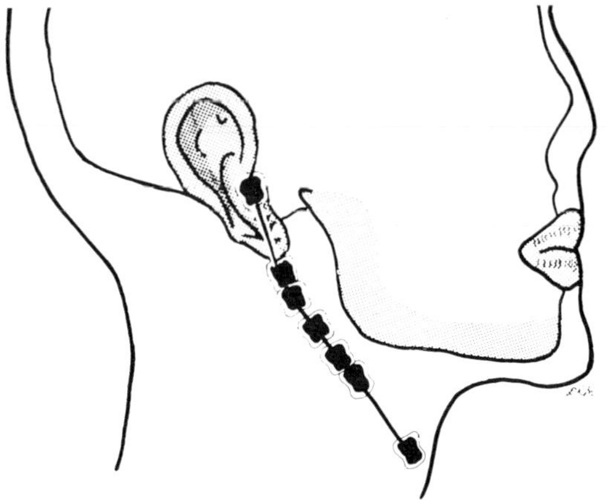

Figure 55. Possible sites for branchial fistulas. (Based on a picture in R. J. Gorlin and H. M. Goldman, *Thoma's Oral Pathology*, 6th ed. St. Louis, The C. V. Mosby Co., 1970.)

Visual Examination

This section includes physical appearance, patient reactions, facial appearance, swellings, oral lesions, gingival appearance, sinus tracts, and teeth.

Physical Appearance

In this category the subjects of height, weight, physical deformity, tremors, exophthalmia, arms, and head are discussed.

Height. Excessive height is indicative of gigantism. A small stature may indicate dwarfism, malnutrition, cherubism, or another genetic and endocrine disorder.

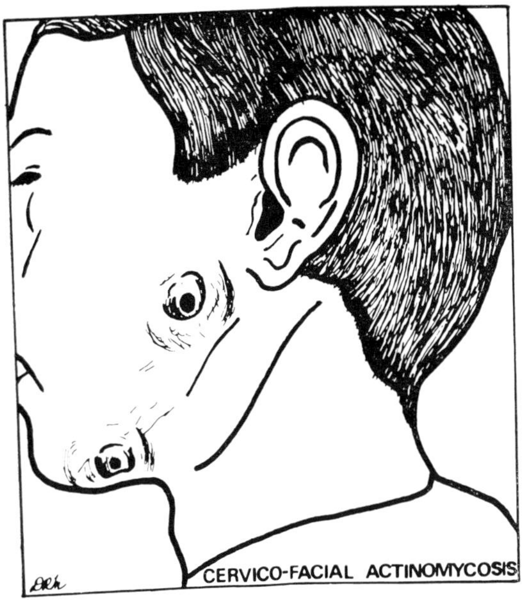

Figure 54. Cervico-facial actinomycosis with discharging sinus tracts.

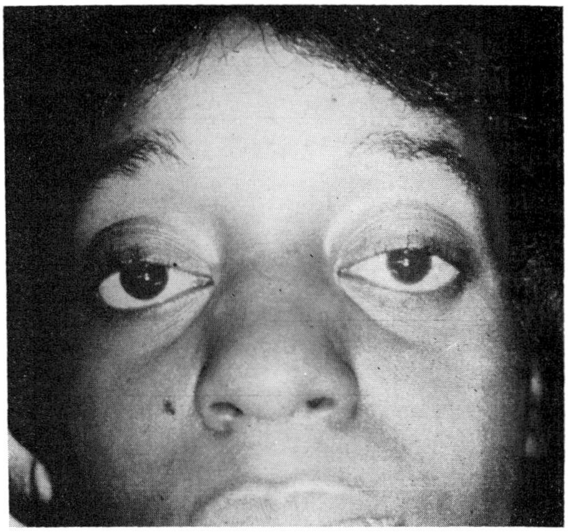

Figure 56. Exophthalmia in a hyperthyroid patient. (Courtesy of Dr. M. Gross, Philadelphia, Pa.)

WEIGHT. Obese individuals are prone to cardiac diseases and diabetes. Thin individuals may be anemic, suffering from degenerative diseases, or normal.

PHYSICAL DEFORMITY AND PATIENTS WITH CASTS, BRACES, SLINGS, AND COLLARS. These patients can be management problems. Treatment sessions should be kept short.

TREMORS. If a patient has tremors, possible causes are Parkinson's disease, cerebral palsy, cerebral lesions, hyperthyroidism, drug abuse (stimulants), and extreme nervousness.

EXOPHTHALMIA. Bulging eyes is pathognomonic for hyperthyroidism (Fig. 56).

HANDS AND ARMS. Patients with scleroderma have a characteristic waxy, atrophic appearance of their hands (Fig. 57). The dentist should look for signs of needle marks (evidence of drug abuse) on patient's arms.

HEAD. An enlarged head is indicative of Paget's disease (Fig. 58). An enlarged mandible is suggestive of acromegaly.

Patient Reactions

The excitable and lethargic patients are discussed in this section.

JITTERY, NERVOUS, IRRITABLE OR EXCITABLE. These patients may be neurotic, nervous, hyperthyroid, on stimulants, have a cerebral lesion, or have some systemic disease with neurological manifestations.

LETHARGIC OR UNRESPONSIVE. These

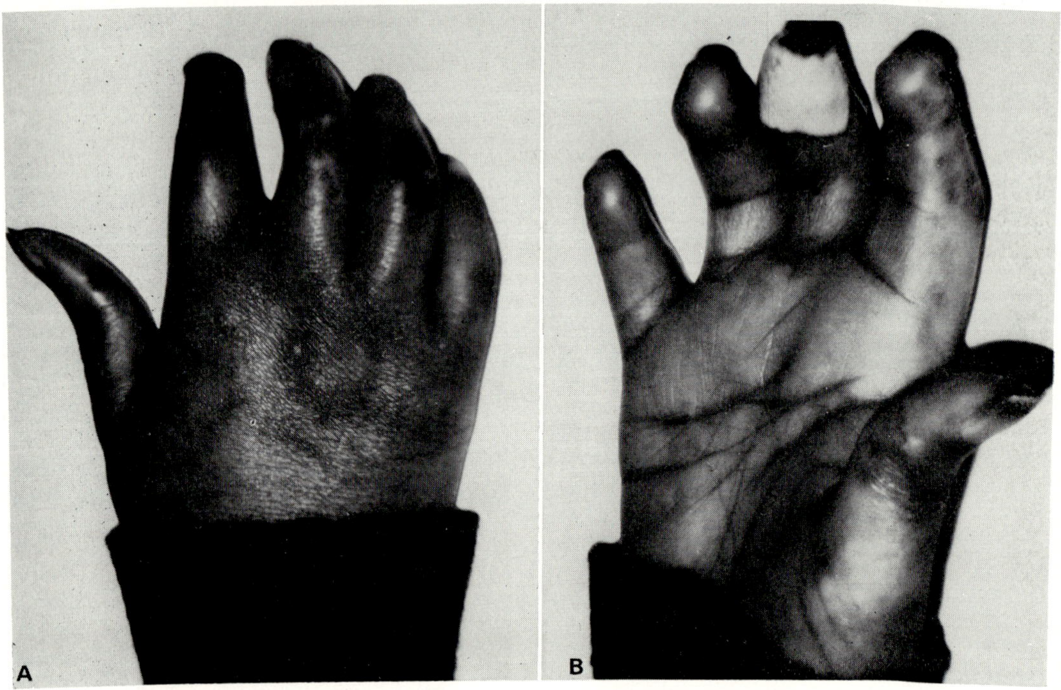

Figure 57. Hands of a patient with scleroderma showing a waxy, taut, atrophic appearance with sparce hairs. A. Dorsal surface. B. Ventral surface. (Courtesy of Dr. L. Muldorf, Philadelphia, Pa.)

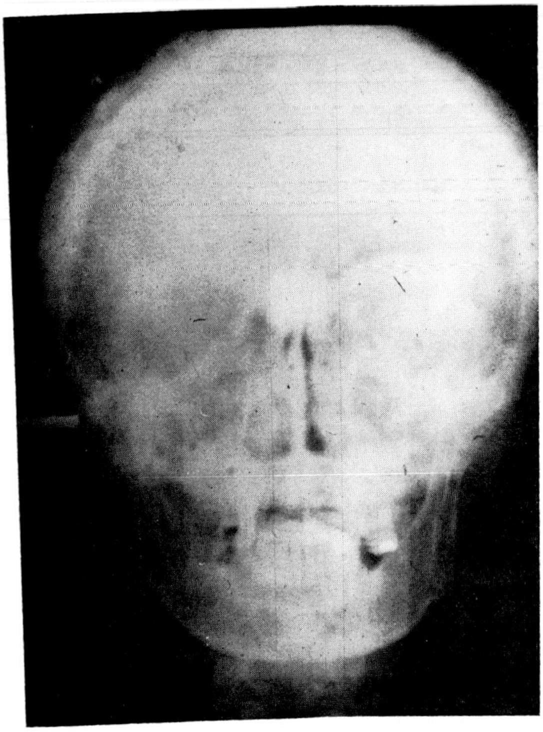

Figure 58. An anterior posterior radiograph of the skull of a patient with Paget's disease, showing enlargement of the skull and generalized radiopacities. (Courtesy of Dr. M. Gross, Philadelphia, Pa.)

patients may be stoic, hypothyroid, on depressant drugs, or have some systemic disease that causes a sluggish metabolism.

Facial Appearance

In this section, the topics of color, asymmetry, scars, and skin sinus tracts are covered.

COLOR.

Pale. The dentist should consider anemias.

Cyanotic. Possibilities are cardiac diseases and respiratory diseases.

Ruddy. This may result from chronic alcoholism, polycythemia vera, disseminated lupus erythematosus, hypertension, sunburn, exercise, embarrassment (blushing), or normal skin coloration.

Pigmented. Addison's disease is one possibility.

Jaundiced. This occurs in liver diseases.

ASYMMETRY. This can occur as the result of swellings, fractures, neuritises (e.g. Bell's palsy), neuralgias, and jaw malformations.

SCARS. This may result from previous sinus tracts among other possibilities.

SKIN SINUS TRACTS. These should be traced to determine the point of origin. Usual cause is a pulpless tooth. Rarer etiologies are actinomycosis, branchial cyst, and tuberculosis.

Swellings

For a description of location and type of swelling, see the section on chief complaints in this chapter.

Oral Lesions in Alveolar Mucosa

For each lesion the dentist should evaluate the following:

(1) The color—yellow is indicative of Fordyce's granules.

(2) Solitary or multiple—if multiple most likely non-endodontic origin.

(3) Attached or not—if attached more likely a tumor.

(4) Firm or fluctuant—if firm more likely a tumor; if fluctuant more likely a parulis.

(5) Discharging or not—if discharging more likely a sinus tract.

Gingival Appearance

A gingivitis or gingival hyperplasia isolated to one tooth may be related to

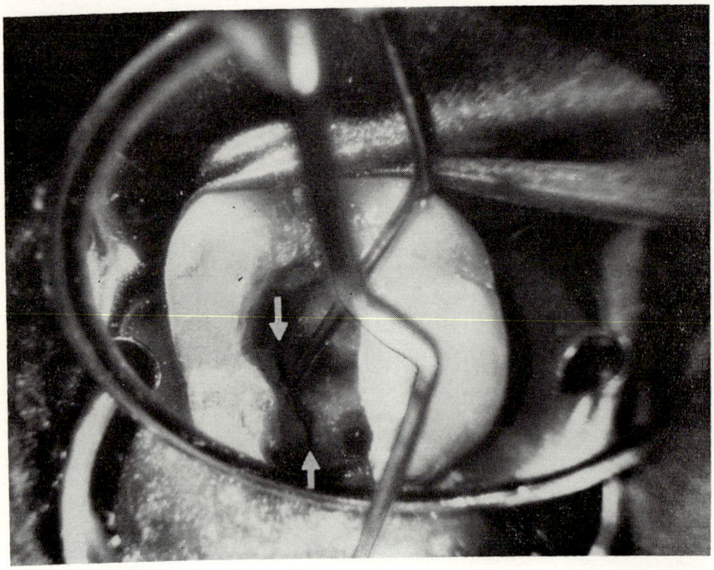

Figure 59. A case of the cracked tooth syndrome. After the restoration was removed, an explorer was used to probe the extent of the fracture. (Courtesy of Dr. L. Muldorf, Philadelphia, Pa.)

an endodontic-periodontic involvement. If more than one tooth is involved, the condition is more likely periodontal. The gingiva should be checked for presence or absence of stippling (absence indicates disease), presence or absence of truncation (latter condition occurs in ANUG), dull or shiny appearance (latter indicates disease), fluid discharge (may result from periodontic or endodontic-periodontic disease), and recent periodontal treatment (look for the presence of healing gingiva or periodontal packs).

Sinus Tracts in Alveolar Mucosa, Floor of the Mouth, Palate, Skin or Nose.

These should be traced to see if they originate from a root apex, furca, gingival sulcus, or periodontal pocket.

Teeth

The dentist should check for several different things.

Crown Fractures (complete or incomplete). These could cause the cracked tooth syndrome.

Combined Crown and Root Fractures. Depending upon the extent of the fracture, these teeth may not be treatable (Fig. 59).

Pulp Exposures. These can result from fractures, dental operative procedures, caries, abrasion (Fig. 60), attrition (Fig. 32), or erosion (Figs. 2, 31, 492).

Hyperplastic Pulp (Pulp Polyp). This could simulate gingival hypertrophy (Fig. 61).

Color Changes. An opaque dull or dark color is evident of a pulpless tooth (Fig. 52). A pink coloration near the cervical margin is indicative of internal resorption (Fig. 62). A pink coloration can also result from hemorrhage into dentinal tubules following a crown preparation. These changes should be differentiated from discolorations caused by metal staining, cigarette smoking, tetracycline ingestion (Fig. 51), fluoridation (Fig. 1), blood diseases, enamel hypoplasia (Fig. 63), and systemic diseases. Generally, all of these nonendodontic cases would show discolorations on more than one tooth.

Defective Restorations and Adjoining Margins. There may be extensive decay beneath the surface.

Improper Tooth Contacts and Embrasures. This may lead to occlusal traumatism.

Occlusal Wear Facets or Shiny Spots on Restorations. These are indicative of occlusal traumatism and

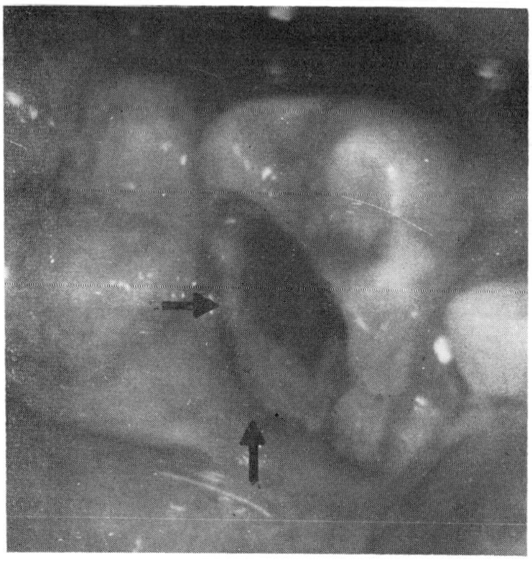

Figure 61. A molar with a hyperplastic pulp *pulp polyp.* (Courtesy of Dr. K. Bomze, Cherry Hill, N. J.)

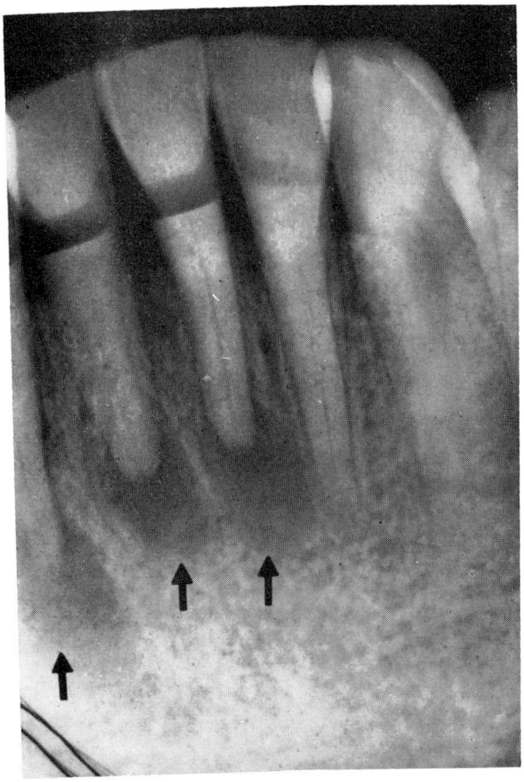

Figure 60. Toothbrush abrasion causing pulp exposures and subsequent development of periapical areas of rarefaction; latter indicated by arrows. (Courtesy of Dr. T. Simpson, Philadelphia, Pa.)

may be a cause of acute apical periodontitis.

Large Restorations. Pulps can become necrotic under large restorations, especially if they have been polished in the mouth.

Silicate or Plastic Restorations. Pulps can become necrotic beneath these restorations, even if the preparations are small.

Porcelain Jackets. These should be checked for evidence of fractures. Pulps often become necrotic as a result of overzealous preparations with inadequate coolants.

Full Crowns. Pulps beneath these restorations can become damaged (Fig. 64). If the tooth in question is a bridge abutment or has a single full crown in position, determination of the location of the root canals may be difficult.

Evidence of Difficult Accessibility

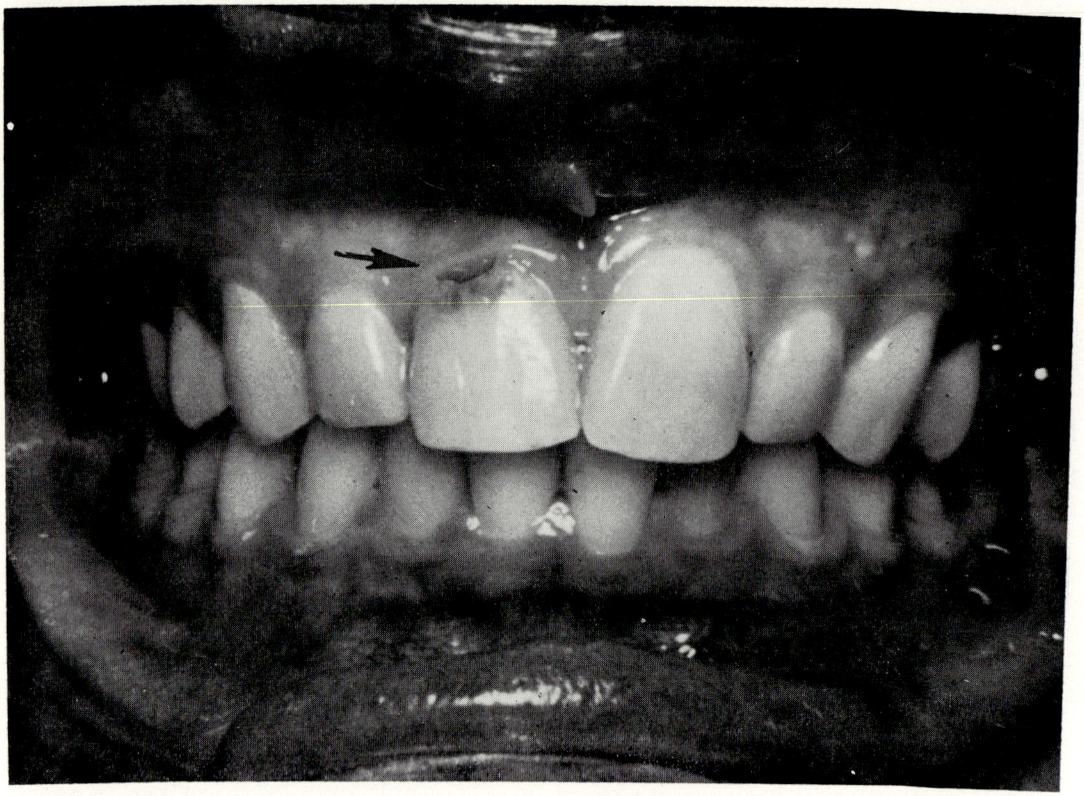

Figure 62. Upper right central incisor shows a *pink spot,* evidence of internal resorption. (From N. Chivian, "Surgical Endodontics—A Conservative Approach," *Journal of the New Jersey Dental Association,* 40:234, 1969.)

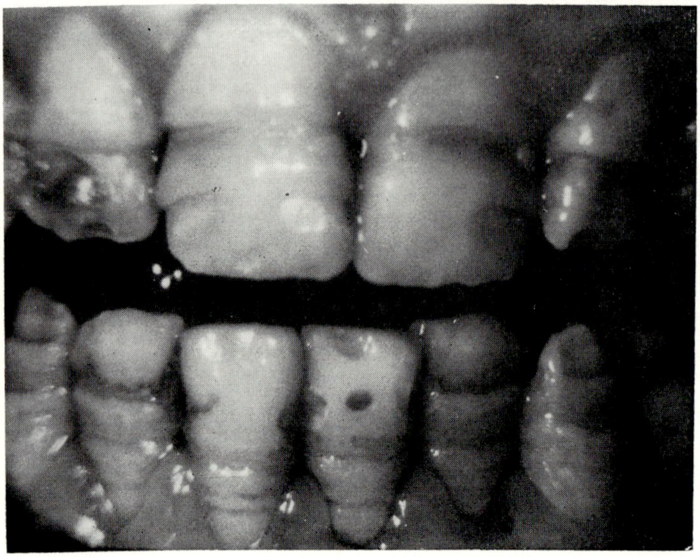

Figure 63. Severe enamel hypoplasia probably resulting from an exanthematous disease during childhood. (Courtesy of Dr. K. Bomze, Cherry Hill, N. J.)

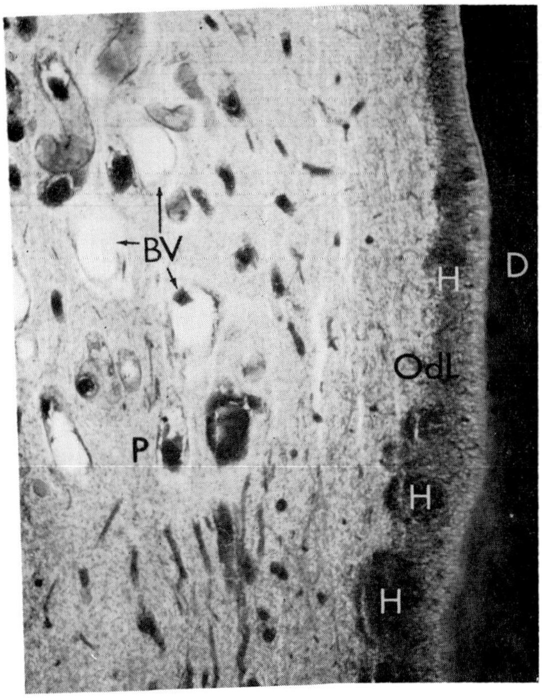

Figure 64. Full crown preparation without water; pulpal blood vessels are engorged and there is hemorrhage in the odontoblastic layer; BV = dilated blood vessels, P = pulp, Odl = odontoblastic layer, H = hemorrhage, D = dentin (×54). (From S. Seltzer and I. B. Bender, *The Dental Pulp*, J. P. Lippincott Co., 1965. Used with permission of J. P. Lippincott Company.)

TO THE PULP. This may result from any of the following:

(1) Inclination of the crown to the root.
(2) Incomplete eruption of the tooth.
(3) Fracture of the tooth beneath the gingiva with subsequent gingival hypertrophy.
(4) Luxation of the tooth into the socket simulating partial eruption.
(5) Extrusion, labial displacement or lingual displacement. In these situations it may be very difficult to put on a rubber dam clamp.

EVIDENCE OF ROOT INCLINATIONS. Sometimes the inclinations of the roots can be seen by a bulging of the alveolar mucosa overlying the roots.

ORTHODONTIC APPLIANCE. This should be checked to see if the tooth in question is banded. Caries may be found beneath bands.

A PARTIAL DENTURE. This should be checked to see if the tooth in question is clasped. There may be decay under the clasp and/or the tooth may be subject to excessive pressures.

THE ABSENCE OF A TOOTH IN THE AREA FROM WHENCE THE PAIN ORIGINATES. This could be a case of *phantom* tooth pain, an acute alveolar osteitis *(dry socket)* or a retained root (cyst or granuloma).

TONGUE ACTION. The patient should be asked to swallow to see if he (or she) pushes the tongue against the teeth in question. This can lead to tooth mobility.

AN OPPOSING TOOTH. It is important to see if the tooth in question has an opponent. If it doesn't, it may not be necessary to perform endodontic therapy.

DAMAGE TO THE OPPOSING ARCH. With anterior teeth involved by trauma, the teeth in the opposite arch should always be checked for evidence of injury.

TEETH WITH DISSIMILAR METALS IN CONTACT. This can occur with a gold crown contacting an amalgam filling. In certain individuals a galvanic current can be set up and pain may result.

OBJECTIVE

This section includes nondental and dental diagnostic tests.

Diagnostic Tests

Nondental, Local and Systemic

These tests help in the determination of whether local or systemic factors or diseases are involved. They are usually prepared in licensed medical laboratories. The tests may be requested by either the dentist or the physician.

When asking for a particular test, the dentist should be aware of the fact that many drugs interfere with the results of medical tests. Therefore the dentist should inform the laboratory of the drugs that he (or she) knows that the patient is taking. Some drugs that interfere with laboratory results are acetohexamide, ACTH, albumin, antacids, aspirin, androgens, barbiturates, corticosteroids, penicillin, erythromycin, tetracyclines, cephalosporins, lincomycin, vitamins A, C, and D, sulfonamides, fluorides, oxalates, phosphates, ammonium compounds, calcium, iron, phenothiazines, and diuretics. Generally, most tests must be taken on an empty stomach.

In this section, the various tests are mentioned and indications are given for what particular conditions they can be used. In the appendix, the blood and urine tests are listed, the normal range of values is shown, and specific diseases with indicated changes, are given.

BLOOD TESTS. In various diseases, there are certain alterations in blood tests. These will be listed for each disease.

Blood Dyscrasias (e.g. leukemias). The values in the following tests are changed in blood dyscrasias.

(1) Erythrocyte Count (usually decreased in leukemias; increased in polycythemia vera)
(2) Leucocyte Count (usually very high in leukemias, and decreased in polycythemia vera)
(3) Thrombocyte Count (usually increased in polycythemia vera)
(4) Differential Leucocyte Count (shift to the left [immature forms] in leukemias, immature leucocytes seen in about one-half polycythemia vera cases)

Anemias. There are various types of anemias and different tests are used for each type. Several general tests are used:

(1) Hemoglobin
(2) Hematocrit
(3) RBC Count
(4) WBC Count
(5) Examination of a Stained Smear
(6) Platelet Count
(7) Reticulocyte Count

The RBC count is used for a determination of the indices, and it is accurate only if done on an electronic counter. There are three indices:

(1) Mean Corpuscular Volume (MCV)
(2) Mean Corpuscular Hemoglobin (MCH) and
(3) Mean Corpuscular Hemoglobin Concentration (MCHC).

Examination of the stained smear determines the morphologic type of anemia (size, shape) and presence of abnormal cells (e.g. sickle cells, spherocytes, target cells) and number and relative type of leucocytes and platelets. Further tests depend upon the particular type of anemia present. An example is the sickle cell test which is a new test available for determination of sickle cell anemia. It can be performed in the dental office and is called the Sickledex test (Johnson & Johnson). The test takes five minutes to read and is reported to be 99 per cent effective.

Inflammation. The following two tests are nonspecific indicators of inflammation.

(1) Sedimentation Rate. This increases in disease and tissue destruction.
(2) C-reactive Protein. This is present during many inflammatory disorders including periodontal and periapical disease (Figs. 126, 127).

Hemorrhagic Disorders. As mentioned previously, hemorrhagic disorders are of three types: (1) Vascular, (2) Platelet, and (3) Coagulation.

For the vascular type, screening tests are the tourniquet test (capillary fragility) and bleeding time. For the platelet deficiencies, screening tests are platelet number evaluation from a stained blood smear, bleeding time, tourniquet test, and clot retraction. Specific tests are the definite platelet count, the ADP-induced platelet aggregation and tests for platelet adhesiveness. For the coagulation defects, screening tests are whole blood clotting time (glass, only gives a gross evaluation), partial thromboplastin time, prothrombin time, and thrombin time. Specific tests are the factor assays and the fibrin-split-products, and euglobulin clot lysis time for acquired fibrinogen deficiencies.

Bone Disorders. There is an alteration of values in these tests in certain bone disorders.

(1) Serum Calcium (e.g. increased in hyperparathyroidism, decreased in hypoparathyroidism)
(2) Serum Phosphorus (e.g. increased in hypoparathyroidism, decreased in hyperparathyroidism)
(3) Alkaline Phosphatase (e.g. increased in Paget's disease, decreased in hypophosphatasia)
(4) Acid Phosphatase (e.g. increased in metastatic carcinoma of the prostate)

Blood Volume Disorders. In blood volume disorders (e.g. edema, dehydration, acidosis, alkalosis), there are changes in the values of these tests.

(1) Serum Potassium
(2) Serum Chloride
(3) Serum Sodium
(4) Total Blood Volume
(5) Nonprotein Nitrogen
(6) Carbon Dioxide Content
(7) pH
(8) Acetone Plasma

Thyroid Diseases. There is a change in the serum iodine values in thyroid diseases. Specific tests used are radioactive iodine uptake (RAI), protein bound iodine^{131} (PBI^{131}), butanol-extractable iodine (BEI), thyroxine measurements, percent free thyroxine, concentration of thyroxine binding globulin (TBG), concentration of unbound TBG, and basic metabolic rate (described later). In hypothyroidism, serum cholesterol is usually increased.

Cardiovascular Diseases. In cardiovascular diseases serum cholesterol is increased and with myocardial infection, there are usually increases in the enzymes, creatine phosphokinase (CPK), glutamic oxaloacetic transaminase (GOT), and the lactic acid dehydrogenases (LDH).

Liver Diseases. The following tests are useful in liver diseases:

(1) Serum Bilirubin Level and Partition
(2) Prothrombin Time
(3) Response to administered vitamin K
(4) Bromsulphalein-Excretion Test
(5) Alkaline Phosphatase (increases in liver diseases)
(6) Transaminases (GOT, GPT, increase in liver diseases)
(7) Serum Protein Level (albumin, globulin, gamma globulin, electrophoretic analysis)
(8) Serum Cholesterol

Diabetes Mellitus. There is an increase in the values of the following tests in diabetes mellitus:

(1) Serum Glucose
(2) Glucose Tolerance Test

Kidney Diseases. There is a change in values in the following blood tests in kidney diseases:

(1) Urea Nitrogen and Nonprotein Nitrogen.
(2) Serum Chloride (high in kidney diseases).
(3) Serum Sodium (low in kidney diseases).
(4) Serum Potassium (increased in renal failure).
(5) Serum Calcium (decreased in renal rickets).
(6) Serum Phosphorus (increased in renal failure).
(7) Serum Proteins (low in nephrosis).

Serum Protein Disturbances. These are seen in agammaglobulinemia fibrinogen deficiency disorders, starvation, liver diseases, kidney diseases, intestinal diseases, dehydration, shock, tuberculosis, acute infections, arteriosclerosis, collagen diseases, malignancies, and macroglobulinemia.

Pancreatic Diseases. In these diseases, there is usually elevated serum amylase and lipase values.

Other Tests for Endocrine Function. Aside from those tests described for thyroid, pancreas, and parathyroid function, there are several possible tests for pituitary and adrenal gland function. These tests are rather detailed and should be prescribed by a physician (usually an endocrinologist).

Muscle Diseases. In muscle diseases such as muscular dystrophy, there is an increase in serum CPK, SGOT, and aldolase.

Other Blood Tests. There are other blood tests that may be used. These include the following:

(1) Blood Cultures; to detect the presence of microbes in the blood stream.
(2) Blood Smears; to detect the presence of normal and abnormal cells and microbes.
(3) Ascorbic Acid; to detect a vitamin C deficiency; this value decreases during stress.
(4) Uric Acid; to detect gout.
(5) Transplantation Antigen Typing; this is important to know prior to transplantations.

Urine Examination. There are changes in values found in bone diseases (calcium and phosphorus level); kidney diseases (albumin, casts, microbes, odor, epithelial cells, polymorph leucocytes), blood, change in volume, pH and specific gravity); tumors (Bence-Jones protein in multiple myeloma), liver diseases (bilirubin, urobilinogen), diabetes mellitus (glucose, ketone bodies, pH change in late stages, increase in volume and specific gravity); diabetes insipidus (volume increase, specific gravity decrease); adrenal cortex disorders (17 keto steroids), cardiac diseases (change in volume, protein in urine); porphyrias (red urine); acid-base disturbances (pH, volume and specific gravity changes).

CARDIAC FUNCTION TESTS. These include blood pressure (Av. 120-150/80), heart rate and pulse (Av. 72/min.), and electrocardiogram (EKG; pattern varies with disease state). There are changes from the normal values of the EKG in hypertension, coronary artery diseases, rheumatic heart diseases, and other systemic diseases.

BODY TEMPERATURE. Normal oral value is 98.6°F. This increases in various infectious diseases.

RESPIRATORY RATE. Normal value is 12 to 20 per minute. This increases with excitement, decreases in respiratory diseases.

BASAL METABOLIC RATE. Normal value is minus 10 to plus 15. This is increased in hyperthyroidism, acromegaly, cardiac diseases, kidney diseases, anemias, leukemias, polycythemias, Cushing's disease, and diabetes mellitus. It is decreased in hypopituitarism, hypothyroidism, Addison's disease, shock, malnutrition and lipoid nephrosis.

GASTRIC ANALYSIS. This is used for the detection of anemias, ulcers, tumors and certain infectious diseases.

STOOL ANALYSIS. This is used for the detection of gastrointestinal and liver diseases. As mentioned previously, knowledge of the patient's diet is important. Various foods can cause stool changes which might simulate changes due to disease processes.

CEREBRAL FUNCTION TESTS. These include electroencephalogram (EEG), analysis of cerebrospinal fluid, reflex tests, pneumoencephalogram, and other specialized tests. The tests are used for suspected cases of tumors, hemorrhages, strokes, meningitis, syphilis, and neuralgias.

SPECIALIZED TESTS. There are specialized tests for eye disorders, ear disorders, nasal and sinus disorders, speech disorders, taste disorders, and throat and bronchial disorders. These tests are usually performed either by ophthalmologists, optometrists (for eye disorders), E.N.T. specialists (for ear, nose, and throat disorders), and neurologists or neurosurgeons (for speech disorders). Certain simple tests for sinusitis can be performed by dentists. These are described in Chapter 2 in the section on frontal and maxillary sinusitis.

BONE MARROW ASPIRATION. This test may be used for suspected cases of leukemias and polycythemia.

TRANS-TRACHEAL ASPIRATION. This procedure is used in severe respiratory infections for direct microbial analysis of bronchial fluids.

SEROLOGICAL TESTS. These are antigen-antibody tests that are used as an aid in identifying microbial pathogens, degrees of host immunity, and in blood typing.

Some of the most important tests are listed below.

(1) *Agglutination Tests*
(2) *Precipitin Tests*
(3) *Toxin-antitoxin Tests.* These first three tests are aids for the identification of microbes and their products and degrees of host immunity.
(4) *Complement Fixation Tests.* These are used in the Wasserman test for syphilis and to identify viruses, fungi and the malaria organism.
(5) *Heterophile Agglutination Test.* This is used for detection of infectious mononucleosis.
(6) *TPI Test.* This is also used in the detection of syphilis.
(7) *Antistreptolysin O Titre.* This is indicative of streptococcal infectious disease. It increases in patients with periapical granulomas and cysts.
(8) *Blood Typing.* Importance is for blood transfusions. Major groups are A, B, AB, O and RH positive and negative.

DIAGNOSTIC SKIN TESTS. These tests are used to help determine whether a host is hypersensitive to a particular microbe, microbial product or specific substance. They can be used to aid in the determination of a specific disease, past history of a specific disease, or immunity to a specific disease.

Some of the more common tests are listed below.

(1) Tuberculin Test for tuberculosis.
(2) The Histoplasmin Test (for histoplasmosis).
(3) The Blastomycin Test (for blastomycosis).
(4) Patch Test for sensitivity to various drugs.

RADIOGRAPHY. This may be used alone or in conjunction with radiopaque drugs, such as Lipiodol® to aid in localization. It is used to help detect lesions, aneurysms, and obstructions.

X-RAY SIALOGRAPHY. This is used for the localization of salivary gland tumors, stones and other disorders.

PROBING OF SALIVARY DUCTS. This is used for the detection of salivary stones (calculi).

ELECTROMYOGRAM. This is used for the determination of the electrical activity of the muscles of mastication. It is an aid in the localization of spasms that can cause dental pain or bruxism.

SPUTUM ANALYSIS. This is used to help differentiate local infectious disease from respiratory and gastrointestinal diseases. It is an aid in the diagnosis of diabetes mellitus.

Dental

The various dental diagnostic tests are discussed in this section. These include radiography, bite registration, periodontal probing, probing of lesions, probing of sinus tract, removal of caries and/or restorations, exploratory flap, exploratory drilling, thermal tests, electric pulp tests, palpation, percussion, mobility tests, anesthetic test, test cavity, tests for the cracked tooth syndrome, biopsy, microbial examination, electrophoretic analysis, exfoliative cytology, transillumination, study models, ultrasonics, thermography, electrical measurements, clinical photography, and auscultation.

RADIOGRAPHY. There is a divergence

of opinion about the types of equipment and techniques to be used for endodontic radiography. There are advocates of right angle and bisection angle techniques and advocates of 90KVP, 70KVP, and 45-50KVP machines. I believe that for endodontic practice the ideal for both diagnostic and treatment considerations is the right angle (long cone) technique. However, a light weight, easily maneuverable 45 to 50 KVP machine, that can be attached to the dental unit has certain advantages. These include ease of use, more economical, and less floor space needed. The right angle technique is preferable because a better differentiation of structures can be obtained with its use. It is also advantageous because of the superior evaluation possible when comparing subsequent radiographs.

Use of a film holder (Fig. 65) aids in obtaining more accurate x-ray images, especially in posterior teeth. The use of a holder also helps in the obtaining of uniform radiographs for comparative purposes. Ultra speed film and one of the rapid developing techniques should be used. Methods for rapid processing of radiographs include use of a more concentrated developer (e.g. Collit's Rapid Developer), warming solutions to 90°F, and use of ultrasonics. With these techniques it is possible to have a readable x-ray film in less than one minute. The automatic dental film processors are the most thorough, the most expensive, and take the longest time (about four minutes). However, they can be used in the treatment room. The exposed film is dropped into a slot and is then developed, fixed, washed, and dried (Fig. 66).

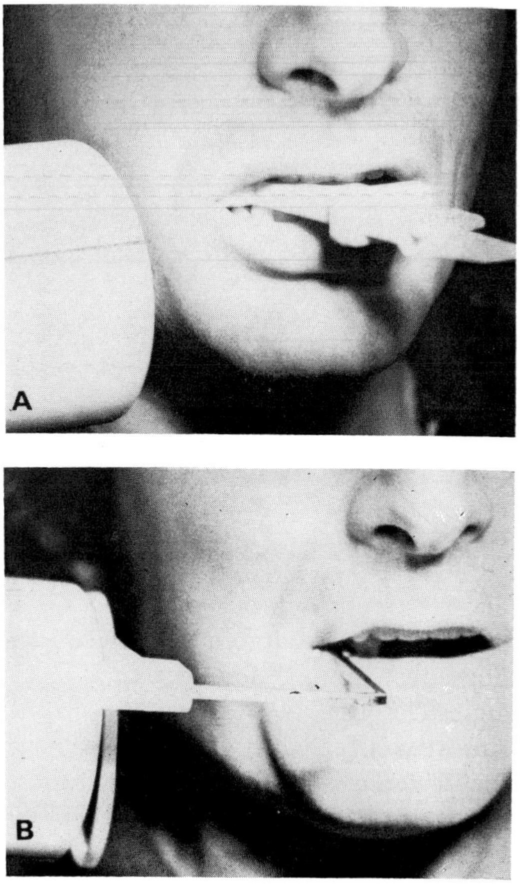

Figure 65. Film holders. A. Rinn snap-a-ray film holder. B. Rinn X-C-P film holder.

A lead apron should be used to protect the gonad region of children and adults in the child-bearing ages. Only as many radiographs as are necessary for good technique should be used. Before taking radiographs, the dentist should be sure that the patient removes all appliances. If not, strange looking radiopacities will be found on the radiograph (Fig. 67).

Single Diagnostic Periapical Radiograph. This is usually all that is neces-

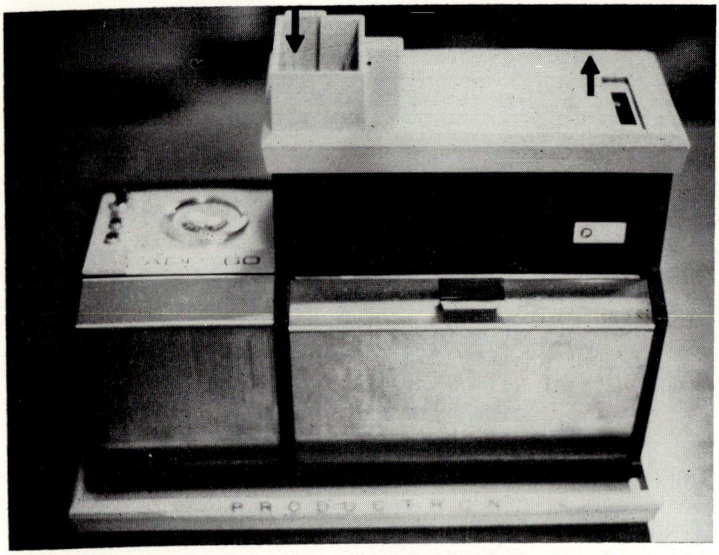

Figure 66. ADP-60 automatic dental film processor (Productron, Inc.); film is placed in left slot (left arrow) and is removed from the right slot (right arrow).

sary for upper anterior teeth. In lower anteriors, it is advisable to take two radiographs from different mesial-distal angles, as often two canals are present. This may also occur in lower premolars. For posterior teeth, bitewings may also be helpful. In cases where there is doubt about where the pain is coming from, radiographs should be taken in the opposite arch. In trauma cases involving the anterior teeth, radiographs should be taken of the opposite arch, because of possible damage to teeth in both arches. When systemic involvement is suspected, x-rays should be taken of all the teeth. The dentist should look for the following when viewing diagnostic radiographs:

(1) *Normal Anatomic Landmarks Which May Simulate Periapical Pathosis.* If the lesion is a pulpally-induced periapical rarefaction, then it will appear to be continuous with the root apex, when a second radiograph from a mesial or distal angulation is taken. If it is a normal anatomic landmark, it will appear to move away from the root apex, when a second differently angled film is taken (Fig. 68).

(2) *Approximate Length of Roots.* This gives the practitioner a guide for the use of root canal instruments.

(3) *Periapical or Lateral Radiolucency.* Lesions are usually larger than their radiographic image. This is because a lesion is not detectable on the radiograph until the cortical bone is reached. If the lesion is confined to the cancellous bone, it will not be visible on the film. Also, the labial (buccal) to lingual (palatal) dimension is not seen on periapical radiographs. Therefore, bone that is destroyed on either of these surfaces, would not be visualized

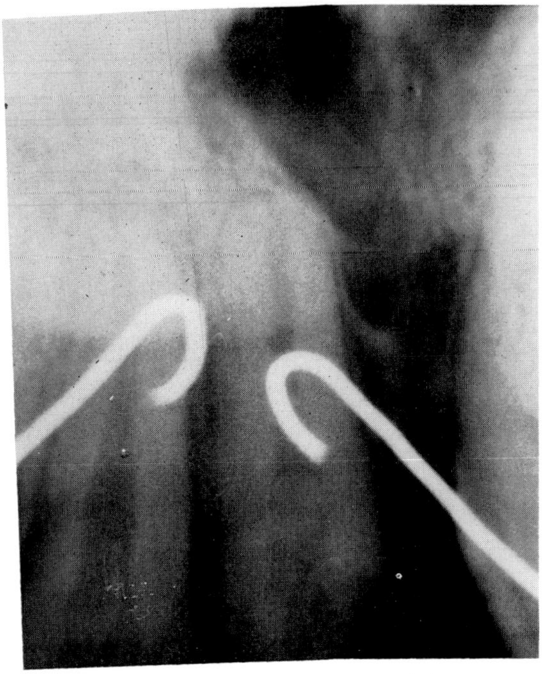

Figure 67. Cleft palate obturator left in position when radiograph is taken shows up as a radiopacity which may interfere with radiograhic interpretation. (Courtesy of Dr. L. Muldorf, Philadelphia, Pa.)

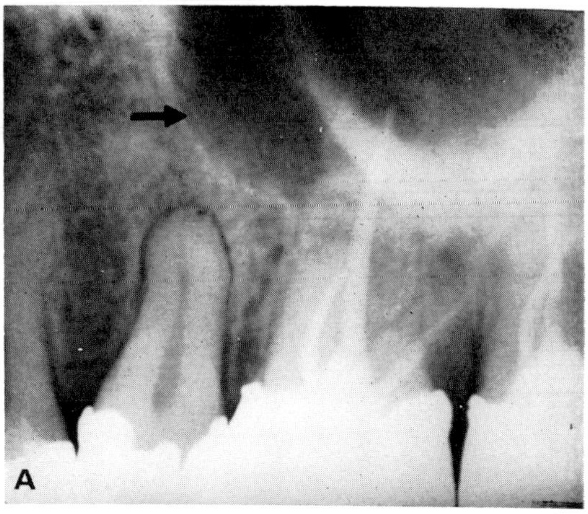

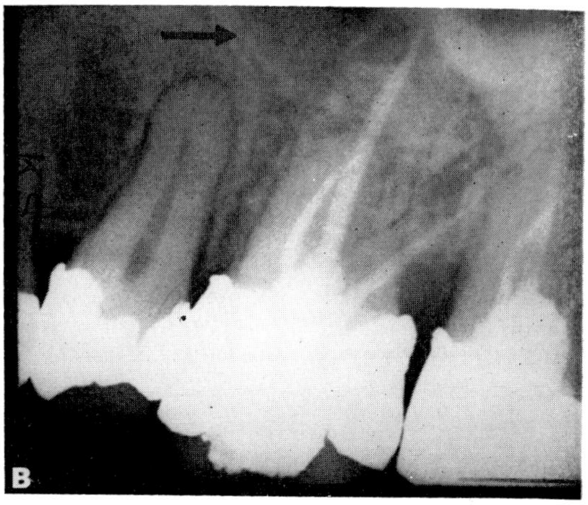

Figure 68. Maxillary sinus or periapical area of pathosis? A. Radiolucency appears as if it was an area of pathosis. B. Taken from a mesial angulation the *area* has moved and the presence of a lamina dura can be detected around the palatal root.

on the radiographs. Another factor concerning periapical and lateral radiolucencies, is the angulation at which the film is taken. Merely by changing the angle, while taking a radiograph, it is possible to superimpose cortical bone over a periapical radiolucency. This would give the illusion that the *area* has disappeared (Fig. 69). If a periapical radiolucency can be seen on one film, and not on another, then it must be present. There are certain teeth in which periapical radiolucencies may fail to show up on a radiograph or may show up later in the disease process. This is because different roots are situated in dissimilar relationships to the cortical plates of bone. In the lower first molar, the mesial root is often closer to the buccal cortex. Therefore, similar sized areas of rarefaction are usual-

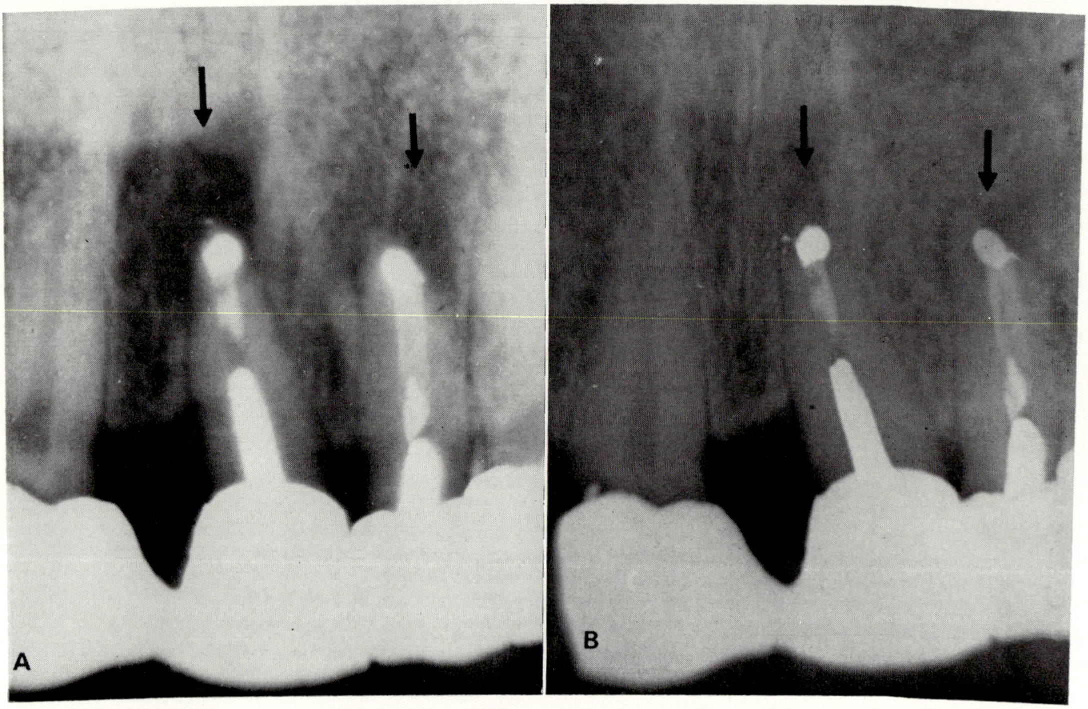

Figure 69. Two views of periapical region of upper right incisors. A. Taken from normal angulation, periapical radiolucencies can be seen. B. Taken from a mesial angulation, periapical radiolucencies have apparently disappeared.

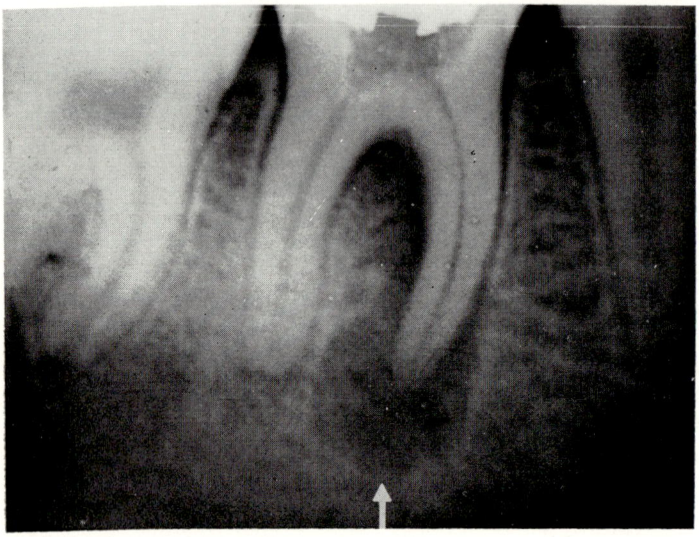

Figure 70. Periapical area of pathosis seen first around the mesial root of lower first molar.

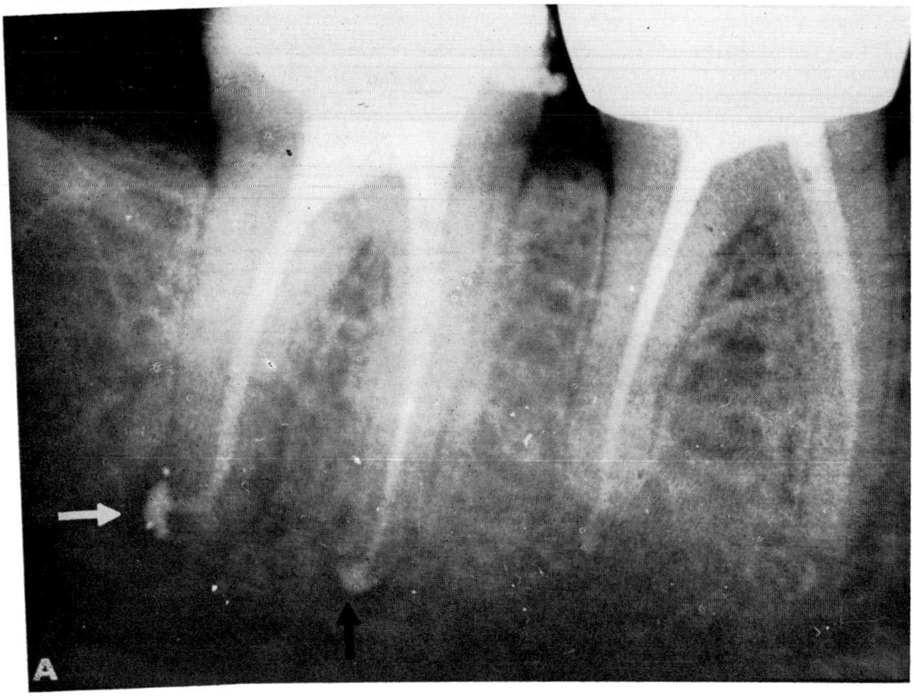

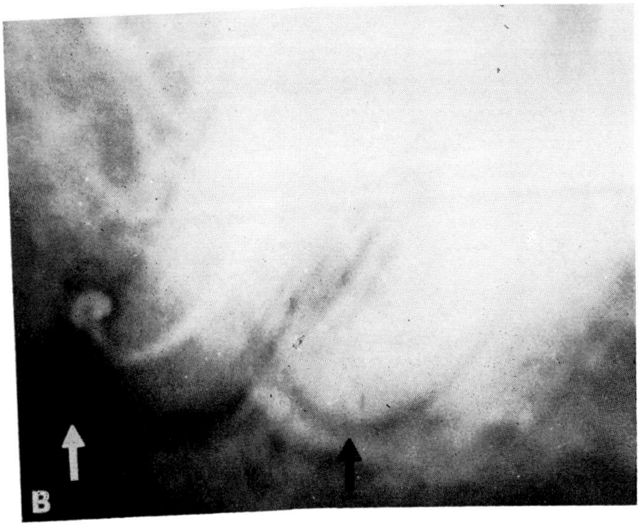

Figure 71A and B. Periapical area of pathosis seen first around the distal root of lower second molar (white arrows).

ly seen around the mesial root before they are visible around the distal root (Fig. 70). In the lower second molar, periapical radiolucencies usually first appear around the distal root in the radiograph, even though both roots are centrally located between the cortical plates (Fig. 71). The probable explanation is that the distal canal often is larger than the mesial canals. It

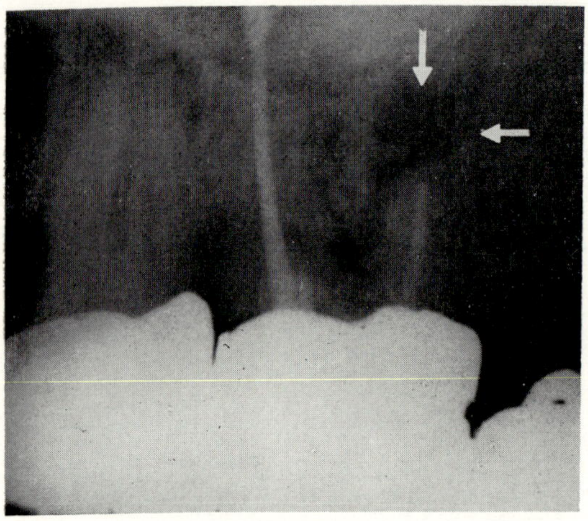

Figure 72. Periapical area of pathosis is seen first around the mesio-buccal root of an upper first molar.

therefore contains a greater concentration of inflammatory products. These products could then diffuse into the periapical bone and cause a greater amount of bone destruction than would be found around the mesial root. Periapical radiolucencies are seen less in upper molars, because these teeth are less frequently involved by caries, and it is difficult to visualize rarefactions because of the usual superimposition of the periapical areas by the maxillary sinus. Areas of rarefaction are less frequently seen around palatal roots, because they are usually embedded in cancellous bone. The distobuccal root is also partially in cancellous bone (most often) and the usual finding for the mesiobuccal root is that it is closest to the buccal cortex. Therefore,

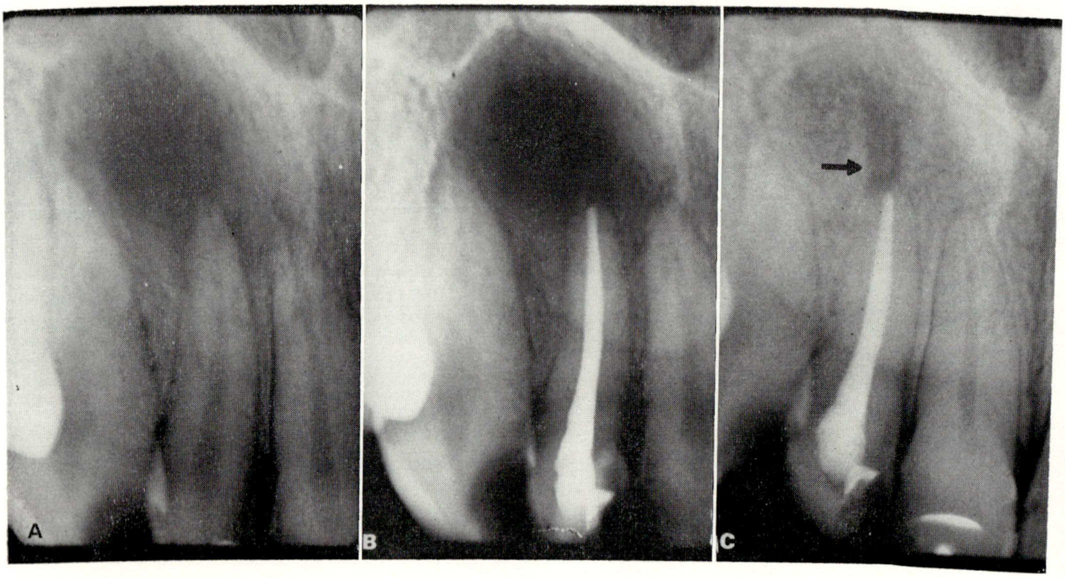

Figure 73. Development of a periapical fibrous scar. A. Periapical area of pathosis present. B. Root canal therapy and periapical curettage performed; bone was destroyed on both labial and palatal plates of bone. C. One year later; periapical healing has occurred except for presence of a fibrous scar.

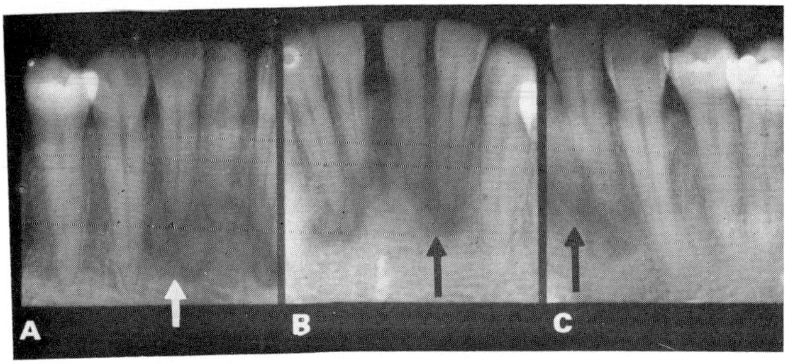

Figure 74. Three different stages of a cementoma seen at the same time. A. Predominantly radiopaque. B. Partially radiopaque and radiolucent. C. Predominantly radiolucent. (Courtesy of Dr. W. Updegrave, Philadelphia, Pa.)

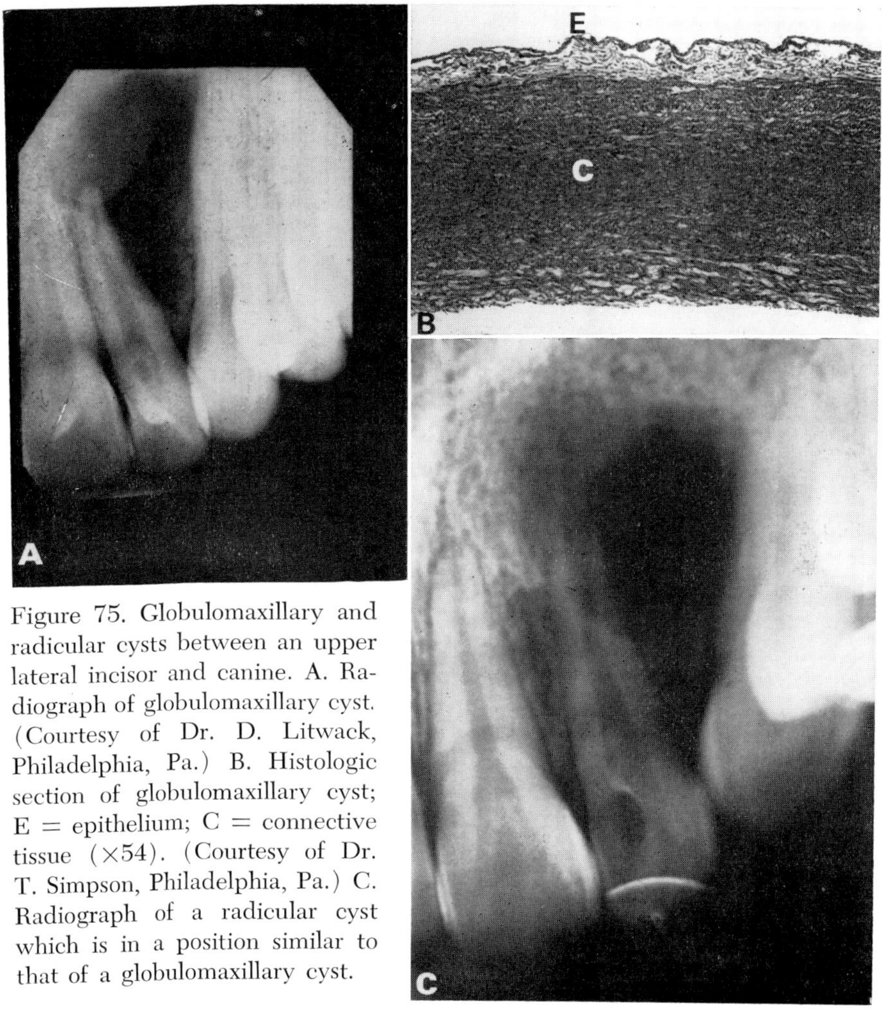

Figure 75. Globulomaxillary and radicular cysts between an upper lateral incisor and canine. A. Radiograph of globulomaxillary cyst. (Courtesy of Dr. D. Litwack, Philadelphia, Pa.) B. Histologic section of globulomaxillary cyst; E = epithelium; C = connective tissue (×54). (Courtesy of Dr. T. Simpson, Philadelphia, Pa.) C. Radiograph of a radicular cyst which is in a position similar to that of a globulomaxillary cyst.

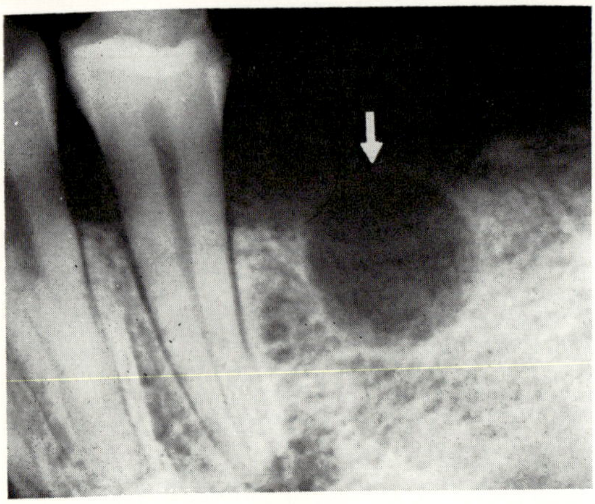

Figure 76. Residual cyst. (Courtesy of Dr. T. Simpson, Philadelphia, Pa.)

the order of visualizing periapical radiolucencies in upper molars is first the mesiobuccal root, second the distobuccal root and third, the palatal root (Fig. 72). The two most common periapical radiolucencies are periapical granuloma and radicular cyst. Other less frequent lesions that can be seen are fibrous scar (Fig. 73), cementoma (Fig. 74), cholesteatoma, globulomaxillary cyst (Fig. 75), residual cyst (Fig. 76), and various bone lesions of both local and systemic origin.

(4) *Osteoporosis.* These are areas of diffuse radiolucency. They can occur in various diseases and conditions including hyperthyroidism, hypothyroidism, hypercortinism, adrenal atrophy, protein malnutrition, acromegaly (hyperpituitarism), cystic fibrosis, diabetes, disuse atrophy, vitamin C deficiency, senility, osteogenesis imperfecta, in the post-menopausal period, ovarian dysgenesis, and osteomalacia.

(5) *Radiopacity.* The most common type seen is from condensing osteitis (Fig. 77). Radiopacities are also seen in late stages of cementoma (Fig. 74A), Garre's osteomyelitis (Fig. 192D), osteo-

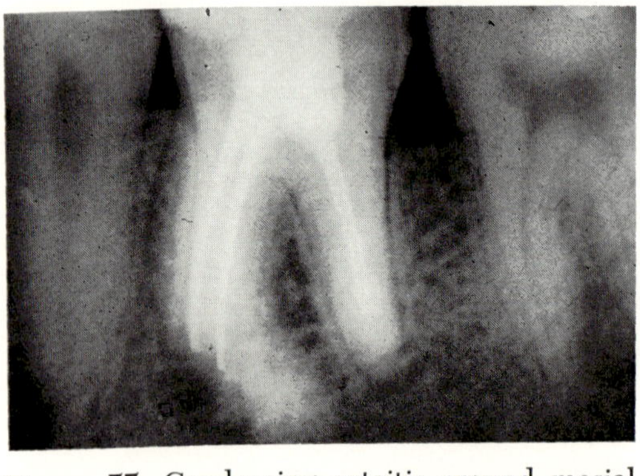

Figure 77. Condensing osteitis around mesial root of lower right first molar. (From S. Seltzer, *Endodontology*, McGraw-Hill, Inc., 1971. Used with permission of McGraw-Hill Book Company.)

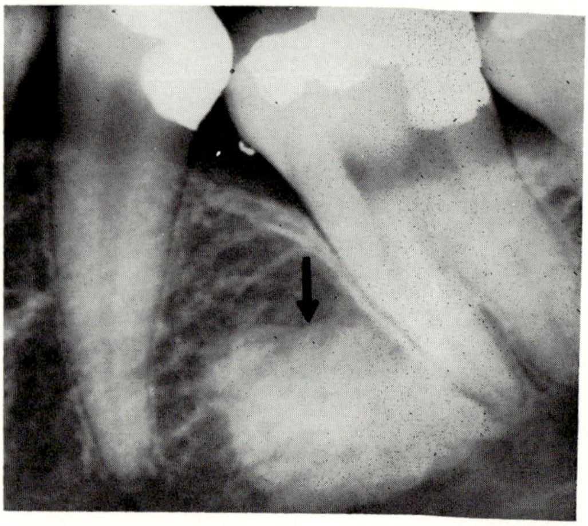

Figure 78. Osteoma; this can be differentiated from condensing osteitis by the presence of the periodontal ligament space around the mesial root. (Courtesy of Dr. W. Updegrave, Philadelphia, Pa.)

sclerosis, ossifying fibroma, osteoma (Fig. 78), late stages of Paget's disease (Fig. 79), osteopetrosis, Leontiasis ossea, and other systemic diseases.

(6) *Root Resorptions, Internal and External.* External root resorption can occur as the result of pulpally-induced periapical inflammation (Fig. 80), orthodontic movement (Fig. 30), pressure from erupting teeth or tumors (Fig. 81), luxation, transplantation and replantation of teeth (Fig. 82), hypothyroidism, other systemic diseases, and unknown causes (Fig. 83). Internal root resorption probably occurs as the result of trauma (Fig. 84), and is seen after

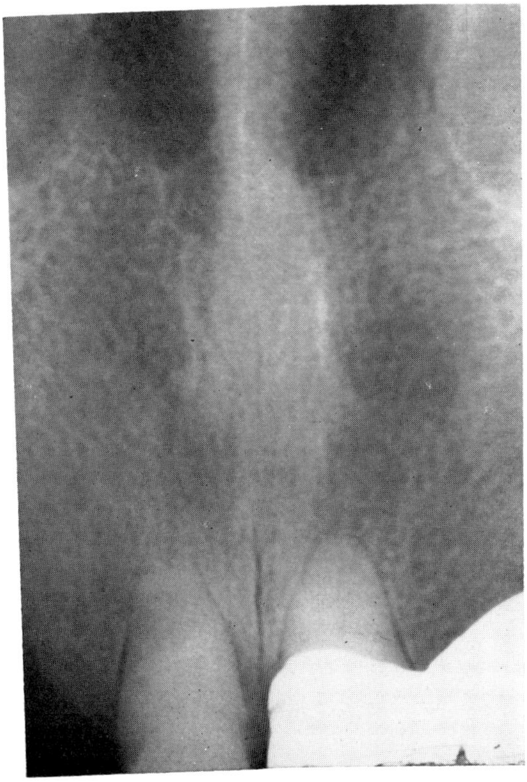

Figure 79. Paget's disease showing ground glass radiopaque appearance and root resorption. (Courtesy of Dr. A. Schlossberg, Philadelphia, Pa.)

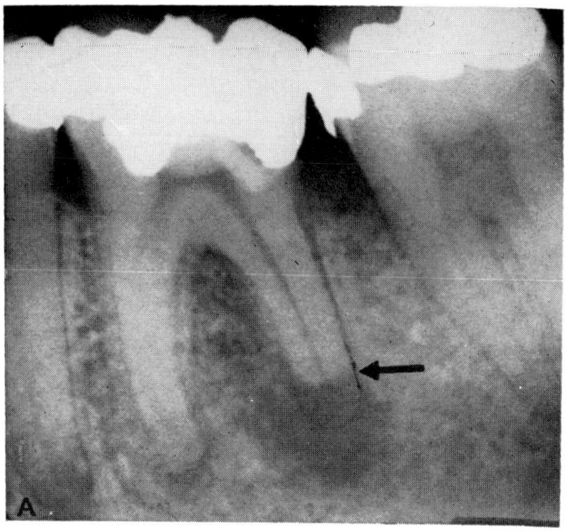

Figure 80A

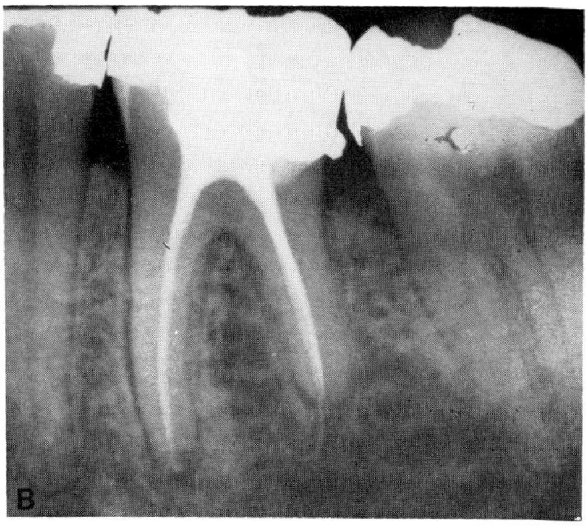

Figure 80B

Figure 80. External root resorption as a result of pulpally-induced periapical inflammation. A. Before; outline of original root is discernible; periapical area of pathosis is present. B. Two years later; root resorption ceased and periapical repair is evident, even though there was overfilling with gutta-percha.

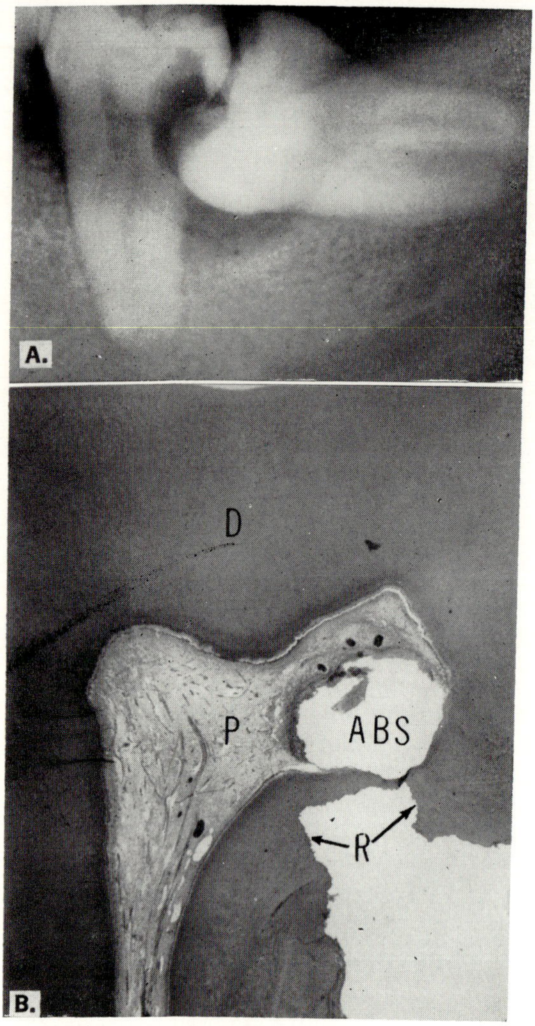

Figure 81. External root resorption of lower second molar caused by pressure from erupting third molar. A. Radiograph. B. Histologic section showing root resorption and chronic pulpitis with liquefaction necrosis; D = dentin, P = pulp, ABS = abscess, R = Root resorption (×8.1). (From S. Seltzer, *Endodontology*, McGraw-Hill, Inc., 1971. Used with permission of McGraw-Hill Book Company.)

pulpotomy and pulp capping procedures (about one third of the cases). In certain cases, there is doubt whether the process began externally or internally (Fig. 84B).

(7) *Alveolar Bone Level.* Taking radiographs at different angulations can give the illusion that the bone has *filled in* (Fig. 85). Also it is possible for a periodontal area of rarefaction to be superimposed over a root apex and this can give the appearance of periapical bone destruction. Another view reveals the true nature of the condition (Fig. 86). Therefore, it is important that radiographs should be taken under standard conditions, in order to compare results without bias. A tooth must have at least 3 mm of supporting bone in order to be treatable with an endodontic implant (Fig. 87). Bone loss in many teeth is indicative of periodontitis or periodontosis (Fig. 88).

(8) *Pulp Exposures.* These can occur as the result of caries, trauma, mechanical exposure, attrition, abrasion, and erosion. Sometimes it is impossible to differentiate an unlined silicate or plastic filling from deep caries. Visual and explorer examination will clarify the issue.

(9) *Depth of Restorations and Presence or Absence of Cavity Liners.*

(10) *Pulp Capping and Pulpotomy.* One should look for the presence or absence of dentin bridges under the area of the

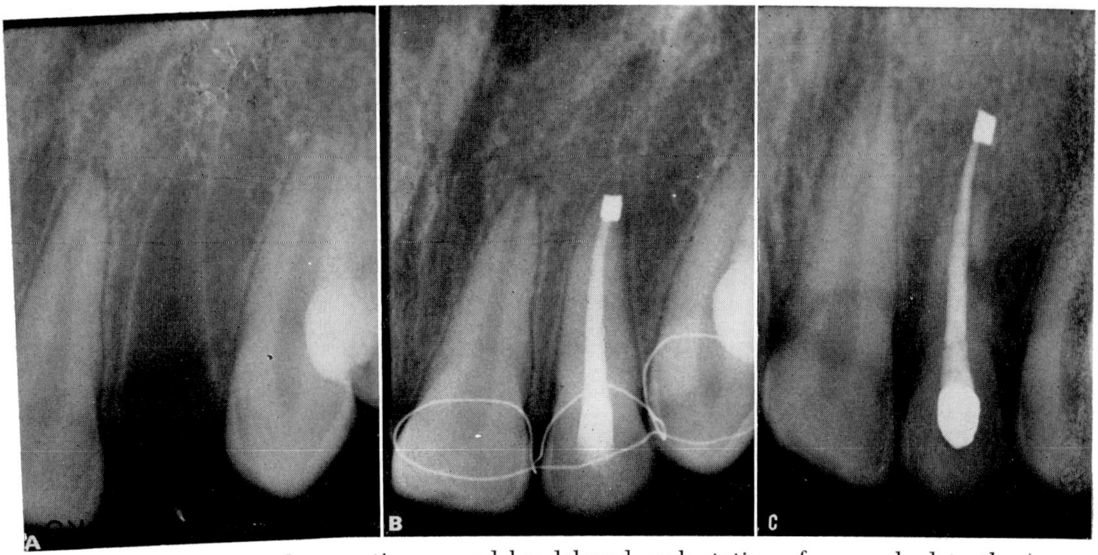

Figure 82. External resorption caused by delayed replantation of an avulsed tooth. A. Tooth socket at time of patient's first office appearance. B. Immediately following replantation; canal had been obturated with gutta-percha-chloropercha, a retrograde amalgam seal was placed, and a wire-acrylic splint was inserted. C. Three years later; external root resorption is apparent on the middle third of the root.

pulp capping or pulpotomy. For indirect pulp capping, the area under the pulp capping paste should be examined for the presence or absence of caries. Also in pulp capping and pulpotomy cases, pulp calcification or internal resorption may be observed.

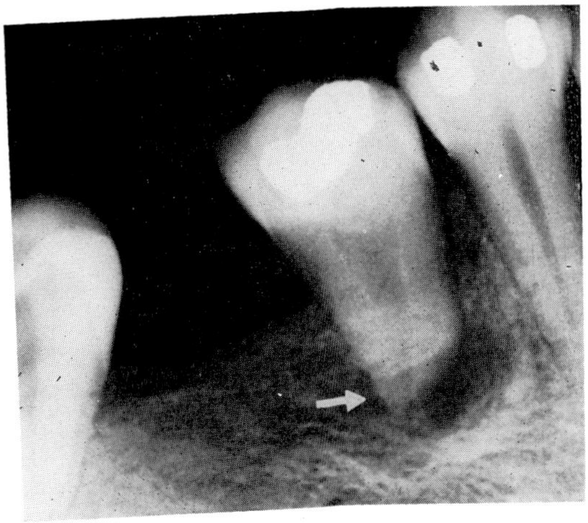

Figure 83. External root resorption of unknown origin. (Courtesy of Dr. A. Schlossberg, Philadelphia, Pa.)

(11) *Cervical Translucencies.* These must be differentiated from root caries. Explorer use can differentiate these possibilities (Fig. 89).

(12) *Root Fractures.* Extent and degree of fracture should be checked (Fig. 90). It may be necessary to take x-rays from different angulations for fracture determination.

(13) *Retained Roots.* These may cause symptoms (Fig. 91).

(14) *Broken Instruments.* This is important to know, before beginning treatment (Fig. 92).

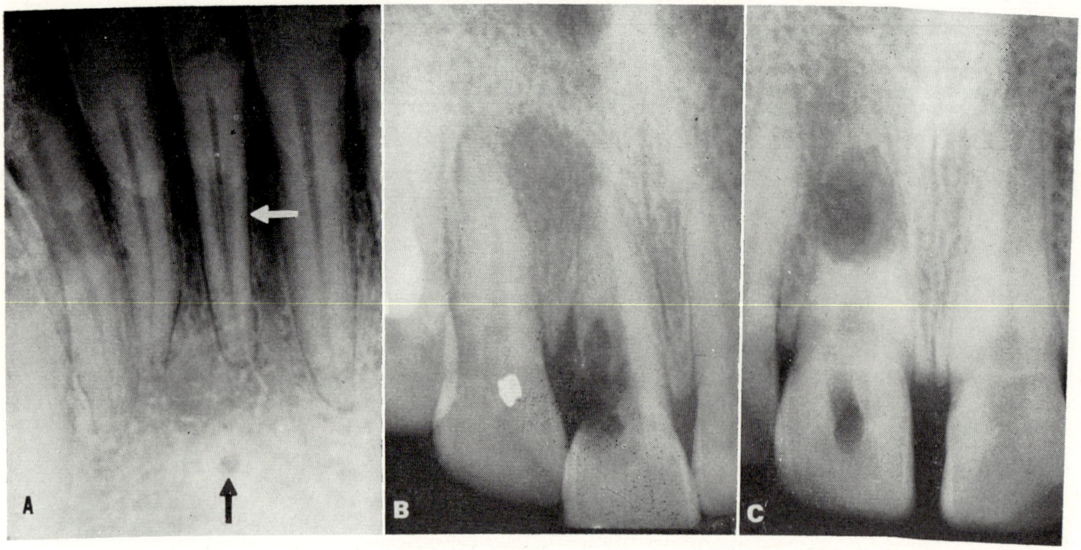

Figure 84. Internal root resorption. A. White arrow shows internal resorption; black arrow indicates the lingual foramen. (Courtesy of Dr. W. Updegrave, Philadelphia, Pa.) B. Internal resorption with perforation on one side of the root. (From D. R. Morse, "The Management of Endodontic Problem Cases," *JDA South Africa,* 27:387, 1972) C. Internal resorption showing complete root perforation (From D. R. Morse, "The Management of Endodontic Problem Cases," *JDA South Africa,* 27:387, 1972)

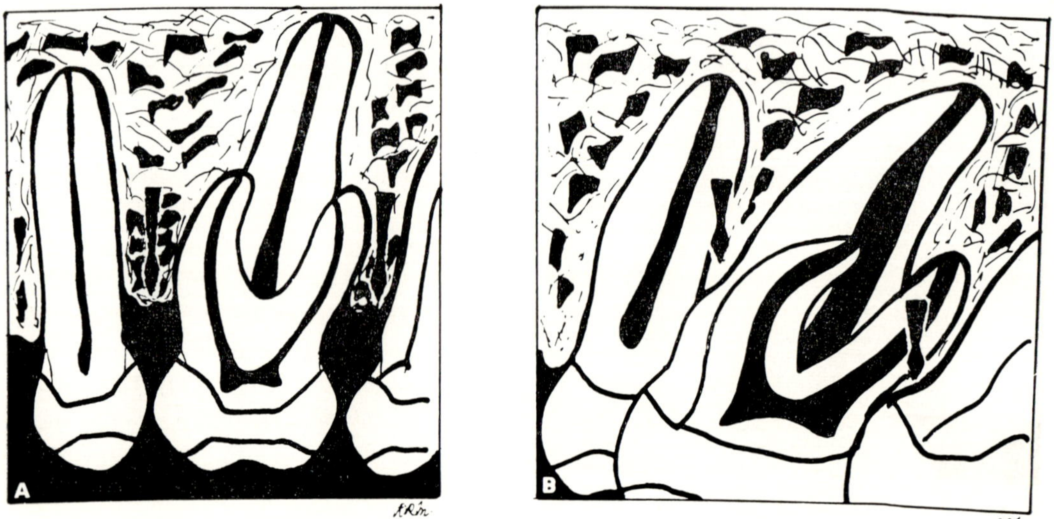

Figure 85. Alveolar bone level, normal X-ray angulation. A. Bone loss is apparent. B. Radiograph taken at a different angle; the bone appears to have *filled in.*

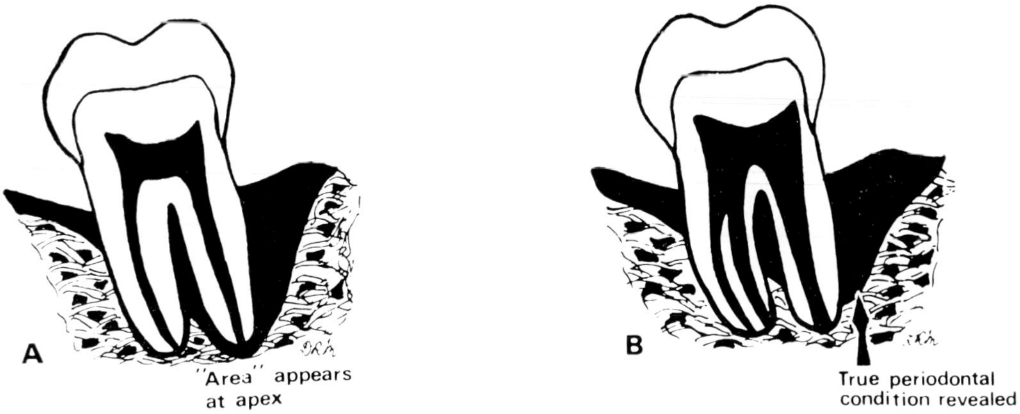

Figure 86. Periodontal *bone loss* simulating periapical area of pathosis. A. Normal angulation. B. Changed angulation.

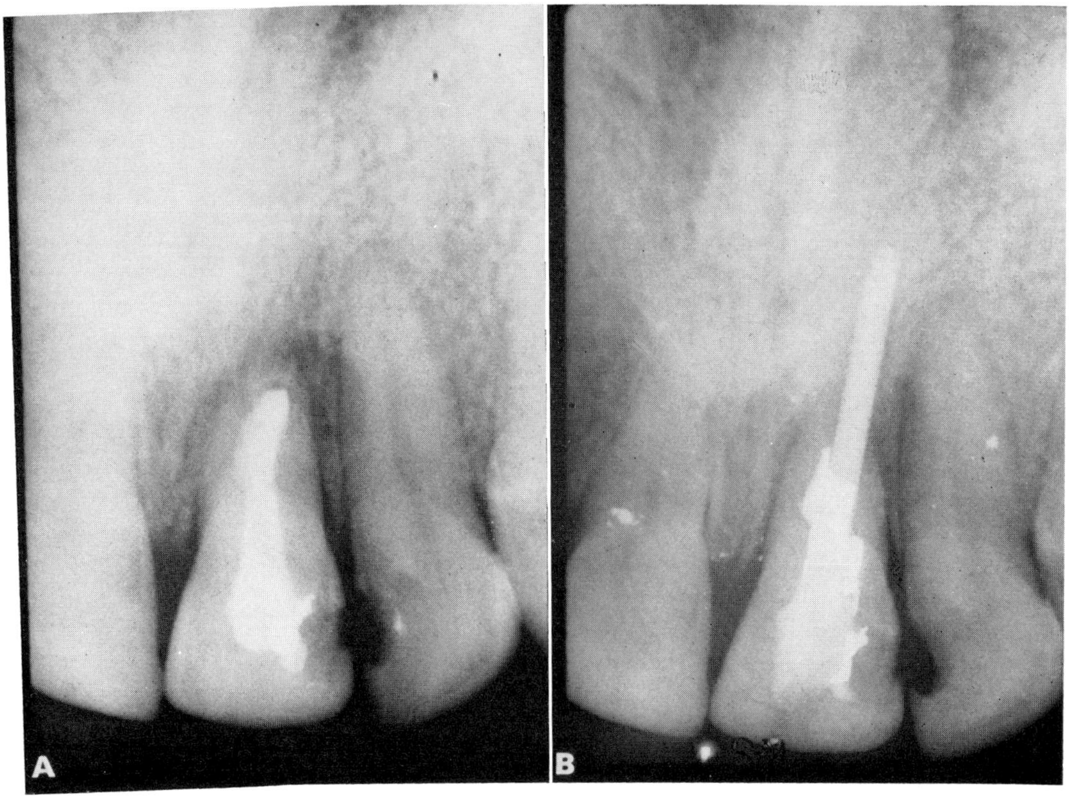

Figure 87. Endodontic implant for a periodontally involved upper right central incisor. (From D. R. Morse, "The Significance of Endodontics in Plantation Procedures," *JDA South Africa*, 26:263, 1971.) A. Before treatment; tooth with Class III mobility, deep pockets, a very short root, and about 5 mm of bony support. B. One year after insertion of a titanium (Plantanium) implant, tooth is firm and periodontal condition has improved.

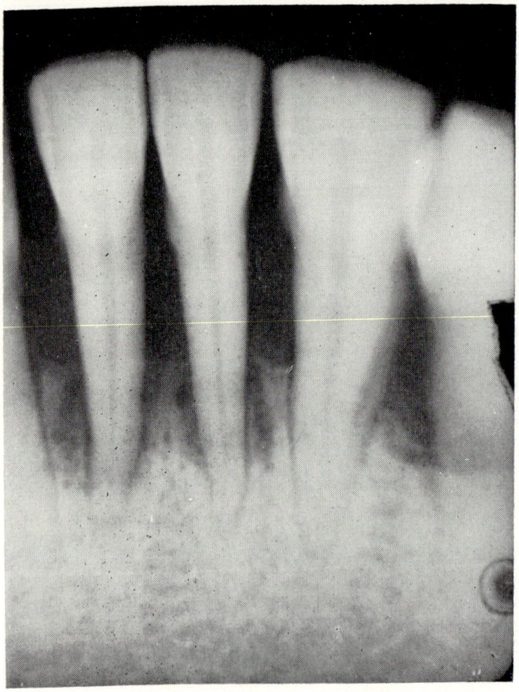

Figure 88. Periodontitis showing extensive *bone loss* on several teeth. (Courtesy of Dr. T. Simpson, Philadelphia, Pa.)

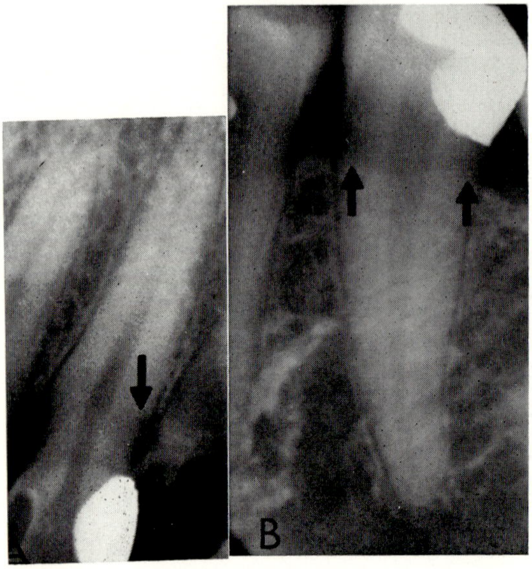

Figure 89. Differentiating cervical translucency from root caries; an explorer examination is necessary. A. Upper premolar. B. Lower premolar.

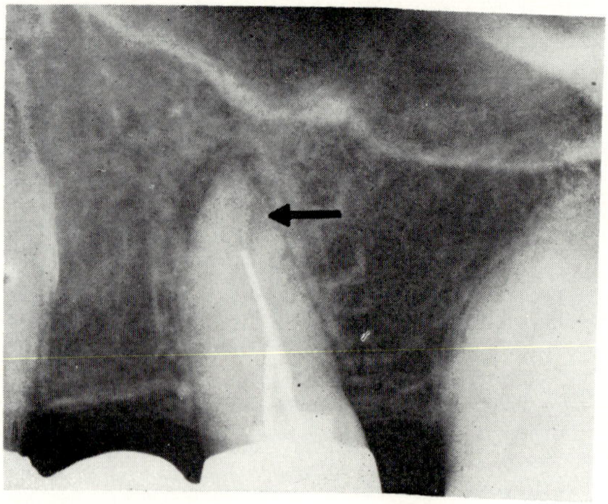

Figure 90. Root fracture at apical region probably causing the periapical rarefaction.

(15) *Root Anatomy.* The number of roots, types of curvatures, and shapes of roots should be checked (Fig. 93).

(16) *Hypercementosis.* This can occur as a result of trauma, Paget's disease (Fig. 17), Cooley's anemia, sickle cell anemia, hyperpituitarism, or for unknown reasons (Fig. 94).

(17) *Root Canal Anatomy.* The number of canals, presence of calcifications, excessively wide or excessively narrow canals and other anatomic variations should be checked. Excessively wide or excessively narrow root canals are signs of pulpal disease (Fig. 95).

(18) *Previous Root Canal Fillings.* The type of filling should be determined. Silver cones are more distinctive and radiopaque than are gutta-percha fillings. Vitallium® implants are more radiopaque than titanium implants (Fig. 96). Presence or ab-

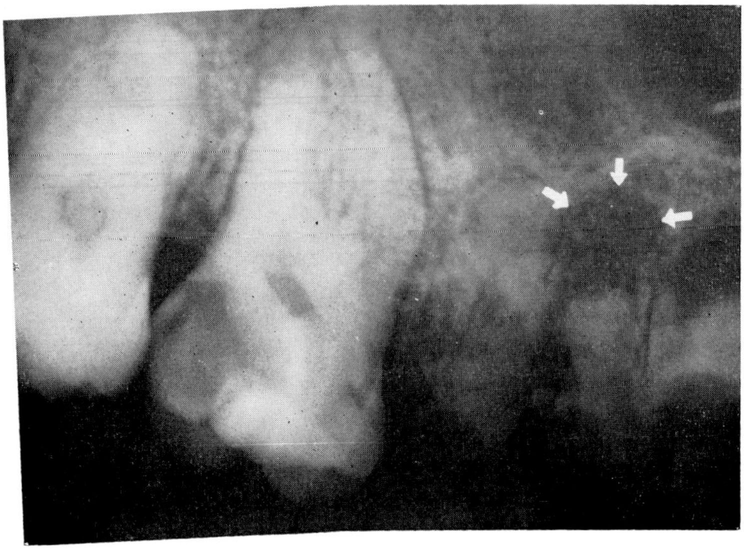

Figure 91. Retained roots and residual area of pathosis; patient's odontalgia could have originated from the cariously involved second molar or the retained roots and periapical area of pathosis (arrows) from the first molar. (Courtesy of Dr. W. Updegrave, Philadelphia, Pa.)

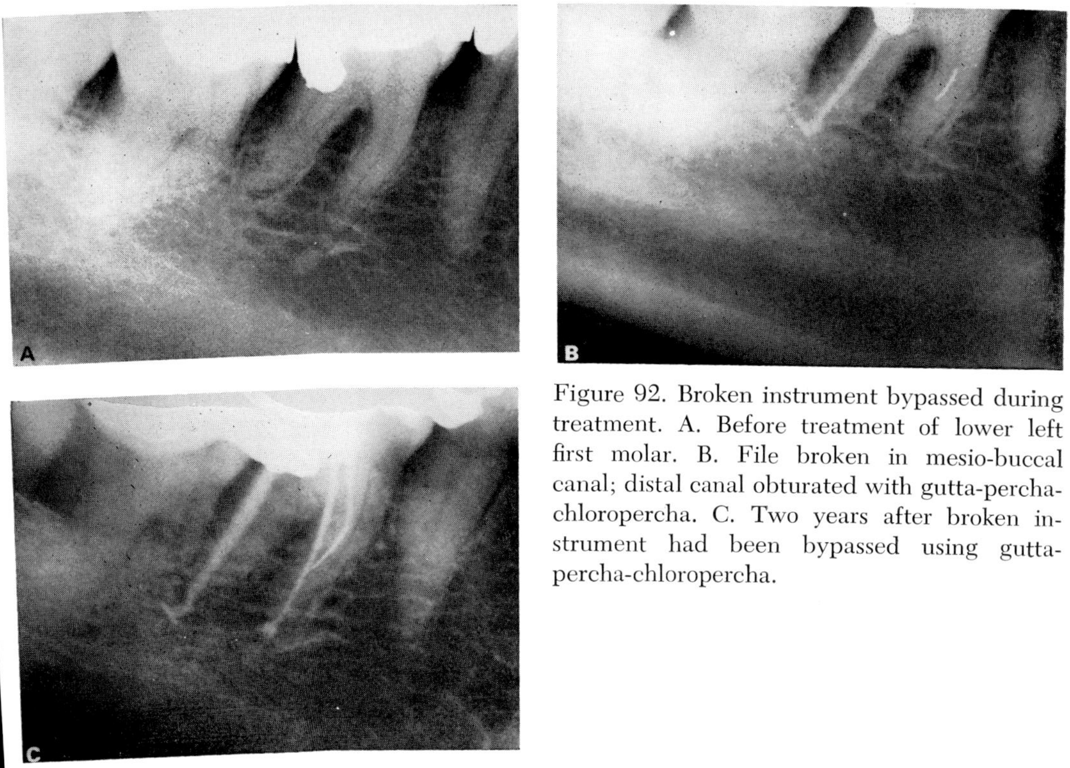

Figure 92. Broken instrument bypassed during treatment. A. Before treatment of lower left first molar. B. File broken in mesio-buccal canal; distal canal obturated with gutta-percha-chloropercha. C. Two years after broken instrument had been bypassed using gutta-percha-chloropercha.

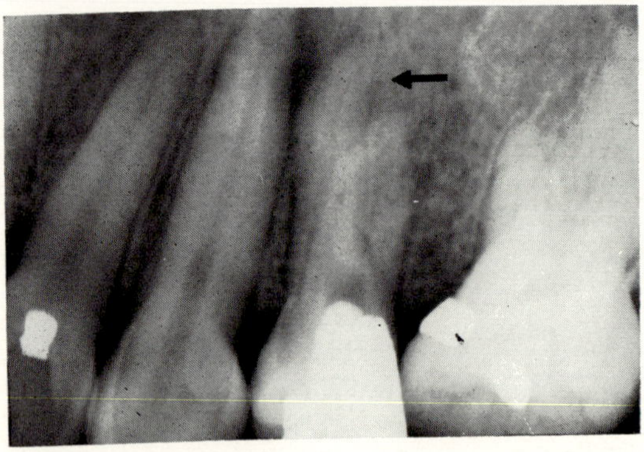

Figure 93. Upper first premolar with three roots.

sence of posts and pins should be determined (Fig. 97). Occasionally retrograde amalgam seals are not placed in the correct location. They may not even be in the root or they may not be at the apex (Fig. 98). Radiographs from more than one mesial-distal angulation will help in the localization. The films should be checked to see if any perforations are involved with previous root canal fillings, posts or pulpotomies (Fig. 98).

(19) *Pulp Stones.* Large pulp stones can interfere with endodontic access and instrumentation (Fig. 99). Large pulp stones may also be indicative of pulp disease and may occasionally cause pulpal pain.

(20) *Width of Periodontal Ligament Space.* An even increase in width (from normal) is indicative of occlusal traumatism (Fig. 100). An abnormal widening is sometimes seen in scleroderma (Fig. 20).

(21) *Lamina Dura.* The lamina dura is lost in some cases of hyperparathyroidism (Fig. 16), Paget's disease, and fibrous dysplasia.

(22) *Furcation Involvements.* If these are seen on more than one tooth, periodontal disease is the usual cause. If the involvement is only on one molar, then the condition is most probably the endodontic-periodontic syndrome (Fig. 101).

(23) *Probing of Sinus Tracts and Pockets.* A radiopaque probe is placed into pockets to see their depth and also to see if they communicate with the apex or a furca. A probe is also placed in a sinus tract to see which root is involved in the disease process or if the tract is non-endodontic in origin (Fig. 102).

(24) *Foreign Bodies.* Occasionally foreign bodies can occur in the soft tissues or periapical regions and this may be visible on a periapical radiograph (Fig. 103).

(25) *Jaw Fractures.* These can be seen as radiolucent lines.

(26) *Embedded Teeth.* If an embedded tooth lies adjacent to the roots of another tooth, pressure from the embedded tooth can cause root resorption and/or pulpal necrosis of the adjacent tooth (Fig. 81).

(27) *Erupting Third Molars.* These can cause pain which may be referred to a tooth anterior to the third molars.

(28) *Artifacts.* Artifacts which can

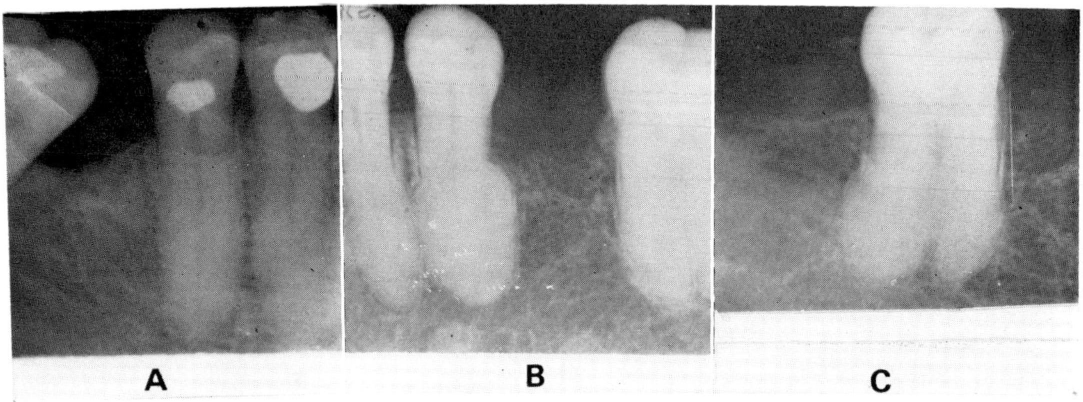

Figure 94. Idiopathic hypercementosis. A. Lower left premolar area. B. Lower right premolar-molar area. C. Lower left molar area. (A, B, and C, Courtesy of Dr. W. Updegrave, Philadelphia, Pa.)

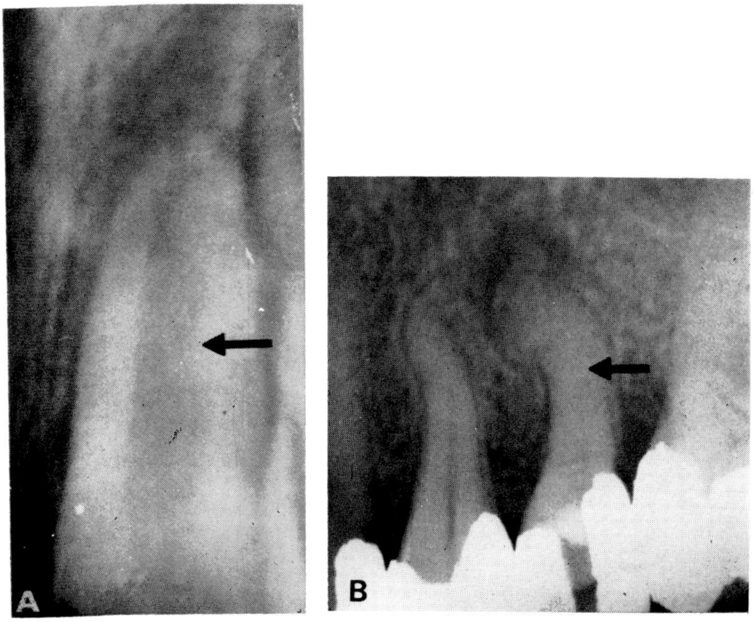

Figure 95. Pulpal necrosis; extremely wide and extremely narrow canals. A. Wide canal. B. Very fine canal.

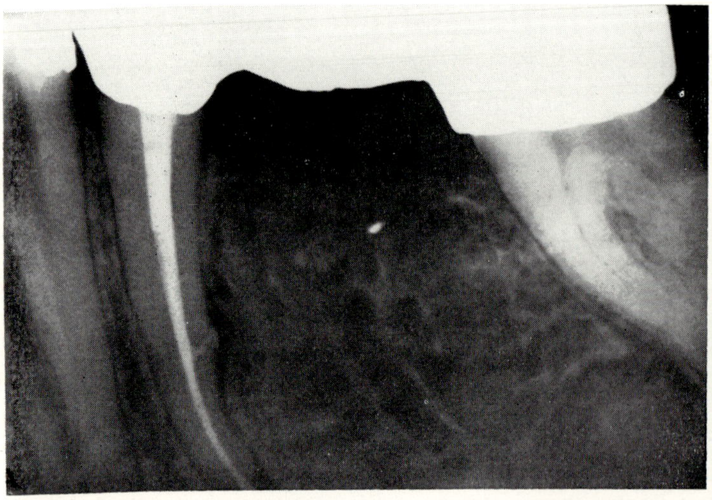

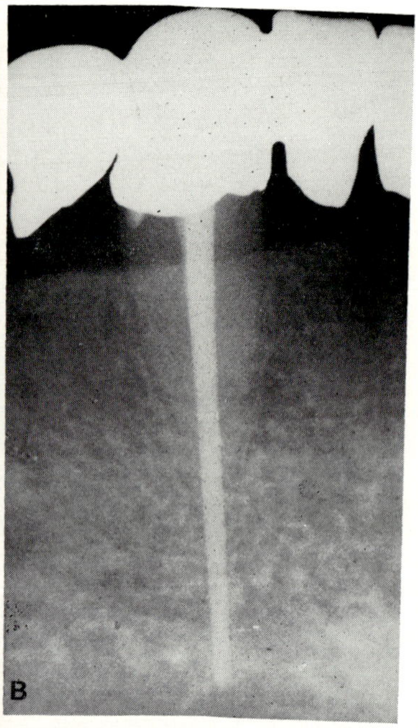

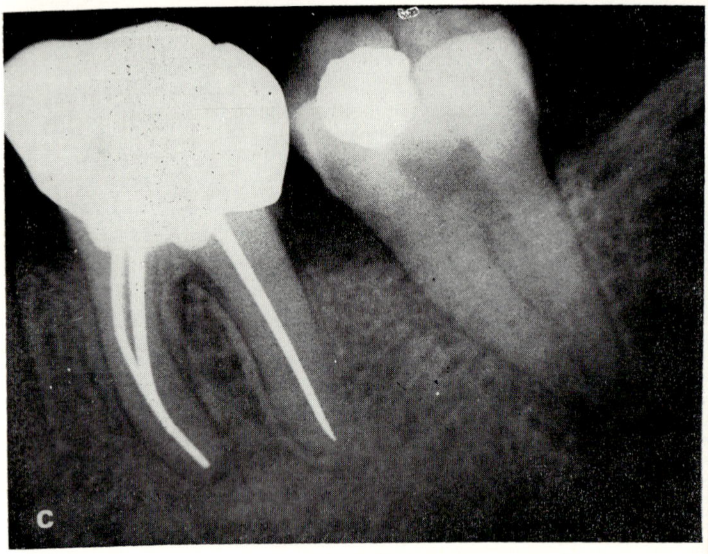

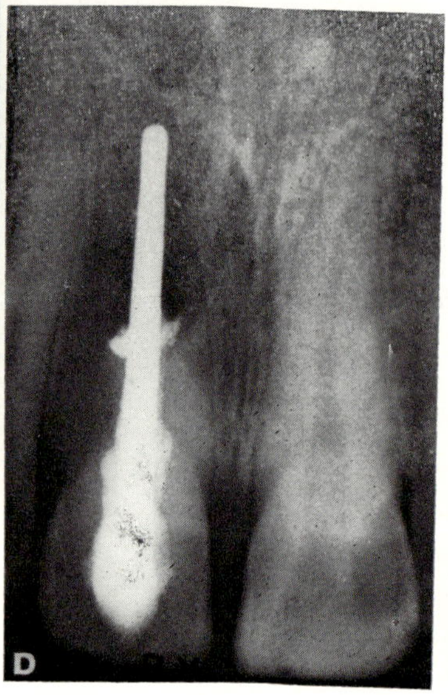

Figure 96. Differences in radiopacity of root canal fillings and endodontic implants; C and D are more radiopaque than A and B. A. Gutta-percha filling. B. Titanium (Plantanium®, Implant Research Corp.), implant. (From D. R. Morse, F. Nislow, and N. Busch, "The Full Arch Splint Using Endodontic Implants: Report of Case," *Journal of the American Dental Association*, 85:351, 1972, Copyright by the American Dental Association. Reprinted by permission.) C. Silver cone filling. (Courtesy of Dr. A. Cetron, Cherry Hill, N. J.) D. Chrome-cobalt alloy (Vitallium, Austinal) implant. (From D. R. Morse, "The Management of Endodontic Problem Cases," *JDA South Africa*, 27:387, 1972)

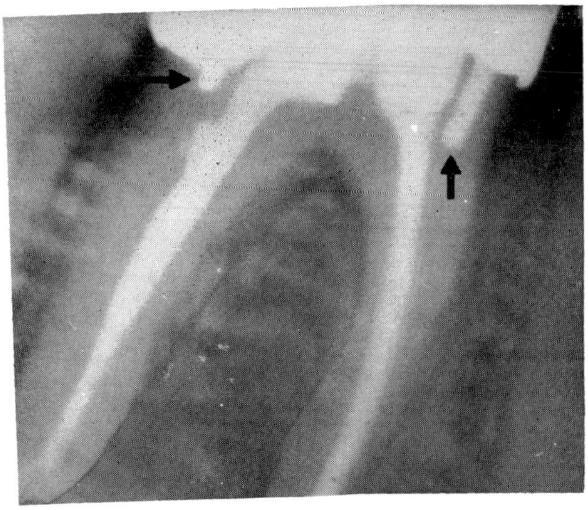

Figure 97. Lower molar with pins.

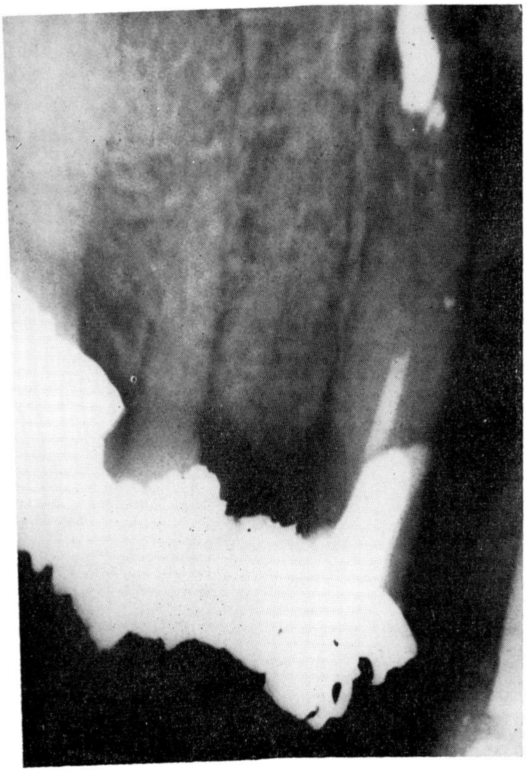

Figure 98. Retrograde amalgam may not have sealed the apex, as there is a periapical *area* present; placement of gold post has caused a root perforation, and the development of a lateral *area*.

simulate fracture lines and periapical lesions can be caused by bending films and developing solution stains (Fig. 104).

Single Treatment Periapical Radiographs. During treatment, the radiographs aid in the following:

(1) *Determining the Length of Roots.* An instrument (file or

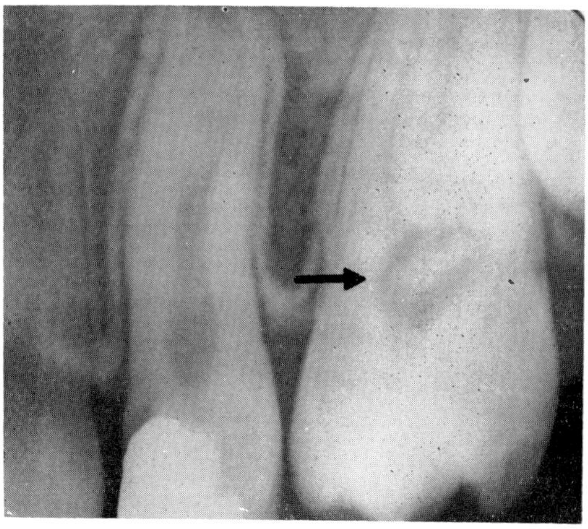

Figure 99. Large pulp stone almost completely occluding pulp chamber.

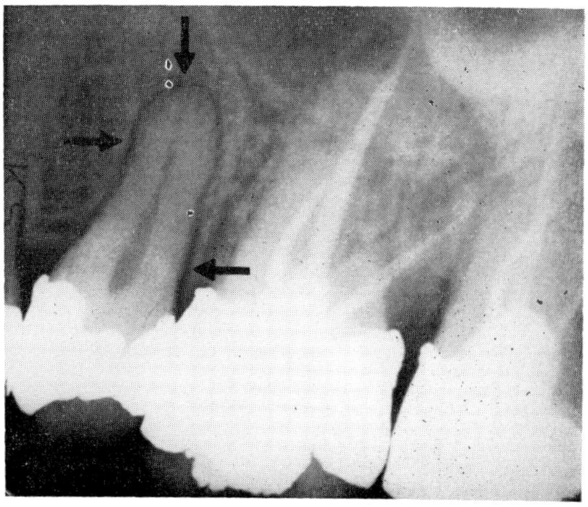

Figure 100. An increased thickening of periodontal ligament space resulting from occlusal traumatism (arrows).

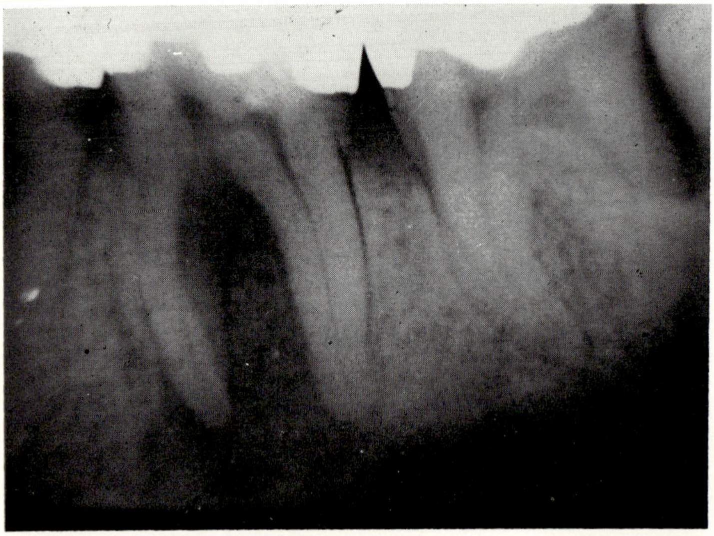

Figure 101. A bifurcation involvement in a lower first molar resulting from the endodontic-periodontic syndrome.

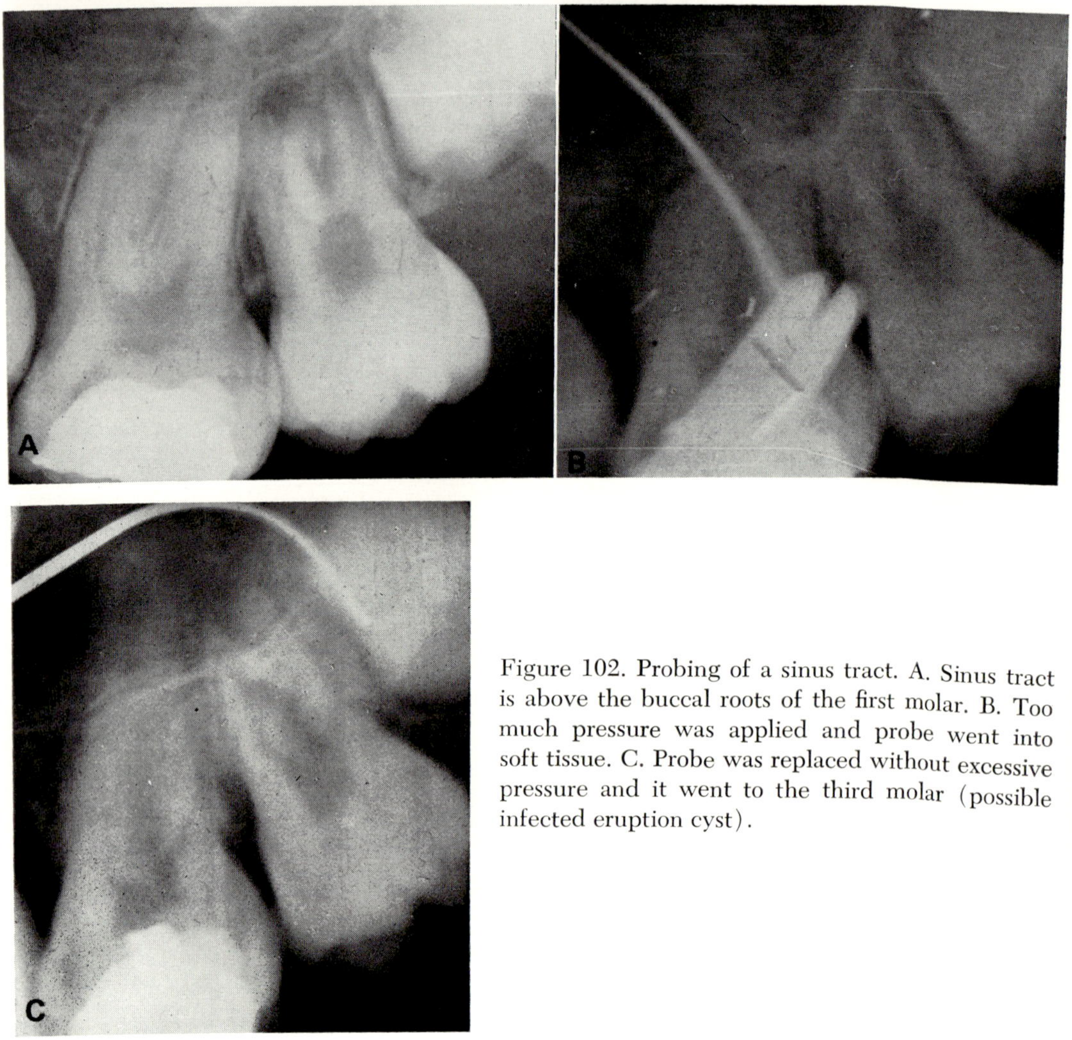

Figure 102. Probing of a sinus tract. A. Sinus tract is above the buccal roots of the first molar. B. Too much pressure was applied and probe went into soft tissue. C. Probe was replaced without excessive pressure and it went to the third molar (possible infected eruption cyst).

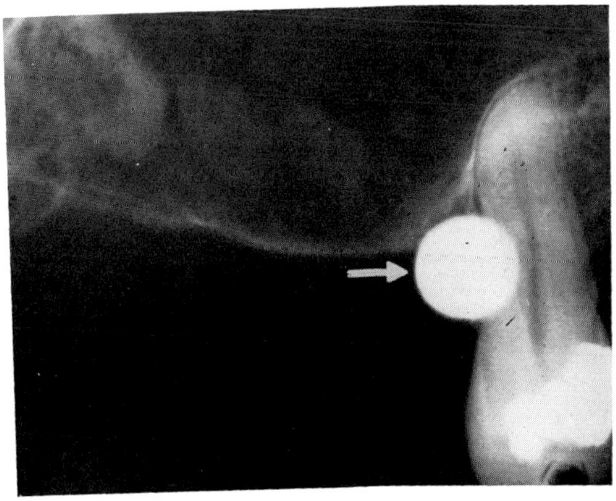

Figure 103. Beebee in cheek is seen on periapical radiograph. (Courtesy of Dr. T. Simpson, Philadelphia, Pa.)

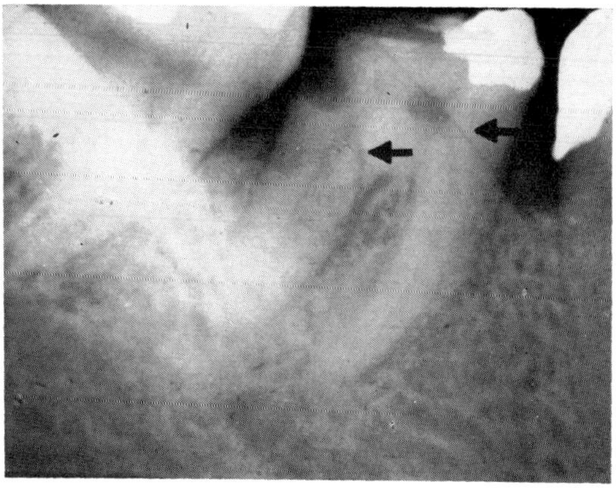

Figure 104. Artifacts simulating fracture lines. (From D. R. Morse, "The Management of Endodontic Problem Cases," *JDA South Africa*, 27:387, 1972)

reamer) is placed into the canal until it reaches the approximate apex. This can be determined by feel (apical bind) or by comparison with the radiographic length of the root of the original diagnostic radiograph. A radiograph is then taken with the instrument in position. The comparison of the instrument to the radiographic apex is made, and necessary adjustments are completed. A more exacting method is the use of the following formula to determine the actual length of the root.

$$\frac{\text{actual length of the instrument (to the tip of cusp)}}{\text{radiographic length of the instrument}} = \frac{\text{actual length of root (X)}}{\text{radiographic length of the root}}$$

Solving for X will give the actual length of the root and then adjustments in the instrument length can be made accordingly.

(2) *Determining the Degree of Penetration of Root Canal Instruments into Root Canals.*

(3) *Visualizing Perforations and Near Perforations.*

(4) *Determining the Fit of Master Filling Cones.*

(5) *Determining the Completeness of Root Canal Filling.* A second radiograph should be taken from the mesial or distal (as compared to the first radiograph). This will help in visualizing the completeness of filling in the buccal-lingual diameter (Fig. 105).

(6) *Determining the Localization of Root Canals.* In teeth with several canals, improved visualization of the individual canals can be made by placing a different instrument in each canal. An example is use of a file in the dis-

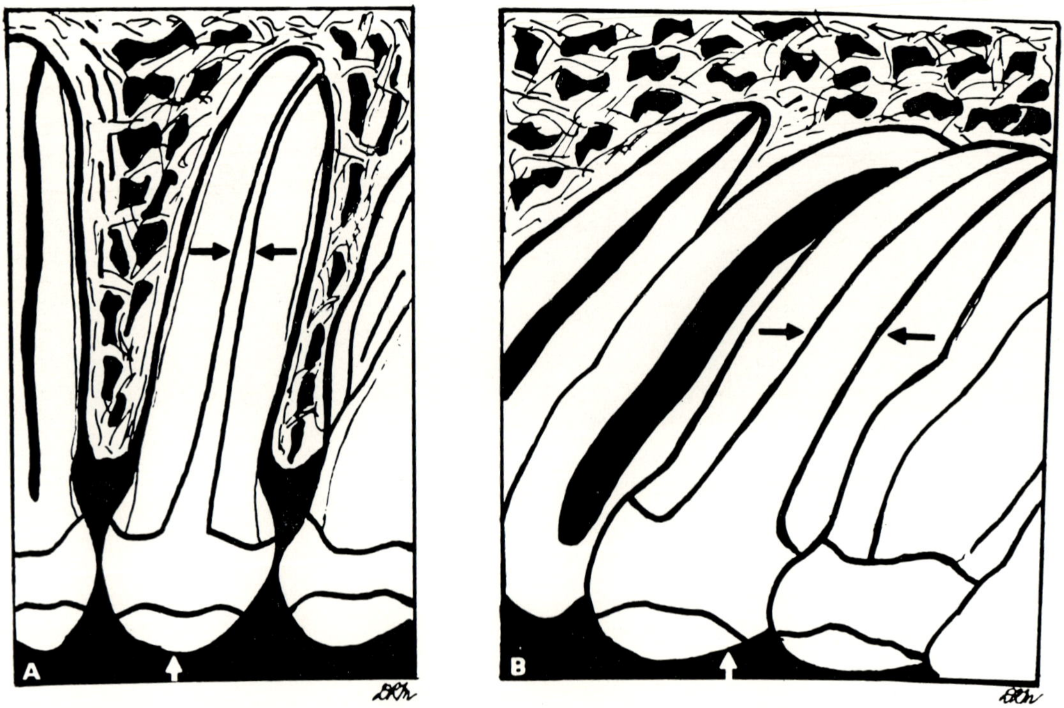

Figure 105. Determining completeness of root canal filling. A. Radiograph taken from normal M-D angulation. B. Radiograph taken from a more mesial angulation.

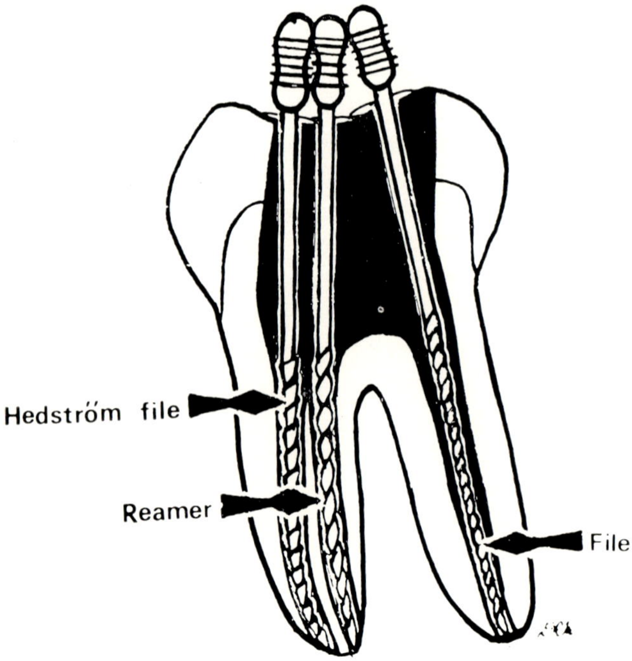

Figure 106. Root canal separation by instruments.

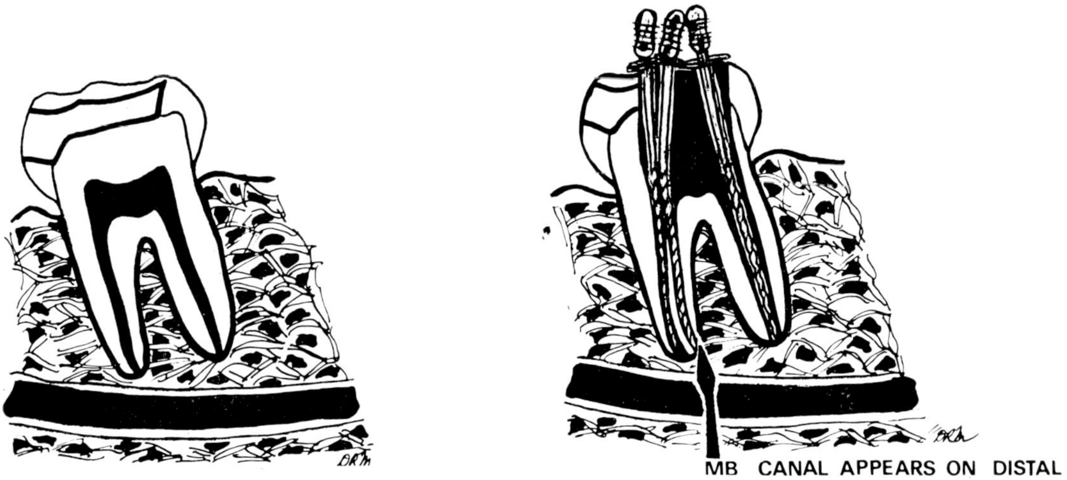

Figure 107. Root canal separation by angulation. A. Normal angulation. B. Mesial angulation.

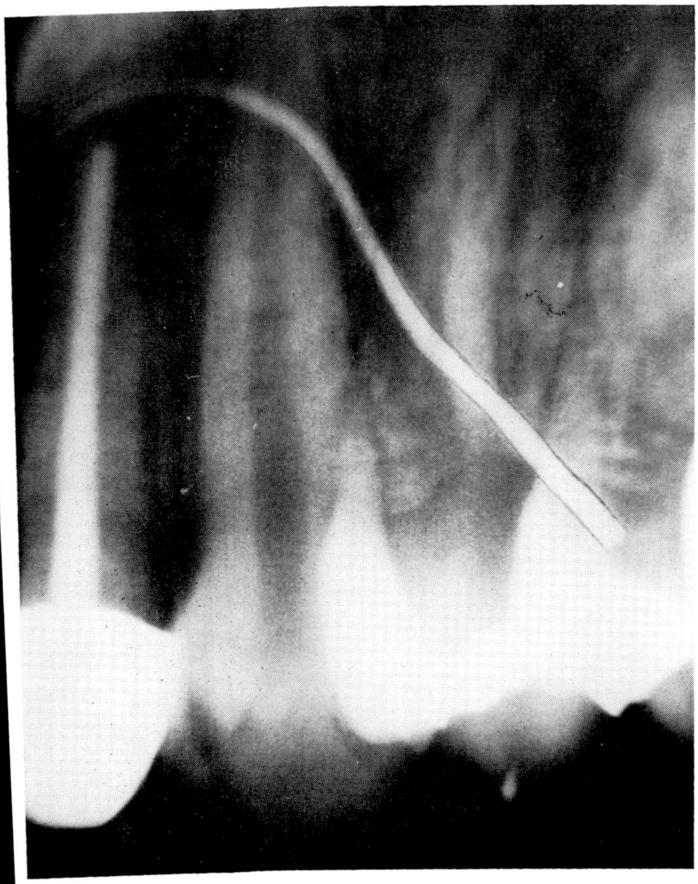

Figure 108. Probing the apex; an explorer is placed in the suspected periapical region and a radiograph is taken to determine if location is correct.

tal canal, a reamer in the mesiobuccal canal, and a Hedström file in the mesiolingual canal of a lower molar. Each one will be visualized differently on the radiograph (Fig. 106). A second method used to identify canals in a multirooted tooth is that the first diagnostic radiograph is taken perpendicular to the long axis of the tooth. The treatment radiograph with the root canal instruments in position is taken from a more mesial direction. On this treatment radiograph, the mesiobuccal canal appears on the distal, and the mesiolingual canal appears on the mesial (Fig. 107). If the treatment radiograph is taken from the distal, then the mesiobuccal canal would appear on the mesial and the mesiolingual canal would appear on the distal.

(7) *Determining Root Apexes, Accessory Roots, Root Perforations, Proximity to Another Root, Proximity to the Maxillary Sinus, and Proximity of the Inferior Alveolar Canal.* An instrument or filling cone is placed into the area that is under investigation. It will then show up as a radiopaque object on the radiograph (Fig. 108).

(8) *Confirming That the Periapical Region Is Free of Excess Filling Material.* It is important to note that materials which are not radiopaque will not be revealed on a radiograph. Therefore, visual and digital examination of the periapical region for materials like cotton, gauze and sponges is essential.

(9) *Determining the Approximate Buccal-lingual Locations of the Inferior Alveolar Canal, Mental Foramen, and the Maxillary Sinus.* Two radiographs are used. An example is given for the inferior alveolar canal localization. The first radiograph is taken with the occlusal surfaces of the lower teeth parallel to the floor. The x-ray beam is parallel to the occlusal plane of the second molar. The x-ray beam is directed so that there is no overlap of the contact points between the first and second molar. For the second radiograph, the factors are the same, except the vertical angle is changed to 25° below the horizontal plane (the tube is tilted upward at a 25° angle). In the second radiograph, if the inferior alveolar canal image moves upward, then the canal lies buccal to the tooth. If the image moves downward, then the canal lies lingual to the tooth (Fig. 109).

Single Recall Periapical Radiograph. Radiographs are essential at the recall visit to answer several questions:

(1) Have periapical *areas* developed in teeth that had no previous *areas?*

(2) Have periapical *areas* either enlarged, stayed the same, or decreased in teeth that had previ-

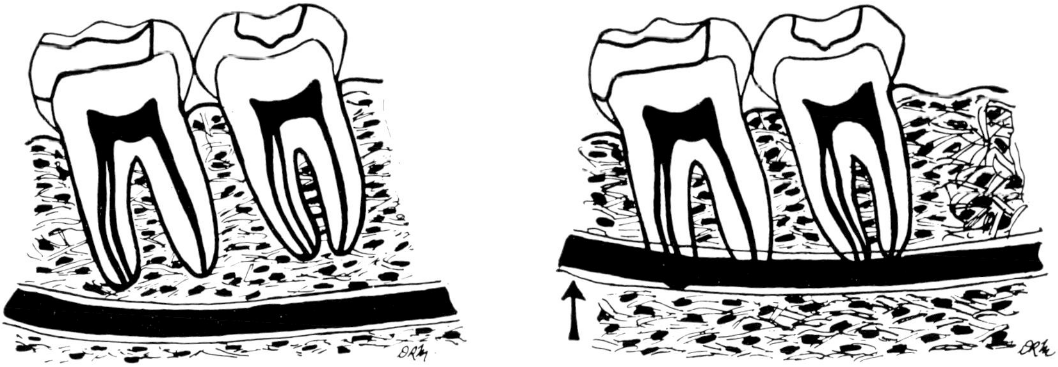

Figure 109. Inferior alveolar canal location. A. Horizontal angulation. B. −25° angulation; See text for explanation.

ous periapical *areas*?

(3) Have periodontal lesions healed in endodontic-periodontic cases?

(4) Have perforations developed from post or pin insertions?

(5) Has periodontal disease developed (alveolar bone loss or thickening of the periodontal ligament)?

(6) Are the margins of coronal restorations satisfactory?

(7) Have caries developed beneath the restorations?

(8) Have root fractures developed?

(9) Have root canal fillings been displaced, especially apical amalgams?

(10) Have rarefactions developed around implants (in implant cases)?

Bite Wing Radiographs. These are useful in posterior teeth for determination of the proximity to pulp horns of the conditions of caries, cavity and crown preparations, abrasion, erosion, and attrition. The radiograph also gives a good view of the anatomy of the pulp chamber (Fig. 110).

Occlusal Films. These films are useful for the following reasons:

(1) Visualization of large lesions.

(2) Examination of several anterior teeth simultaneously.

(3) Concomitant examination of the teeth and nasal fossae or sinuses.

(4) To determine anterior jaw fractures.

(5) Examination of foreign bodies that are outside the range of the periapical radiograph.

(6) Visualization of the buccal-lingual diameter.

(7) Diagnostic radiograph for patients who have difficulties in opening their jaws.

The technique is as follows. The occlusal plane of the teeth is held parallel to the floor. The film is placed in the mouth with the rough side facing the occlusal and incisal surfaces. The patient then bites down on the film. The x-ray tube is placed perpendicular to the

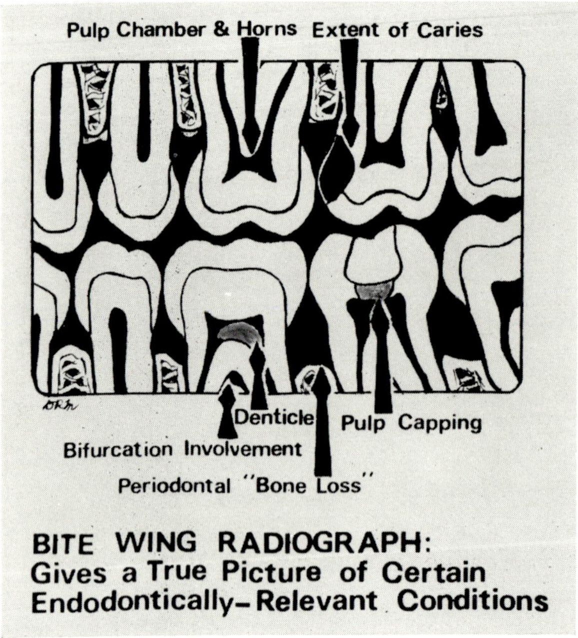

Figure 110.

film; for uppers at the tip of the nose; for lowers at the bottom of the chin.

Other Techniques. There are certain types of radiographs that may be of occasional use. The dentist can take them himself if he has the facilities and is competent in the method. If not, he can refer the patient to an oral radiologist. The most common ones are listed below:

(1) *Panograph.* With the use of this relatively new type of dental x-ray equipment, a full mouth radiograph can be taken with one exposure. This film is helpful in determining the extent of lesions, the presence of maxillary sinusitis, and to observe if lesions or conditions are bilateral. In the latter case, systemic involvement is probable.

(2) *Lateral Jaw Film.* This is also helpful in determining extent of lesions and to see if adjacent bony structures are also affected (Fig. 111).

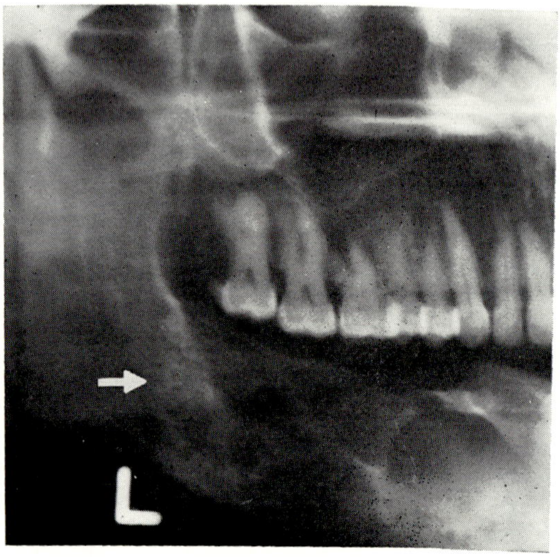

Figure 111. Lateral jaw film showing extent of ameloblastoma. (Courtesy of Dr. W. Updegrave, Philadelphia, Pa.)

(3) *Water's View.* This is useful in the detection of sinus disease.

BITE REGISTRATION. This is used to see if there are occlusal imbalances on the tooth in question.

Bite Tab. The patient bites in centric occlusion on a heated wax-filled tab. If there are occlusal imbalances, a hole will be seen through the wax.

Articulating Paper. The patient bites on a sheet of thick articulating paper and goes through various excursions. High spots on the tooth will show up as a purplish mark. Pain resulting from acute apical periodontitis is usually alleviated by occlusal adjustment.

PERIODONTAL PROBING. A calibrated periodontal probe is placed into all aspects of the pocket. Depth of the pocket is charted (Fig. 112). As stated in the radiography section, the use of a probe along with a radiograph can show pocket depth and whether the apex or a furca is involved.

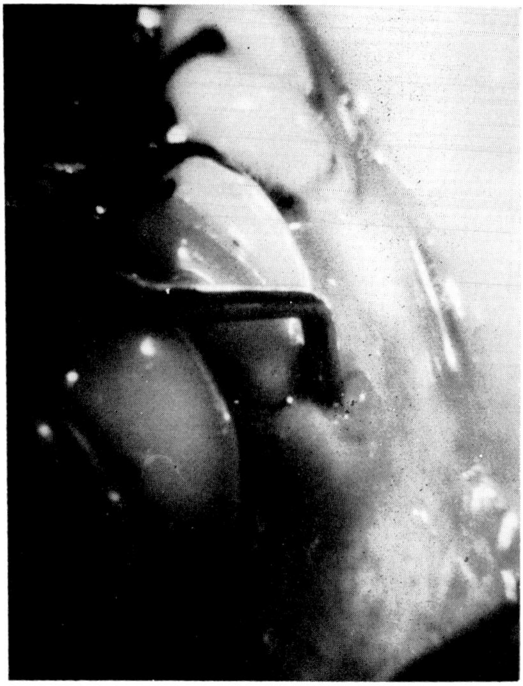

Figure 112. Probing a pocket in a suspected endodontic-periodontic case.

PROBING OF LESIONS. This includes probing for caries, attrition, erosion, abrasion, crown or cavity preparations, margins of restorations, and fracture margins to determine if the pulp is vital and to give an indication of the depth of the lesion.

PROBING OF SINUS TRACT OR FISTULA. This is done in order to determine which tooth is involved in the disease process or whether a non-endodontic condition is the causative factor. A radiopaque probe such as a silver cone or gutta-percha cone is placed through the sinus opening until it meets with resistance. A periapical radiograph is then taken and the tooth or other causative factor is determined by the termination of the probe. It is important that pressure is not exerted during probe insertion, as normal tissue may be penetrateed, thus giving a false result (Fig. 102).

REMOVAL OF CARIES AND/OR RESTORATIONS (IF UNDERMINED). This is used to determine restorability of the involved tooth, if the pulp is affected, and if a dentinal fracture is present (Fig. 59).

EXPLORATORY FLAP. In cases where there is doubt about location of a resorptive defect or the possible presence of a fracture, an exploratory flap can be made. The flap helps to determine the location of these conditions.

EXPLORATORY DRILLING. In cases where there is doubt about the presence of a root canal in an anterior tooth (is the canal calcified?), it may be necessary to perform exploratory drilling. The result of this test determines whether endodontics is feasible or whether periapical surgery has to be performed.

THERMAL TESTS. These are used to detect deviations from controls. There are two types, heat and cold.

Heat. Heat is used in the form of hot air, a hot burnisher, hot gutta-percha, hot gutta-percha on the tip of a burnisher, or a thermal stimulation pulp tester (Parkell). The heat is applied to the tooth, first on the incisal or occlusal edge and then over the other surfaces (Fig. 113). Excess heat is avoided as pulpal damage can occur. In cases of chronic total pulpitis (some cases), coagulation necrosis, gangrene, granuloma and radicular cyst, there is usually no response.

A normal contra-lateral tooth should be tested first. A slight feeling of warmth or pain may be generated, but it stops once the stimulus is removed. However, this may vary with the individual, the time of day, or the individual's mood. An intensely painful, more prolonged response indicates irreversible pulpal or periapical disease, usually with liquefaction necrosis present. Generally, when a crown is present, it is not possible to obtain a true response. However, it has been reported that with the use of a rubber wheel rotated on the lingual aspect of the crown, a response to heat can be generated.

Cold. Cold is applied in the form of cold air, ice, ethyl chloride spray, an electrical impulse, or carbon dioxide snow. Ice can be in the form of a piece of ice wrapped in gauze or an anesthetic carpule filled with ice (Fig. 114). Ice is applied to the labial or buccal surfaces of the teeth. Other methods of applying cold are listed below:

(1) Ethyl chloride spray directed against the tooth or a cotton pledget saturated with ethyl chloride and applied to the tooth. The tooth is first isolated under the rubber dam to prevent systemic absorption.

(2) Compressed air directed against

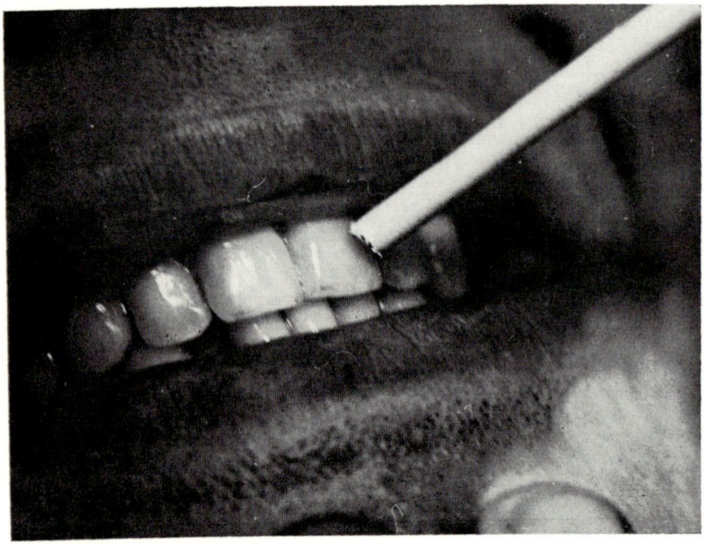

Figure 113. Pulp testing by heat; warm gutta-percha being applied to the labial surface of an upper central incisor.

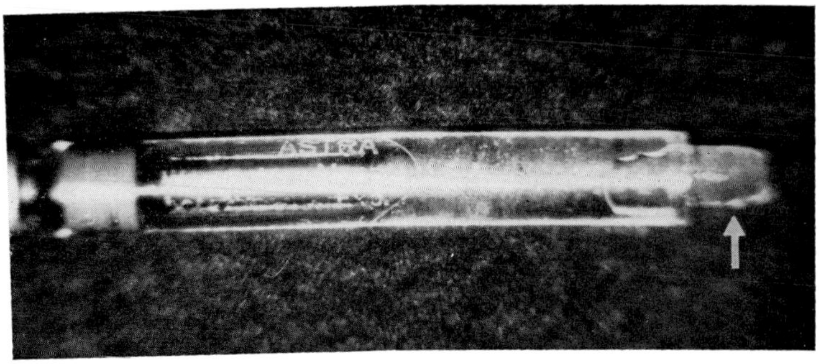

Figure 114. An anesthetic carpule filled with ice for use in pulp testing by cold.

solid tooth structure.

(3) Carbon dioxide snow applied directly to the teeth to be tested.

(4) A new cold-generating unit (Union Broach) is purported to be effective in cases with full coverage.

A normal contra-lateral tooth is tested; then the tooth in question is tested. There is usually no response from teeth with chronic total pulpitis (some cases), coagulation necrosis, gangrene, granuloma, and radicular cyst. With normal teeth, patients usually feel slight pain or a cold sensation that stops once the stimulus is removed. Often a severe, prolonged, painful response is felt by the patient if the tooth is involved with irreversible pulpal or periapical disease with liquefaction necrosis.

Electric Pulp Tests. These are also used to detect deviations from controls. Four types that have been used are high frequency, low frequency, faradic and galvanic. However, the most commonly used type is the small portable transistorized battery-operated pulp tester. It is entirely operated by the dentist. It has an easily movable dial with gradations from 0 through 10. The batteries generally last for at least one year. As with the thermal tests, a normal contra-lateral tooth is used as a control and is tested first. If there is no available contra-lateral tooth, then a normal adjacent tooth should be used as a control. The teeth to be tested should be isolated and then dried with cotton rolls and/or air. If not, tissue fluids could conduct the impulse to the periodontal ligament and yield a false positive response. The tip of the pulp tester is moistened with toothpaste or vaseline and is applied to the incisal edge or labial surface (or both) of anterior teeth and to the occlusal, buccal, or lingual surface of posterior teeth (Fig. 115). The tip should not be placed on metal restorations, as the metal will conduct the electrical current, and give a false positive response. The tip should be placed on surfaces where no metal is evident. In full crowns, it is necessary to drill an opening through the occlusal surface of the crown into normal tooth structure. The electrode tip should not be placed on silicate, acrylic or porcelain restorations, as these conduct the electric current poorly resulting in a false negative response. After the tip is placed in contact on the tooth, the dial is slowly turned upward from the 0 position. It is increased by gradations of 1 until the patient feels a twinge of pain in the

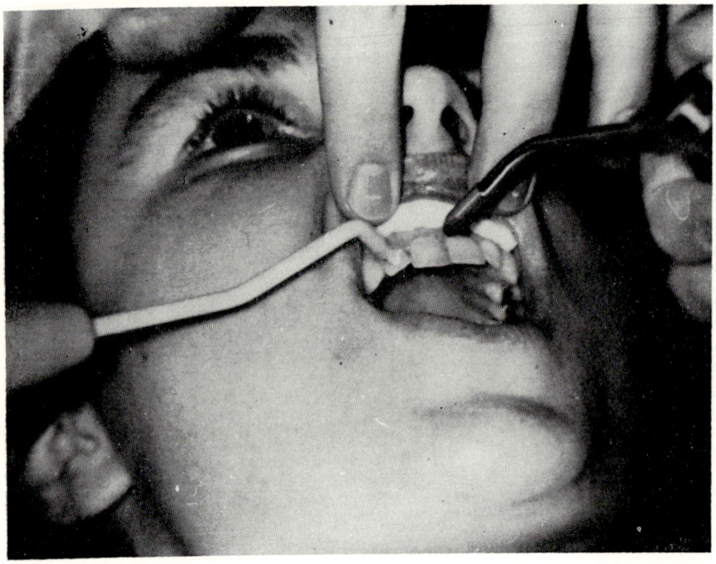

Figure 115. Upper right central incisor is being tested with a portable, battery-type electric pulp tester; air syringe is used to dry the area.

tooth. The number at which the patient first responds is entered on the patient's chart. The test is repeated two or three times and the average response is charted. Teeth with chronic total pulpitis (some cases), coagulation necrosis, granulomas, and cysts usually give no response. Teeth with a chronic pulpitis and a pulpless tooth with liquefaction necrosis may give a response at a higher value than the control but this is not necessarily true. Normal teeth show a range of vital responses. There are many pitfalls with the electric pulp tester. These are as follows:

(1) Pulp responses may differ according to the emotional outlook of the patient. They may also vary if the patients are taking sedatives, antianxiety agents or analgesics. Patient fear of electric pulp testing may prevent the use of this modality.

(2) In multirooted teeth, there may be two pulpless canals, and one with a vital pulp, and a vital response will be obtained by the pulp tester. In this case, one should try to test each canal individually by placing the point over the tip of each cusp. This is not always easy to do.

(3) Teeth with thick layers of secondary or reparative dentin may block impulses to the pulp and yield a false negative response.

(4) Necrotic pulps with liquefaction necrosis, teeth with periapical *areas* and liquefaction necrosis, and teeth with partial pulpitis all can give a vital response to the electric pulp tester.

(5) Immediately following a traumatic shock, a tooth can register no response, which at a later date can change to a normal one. The same result can occur after recent orthodontic movement. This may be related to neural damage

without concomitant blood vessel damage.

(6) Immature teeth often give a delayed or negative response to the electric pulp tester.

(7) Findings in electric pulp testers cannot be compared using different units. With battery-type units, if the batteries are old, the responses may be prolonged.

(8) In patients with pacemakers, the use of the pulp tester may interfere with the action of the pacemaker.

(9) The pulp tester might act as a pulpal irritant and contribute to the development of a pulpitis, although this has not been proven.

(10) Even without salivary contamination, it is possible to obtain a vital response solely from periodontal ligament stimulation.

Even with these drawbacks, the pulp tester is still fairly accurate in the diagnosis of a pulpless tooth. It should be used along with other tests described. It is important to note that in trauma cases involving the anterior teeth, teeth aside from the one in question should be tested. This includes teeth in the opposite jaw. The results should be recorded for future reference.

PALPATION. Palpation is a procedure utilizing finger tip pressure in order to determine the consistency of tissues and the extent of lesions. In endodontic diagnosis, palpation is used both intraorally and extraorally.

Extraoral Palpation

(1) *The Consistency and Extent of Lymph Node Enlargement (if any).* When the upper anterior and the posterior teeth are infected, the submaxillary lymph nodes may become involved. When the lower anteriors are infected, the submental nodes may become involved. The parotid nodes are involved in mumps and other salivary gland infections. The submaxillary nodes can also be involved as a result of salivary gland infections, tonsillitis, streptoccal sore throat, infectious mononucleosis, oral malignancies, ear infections, and other oral diseases. Inflammatory nodes are usually soft, painful and not fixed to the underlying tissue; whereas tumorous nodes are often painless, firm, and well attached to the underlying tissue. The lymph nodes can be palpated from in front of the patient (Fig. 116A and B), or from behind the patient (Fig. 116C).

(2) *Muscle Spasms.* Spasms in the muscles of mastication can cause referred dental pain. Extreme tension in the muscles indicates spasms.

(3) *Jaw Fractures.* Movement can be felt if there are jaw fractures.

(4) *Temporo-mandibular Joint Disease.* Placement of the doctor's fingers in the patient's ears (palpation in external auditory canals) with forward pressure, while the patient opens and closes his (or her) jaw, should accentuate any pain that may be present (Fig. 117). This helps in the differential diagnosis of a

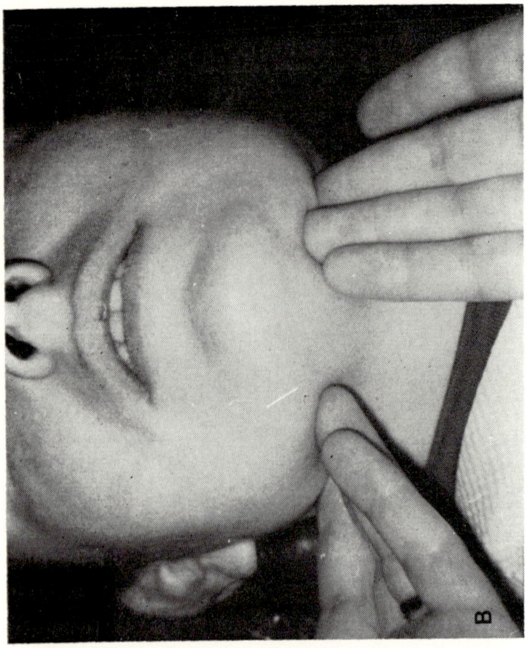

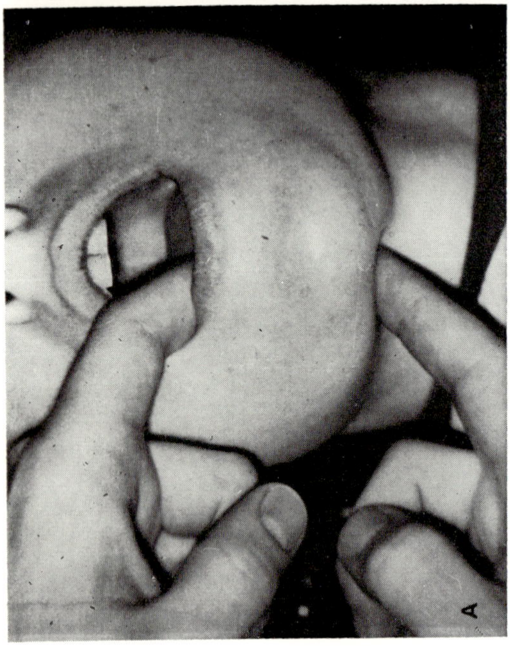

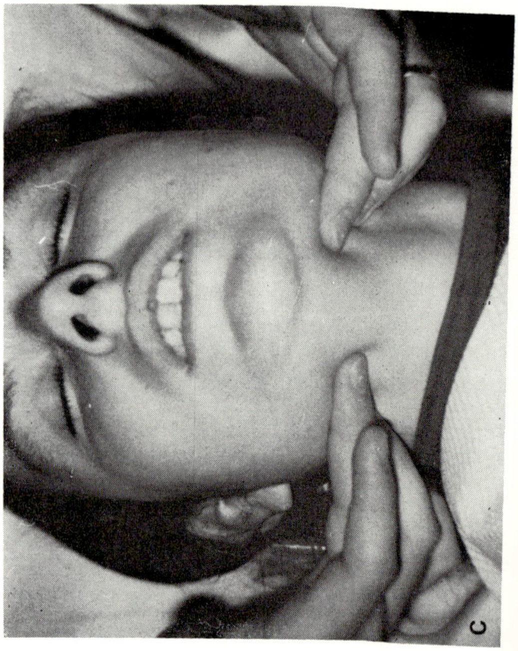

Figure 116. Lymph node palpation. A. Palpating the submental nodes. B. Palpating the submaxillary nodes from in front. C. Palpating the submaxillary nodes from behind.

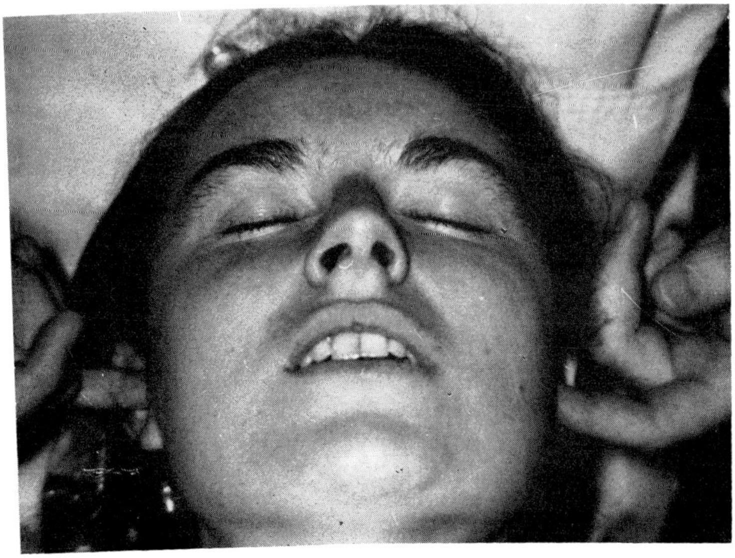

Figure 117. Testing for TMJ dysfunction; see text for explanation.

vague pain that may be referred to the teeth.

(5) *Neurological Disease.* To help in differentiating neurological pain from dental pain, a cotton wisp can be gently placed along the face at the sites of the patient's painful symptoms. The patient is asked to keep his (or her) eyes closed. As a control, the contra-lateral side of the face is checked. Relative hyper- or hypo-sensitivity may indicate a neurological problem. If this is the case, a neurological consultation is necessary.

(6) *The Presence of Sinusitis.* A sign of maxillary sinusitis is pain upon palpation of the infraorbital area. A sign of frontal sinusitis is pain upon palpation of the inferior surfaces of the supraorbital ridges.

Intraoral Palpation

(1) *Lesions.* The size, relative firmness, and attachment of lesions in various sites can be determined.

(2) *Apical Sensitivity.* The operator's index finger is placed in the alveolar mucosa near the mucobuccal fold of the tooth in question. Gentle pressure is exerted (Fig. 118). Pain is indicative of pulpally-induced periapical disease. However, other tests must be performed as pain is also a symptom of acute apical periodontitis caused by occlusal traumatism. If a movable mass is felt, this may be the result of periapical disease. There are other possibilities, which have been previously discussed in the section on swelling. It is important to test the periapical region of

adjoining teeth for comparative purposes.

PERCUSSION. Percussion is the act of gently tapping a tooth by means of a blunt instrument, either on the incisal (occlusal), labial (buccal), or lingual (palatal) surface (Fig. 119). All three surfaces should be percussed. Pain is indicative of acute apical periodontitis, pulpally-induced periapical disease, or a fractured tooth. Maxillary sinusitis is probably involved when several upper posterior teeth are sensitive. In periodontal disease, several teeth may also be sensitive to percussion. With a severe periapical inflammation, teeth adjacent to the involved tooth may also be sensitive to percussion. In performing the percussion test, it is practical to change the order of testing each time the teeth are tested. In this way, the patient would be less apt to give a predetermined response. A tooth that is extremely sore should not be percussed, as the procedure can initiate a severe odontalgia.

MOBILITY TEST. This is a test that is used for the determination of the degree of attachment of a tooth to its alveolus. In this test, the operator tries to move the tooth in question in a labial (buccal) to lingual (palatal) direction. The usual method is by the use of two tongue blades held between the thumb and index finger of each hand (Fig. 120). Just discernible motion indicates one degree mobility. If the arc of motion approximates one mm in distance, this is considered two degree mobility. Greater than the one mm range is three degree mobility. If a tooth can be depressed or elevated in its socket to a noticeable degree, this is also three degree mobility. Teeth adjacent to the involved one must be checked to aid in the etiology determination. Tooth mobility can result from any of the following:

(1) *Acute Apical Periodontitis Re-*

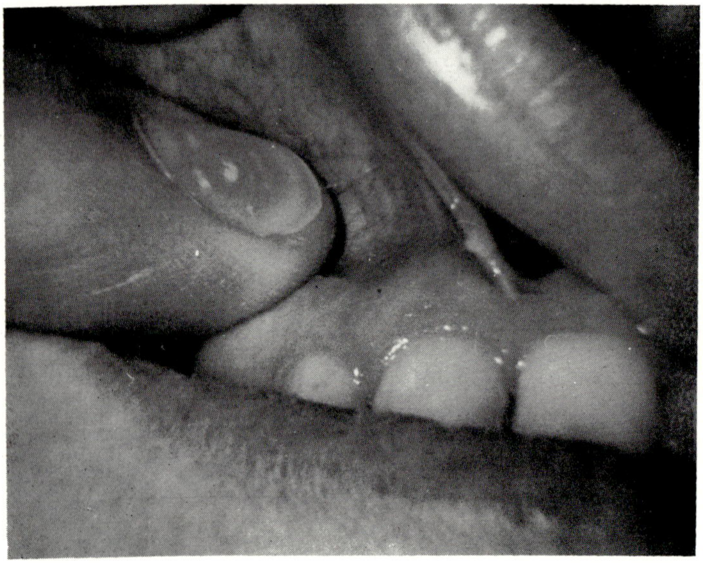

Figure 118. Apical palpation.

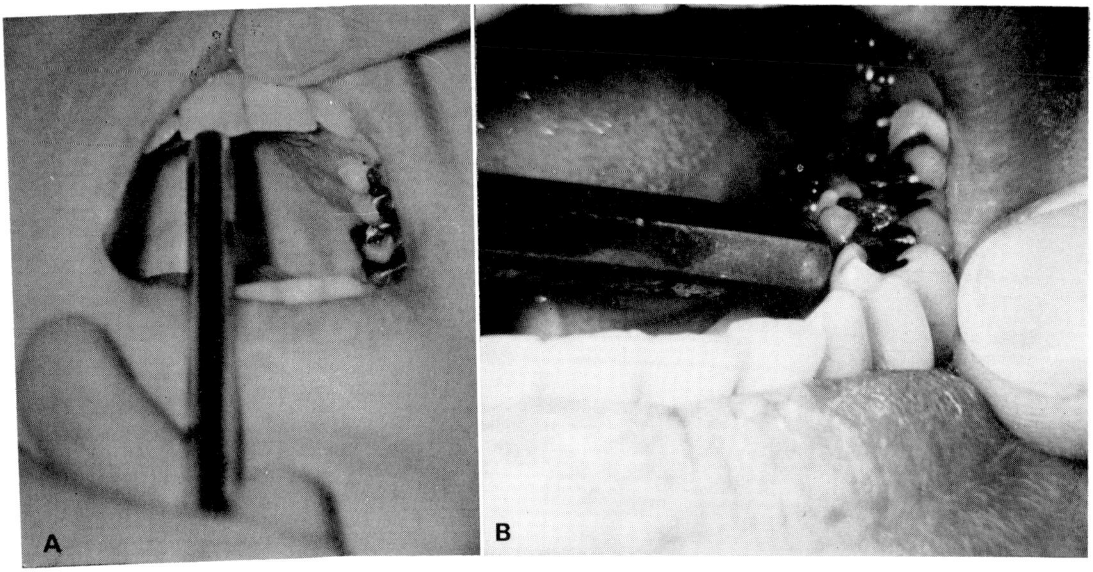

Figure 119. Percussion by means of a mirror handle. A. Vertical percussion. B. Horizontal percussion.

sulting from Occlusal Trauma. In this case, the mobility should stop once the occlusion is adjusted.

(2) *Periodontal Disease.* It is difficult to affect bone regeneration and loss of mobility, when the mobility is caused by alveolar bone loss. If the mobility is caused by a combination of local etiologic agents that are amenable to periodontal treatment, then a certain degree of fixation can be achieved. A good diagnostic sign is that mobility occurs on more than one tooth (usually) when periodontal disease is present.

(3) *Acute Apical Abscess, Acute Exacerbation of a Radicular Cyst or Granuloma, and Cellulitis.* In these cases, pulpal disease is the original etiological factor responsible for the mobility. The mobility should be markedly reduced, once the acute condition is alleviated by the inception of endodontic therapy. With chron-

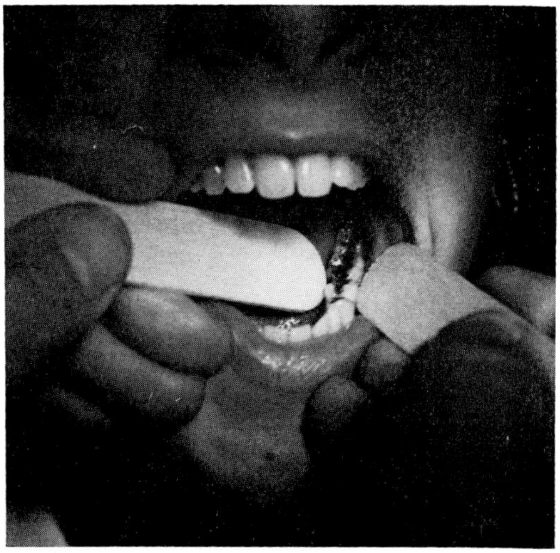

Figure 120. Tooth mobility tested by means of tongue blades.

ic conditions, a slight amount of mobility may be present (depends upon amount of bone loss).

(4) *Root or Crown Fracture.* The dentist should determine if different sections of the tooth are independently mobile to ascertain whether a fracture is involved. Treatment is dependent upon the amount of remaining tooth structure for restoration (coronally) or support (radicular region).

(5) *Bone Lesions.* There are various types of bone lesions that can cause pressure on roots leading to resorption and mobility.

(6) *Trauma from a Blow or Fall.* Once the inflammation decreases, the tooth should become firm in its socket.

(7) *Orthodontic Therapy.* Too rapid movement can cause mobility. Once stabilization has been achieved, the mobility should decrease.

(8) *Tongue Habits.* Excessive pressure by the tongue can cause tooth mobility. Return to normalcy depends upon the extent of the alveolar bone loss and whether the habit can be corrected.

ANESTHETIC TEST. This test involves the injection of a local anesthetic agent into various jaw segments. It is used for those cases in which there is doubt about the origin of the patient's oral pain. An example is when the patient has pain in the posterior oral region, but is unable to localize it to a particular jaw. An inferior alveolar injection is given. If the patient's painful symptoms are alleviated, then the presumption is that the pain had originated in the lower jaw. However, if the pain persists, injections are given in the upper posterior jaw, starting with one tooth at a time. If the pain abates after an injection in the upper second molar region, then this tooth is most probably the culpable one.

TEST CAVITY. The test entails the drilling of a small cavity preparation into a gold, porcelain, plastic, or amalgam restoration in order to determine the pulp viability. It is used for those cases where, because of the extensive restoration present, it is not possible to pulp test normal tooth structure. It can also be used for cases with extensive secondary or irregular dentin in which the pulp tests fail to elicit a response.

TESTS FOR THE CRACKED TOOTH SYNDROME. These tests are used for the determination of a possible crown and/or root fracture.

Occlusal Test. Small ball bearings or a wooden applicator is placed on the occlusal surface of the tooth to be tested. The patient is asked to bite (Fig. 121). Pain is an indication of a fracture. A periapical radiograph is taken while the patient is biting. It may then be possible to see the fracture as a result of the separation of the parts by the pressure. After this test, the iodine test should then be used.

Iodine Test. A couple of drops of tincture of iodine are placed on the occlusal (or incisal) surface of the tooth in question. A fracture shows up as a dark stain. The dentist should then place an explorer into the crack to determine if the patient has pain and to verify the degree of fracture (Fig. 59).

BIOPSY. This is the process of surgical removal of a lesion, for the purpose of histopathological examination of sections of the lesion (Fig. 122). The excised lesion is fixed, stained, sectioned, and slides are made and examined microscopically by a histopathologist. The examination is used to determine the histopathological nature of the lesion as an aid in differential diagnosis. The principal means of differentiating a radicular cyst from a periapical granuloma is by means of histopathological examination. A recent innovation is the use of biopsy of the dental pulp for diagnosis of systemic conditions. An example is the examination for sulfatide granules in the nerve fibers of the dental pulp for the diagnosis of metachromatic leukodystrophy.

MICROBIAL EXAMINATION OF ROOT CANAL OR PERIAPICAL FLUID. An exudate from a root canal, draining sinus tract, or fluctuant swelling can be used for Gram stain, microbial culture tests,

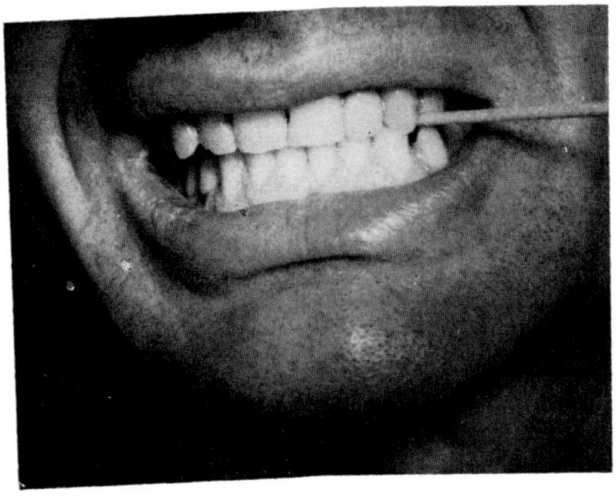

Figure 121. Occlusal test for cracked tooth syndrome; use of a wooden applicator.

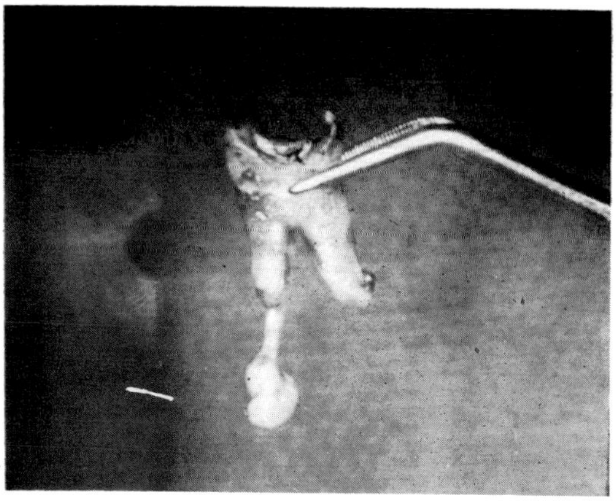

Figure 122. Nonrestorable; nontreatable tooth extracted with its attached periapical lesion; histopathological examination of the sectioned tissue revealed a radicular cyst.

antibiotic sensitivity testing, and phase microscopy.

Gram Stain. The material is wiped on a clean, dry slide. The slide is heat fixed for a few seconds over a bunsen flame and then is stained by Gram's method. Gram stain examination will reveal the presence or absence of microorganisms (Gram positive or negative), epithelial cells, erythrocytes, and polymorph leucocytes (Fig. 123). As endodontic diseases can show the presence of practically any strain of oral microbe, this test, and the culture tests are not specific for diagnosis of any type of endodontic disease or symptom. The Gram stain slide also does not differentiate live from dead microbes, but it does give an indication of the microbial flora involved in the particular condition. Also in rare diseases such as leprosy, yaws, and actinomycosis, it may be possible to detect these organisms in both Gram stained slides and cultures. One advantage of the Gram stain examination is that it

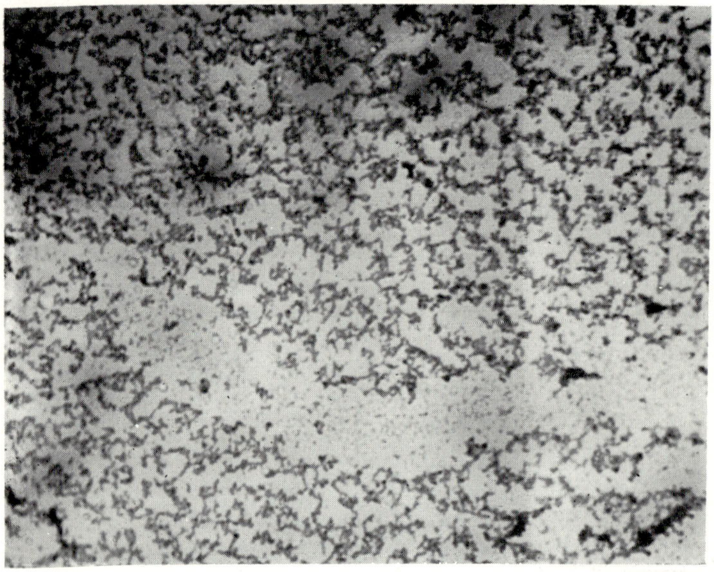

Figure 123. Gram stained root canal exudate reveals various microbes.

gives an indication of host response. Detection of large numbers of polymorph leucocytes with few or no microbes indicates a good host response. The presence of many microbes and no polymorphs is indicative of salivary contamination.

Microbial Culture Tests. Although it is felt that microbial culture tests are not useful for the determination of when to fill a root canal, they may have some function in diagnosis. However, even in this aspect, it is imperative that no single culture medium be used, as most commonly used culture media such as trypticase soy broth with agar, brain-heart-infusion broth, glucose ascites medium, and thioglycollate broth, do not allow for good growth of all the various possible microbes that might be present. Rather, an overgrowth of Gram positive cocci is the usual result of culturing in these media. Another important problem is that some strains

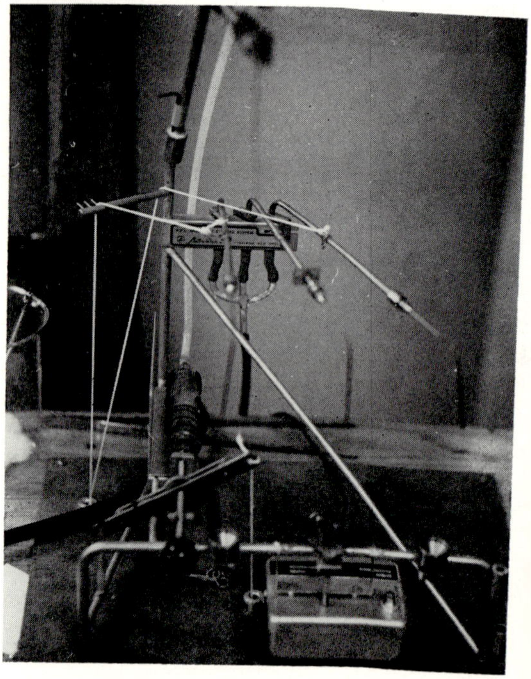

Figure 124. VPI Anaerobe Culture System (Bellco Glass Co.); this is used for the detection of obligate anaerobes; it is currently in use at Temple University School of Dentistry for research into the root canal flora.

of obligate anaerobes would not grow in these media, even if the culture tubes were incubated under anaerobic conditions. It has been found that many infectious diseases, and most blood infections are caused by obligate anaerobes. There are now available methods to detect obligate anaerobes from root canals (Fig. 124). However, currently these methods are not readily available in commercial laboratories. Hence, the practitioner who is interested in the determination of root canal infection must rely on the not too effective culture media that are presently available. The determination of the microbes *in situ* only has importance in differential diagnosis if some rare microbe is uncovered (as discussed under Gram stain).

Antibiotic Sensitivity Testing. Some endodontists advocate taking a culture at the initial visit of each endodontic case. The culture is then incubated and sent to a microbiological laboratory for identification and antibiotic sensitivity testing. The rationale is that in case of a treatment flare-up, the dentist will be able to prescribe a specific antibiotic that will be effective against the microbes present in the particular root canal(s). The fallacies of this concept and some problems with antibiotic sensitivity testing are the following:

(1) The microbes that are present at the initial visit may have no relationship to the microbes that can cause a flare-up later in the treatment regimen. Studies have shown that there are changing microbial populations during treatment. To determine which microbe might be responsible for the clinical condition, it would be necessary to do antibiotic sensitivity testing at the initial visit and then at the flare-up visit.

(2) As stated before, detection of microbes using only one culture medium is very difficult. There may be more than one microbial species present in the root canal, but the species that grows best in a particular medium will overgrow the other species. This has been shown to occur often with alpha streptococci. Therefore, when antibiotic sensitivity testing is performed, only one microbial population may be present, and that population may not necessarily be the one responsible for the clinical condition.

With the use of transport media (available in most commercial laboratories), it may be possible to maintain microbial viability, while preventing overgrowth by one species. In the laboratory, plating and antibiotic sensitivity testing can be carried out, both aerobically and anaerobically.

(3) Antibiotic sensitivity testing is usually performed in clinical laboratories by the agar disc method (Fig. 125). This method is not completely reliable because some antibiotics diffuse better than others in the medium, thereby producing larger zones of inhibition. This may not correlate with the *in vivo* action. This factor

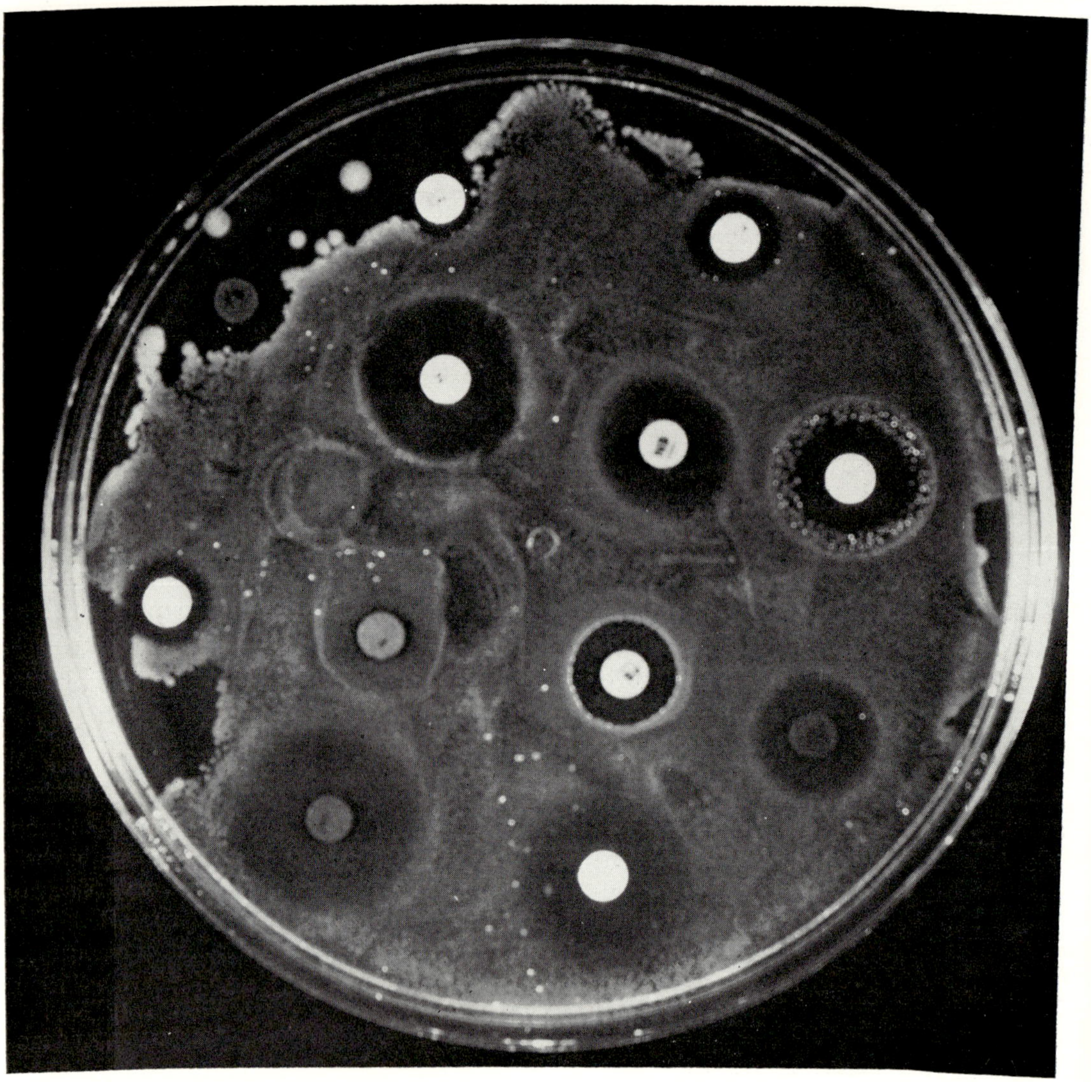

Figure 125. Antibiotic sensitivity testing; various zones of inhibition are shown, using different antibiotics with the agar disc method.

is taken into consideration with most standardized test interpretations. The agar disc method does not provide information regarding bacteriocidal or bacteriostatic action.

A better determination of antibiotic sensitivity is the use of the tube dilution method, and not all laboratories are equipped to use this method. With this modality, the actual antibiotic concentration needed can be evaluated by incubating the microbial culture in a series of test tubes containing different quantities of the antibiotic.

(4) As previously stated, an impor-

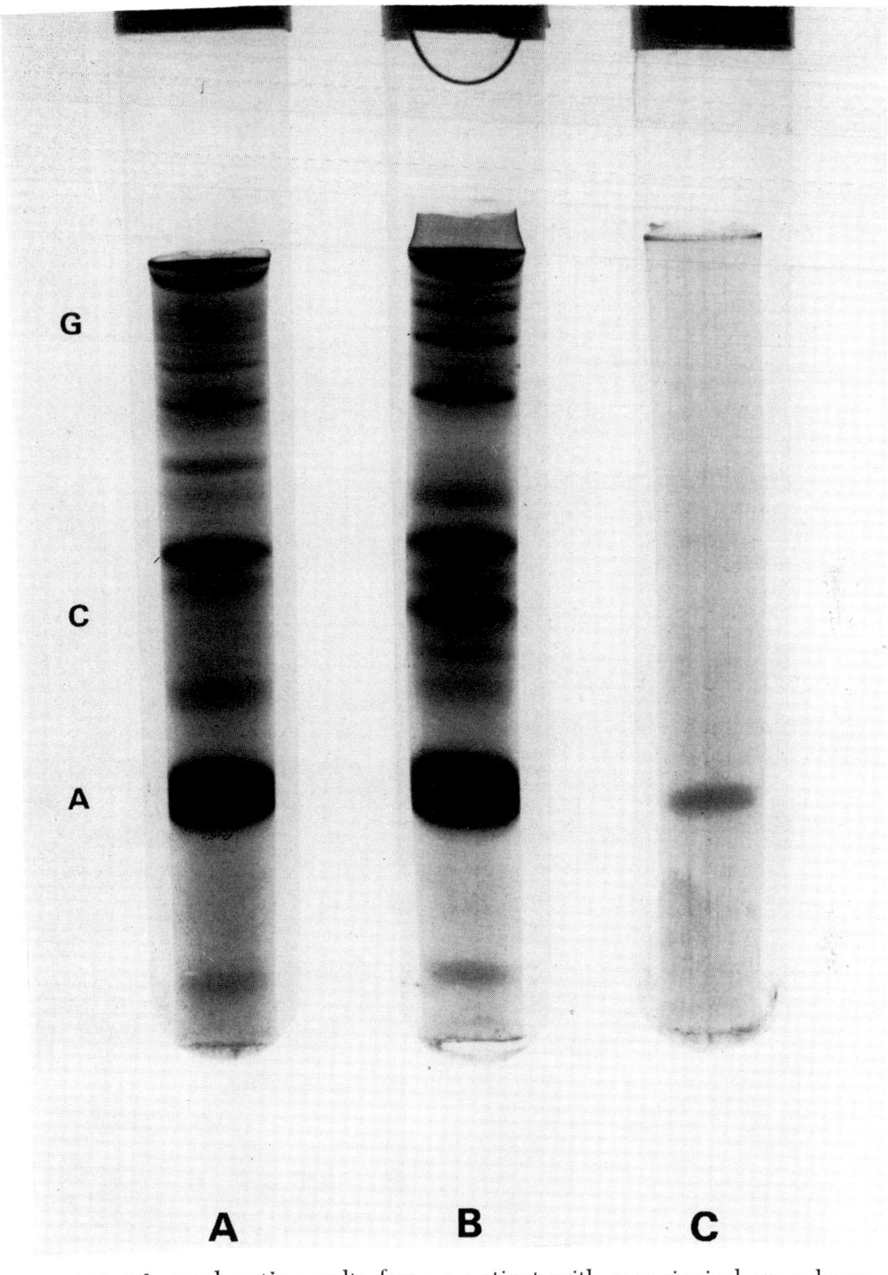

Figure 126. Electrophoretic results from a patient with a periapical granuloma; A = albumin zone, C = ceruloplasmin zone, G = gamma globulin zone. A. Finger tip serum. B. Periapical serum. C. Root canal fluid.

tant consideration is the detection of obligate anaerobes. Preliminary studies in our laboratory using special equipment have shown the presence of these species in root canals. Most microbiological laboratories associated with dental schools do not have this type of equipment. Also, antibiotic sensitivity for obligate anaerobes must be performed under different conditions than is currently used for aerobes and faculative anaerobes.

(5) The clinical manifestation (cellulitis) may be the result of a hypersensitivity reaction. As antibiotic sensitivity testing doesn't take into consideration the virulence of the microbes, it is possible that the microbes may only be *innocent bystanders* and not directly involved in the disease process.

(6) Interpretations must consider the actual clinical dose range which may be modified by the toxicity, allergenicity and routes of administration of the antibiotic, and the host's condition.

Phase Microscopy. The phase microscope is an optical microscope that, because of special properties, allows for direct visualization of living, unstained microorganisms. It can be used to demonstrate to patients, the presence of living microorganisms from within their root canals. This can show the patients the importance of techniques such as instrumentation and irrigation for the removal of microbes. It can also be used to detect motile microbes, such as spirochetes.

ELECTROPHORETIC ANALYSIS OF ROOT CANAL FLUID. This is a recent test devised in the Endodontology Department of Temple University School of Dentistry for use as an adjunct in the differential diagnosis of radicular cysts and granulomas. Fluid is withdrawn from a root canal after instrument penetration has been made into the periapical area of rarefaction. The fluid is then subjected to polyacrylamide gel electrophoresis. There is a different electrophoretic pattern observed for complete radicular cysts as compared to periapical granulomas (Fig. 126, 127). As far as treatment is concerned, we are currently investigating whether electrophoretically-diagnosed cysts can heal after nonsurgical endodontic therapy. Preliminary results indicate that radicular cysts may heal following nonsurgical treatment (Fig. 128).

EXFOLIATIVE CYTOLOGY OF ROOT CANAL FLUID. This is another test that has been used for the differentiation of radicular cysts and granulomas. The fluid is withdrawn from the root canals and placed on a slide which is then stained by the Papinicolau method. An examination is made for epithelial cells. The presumption is that presence of epithelial cells is equated with the diagnosis of a radicular cyst. As many granulomas also contain epithelium, this method may have some pitfalls. However, preliminary studies have shown correlation between the presence of epithelial cells with the histopathological diagnosis of a radicular cyst.

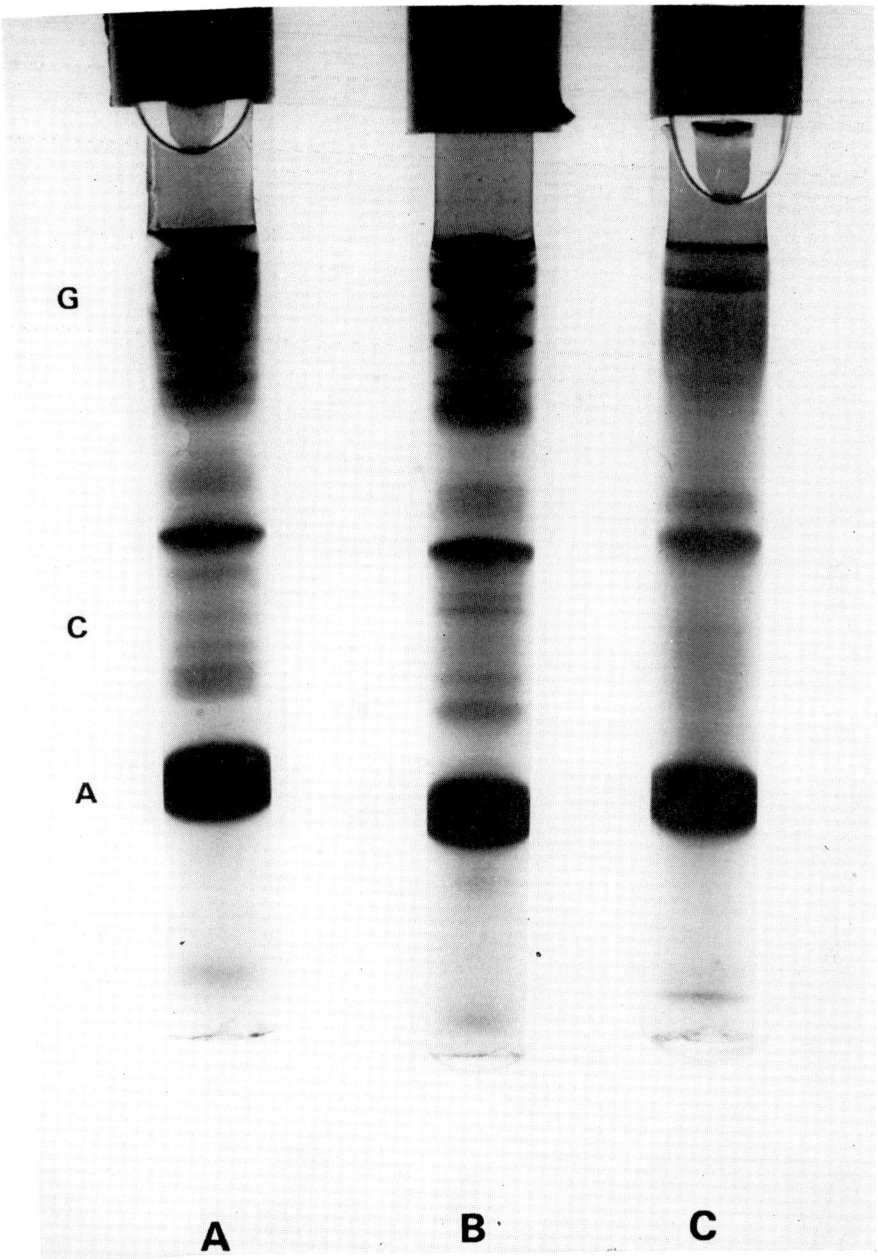

Figure 127. Electrophoretic results from a patient with a radicular cyst; A = albumin zone, C = ceruloplasmin zone, G = gamma globulin zone. A. Finger tip serum. B. Periapical serum. C. Root canal fluid.

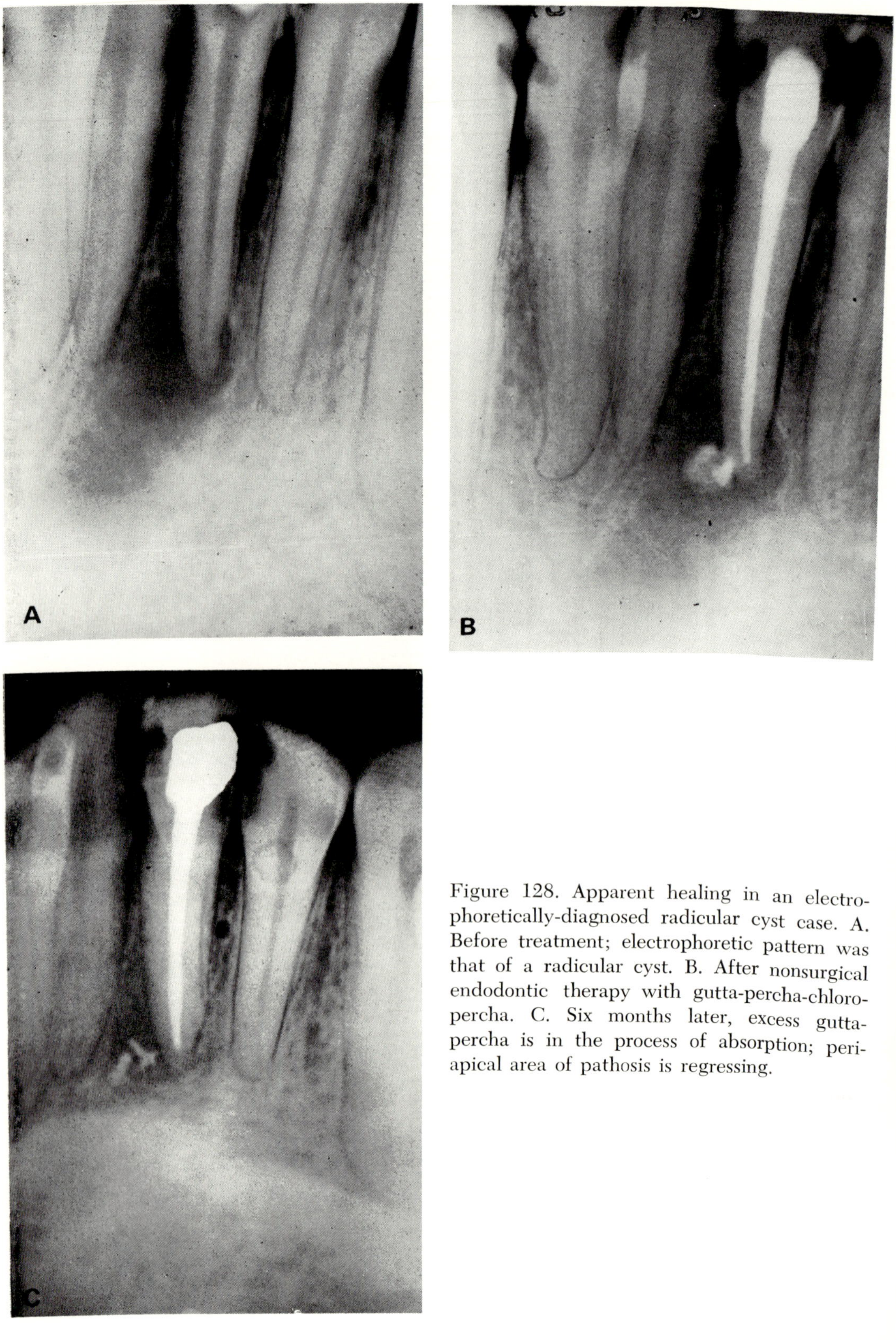

Figure 128. Apparent healing in an electrophoretically-diagnosed radicular cyst case. A. Before treatment; electrophoretic pattern was that of a radicular cyst. B. After nonsurgical endodontic therapy with gutta-percha-chloropercha. C. Six months later, excess gutta-percha is in the process of absorption; periapical area of pathosis is regressing.

Transillumination. In this test, a bright light is shown from the lingual (palatal) aspect of a tooth, in a partially darkened room. It is used to differentiate a vital from a pulpless tooth. The light source that is generally used is the fiber optic unit (Fig. 129). In pulpless teeth, there is a darkened appearance in the vicinity of the pulp chamber; in vital teeth the region appears light. It is also possible to transilluminate the alveolar mucosa in the periapical regions. A lesion close to the cortical plate of bone will show up as a darkened area. Normal periapical bone will not give this appearance. Fracture lines can also be visualized with the use of fiber optic transillumination.

Study Models. Although endodontists rarely have the need to take impressions for study models, general practitioners usually do. Study models will aid in endodontic treatment planning for the following reasons:

(1) To help to determine the strategic and esthetic value of the tooth in question.

(2) To give an index to the periodontal health of the tooth under consideration and the adjoining teeth.

(3) To determine whether the tooth in question is in normal or traumatic occlusion.

Ultrasonics. This is a method currently being investigated in the use of sound to determine pulp vitality. Preliminary studies show that the transmission and reflection of sound from the dentin enamel junction and from the dentin pulp interface varies with the pulp vitality.

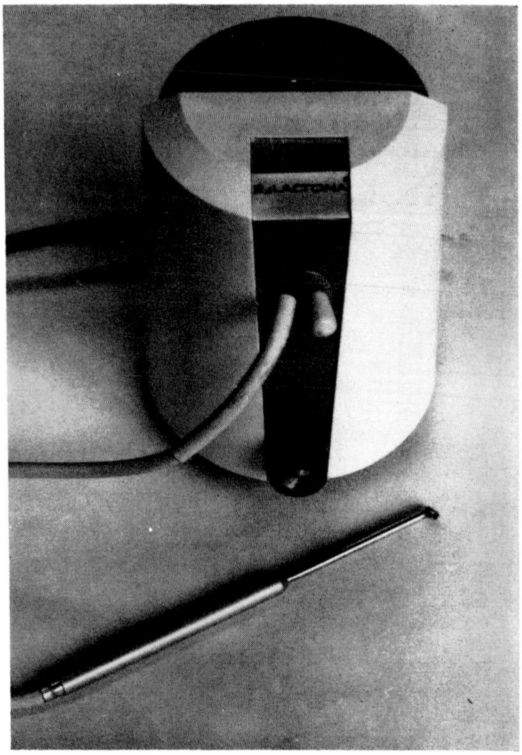

Figure 129. Lactona fiber optic unit, used for transillumination.

Thermography with Cholesteric Liquid Crystals. This method is based on the use of cholesteric liquid crystals to determine the surface temperature of teeth, as an aid in the detection of pulp vitality. The rationale is that in a pulpless tooth, because of the absence of an internal blood supply, the tooth would have a lower surface temperature. Preliminary studies have shown that this method may have some merit.

Electrical Measurements. The use of electrical impedance measurements reveals information about blood flow. It appears that electrical impedance measurements differ when testing is performed on vital and pulpless teeth. Another method under investigation is the measurement of the electrical properties of a tooth under both normal and diseased states. The results can be visually analyzed on an EKG-type recorder. These methods are also just in the preliminary stages.

CLINICAL PHOTOGRAPHY. Photographs should be taken of unusual lesions, swellings, malformations, fractures, etc. before the start of treatment, and then again at the conclusion of therapy and/or when the condition has been resolved. The pictures will aid in the determination of the effect of the treatment rendered (Fig. 130).

AUSCULTATION. This is the use of hearing to determine pathologic conditions. This is used in conjunction with the stethoscope for determination of blood pressure, and heart and lung sounds. In dental testing, it can be used to aid in the determination of fractures and emphysema. In the latter conditions, upon palpation, a crackling sound or crepitus can be heard. Some investigators state that upon percussing pulpless teeth, they hear a dull sound which is not heard when percussing vital teeth. Teeth involved with a maxillary sinusitis are stated to produce a *tinny* sound

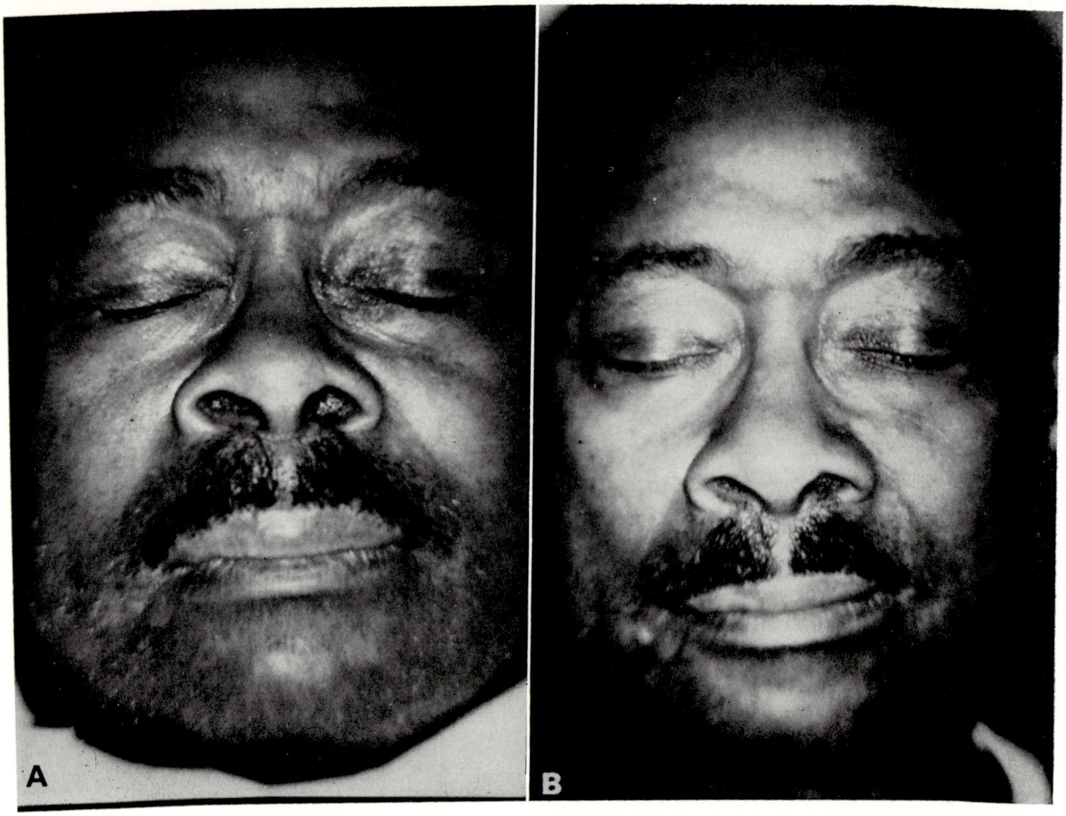

Figure 130. Use of photography to show the results of treatment; case of submaxillary space cellulitis. A. Submaxillary space cellulitus. B. At conclusion of treatment, swelling has resolved.

upon percussion. It has also been claimed that ankylosed teeth sound dull upon percussion as compared to teeth with a normal periodontal ligament. These last few uses of auscultation are too subjective to be reliably employed.

BIBLIOGRAPHY

Systemic History

American Dental Association: *Accepted Dental Therapeutics 1973/1974,* 35th ed. Chicago, American Dental Association, 1973.

American Heart Association: Prevention of bacterial endocarditis. *JADA, 85:*1377, 1972.

Battistone, G. C., Posey, W. R., Barone, J. J., and Cutright, D. E.: Zinc and bone healing: The effect of zinc cysteamine-n-acetic acid on the healing of extraction wounds in rats. *Oral Surg, 34:*704, 1972.

Beeson, P. B., and McDermott, W.: *Cecil-Loeb Textbook of Medicine,* 13th ed. Philadelphia, Saunders, 1971.

Bourquin, A., and Musmanno, E.: Preliminary report on the effect of smoking on the ascorbic acid content of whole blood. *Am J Dig Dis, 20:*75, 1953.

Briggs, M., and Briggs, M.: Vitamin C requirements and oral contraceptives. *Nature, 238:*277, 1972.

Bulletin Trenton Bureau: State closes Camden Well: Cites chromium. In *The Evening Bulletin, New Jersey News,* Dec. 29, 1972.

Burket, L. W.: *Oral Medicine: Diagnosis and Treatment,* 6th ed. Philadelphia, Lippincott, 1971.

Davidsohn, I., and Henry, J. B.: *Todd-Sanford Clinical Diagnosis by Laboratory Methods,* 14th ed. Philadelphia, Saunders, 1969.

Donaldson, D.: Homologous serum hepatitis and the dental treatment of renal dialysis and kidney transplant patients. *Br Dent J, 132:*391, 1972.

Ellison, R.: *Drug Considerations in Endodontics.* Presented at the Louis I. Grossman Endodontic Study Club Meeting, Oct. 1972, Philadelphia, Pennsylvania.

Göransson, K.: Possibility of iodine resorption by the pulp. *Dent Abst, 3:*277, 1958.

Guyton, J. S., and Woods, A. C.: Etiology of uveitis: A clinical study of 562 cases. *Arch Ophthalmol, 26:*983, 1941.

Harvey, A. M., Johns, R. J., Owens, A. H., Jr., and Ross, R. S.: *The Principles and Practices of Medicine,* 18th ed. New York, Appleton-Century-Crofts Educational Division/Meredith Corp., 1972.

Ingle, J. I.: *Endodontics.* Philadelphia, Lea & Febiger, 1965.

Knapp, A. A.: Healing of eye diseases by cure of oral foci. *Oral Surg, 5:*799, 1952.

Martin, E. W.: *Hazards of Medication: A Manual of Drug Interactions, Incompatibilities, Contraindications, and Adverse Effects.* Philadelphia, Lippincott, 1971.

Medical News: Smoking interferes with ability to utilize vitamin C. *JAMA, 208:*626, 1969.

Miller, S. C.: *Textbook of Periodontia (Oral Medicine),* 3rd ed. Philadelphia, Blakiston, 1950.

Mitchell, D. F., Standish, S. M., and Fast, T. B.: *Oral Diagnosis/Oral Medicine,* 2nd ed. Philadelphia, Lea & Febiger, 1971.

Rubin, E., and Lieber, C. S.: Alcoholism, alcohol, and drugs. *Science, 172:*1097, 1971.

Sahud, M. A., and Cohen, R. J.: Effect of aspirin ingestion on ascorbic-acid levels in rheumatoid arthritis. Lancet, 1:937, 1971.

Schuck, P. H., and Wellford, H.: Botulism and nitrites. *Science, 180:*1322, 1973.

Seltzer, S.: *Endodontology: Biologic Considerations in Endodontic Procedures.* New York, McGraw, 1971.

Slocumb, C. H., Binger, M. W., Barnes, A. R., and Williams, H. L.: Focal infection. *JAMA, 117:*2161, 1941.

Stanley, H. R.: The effect of systemic diseases on the human pulp. *Oral Surg, 33:*606, 1972.

Stern, M. H., and Cole, W. C.: Radiographic changes in the mandible associated with leukemic cell infiltration in a case of acute myelogenous leukemia. *Oral Surg, 36:*343, 1973.

Stones, H. H.: *Oral and Dental Diseases: Aetiology, Histopathology, Clinical Features and Treatment,* 4th ed. Baltimore, Williams and Wilkins, 1962.

Tice, L. F., Chairman: Parameters Influencing Drug Interactions. Presented at the Annual Meeting of the AAAS, Dec. 1972, Washington, D. C.

Uthman, A. A., and al-Shawaff, M.: Paget's disease of the mandible: report of a case. *Oral Surg, 28:*866, 1969.

Waldrep, A. C., Jr., and McKelvey, L. E.: Oral surgery for patients on anticoagulant therapy. *J Oral Surg, 26:*374, 1968.

Walker, R. D., and Schenck, K. L., Jr.: Infarct of the mandible in sickle cell anemia. report of case. *JADA, 87:*661, 1973.

White, E.: Ethnic variation in root morphology: anticipated endodontic and surgical problems, *JSCDA, 40:*994, 1972.

Xhonga, F. A., and Van Herle, A.: The influence of hyperthyroidism on dental erosions. *Oral Surg, 36:*349, 1973.

Oral History

Abramson, I. I., and Norris, J. P.: *Atlas of Endontic Technique: A Clinical Guide,* St. Louis, Mosby, 1966.

Bell, W. E.: Clinical diagnosis of the pain-dysfunction syndrome. *JADA, 79:*154, 1969.

Birn, H.: Spread of dental infections. *Dent Pract, 22:*347, 1972.

Burton, R. C.: The problem of facial pain. *JADA, 79:*93, 1969.

Chasens, A.: Facial pain—part 1. *J Oral Med,* 27:43, 1972.

Clark, H. B., Jr.: *Practical Oral Surgery,* 2nd ed. Philadelphia, Lea & Febiger, 1959.

Friend, L. A., and Glenwright, H. D.: An experimental investigation into the localization of pain from the dental pulp. *Oral Surg, 25:*765, 1968.

Glick, D.: Locating referred pulpal pains. *Oral Surg, 15:*613, 1962.

Grossman, L. I.: *Endodontic Practice,* 7th ed. Philadelphia, Lea & Febiger, 1970.

Herman, J. L.: Case report: odontalgia resulting from prodromal herpes zoster. *J Mich Dent Assoc, 54:*102, 1972.

Ingle, J. I.: *Endodontics.* Philadelphia, Lea & Febiger, 1965.

Landay, M. A., Nazimov, H., and Seltzer, S.: The effects of excessive occlusal force on the pulp. *J Periodontol, 41:*3, 1970.

Lawrence, T. S.: Case report: Unusual galvanic response during endodontic therapy. *Dent Surv, 49:*32, 1973.

McGehee, W. H. O., True, H. A., and Inskipp, E. F.: *A Textbook of Operative Dentistry,* 4th ed. New York, McGraw, 1956.

Schuchard, A., and Reed, O. M.: Pulpal response to pin placement. *J Prosthet Dent,* 29:292, 1973.

Seltzer, S., and Bender, I. B.: *The Dental Pulp: Biologic Considerations in Dental Procedures.* Philadelphia, Lippincott, 1965.

Sommer, R. F., Ostrander, F. D., and Crowley, M. C.: *Clinical Endodontics: A Manual of Scientific Endodontics,* 3rd ed. Philadelphia, Saunders, 1966.

Stones, H. H.: *Oral and Dental Diseases: Aetiology, Histopathology, Clinical Features and Treatment,* 4th ed. Baltimore, Williams and Wilkins, 1962.

Tarsitano, J. J.: The use of antibiotics in dental practice. *Dent Clin North Am, 14:*697, 1970.

van Gool, A. V.: Injury to the permanent tooth germ after trauma to the deciduous predecessor, *Oral Surg, 35:*2, 1973.

Weine, F. S.: *Endodontic Therapy,* St. Louis, Mosby, 1972.

Diagnostic Tests

Abramson, I. I., and Norris, J. P.: *Atlas of Endodontic Technique: A Clinical Guide.* St. Louis, Mosby, 1966.

Barber, F. E., Lees, S., and Lobene, R. R.: Ultrasonic pulse-echo measurements in teeth. *Arch Oral Biol, 14:*745, 1969.

Barker, R. B.: Paired culture interactions of the oral microbiota. *J Dent Res, 49:*804, 1970.

Bartels, H. A., Naidorf, I. J., and Blechman, H.: A study of some factors associated with endodontic "flare-ups." *Oral Surg, 25:*255, 1968.

Bhaskar, S. N., and Rappaport, H. M.: Dental vitality tests and pulp status. *JADA, 86:* 409, 1973.

Civjan, S., Barone, J. J., and Vaccaro, G. J.: Electric pulp vitality testers. *J Dent Res, 52:*120, 1973.

Council on Dental Materials and Devices: Possible electromagnetic interference with cardiac pacemakers from dental induction casting machines and electrosurgical devices. *JADA, 86:*426, 1973.

Cundy, K. R., Finegold, S. M., Randall, E. L., and Sutter, V. L.: New Applied Techniques in Anaerobic Clinical Microbiology. Presented at the Meeting of the Clinical Microbiology Section of the Eastern Pennsylvania Chapter of the American Society for Microbiology, Oct. 1971, Philadelphia, Pennsylvania.

Davidsohn, I., and Henry, J. B.: *Todd-Sanford Clinical Diagnosis by Laboratory Methods,* 14th ed. Philadelphia, Saunders, 1969.

Editorial: Researchers test dental diagnostic aids. *Dent Surv, 49:*15, 1973.

Frank, V. H.: Mandibular canal localization. *Oral Surg, 21:*312, 1966.

Friedman, J., and Marcus, M. I.: Transillumination of the oral cavity with use of fiber optics. *JADA, 80:*801, 1970.

Goldman, M., and Pearson, A. H.: Post-debridement bacterial flora and antibiotic sensitivity. *Oral Surg, 28:*897, 1969.

Grossman, L. I.: *Endodontic Practice,* 7th ed. Philadelphia, Lea & Febiger, 1970.

Harvey, A. M., Johns, R. J., Owens, A. H., Jr., and Ross, R. S.: *The Principles and Practice of Medicine,* 18th ed. New York, Appleton-Century-Crofts Educational Division/Meredith Corporation, 1972.

Holmberg, K., and Hallander, H. O.: Interference between gram positive microorganisms in dental plaque. *J Dent Res, 51:* 588, 1972.

Howell, F. V., de la Rosa, V. M., and Abrams, A. M.: Cytologic evaluation of cystic lesions of the jaws: a new diagnostic technique. *JSCDA, 36:*161, 1968.

Howell, R. M., Duell, R. C., and Mullaney, T. P.: The determination of pulp vitality by thermographic means using cholesteric liquid crystals: a preliminary study. *Oral Surg, 29:*763, 1970.

Ingle, J. I.: *Endodontics.* Philadelphia, Lea & Febiger, 1965.

Ingle, J. I. (Interview): Screening for the medical links to facial pain. *Clin Dent, 1:* 6, 1973.

Johns, R. B., and Boyde, E.: Demonstration at Guys Hospital dental clinic meeting. In Rowe, A. H.: Endodontics 1972. *J Br Endo Soc, 6:*13, 1972.

Kantz, W. E., and Henry, C. A.: Isolation and classification of anaerobic bacteria from non-vital teeth with intact pulp chambers. *Arch Oral Biol.* In Print.

King, D. R.: Pulp vitality tests. *J Acad Gen Dent, 20:*35, 1972.

Martin, H., Ferris, C., and Mazzella, W.: An evaluation of media used in electric pulp testing. *Oral Surg, 27:*374, 1969.

McCall, J. O., and Wald, S. S.: *Clinical Dental Roentgenology: Technic and Interpretation,* 4th ed. Philadelphia, Saunders, 1957.

McDaniel, K. F., Rowe, N. H., and Charbeneau, G. T.: Tissue response to an electric pulp tester. *J Prosthet Dent, 29:*84, 1973.

McGehee, W. H. O., True, H. A., and Inskipp, E. F.: *A Textbook of Operative Dentistry,* 4th ed. New York, McGraw, 1956.

Mitchell, D. F., Standish, S. M., and Fast, T. B.: *Oral Diagnosis/Oral Medicine,* 2nd ed. Philadelphia, Lea & Febiger, 1971.

Morse, D. R.: The endodontic culture technique: an impractical and unnecessary procedure. *Dent Clin North Am, 15:*793, 1971.

Morse, D. R.: Resolved That Culturing Is Contributory to Endodontic Success: Con. Trans. Fifth Inter. Conf. Endo., Philadelphia, Univ. Penn., 1974. In Print.

Morse, D. R., Patnik, J. W., and Schacterle,

G. R.: Electrophoretic differentiation of radicular cysts and granulomas. *Oral Surg, 35:*249, 1973.

Morse, D. R., Spott, R., and Farber, P.: *In Vitro* Antagonism of Root Canal Microorganisms. In Preparation.

Parker, W. A., and Hutchins, D. W.: Periapical localization using fiber optics. *J Oral Med, 26:*17, 1971.

Poyton, H. G.: Maxillary sinuses and the oral radiologist. *Dent Radiogr Photogr, 45:*43, 1972.

Schlagel, E., Seltzer, R. J., and Newman, J. J.: Apicoectomy as an adjunct to diagnosis. *NY State Dent J, 39:*156, 1973.

Simring, M., and Goldberg, M.: The pulpal pocket approach: retrograde periodontitis. *J Periodontol, 35:*22, 1964.

Sommer, R. F., Ostrander, F. D., and Crowley, M. C.: *Clinical Endodontics: A Manual of Scientific Endodontics,* 3rd ed. Philadelphia, Saunders, 1966.

Tarsitano, J. J.: The use of antibiotics in dental practice. *Dent Clin North Am, 14:*697 1970.

Teitler, D., Tzadik, D., Eidelman, E., and Chosack, A.: A clinical evaluation of vitality tests in anterior teeth following fracture of enamel and dentin. *Oral Surg, 34:* 649, 1972.

Weine, F.: *Endodontic Therapy.* St. Louis, Mosby, 1972.

CHAPTER 2

DIFFERENTIAL DIAGNOSIS

In this chapter, a discussion is given of the differential diagnosis of endodontic conditions and lesions from normal anatomic landmarks, normal physiological conditions, and non-endodontic lesions, diseases, and symptoms.

ENDODONTIC CONDITIONS, LESIONS AND SEQUELAE TO ENDODONTIC LESIONS

For each of these entities is given the definition, causative factors, symptoms, signs, results of tests, histologic appearance, prognosis, and possible treatments.

Hypersensitive Dentin

This is a state in which the dentin is unusually sensitive to external irritants. This condition can result from any of the following:

(1) The loss of the external enamel or cementum by a process of abrasion, erosion, attrition, or fracture. In certain cases, cementum does not form in the cervical area.

(2) Microbes and their products (result of caries).

(3) Mechanical and thermal irritation resulting from crown and cavity preparation, gold foil insertion, or periodontal treatment.

(4) Chemical irritation resulting from products placed on cavity floors and coronal surfaces; examples are phenol, alcohol, silver nitrate, hydrogen peroxide, and zinc phosphate cements.

(5) Chemical irritation resulting from filling materials such as silicate cements and acrylic fillings.

(6) Air blown into a cavity or crown preparation.

(7) Hypersensitivity has also been reported as occurring as the result of thiamine (vitamin B_1) deficiency.

The usual symptom of this condition is pain of a sharp character that is provoked by external irritants such as cold, sweet, sour, air and touch, applied to the exposed cervical margin. The painful response ceases as soon as the irritant is removed. This is considered to be dentin-type pain mediated by odontoblasts. Certain investigators consider that a tooth in this condition has a hyperemic condition of the pulp, in which there is a vasodilatation of the blood vessels. There has never been any incontrovertible histological proof to reinforce this contention.

A tooth in this condition can remain in this state, or if further pulpal irritation occurs, then a pulpitis can result.

Treatment depends upon the etiology. For exposed dentin, many procedures have been tried including applications of sodium fluoride, sodium silicofluoride, ionization with or without fluoride solutions, calcium biphosphate, corticosteroid pastes, stannous fluoride, strontium chloride toothpaste (Sensodyne®), Thermodent® toothpaste (a formalin based formula), Colgate® toothpaste (with sodium monofluorophosphate), silver nitrate impregnation with or without eugenol, zinc chloride-potassium ferrocyanide impregnation (Gottlieb's technique) and calcium hydroxide application. Periodontal treatment may either cure or cause dentin and/or cementum hypersensitivity. Removal of cementum can expose dentinal tubules and lateral canals to the external environment, thus causing hypersensitivity. It has also been theorized that acids in plaque permeate through dentinal tubules, thus causing pain. The removal of the plaque allows the tubules to be sealed, thus inhibiting hypersensitivity.

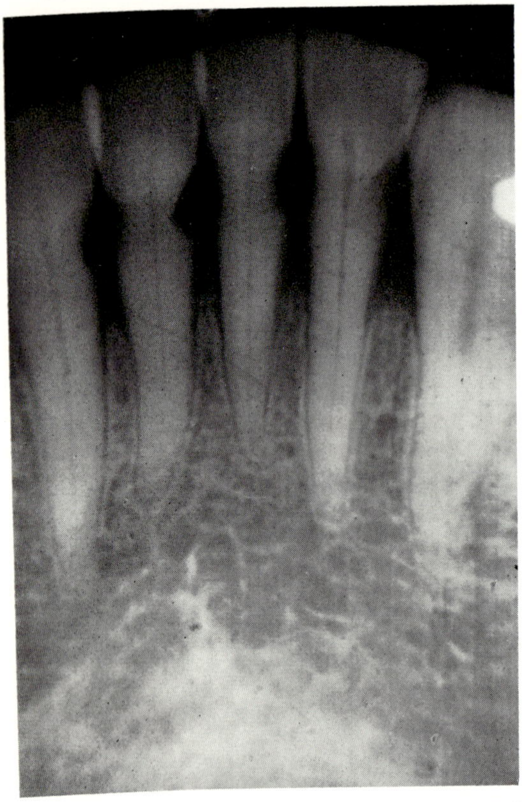

Figure 131. Toothbrush abrasion and gingival recession; roots exposed with resultant hypersensitive cementum. (Courtesy of Dr. T. Simpson, Philadelphia, Pa.)

Some investigators have achieved good results in treatment from the application of an orangewood stick, at several intervals, to the exposed root surfaces. The possible mechanism is by an increase in reparative dentin and peritubular dentin, with a decrease in sensation reaching the odontoblasts.

For carious lesions, the caries should be removed without exposing the pulp and a zinc oxide eugenol or calcium hydroxide base should be inserted, followed by a permanent restoration.

Hypersensitive Cementum

This condition is analogous to cervical dentin hypersensitivity, except that the cause is gingival recession with concomitant exposure of the root to the oral fluids (Fig. 131). Symptoms are the same as for hypersensitive dentin and treatment is the same as was described for exposed dentin.

Transitional Pulp (Stage)

A tooth in this condition has a pulp in which there are scattered chronic inflammatory cells but no overt inflammation. The causative factors may be caries, abrasion, attrition, erosion, periodontal disease, and mechanical, thermal, and chemical irritation from the prepa-

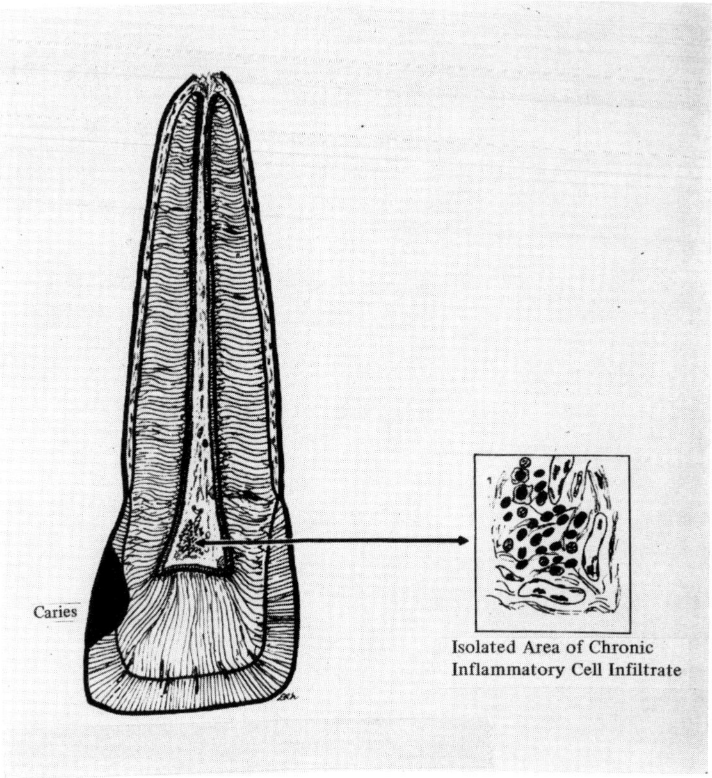

Figure 132. Tooth with a transitional pulp; showing low power and high power views.

ration and insertion of restorations. There are no clinical signs or symptoms pathognomonic of this state. The histological appearance shows scattered lymphocytes, macrophages, occasional plasma cells, and some dilated blood vessels (Fig. 132). The prognosis is good if no further irritation intervenes. However, subsequent caries or operative procedures can cause the development of pulpitis. For the state of transitional pulp without clinical manifestations, there is no treatment necessary.

Acute Pulpitis

Acute pulpitis is an acute inflammation of the pulp. It can be caused by various mechanical, thermal and chemical operative procedures such as cavity and crown preparations, impression taking, cavity sterilization, chip blowing, cementation, and insertion of restorations. It can also occur following mechanical pulp exposures, vital pulpotomies, exposure of lateral canals in periodontal disease or as the result of scaling, curettage and periodontal surgery, rapid orthodontic movement, extraction of adjoining teeth, galvanism (contact of dissimilar metals), nasal and sinus operations, oral intubation procedures during general anesthesia, and sudden trauma to the tooth. Contrary to the impression of many clinicians, acute pulpitis is usually not correlated with painful symptoms. The patient may have slight tenderness or pain following the operative procedures, which soon disappears. The histologic appearance shows an acute inflammation consisting primarily of polymorph leucocytes and engorged capillaries, in that portion of the pulp subjacent to the involved dentinal tubules (Fig. 133). The prognosis is usually good, except for the cases involving a large contaminated exposure, untreated periodontal disease, and severe trauma. A chronic pulpitis can develop in these cases. The treatment depends upon the etiology. If the condition results from operative procedures, usually no treatment is necessary. With a large contaminated pulpal exposure, complete endodontic therapy is necessary. Complete endodontic therapy is also necessary if a symptomatic chronic pulpitis develops

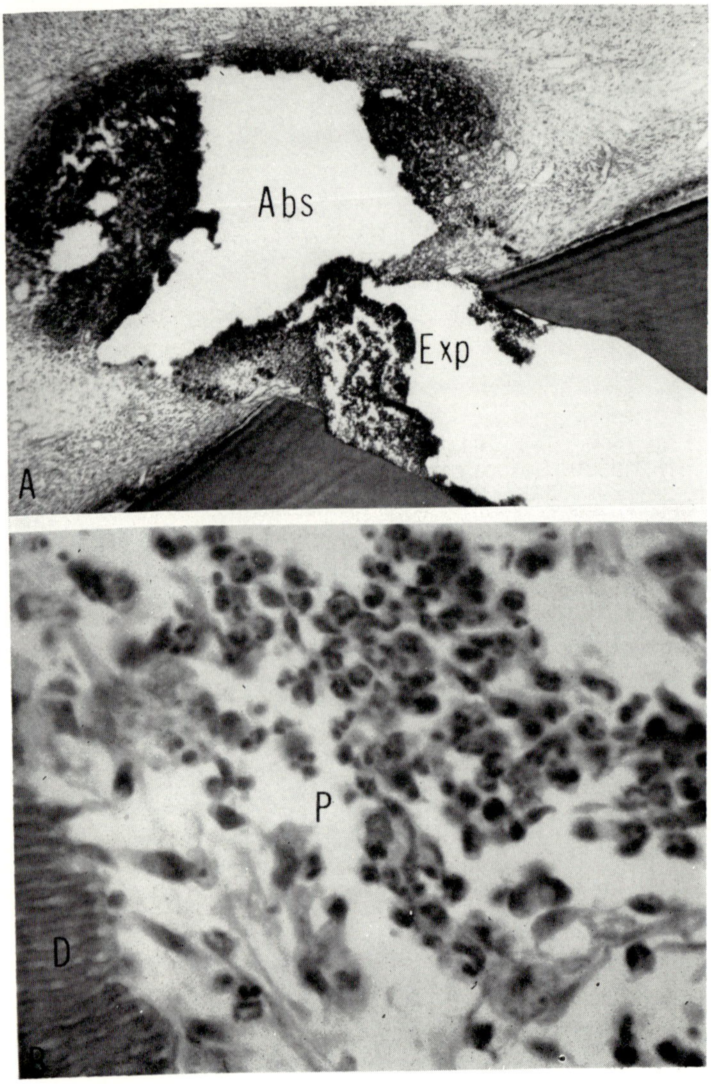

Figure 133. Acute pulpitis with acute abscess under a mechanical exposure. A. Abs = abscess, Exp = exposure (×54). B. D = Dentin, P = pulp containing many polymorph leucocytes (×960). (From S. Seltzer and I. B. Bender, *The Dental Pulp*. J. B. Lippincott Co., 1965. Used with permission of J. P. Lippincott Company.)

from subsequent periodontal disease, periodontal treatment, or trauma.

Chronic Pulpitis

Chronic pulpitis is a chronic inflammation of the pulp. There are several types including chronic partial pulpitis, chronic partial pulpitis with liquefaction or coagulation necrosis, and chronic total pulpitis. In chronic partial pulpitis, only a portion of the pulp is involved by a chronic inflammation. This is usually that portion of the pulp subjacent to the involved dentinal tubules. It may also be that portion of the pulp approximating a lateral canal, exposed by periodontal disease (Fig. 134). In chronic partial pulpitis with necrosis, there is a portion of the inflammation in which coagulation necrosis or liquefaction necrosis (pus) has occurred. In chronic total pulpitis, the chronic inflammation reaches the entire extent of the pulp and even spreads into the periodontal ligament. Coagulation or liquefaction necrosis is present, usually in the coronal pulp. The chronic pulpidities can also be subdivided into either chronic hyperplastic pulpitis (pulp polyp) or chronic ulcerative pulpitis. The latter two divisions can show any degree of partial or total pulpitis, but they are differentiated by the presence or absence of a proliferative response. In chronic hyperplastic pulpitis, there is a proliferation of granulomatous pulpal tissue, caused by irritating cavity margins. This tissue overgrows the pulp chamber and it simulates gingival hyperplasia (Fig. 61). It generally occurs in young children who have a maximal blood supply to the pulp. In chronic ulcerative pulpitis, the overlying dentin has been destroyed by the carious process leaving a layer of necrotic material. This occurs in older individuals (Fig. 135).

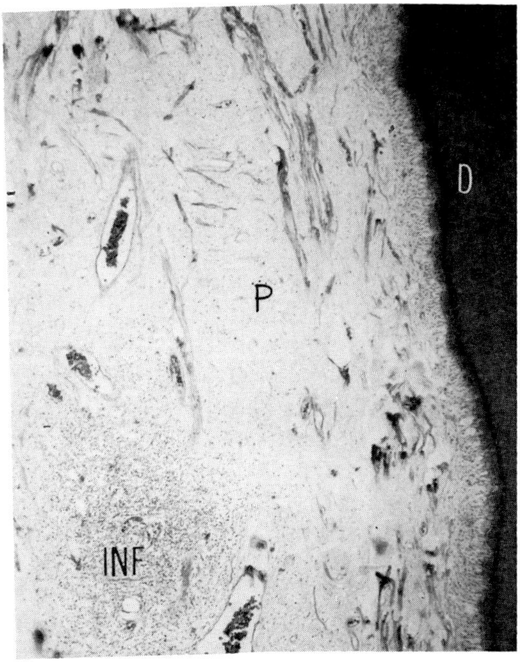

Figure 134. Pulp inflammation (chronic pulpitis) in a periodontally involved tooth in which there is no caries or restoration present; Inf = inflammation, P = pulp, D = dentin (×54). (From S. Seltzer and I. B. Bender, *The Dental Pulp*, J. P. Lippincott Co., 1965. Used with permission of J. P. Lippincott Company.)

The etiological factors are caries (coronal or root), with or without pulp exposures, attrition, abrasion, erosion, periodontal disease, and secondarily to operative dentistry procedures, periodontal treatment, trauma (cracked tooth), and excessive or rapid orthodontic tooth movement.

The signs and symptoms of chronic pulpitis depends upon the degree of the

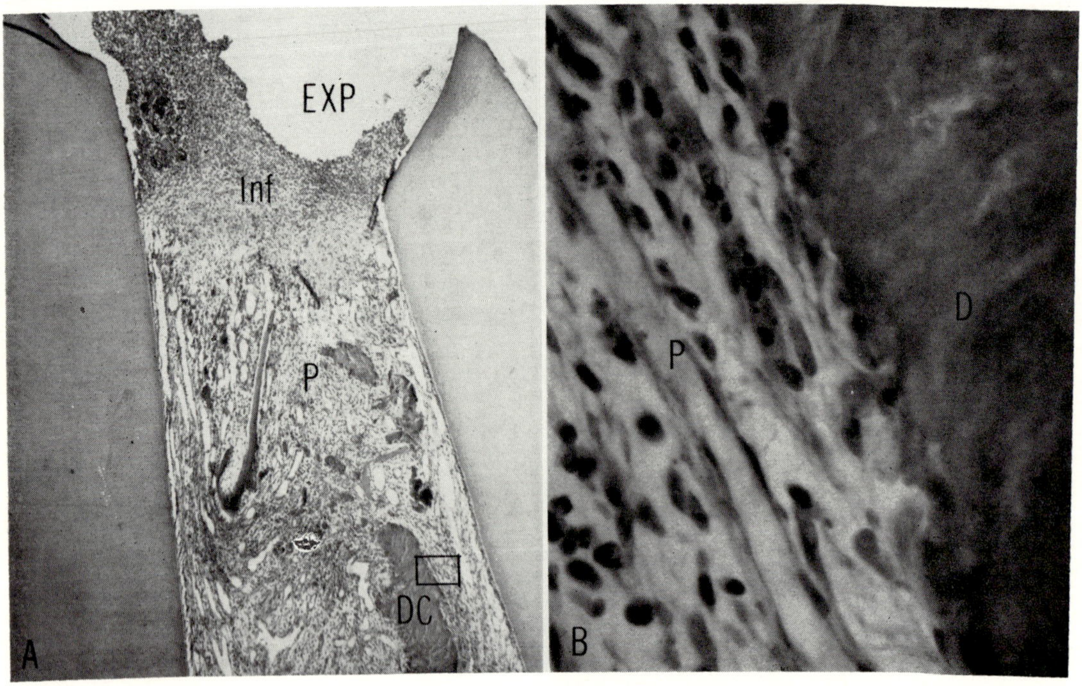

Figure 135. Chronic pulpitis under an exposure that was capped with chrondroitin sulfate. A. Exp = exposure, Inf = inflammation, P = pulp, DC = dentin chip (×54). B. Higher magnification of area within the rectangle; P = pulp, D = dentin chip (×960). (From S. Seltzer and I. B. Bender, *The Dental Pulp*, J. P. Lippincott Co., 1965. Used with permission of J. P. Lippincott Company.)

pulp involvement. Pain incidence increases with the severity of the disease, being least in chronic partial pulpitis and the most in chronic total pulpitis. Intensity of pain is greatest with chronic partial pulpitis with necrosis. There is less pain associated with chronic partial pulpitis without necrosis and chronic total pulpitis. There appears to be no correlation between the type of chronic pulpitis and the character of the pain (e.g. sharp, dull, lancinating, throbbing, etc.). Referred pain can often occur with chronic partial pulpitis. Pain on percussion is more frequently found in chronic partial pulpitis with necrosis. There is no correlation between the type of chronic pulpitis and the reaction to the electric pulp tester or thermal tests. All ranges of responses can be elicited. Usually, a more intense response to heat or cold, apical palpation, eating sweet or sour foods, or lying down, indicates a more severe pathologic state of the pulp. The histologic appearance of chronic pulpitis shows the presence in the pulp of granulomatous tissue. This tissue contains abundant capillaries, fibroblasts, collagen fibers, lymphocytes, macrophages, plasma cells, and occasionally polymorph leucocytes (Fig. 136). A cheesy type material is found when regions of coagulation necrosis are present (Fig. 137). In re-

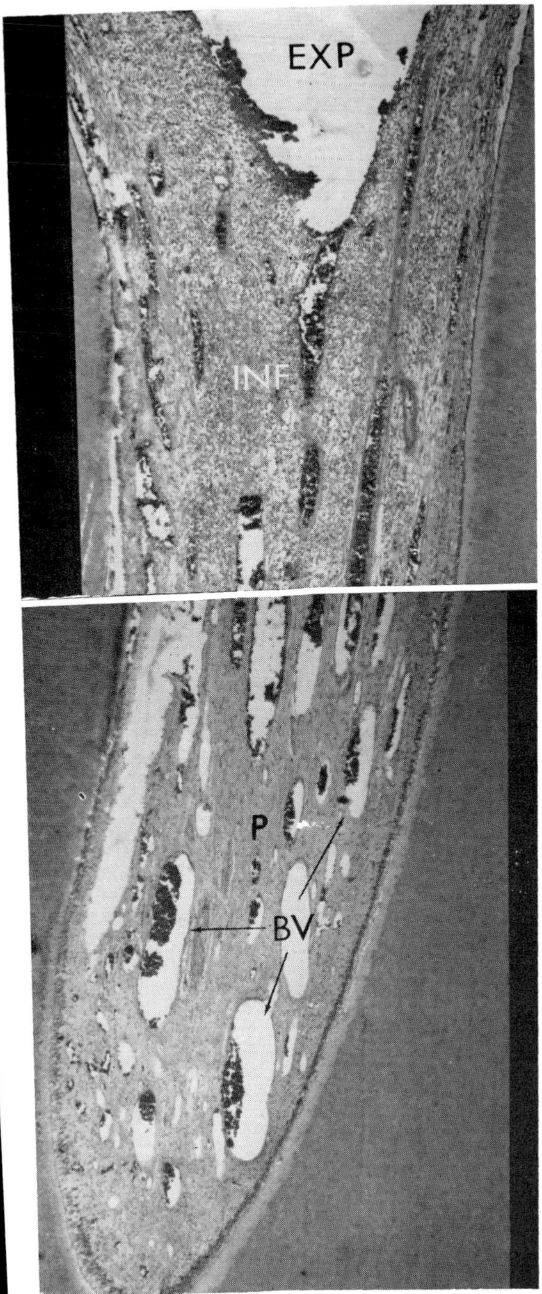

Figure 136. Chronic pulpitis; Exp = carious exposure, Inf = inflammation, P = pulp, BV = widely dilated blood vessels (×54). (From S. Seltzer and I. B. Bender, *The Dental Pulp*, J. P. Lippincott Co., 1965. Used with permission of J. P. Lippincott Company.)

gions of liquefaction necrosis, pus is present (Figs. 137, 138). This consists of dead or dying polymorph leucocytes with their decomposition products and breakdown products of cells and/or microorganisms. If there is a sensitivity to percussion, this indicates edema in the apical periodontal ligament space.

The prognosis and treatment for chronic pulpitis depends upon the state of the disease and causative factors. In chronic partial pulpitis without necrosis, the prognosis for pulp conservation is good. For deep caries cases, the treatment of choice is indirect pulp capping. Chronic partial pulpitis may be present beneath restorations. If the patients have no signs or symptoms, then no treatment is necessary. However, it is possible that the teeth may require endodontic therapy at a future date. In chronic partial pulpitis with partial coagulation necrosis, it is possible that indirect pulp capping would be successful, but the chances are not as good as with simple chronic partial pulpitis. In chronic partial pulpitis with liquefaction necrosis and chronic total pulpitis, the pulp must be extirpated followed by complete endodontic therapy. In chronic hyperplastic pulpitis, the excess granulomatous tissue must first be removed either by electrocautery or the use of a scalpel. Then complete endodontic therapy should be performed.

Acute Exacerbation of Chronic Pulpitis

This condition is an acute inflammation superimposed upon a chronic pulpitis. This can occur following operative procedures on a tooth that had previous

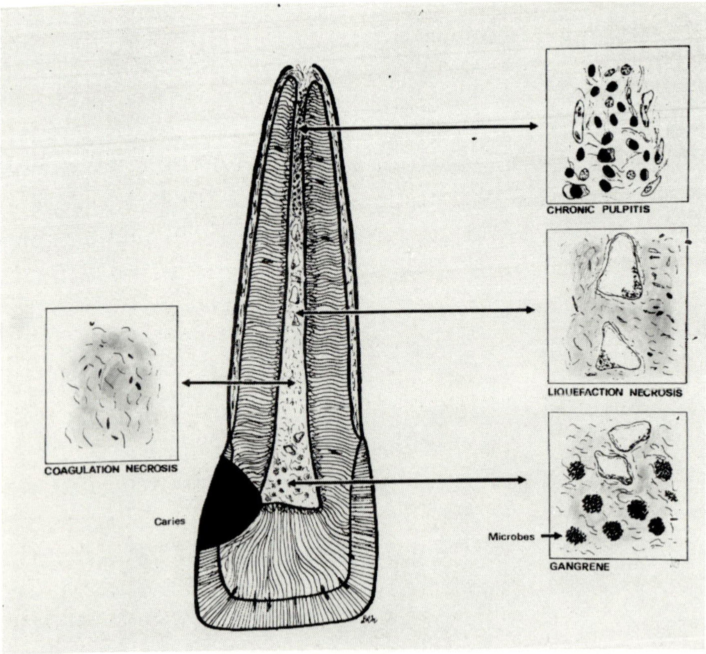

Figure 137. Hypothetical case showing various types of pulpal disease including chronic pulpitis, coagulation necrosis, liquefaction necrosis, and gangrene.

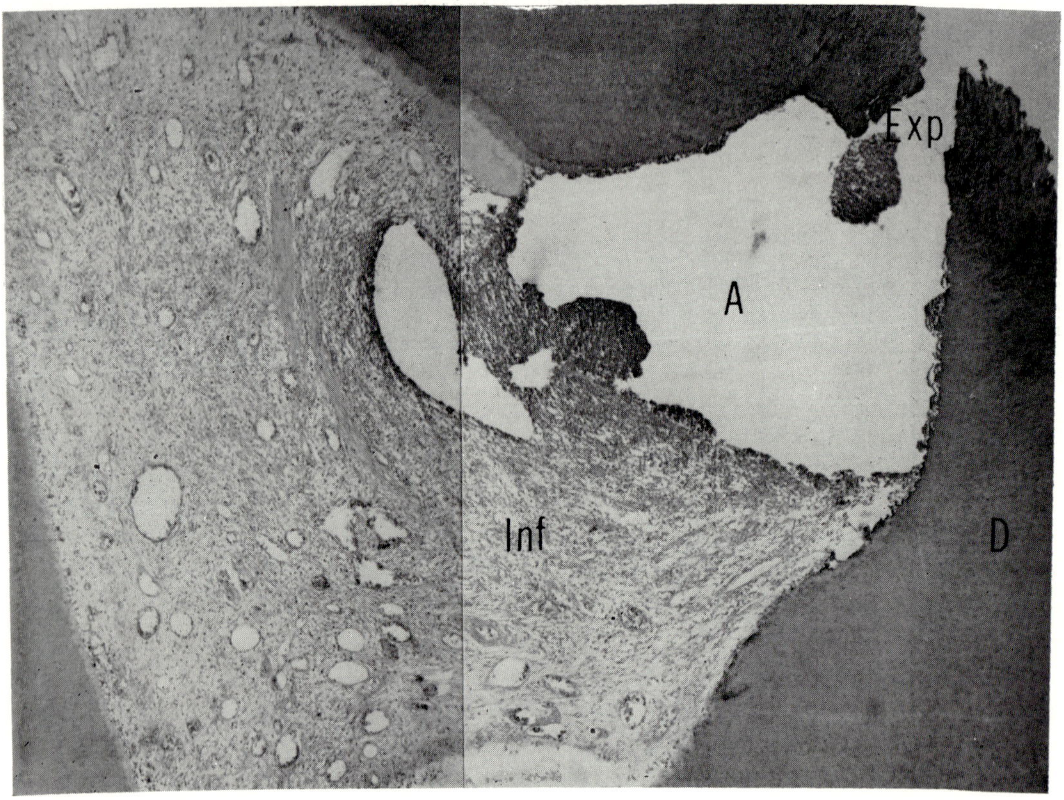

Figure 138. Chronic pulpitis with liquefaction necrosis; Exp = carious exposure, A = abscess, Inf = inflammation (chronically inflamed pulp tissue), D = dentin (×54). (From S. Seltzer and I. B. Bender, *The Dental Pulp*, J. P. Lippincott Co., 1965. Used with permission of J. P. Lippincott Company.)

caries, abrasion, erosion, attrition, restorations, periodontal disease, periodontal treatments, orthodontic movement, or trauma. It may also occur spontaneously and for no apparent reason in a tooth that had a restoration placed in, many years previously. This is the condition that is often referred to by clinicians as an acute pulpitis. However, as described previously pain is not a usual symptom of acute pulpitis. Severe pain does often accompany an acute exacerbation. These patients may give a history of sensitivity or slight pain resulting from a previous restoration on the involved tooth. The particular tooth is often painful to percussion. Heat, cold, lying down, and other external stimulants usually intensify the pain. Electrical pulp test results are equivocal. The histologic appearance shows a tremendous increase in polymorph leucocytes as well as dilated blood vessels superimposed on a background of chronic inflammatory cells (Fig. 139).

The pulp must be extirpated, followed by complete endodontic therapy if the tooth is to be saved.

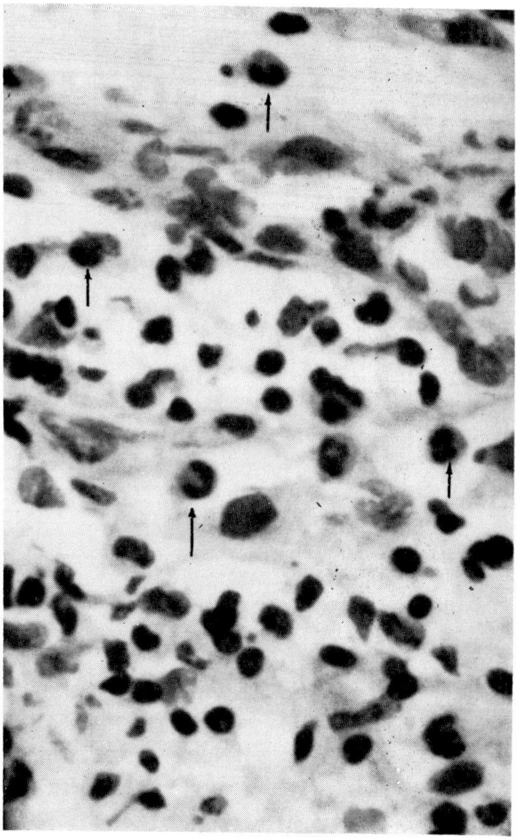

Figure 139. Acute exacerbation of a chronic pulpitis; arrows point to polymorph leucocytes; these are superimposed on a background of chronic inflammation (×960). (From S. Seltzer and I. B. Bender, *The Dental Pulp*, J. P. Lippincott Co., 1965. Used with permission of J. P. Lippincott Company.)

Acute Apical Periodontitis (Acute Pericementitis)

This condition is an acute inflammation of the apical periodontal ligament space. It can be caused by occlusal traumatism, usually resulting from a high restoration. It may occur as a result of apical extension of a chronic pulpitis or acute pulpitis. Acute apical periodontitis can follow pulp extirpation, instrumentation, intracanal medication placement, or a temporary restoration inserted in supraocclusion. The cardinal symptoms are painful responses to percussion, chewing or biting. If the patient gives a history of recent placement of a restoration, and there is a high shiny spot on the restoration, this is generally pathognomonic of acute apical periodontitis. Patients who have had teeth that have recently been moved orthodontically can also have temporary symptoms of acute apical periodontitis. The involved tooth usually responds

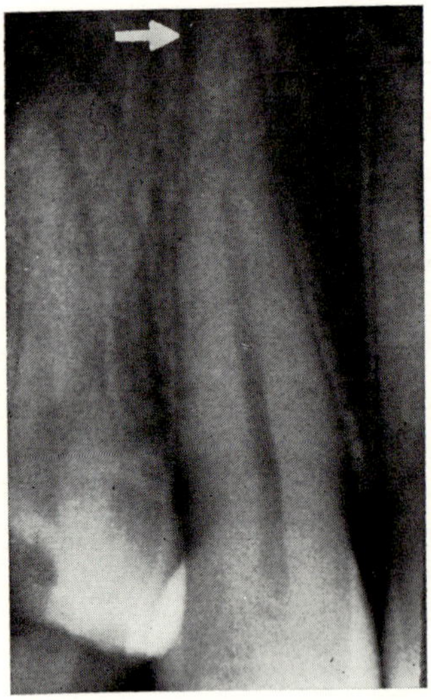

Figure 140. Acute apical periodontitis; condition is manifested by thickening of the apical periodontal ligament space.

normally to the electric pulp tester, and to thermal tests. The region around the apex at the mucobuccal fold may be sensitive to palpation.

A periapical radiograph often shows a thickening of the apical periodontal ligament space (Fig. 140). As stated previously, acute apical periodontitis can also occur concurrently with chronic pulpitis, and this can be diagnosed by the symptoms of the latter disease plus the sensitivity to percussion and palpation.

The histologic appearance may show a polymorph infiltration, dilated blood vessels, and edema in the apical periodontal ligament region, although this has not been definitely ascertained. The prognosis and treatment depends upon the etiology. If the periodontitis is caused by occlusal traumatism, reducing the *high* spot should relieve the condition. If the etiology is an apical extension of a chronic pulpitis, then the prognosis for saving the pulp is poor. However, the prognosis is good for saving the tooth, provided that complete endodontic therapy is performed. If acute apical periodontitis occurs during endodontic therapy, then removing or preventing the etiologic factors must be done. This includes not over-instrumenting, using a slight amount of a nonirritating dressing, and relieving the occlusion.

Chronic Apical Periodontitis and Periodontal Ligament Thickening

Radiographically, chronic apical periodontitis is similar in appearance to acute apical periodontitis (Fig. 141). Histologically, it is characterized by the presence of lymphocytes, plasma cells and macrophages. It is a short-lived in-

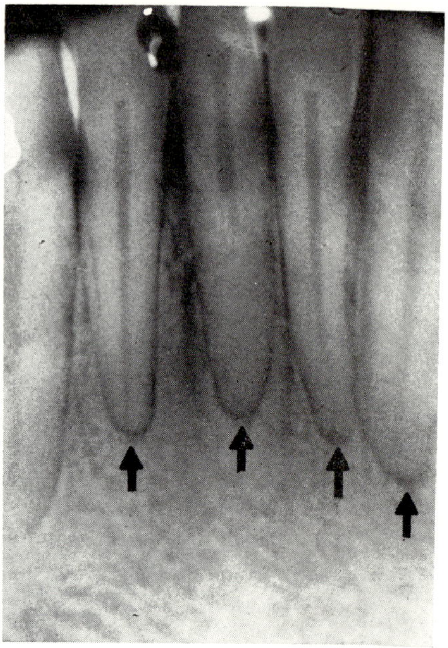

Figure 141. Chronic apical periodontitis; apical periodontal ligament thickening on several lower anterior teeth. (From D. R. Morse, "The Management of Endodontic Problem Cases," *JDA South Africa*, 27:387, 1972)

terim stage between chronic pulpitis or pulpal necrosis and a periapical granuloma or radicular cyst. Periodontal ligament thickening is not an endodontic condition, but it is included here because of its similarity to apical periodontitis. However, the response is not confined to the apical region but can include the entire periodontal ligament. This response is also more chronic in nature, as the etiological factor is generally continuous occlusal traumatism. The tooth is usually sensitive to percussion and responds vitally to electric and thermal tests. It may have a certain degree of mobility. A periapical radiograph shows a widening of the periodontal ligament space, loss of the lamina dura, possible root resorption, and loss of supporting bone as evidenced by a radiolucent appearance (Fig. 100). The histologic findings reveal edema and there may be a chronic inflammatory infiltration of the periodontal ligament space, although this has never been proven. Prognosis is generally good if the occlusion can be balanced, the mobility can be lessened and periodontal therapy can be successfully performed. There are other causes of loss of the lamina dura and widening of the periodontal ligament space. Loss of the lamina dura can occur in hyperparathyroidism (Fig. 16), Paget's disease, and fibrous dysplasia. Widening of the periodontal ligament space can occur in diffuse scleroderma (Fig. 20), and occasionally in malignant bone tumors, such as osteogenic sarcoma.

The Cracked Tooth Syndrome

In this condition, there is an incomplete fracture of the tooth. The split is very difficult to find. The cause may be the biting of a hard object, but the time of the actual occurrence is difficult to trace. The patient may have a whole range of symptoms including pain during chewing, sensitivity to thermal changes, and symptoms of hypersensitive dentin, chronic pulpitis, or acute apical periodontitis. In diagnosis of the fracture, the occlusal tests and the iodine test should be used. The results of other clinical tests, such as x-ray, electric pulp test, thermal tests, percussion, palpation, and probing (Fig. 59) depend upon the extent of the fracture (e.g. whether the enamel, dentin or pulp is involved). Histologic appearance depends upon the underlying disease process (e.g. whether it is hypersensitive dentin, chronic pulpitis and/or acute apical periodontitis). The prognosis also depends upon the extent of the fracture. If a vertical fracture occurs, then the chance of saving the tooth is practically nil. If the pulp is involved and there is enough remaining tooth structure for a restoration, then the prognosis is good for retention of the tooth. This occurs, provided that complete endodontic therapy is successfully performed. With an incomplete fracture, only through the enamel and or dentin, there is the possibility of saving the pulp as well as the coronal tooth structure. It is possible to cement a crown on the occlusal surfaces and bind the fractured parts together.

Aerodontalgia

Aerodontalgia is a syndrome in which odontalgia occurs at high altitudes or under other conditions of low atmospheric pressure, such as during flight

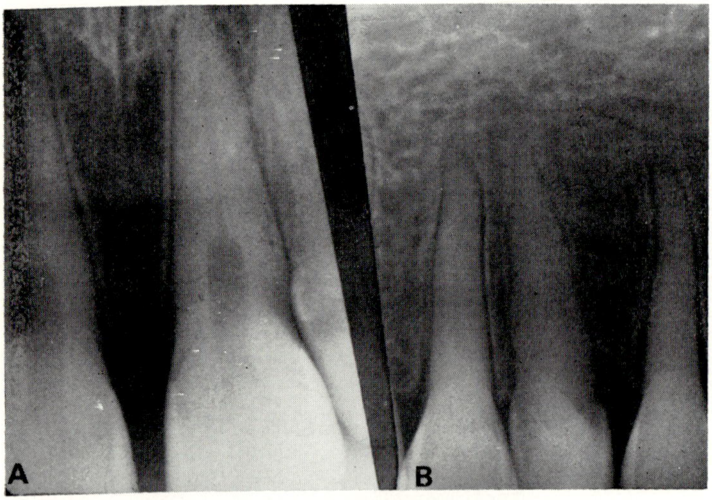

Figure 142. Hereditary opalescent dentin. A. Pulp chambers are evident; root canals are narrow. B. Pulp chambers are calcified, root canals are almost obliterated. (Courtesy of Dr. T. Simpson, Philadelphia, Pa.)

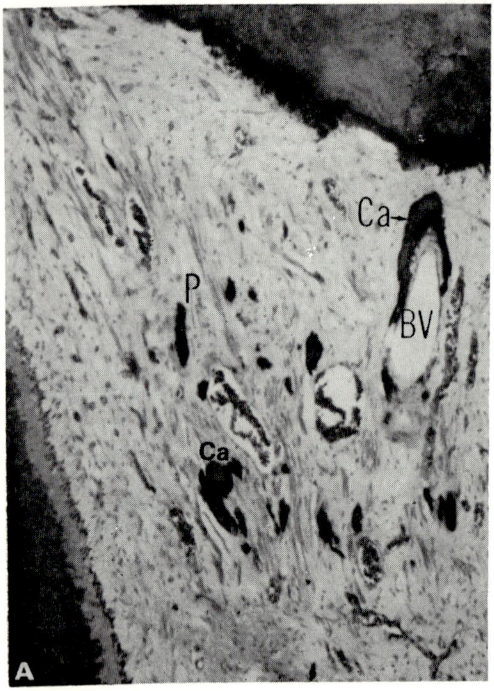

Figure 143. Dystrophic calcification of the pulp. A. Calcification of collagen fibers (left) and in the wall of blood vessel (right) in a periodontally involved tooth; CA = calcification, BV = blood vessel, P = pulp (×96). B. Calcification of nerves; N = myelin sheath, CF = collagen fibers, D = dentin, BV = blood vessels (×135). C. Higher magnification of area within rectangle in B; N = myelinated nerve, CA = calcification (×540). (From S. Seltzer and I. B. Bender, *The Dental Pulp*, J. P. Lippincott Co., 1965. Used with permission of J. P. Lippincott Company.)

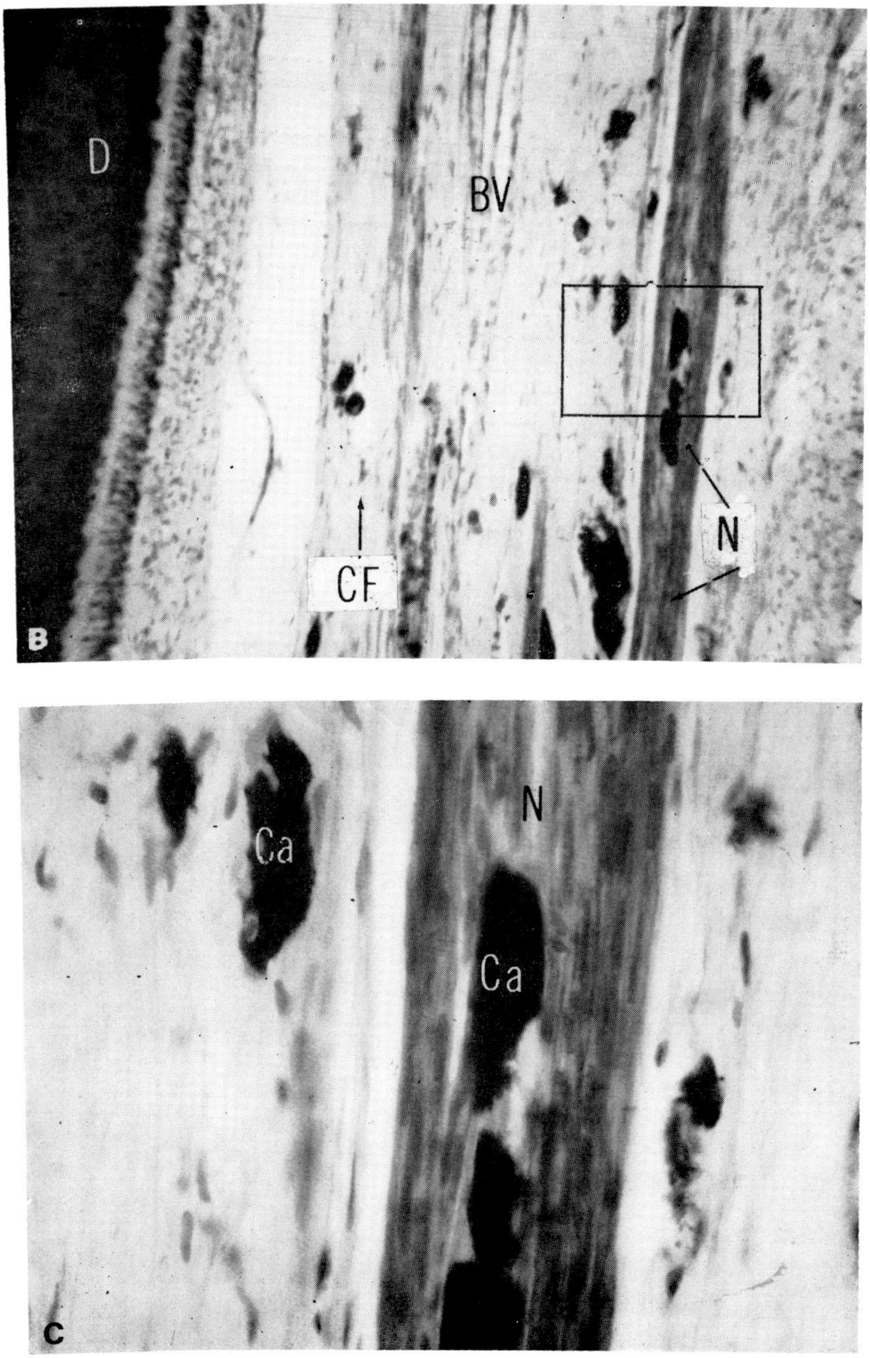

Figure 143

or in a decompression chamber. The teeth involved usually have a history of having been restored within twelve months prior to the onset of the painful condition. Patients with this condition usually do not have painful symptoms when they are at ground level (below 5000 feet). The pain can range from slight and transient to intense and of long duration. Apparently these teeth have a chronic partial pulpitis in which an exacerbation occurs under the described conditions. It is possible that an occasional flight will not cause any further pulpal damage. However, continuous flights could conceivably cause severe enough pulpal injury to necessitate complete endodontic therapy in order to save the involved tooth. Tests, histological appearance, prognosis and treatment all depend upon the type of chronic pulpitis that is present. Teeth with apparently well filled, or even poorly filled, root canals may be painful under conditions of high altitude or low atmospheric pressure. At ground level, the teeth may be symptomless. These cases have a mild chronic periapical inflammation that flares up only when relative anoxia occurs. There have also been cases of restorations fracturing or dislodging under conditions of high altitude.

Pulposis (Atrophy of the Pulp)

This is a fibrous and calcific degeneration of the pulp. It can occur naturally by aging or as the result of insults to the pulp such as operative procedures, caries, abrasion, erosion, attrition, periodontal diseases, periodontal treatment, orthodontic treatment, and trauma. It may also be found in hereditary opalescent dentin (Fig. 142), dentin dysplasia, atypical dentine dysplasia with typical facies, pulpal dysplasia and in systemic diseases such as progeria, osteogenesis imperfecta with dentinogenesis imperfecta, and hypervitaminosis D.

There are no clinical symptoms or signs. Responses to the electric pulp tester and thermal tests may be normal, but often the responses are slightly less than normal. Histologic appearance shows a decrease in the number and size of fibroblasts and an increase in the number and a wider distribution of collagen fibers. There is also an increase in pulpal calcifications (Fig. 143). Prognosis is good and no treatment is necessary. Occasionally, pulposis becomes so severe that the nerve fibers become completely calcified. In these cases, there may be no response to electric and thermal pulp testing. As there is no diagnostic method to differentiate this condition from symptomless complete pulpal necrosis, the best treatment is no treatment. Should manifestations of pulpal or periapical disease develop, the appropriate endodontic therapy can be performed.

Total Pulpal Necrosis

Total necrosis is complete pulp death and can be of three kinds, coagulation, liquefaction, or gangrene. In coagulation necrosis, the cellular protoplasm is fixed into a solid, cheesy-type material consisting of coagulated proteins, fats, and water. In liquefaction necrosis, the pulp is converted into a liquid media consisting of edematous fluid surrounded by inflammatory cells. In gangrene, there is a rapid complete necrosis of the pulp with a concomitant microbial invasion. The gangrene can be dry (dessication) or wet (liquefaction). There is putrescence present, with protein decomposition products and other breakdown substances found. These products include indole, skatole, putrescene, cadavarine, ammonia, hydrogen sulfide, carbon dioxide, fatty break-down products, indican, ptomaines, and water. The causative factors can be any of those listed under chronic pulpitis. Pulps may also become necrotic following mummification procedures with drugs such as paraformaldehyde, formocresol, phenol and arsenic. In necrosis, the patient generally has no symptoms and pulp test results are negative. However, if liquefaction necrosis or moist gangrene is present, the tooth may be sensitive to hot and respond to the electric pulp tester. This may result from expansion of gases and the conducting possibilities of the liquefied mass (although this has never been proven). The patient may give a history of a previous blow or fall, pulp capping, deep filling, pain after insertion of a restoration, orthodontic movement, pain after periodontal treatment, or a habit that traumatized the tooth. Teeth with necrotic pulps often appear darker than the adjoining teeth. When viewed with transillumination, the shadow of the pulp chamber appears darker than the adjacent vital teeth. Pain is usually not present in these conditions. In coagulation necrosis, there

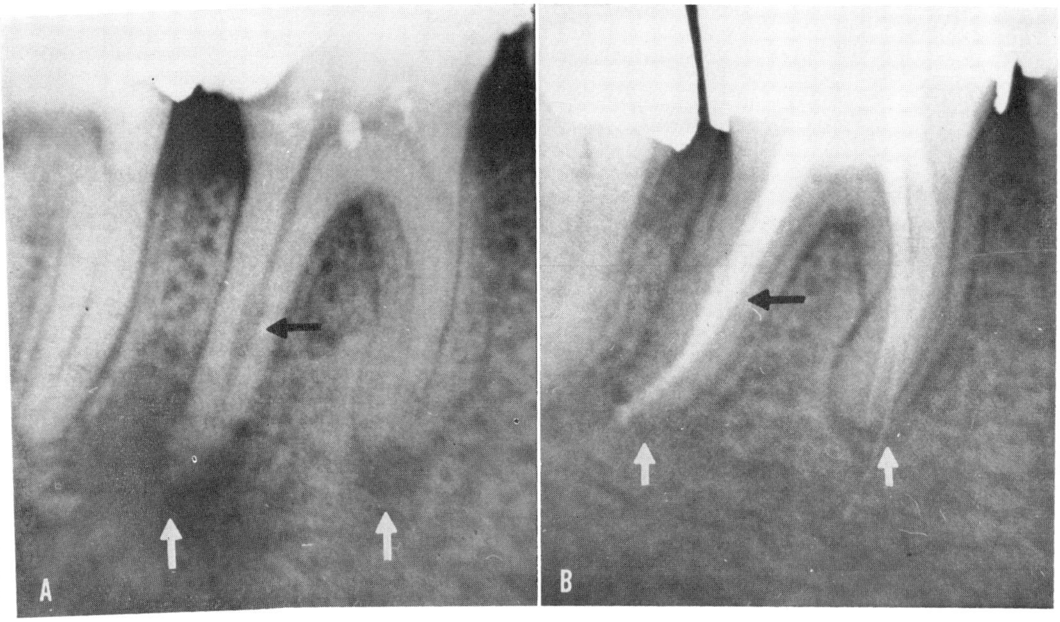

Figure 144. Lower first molar showing internal resorption and periapical areas of pathosis. A. Before treatment. B. One year after obturation with gutta-percha-chloropercha, internal resorption defect is sealed and periapical *areas* are healing; excess of gutta-percha on M-B root is being absorbed.

is a recognizable coagulated cell mass, but the intracellular detail is missing (Fig. 137). In liquefaction necrosis, an empty space is seen (where the fluid was) surrounded by a zone of polymorph leucocytes in varying stages of viability, plus chronic inflammatory cells (Figs. 137, 138). In gangrene, the picture is similar for the dry (coagulation necrosis) and wet (liquefaction) types, except that there may also be seen microorganisms and microbial fragments (Fig. 137).

The prognosis is good for retention of the tooth provided that complete endodontic therapy is performed.

Internal Resorption and Pulp Canal Enlargements

Internal resorption is a pulpal degeneration in which the pulpal tissue is replaced by granulomatous tissue. There is an active clastic activity by multinucleated giant cells that causes dentinal, and if left unchecked, cemental and/or enamel resorption. Eventually complete crown or root perforation can occur. The cause is unknown but trauma has been implicated and internal resorption often follows direct pulp capping. As internal resorption is a form of chronic pulpitis, the symptoms and signs can mimic those of that disease. Often the patients have no symptoms, and the first indication of the presence of resorption is a localized increase in diameter of the pulp cavity as seen on a diagnostic periapical radiograph (Fig. 144). If internal resorption occurs in the coronal region, a pink spot can be seen near the cervix (Fig. 62).

Histologically, the pulp is converted to granulomatous tissue (Fig. 27). Multinucleated clastic type giant cells and resorptive lacunae can be observed (Fig. 145). The prognosis depends upon the stage of the resorption. If complete endodontic therapy can be performed with sealing of the resorptive defect, then the prognosis for the retention of the tooth is good.* With a completely perforated root, it may be possible to

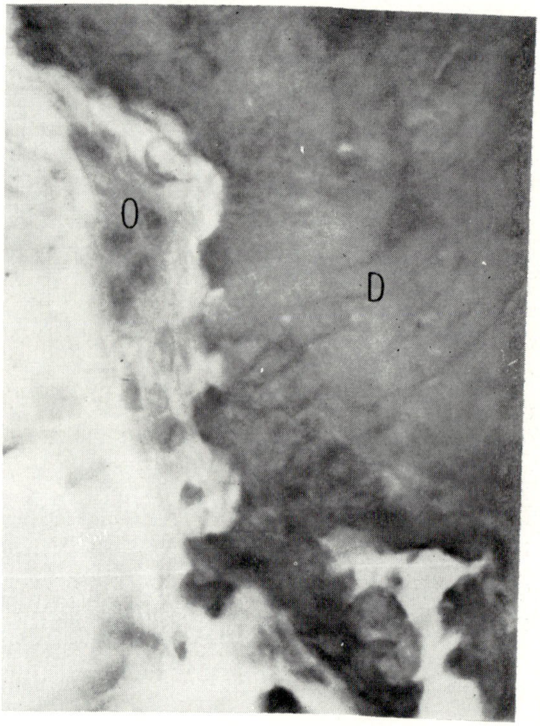

Figure 145. Multinucleated cell resorbing dentin; O = multinucleated resorbing cell, D = dentin (×960). (From S. Seltzer and I. B. Bender, *The Dental Pulp*, J. P. Lippincott Co., 1965. Used with permission of J. P. Lippincott Company.)

* Recent findings have shown that following instrumentation, use of a calcium hydroxide paste within the root canal may arrest internal resorption and cause the formation of a hard tissue barrier that would allow for subsequent obturation with gutta-percha.

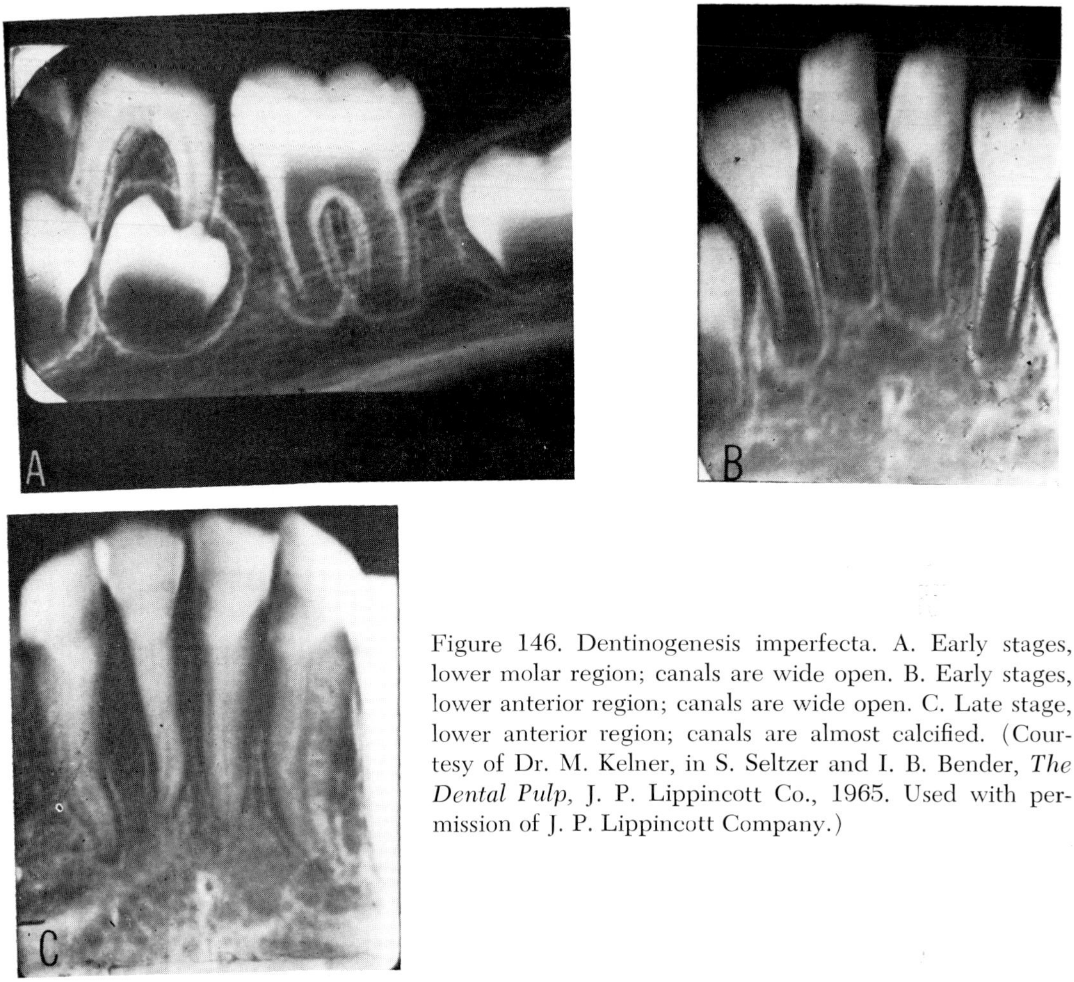

Figure 146. Dentinogenesis imperfecta. A. Early stages, lower molar region; canals are wide open. B. Early stages, lower anterior region; canals are wide open. C. Late stage, lower anterior region; canals are almost calcified. (Courtesy of Dr. M. Kelner, in S. Seltzer and I. B. Bender, *The Dental Pulp,* J. P. Lippincott Co., 1965. Used with permission of J. P. Lippincott Company.)

remove the apical section of the root and insert an endodontic implant. However, the prognosis with this treatment is not as good as for the previous situation.

Pulp canal enlargements may result in some cases from pulpal death while the root is in an immature state (Fig. 95A). This occurs often when the pulp is injured by trauma. Other conditions in which there are large pulp cavities are hereditary opalescent dentin (early stages), osteogenesis imperfecta with dentinogenesis imperfecta (early stages) (Fig. 146), taurodontism (Fig. 147), hypophosphatemic vitamin D resistant rickets, Fanconi's syndrome, hypophosphatasia, and odontodysplasia.

Acute Apical Abscess (Acute Alveolar Abscess)

An acute apical abscess is a localized periapical inflammation characterized by a purulent exudate with an abundance of polymorph leucocytes. It occurs as a sequel to pulpal necrosis and

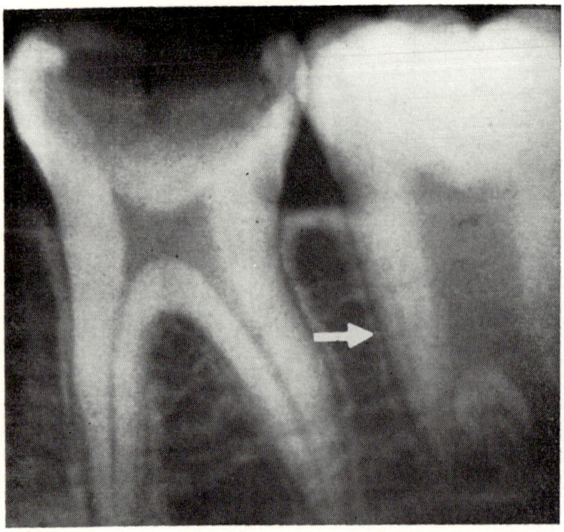

Figure 147. Taurodontism of lower second molar; long crown with enlarged pulp chamber, and short roots can be seen. (Courtesy of Dr. T. Simpson, Philadelphia, Pa.)

acute apical periodontitis and is manifested when the inflammation reaches the periapical bone. The condition can result from caries, trauma, operative procedures and other pulpitis-inducing factors. The immediate cause is usually microbial (or microbial products) invasion of the periapical tissues. It has been stated that an abscess is more likely to be caused by staphylococci than streptococci, but any oral microbes can be involved. More important in the determination of the type and path of the infectious process is the resistance of the host, the virulence of the microbes, and the tissue barriers present. Symptoms are tenderness to biting, mastication, or touch, which get progressively worse with time. The tooth usually becomes mobile and feels elongated. The adjoining teeth may also become mobile and feel sensitive to biting or touch. Pain is generally of an intense, throbbing type. Swelling occurs in the mucobuccal fold and can extend into the soft tissues of the cheeks. If the disease remains unabated, a cellulitis, or osteomyelitis can occur. It may also become quiescent and form a granuloma.

Clinical tests show no response to electric or thermal tests, although occasionally, because of the inflammatory exudate, there may be a painful response to heat. The involved tooth is tender to percussion, palpation and is usually quite mobile. Depending upon the stage of the disease, a periapical radiograph may show no periapical change, a thickening of the apical periodontal ligament space, or a definite periapical radiolucency. The tooth is dark in appearance and opaque to transillumination. The patient may have a fever of 100° F or higher, be in a state of malaise, and feel weak.

The histological appearance shows

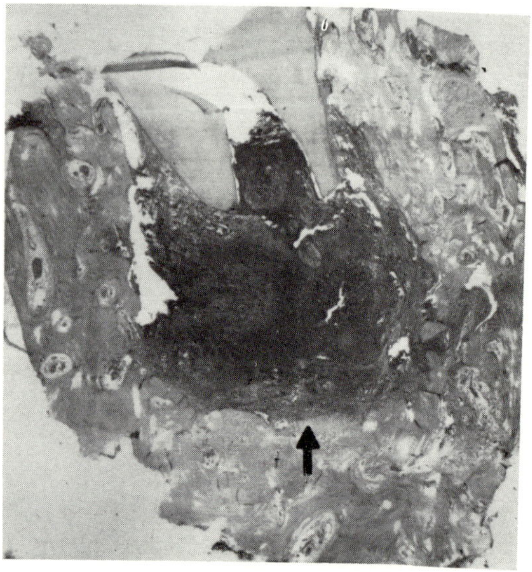

Figure 148. Acute apical abscess in a lower molar (×9.6). Courtesy of Dr. S. Seltzer, Philadelphia, Pa.)

the following. The root canal is usually devoid of tissue and may contain cellular debris and microorganisms. The periapical area is the site of an acute inflammatory response, characterized by numerous polymorph leucocytes, a purulent exudate, destruction of the apical periodontal ligament fibers, and destruction of the apical alveolar bone (Fig. 148). In addition to the *polys,* macrophages, lymphocytes and osteoclasts can later be found. Microbes may also be present.

Provided drainage can be established,

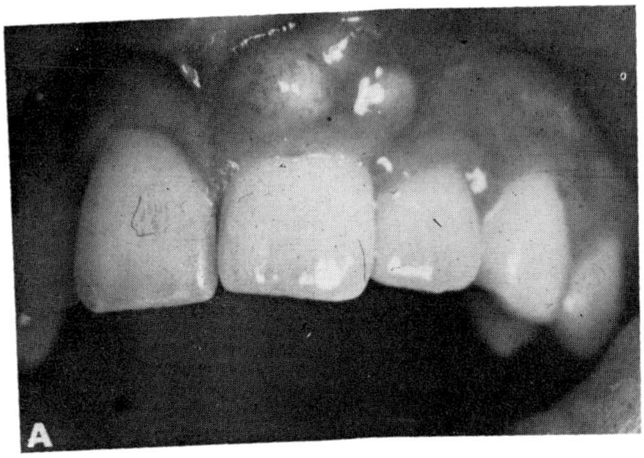

Figure 149. Parulis (stoma, *gum boil*), two examples: A. Upper central. (From S. Seltzer and I. B. Bender, *The Dental Pulp,* J. P. Lippincott Co., 1965. Used with permission of J. P. Lippincott Company.) B. Upper molar.

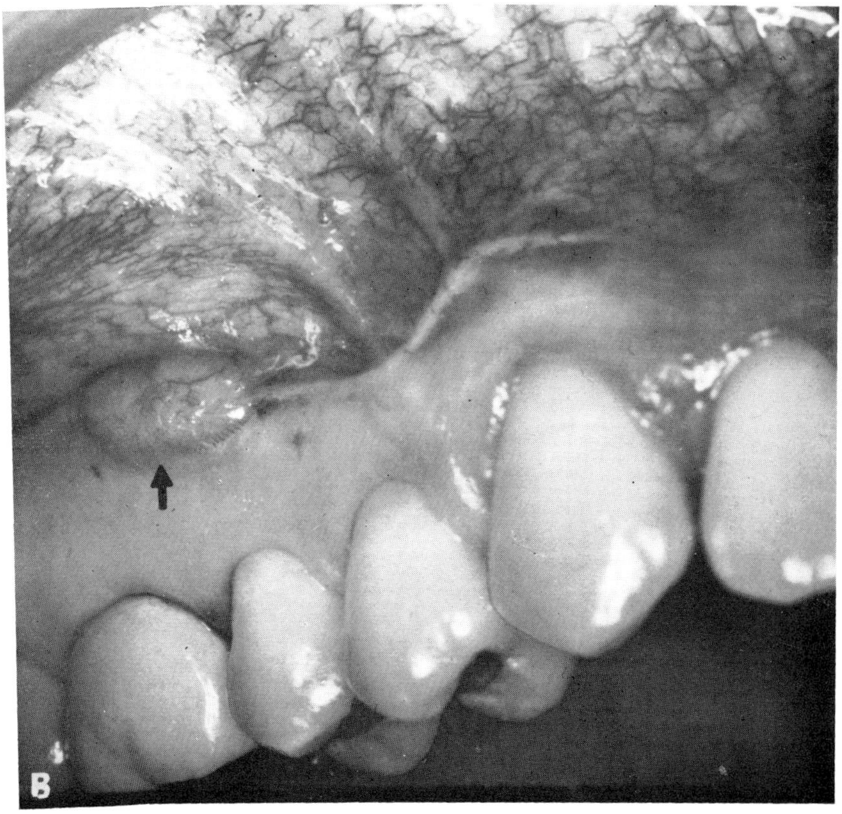

the prognosis is good for retention of the tooth. Treatment consists of establishing drainage either through the root canal, alveolar mucosa, or systemically after the administration of antibiotics. This then is followed by complete endodontic therapy.

Periapical Granuloma

This lesion is a tumor-like accumulation of granulomatous tissue in the periapical region. It occurs as a sequela to pulpal necrosis, chronic pulpitis, or an acute apical abscess. It results from the diffusion of toxic microbial products and cellular break-down products from the root canal into the periapical region. A granuloma is, in essence, a defensive reaction to the presence of a low grade irritant in the root canal. There are several types of granulomas. The first is the simple granuloma, the second the granuloma with proliferating epithelium, and the third the granuloma with liquefaction necrosis. The latter is termed a chronic alveolar abscess by some authorities. The granuloma with liquefaction necrosis may be accompanied by a draining sinus tract. The latter is also known as a fistula, but most tracts are not lined by epithelium as the term fistula implies. Rather, they are lined by granulomatous tissue. Instead of just being a draining opening, the sinus tract can close up temporarily and then a proliferation of granulomatous tissue can occur. This takes the form of a soft tissue lesion that is often raised, reddish and fluctuant. It is known as a parulis, stoma, or *gum boil* (Fig. 149). It may be located a distance away from the vicinity of the root apex. Probing of the lesion by a silver or gutta-percha cone, followed by a ra-

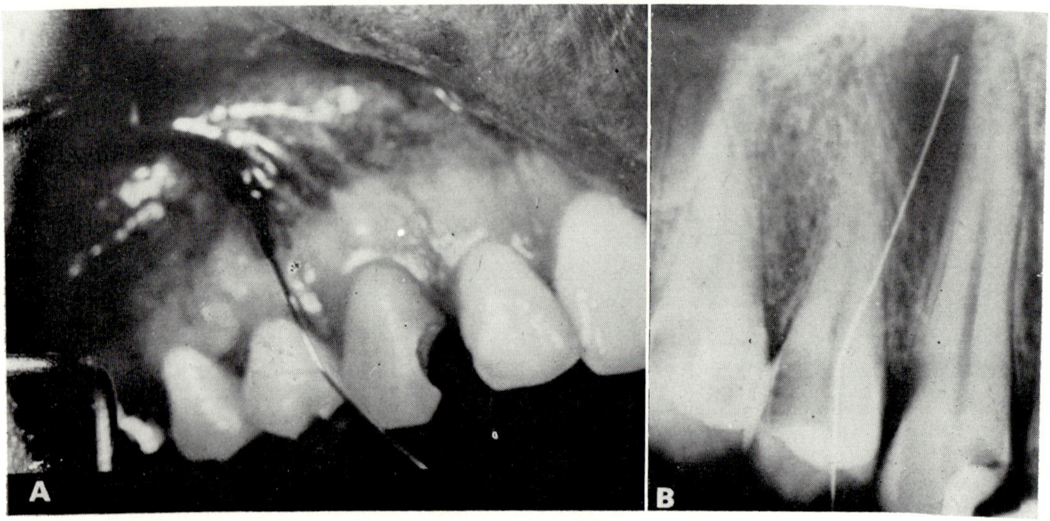

Figure 150. Tracing a sinus tract; use of a diagnostic wire. A. Clinical. B. Radiographic; upper canine is the involved tooth. (From I. B. Bender and S. Seltzer, "The Oral Fistula: Its Diagnosis and Treatment," *Oral Surgery, Oral Medicine and Oral Pathology*, 14:1367, 1961.)

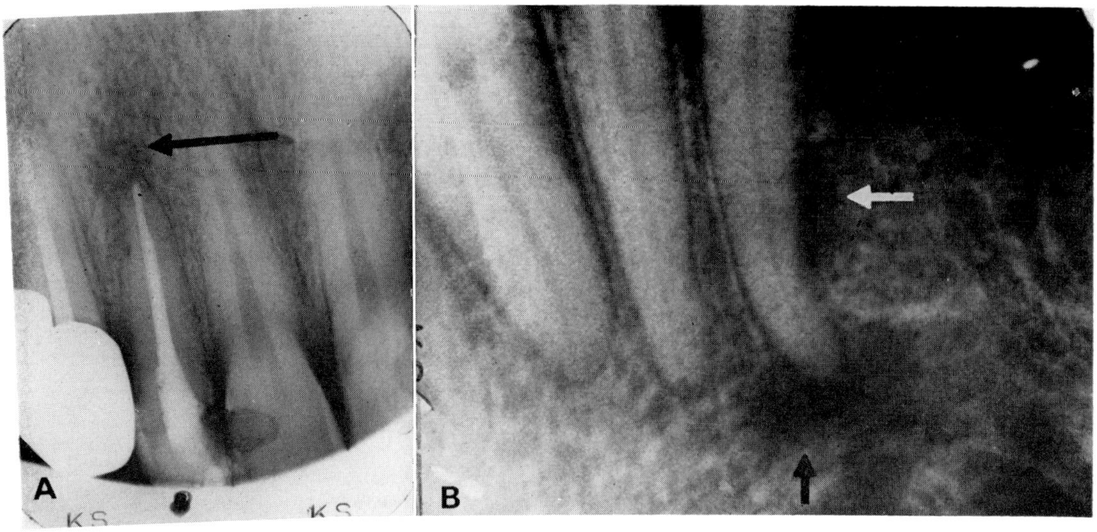

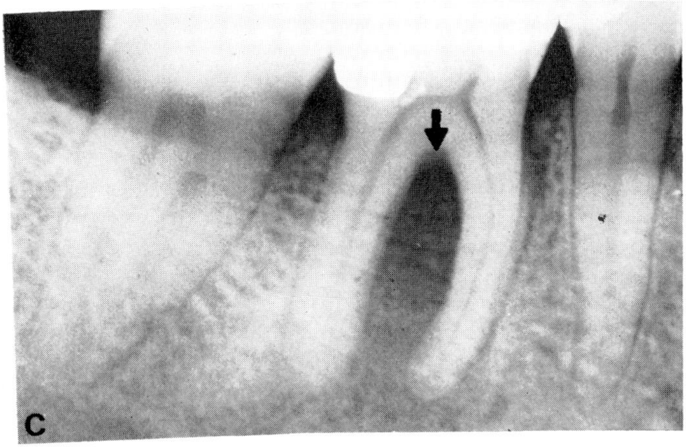

Figure 151. Various granulomas related to pulpless teeth: A. Periapical. B. Lateral (white arrow), periapical (black arrow). C. Furcation.

diograph, is helpful in location of the involved apex, and in differentiating the parulis from a non-endodontic lesion (Fig. 150). The causes are any of the previously mentioned factors leading to chronic pulpitis and necrosis. The immediate cause is a chronic low grade irritant in the root canal (usually microbial) leading to an alternating proliferative and destructive periapical response. Usually, the patients have no symptoms. There is no response to either the electric pulp tester or thermal tests. The diagnosis of periapical granuloma is aided by the discovery of a radiolucent area of rarefaction in the periapical region (Fig. 151A, B). The radiolucency may also be present along the lateral aspect of the root (Fig. 151B) or in the furcation area (Fig. 151C). Although there have been contrary claims, there is no definite radiographic method to differentiate a periapical granuloma and radicular cyst. Another diagnostic aid is the presence of a sinus tract, in certain cases of

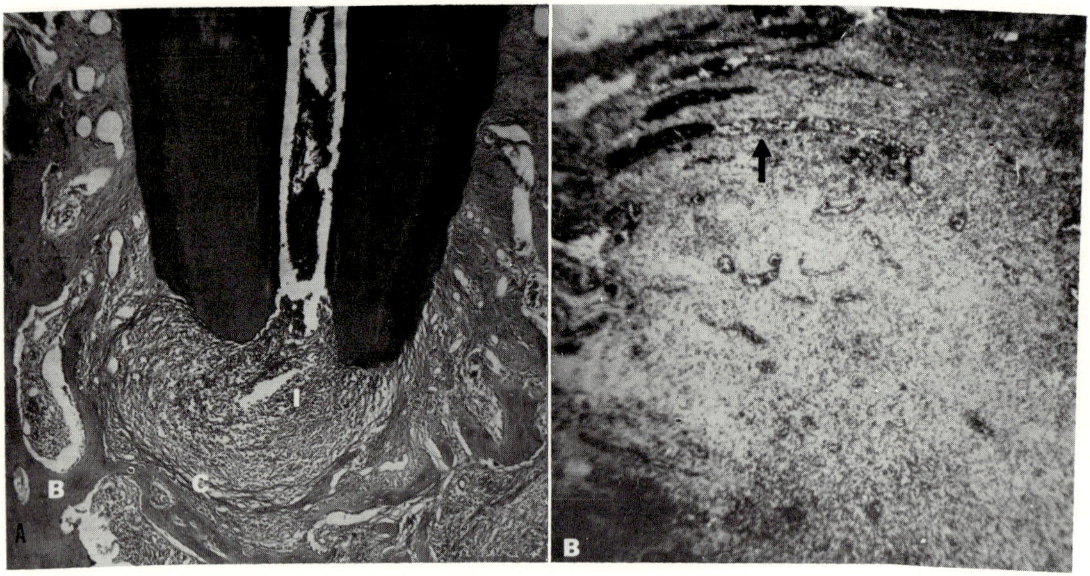

Figure 152. Granulomas. A. I = inflammation, C = connective tissue capsule, B = bone (×42). (From S. Seltzer, *Endodontology*, McGraw-Hill, Inc., 1971. Used with permission of McGraw-Hill Book Company.) B. Arrow points to capillary (×96).

granulomas with liquefaction necrosis. The tooth is dark in appearance and to transillumination. Transillumination usually reveals a shadow at the periapex. Very rarely, the bone around the lesion bulges out.

Histological appearance shows the presence of granulomatous tissue consisting of lymphocytes, macrophages, some plasma cells, abundant capillaries, fibroblasts, osteoclasts, and collagen fibers. Surrounding the granulomatous tissue is a fibrous connective tissue capsule which is surrounded in turn by alveolar bone (Fig. 152). In granulomas with epithelial proliferation strands or nests of epithelium with connective tissue cords are found (Fig. 153). In granulomas with liquefaction necrosis, empty spaces are present (formerly filled with purulent exudate) and a polymorph leucocyte infiltration surrounds these zones (Fig. 154). The pulp is either empty or contains debris and possibly some microbes. The prognosis is good provided that complete endodontic therapy can be successfully completed. Regardless of the size of the lesion, periapical surgery is not necessary.

Radicular Cyst (Periapical Cyst, Dental Cyst)

A radicular cyst is a periapical lesion consisting of an epithelially-lined, fluid-filled sac surrounded by granulomatous tissue. The latter tissue is covered by a fibrous capsule which is surrounded by alveolar bone. The radicular cyst occurs as a sequela to pulpal necrosis or a periapical granuloma. It results from the diffusion of products into the periapex. Direct cause of the cyst is stimulation of the epithelial cells in the area (cell rests of Malassez, which are presumably remnants of Hertwig's epithelial root sheath) by these products. A radicular cyst can also be caused iatrogenically by overinstrumentation of the root canal

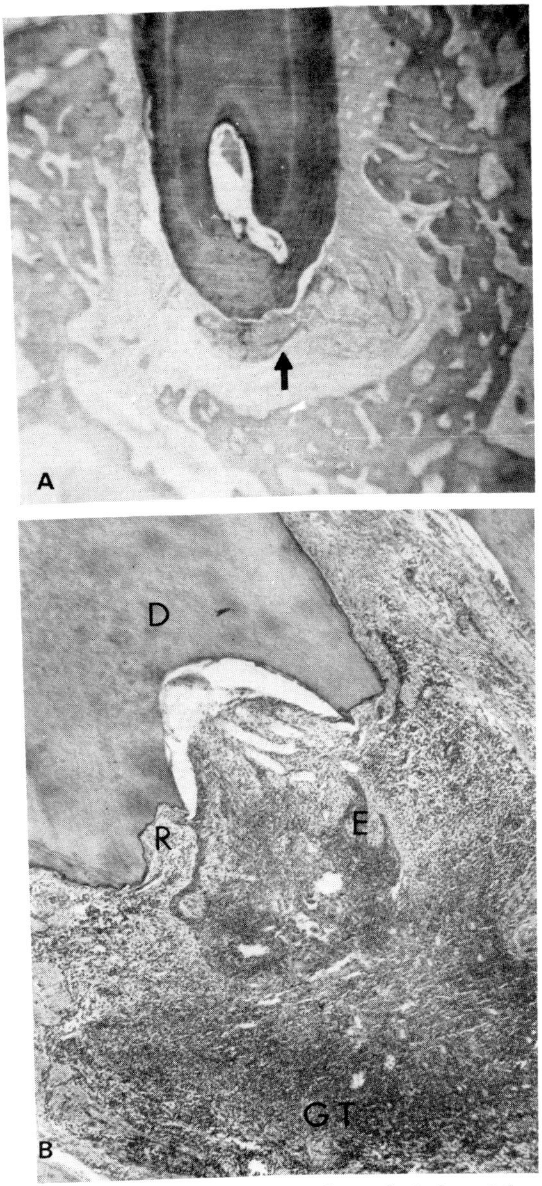

Figure 153. Granuloma with epithelial proliferation. A. Arrow points to epithelium (×42). B. D = dentin, R = root resorption, E = epithelium, GT = granulomatous tissue (×58.5). (Courtesy of Dr. S. Seltzer, Philadelphia, Pa.)

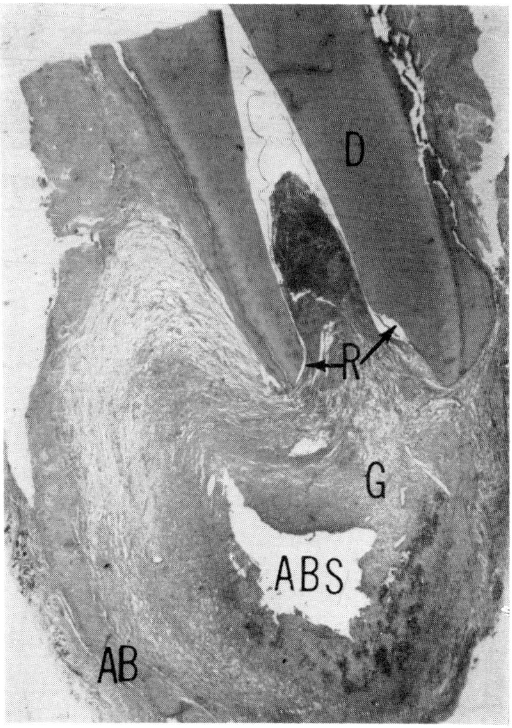

Figure 154. Granuloma with liquefaction necrosis; D = dentin, R = root resorption, G = granuloma, ABS =abscess, AB = alveolar bone (×6.3). (From S. Seltzer, *Endodontology,* McGraw-Hill, Inc., 1971. Used with permission of McGraw-Hill Book Company.)

during endodontic therapy of a vital case (Fig. 155). There is some evidence to indicate that there is a genetic tendency toward the development of radicular cysts. When a cyst is small or confined to the alveolar bone, there are usually no symptoms. If it causes pressure on adjoining teeth, then mobility of the teeth can occur and the teeth can change their alignment. If a cyst enlarges enough, it can cause swelling of the alveolar bone and the associated alveolar mucosa as well as external root resorption. The involved tooth does not respond to thermal and electrical pulp

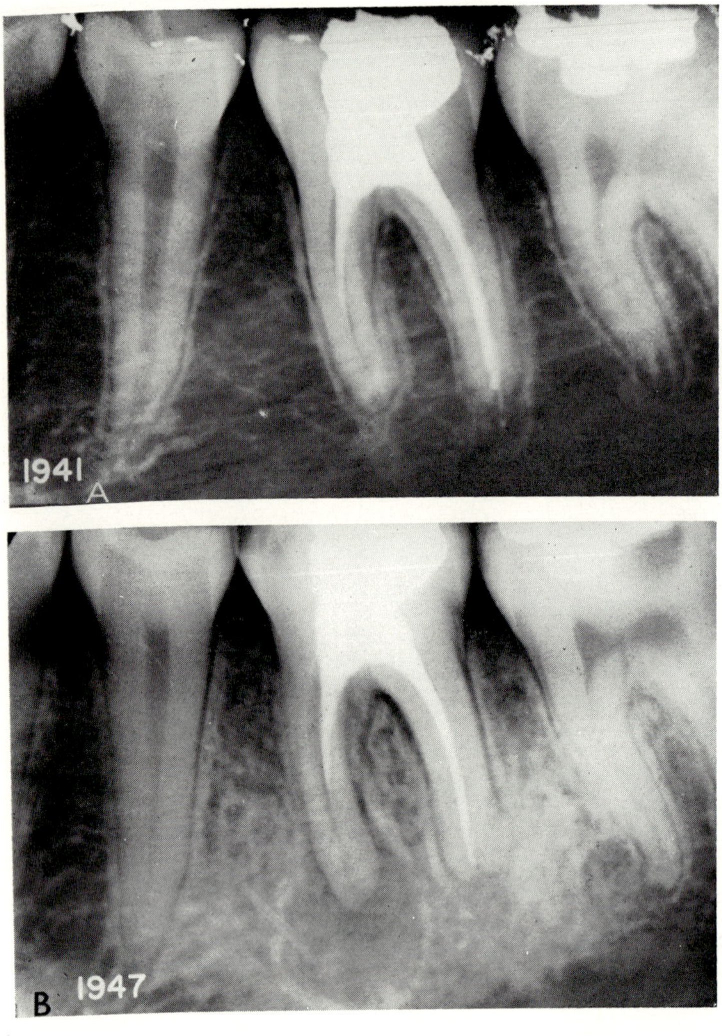

Figure 155. Iatrogenic (dentistogenic) development of a radicular cyst. A. Immediately after incomplete endodontic therapy. B. Several years later; large periapical *area* developed which was histopathologically verified to be a radicular cyst. (Courtesy of Dr. W. Updegrave, Philadelphia, Pa.)

testing. It is darkened in appearance and transillumination results are the same as with a granuloma. The radiographic appearance is not pathognomonic, but often there is a large circumferential periapical radiolucent rarefaction (Fig. 156), and if untreated a cyst can become quite extensive (Fig. 157). The roots of the adjacent teeth may be deflected. Occasionally, a radiograph may reveal a residual radicular *cyst* that remained after the extraction of a tooth or the loss of a primary tooth (Fig. 76). If the *cyst* lies near the apex or the lateral aspect of the tooth in question, it may appear to be related to that tooth. Electrical pulp testing or thermal tests should be normal for that tooth, and then the diagnosis of residual area of pathosis can be made. A definitive diagnosis of a cyst requires a histopathological examination (Fig. 158). A residual lesion may also discharge fluid to the oral cavity via a si-

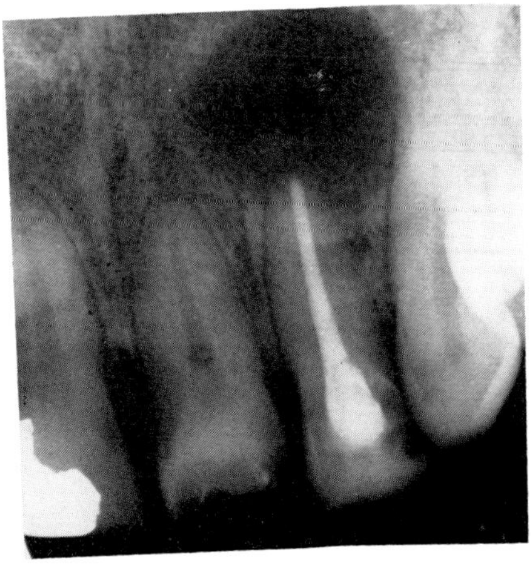

Figure 156. Radicular cyst; periapical lesion was determined to be a radicular cyst by histopathological examination.

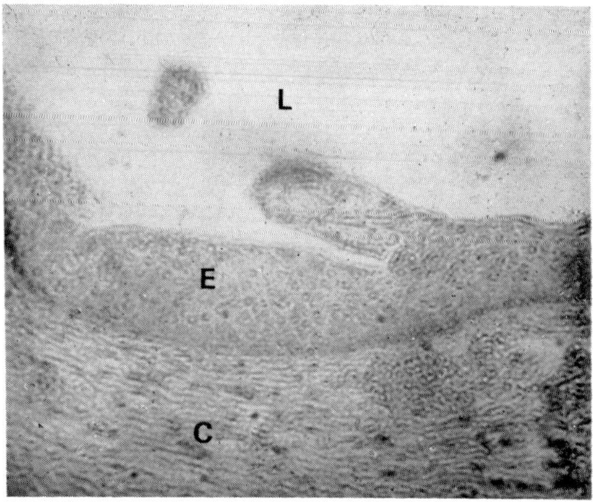

Figure 158. A residual cyst; L = lumen, E = epithelium, C = connective tissues (×540). (Courtesy of Dr. T. Simpson, Philadelphia, Pa.)

nus tract. Electrophoretic analysis of cyst fluid shows a typical appearance with an increase in the albumin and gamma globulin zones, as contrasted to granulomas. The latter shows a slight pattern in the albumin zone of the gel (Figs. 126, 127). Histological examination shows the following. An epithelial lining is present. It is of several cells thickness, and it surrounds a lumen. The lining may be complete or incomplete. In expanding cysts, numerous polymorph leucocytes are found in the epithelial lining and in the surrounding granulomatous tissue. The latter tissue consists of abundant lymphocytes and plasma cells, capillaries, fibroblasts and collagenous fibers. In the lumen, debris may be found, as well as chronic inflammatory cells and cholesterol crystals. Surrounding the granulomatous tissue is a fibrous tissue capsule, which is covered in turn by alveolar bone. There may be pockets of liquefaction necrosis throughout the lesion (Fig. 159). The pulp is empty or filled with debris. The prognosis for saving the tooth is good,

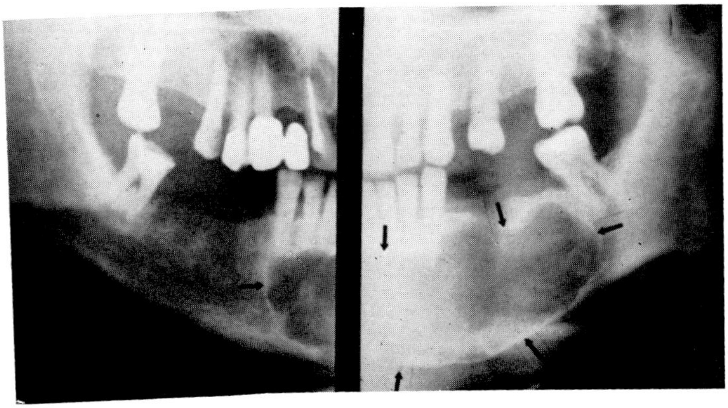

Figure 157. Extensive radicular cyst; huge defect in mandible created by expansive radicular cyst (verified by histopathological examination). (Courtesy of Dr. W. Updegrave, Philadelphia, Pa.)

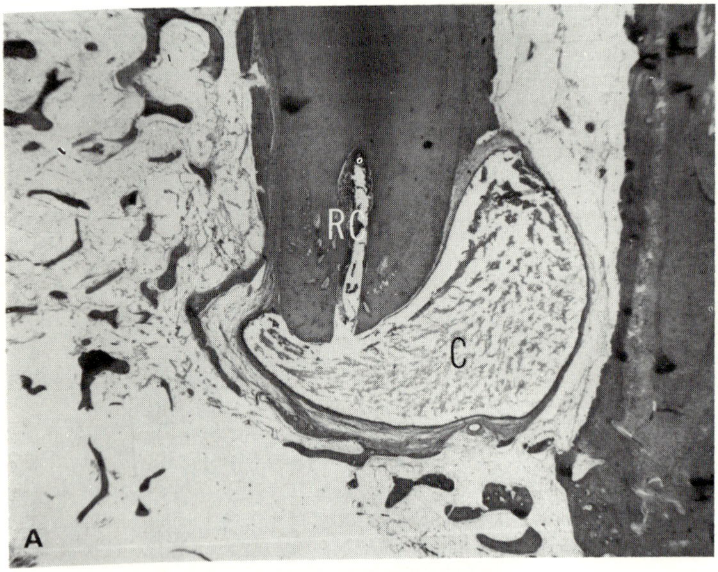

Figure 159. Radicular cysts: A. From a lower molar in a dog; RC = root canal, C = cyst (×6.8). (From S. Seltzer, *Endodontology*, McGraw-Hill, Inc., 1971. Used with permission of McGraw-Hill Book Company.) B. From a human; arrow points to epithelium (×96). C. From a human; inflammation is present (×96).

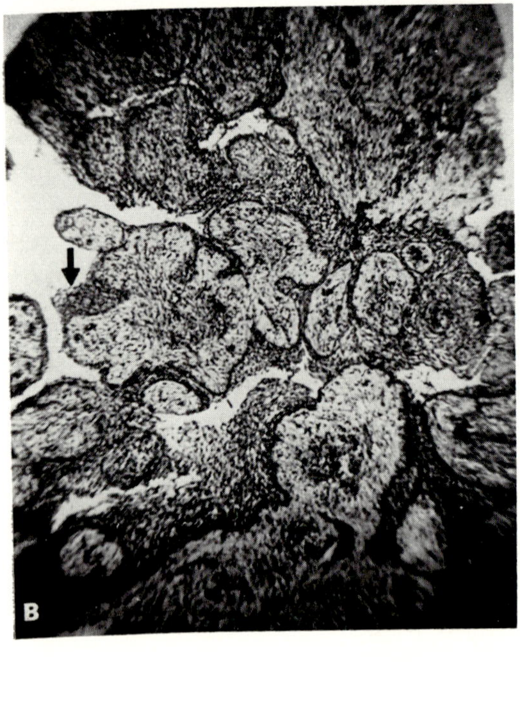

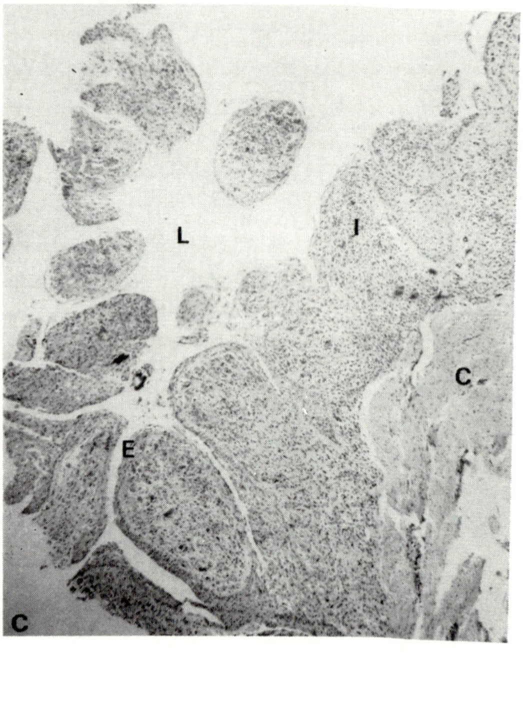

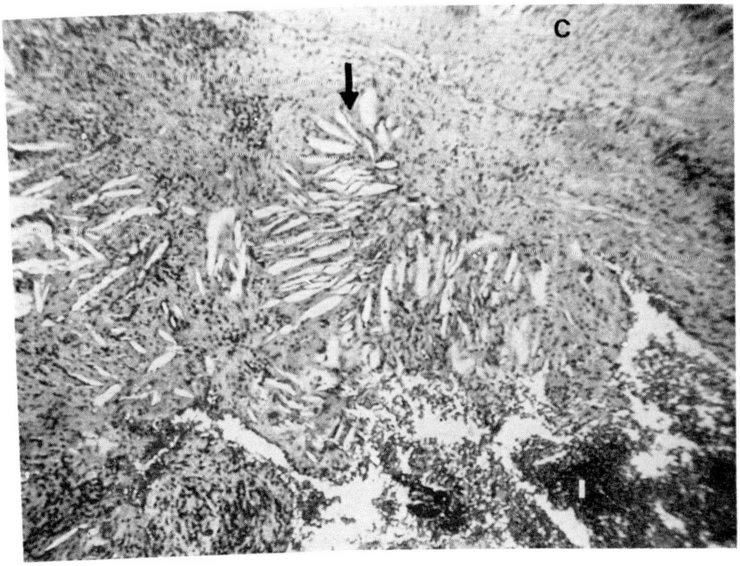

Figure 160. Cholesteatoma; C = connective tissue, I = inflammation; arrow indicates *cholesterol* slits (×96).

if successful complete endodontic therapy can be performed. The indirect evidence to date supports the contention that periapical surgery is not necessary for healing of periapical cysts (Fig. 128).

Cholesteatoma

This lesion is either a radicular cyst or periapical granuloma in which there is a large accumulation of lipids. Some investigators do not consider this as a separate lesion. The histologic appearance shows a large accumulation of slit-like spaces which had been filled *in vivo* with cholesterol or other lipids (Fig. 160). All other factors are the same as those described under radicular cyst and periapical granuloma.

Acute Exacerbation of Periapical Granuloma or Radicular Cyst (Phoenix Abscess)

In this condition, there is an acute inflammatory response superimposed upon a chronic inflammatory periapical lesion. The precipitating causes may be increased virulence of the microorganisms, decreased resistance of the host, or changing of the host-parasite relationship. The interaction between host and parasite can be modified by opening into the root canal of a periapically involved pulpless tooth, instrumentation into such a canal, or using an irritating medicament. Trauma to a tooth with a quiescent periapical lesion can also cause an acute exacerbation.

The patient's symptoms are similar to those described for acute apical abscess, although this condition is much more common than the latter. Clinical test results are also similar, except the periapical radiograph shows the presence of a periapical rarefaction. The histologic appearance reveals an acute infiltration of polymorph leucocytes surrounding areas of liquefaction necrosis. This is superimposed upon a background of granulomatous tissue (Fig. 161). In the case of a radicular cyst, disruption

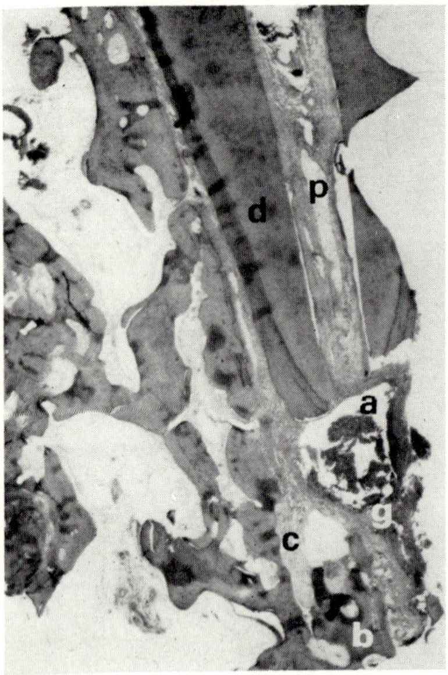

Figure 161. Acute exacerbation of granuloma; d = dentin, p = pulp, a = abscess, g = granulomatous tissue, c = connective tissue capsule, b = bone (×40). (Courtesy of Dr. S. Seltzer, Philadelphia, Pa.)

of the epithelial lining is evident (Fig. 159C). Microorganisms may also be found. Provided that drainage can be established and successful endodontic therapy can be performed, the prognosis is good for saving the tooth.

Condensing Osteitis (Periapical-Pulpo-Osteosclerosis)

This lesion results from a proliferative osteoblastic response in the periapical bone to the presence of low grade irritants in the root canal. It occurs primarily around the apexes of lower molars in young individuals. The root canal microbes are considered to have low virulence and the host resistance is believed to be high. The causative factors are the same as those responsible for cyst and granuloma formation. The pulp may be completely necrotic, but generally there is a chronic pulpitis present. Signs and symptoms are those of the underlying pulpal condition. Occasionally, condensing osteitis can cause pressure on the inferior alveolar nerve and pain can result. The radiographic appearance shows a radiopaque lesion present in the periapical region, surrounding one or both roots of a lower molar (usually). There is a loss of the apical lamina dura with a consequent widening of the periodontal ligament space (Figs. 77, 162). This ap-

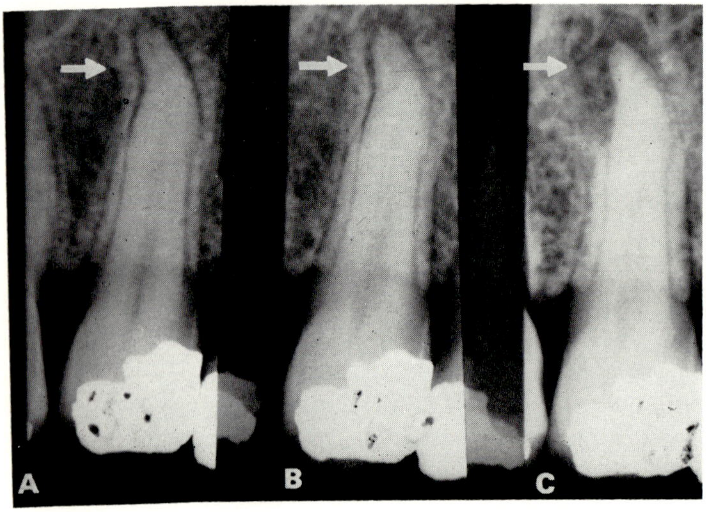

Figure 162. From condensing osteitis to periapical area of pathosis. A. Condensing osteitis with loss of apical lamina dura and widening of the periodontal ligament space. B. A few months later; more periapical bone destruction is occurring. C. Over one year later; periapical area of pathosis is now present. (Courtesy of Dr. W. Updegrave, Philadelphia, Pa.)

pearance helps in differentiating the condition from other osteosclerotic bone lesions in which the lamina dura is intact. The histologic appearance shows the overall presence of extremely dense alveolar bone with almost complete elimination of marrow spaces. There may also be present some pockets of bone destruction and areas filled with granulomatous tissue (Fig. 163). Following successful endodontic therapy, the lesion usually heals and normal trabeculated bone reappears.

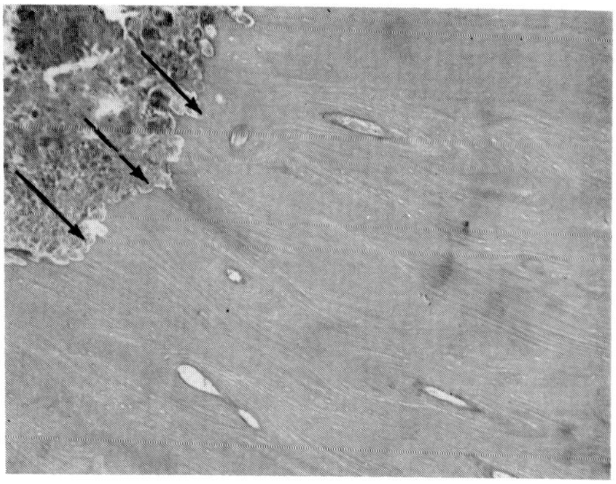

Figure 163. Condensing osteitis histological section; arrows point to areas of bone destruction (×32). (From S. Seltzer, *Endodontology*, McGraw-Hill, Inc., 1971. Used with permission of McGraw-Hill Book Company.)

External Root Resorption

The condition of external root resorption may result from endodontic

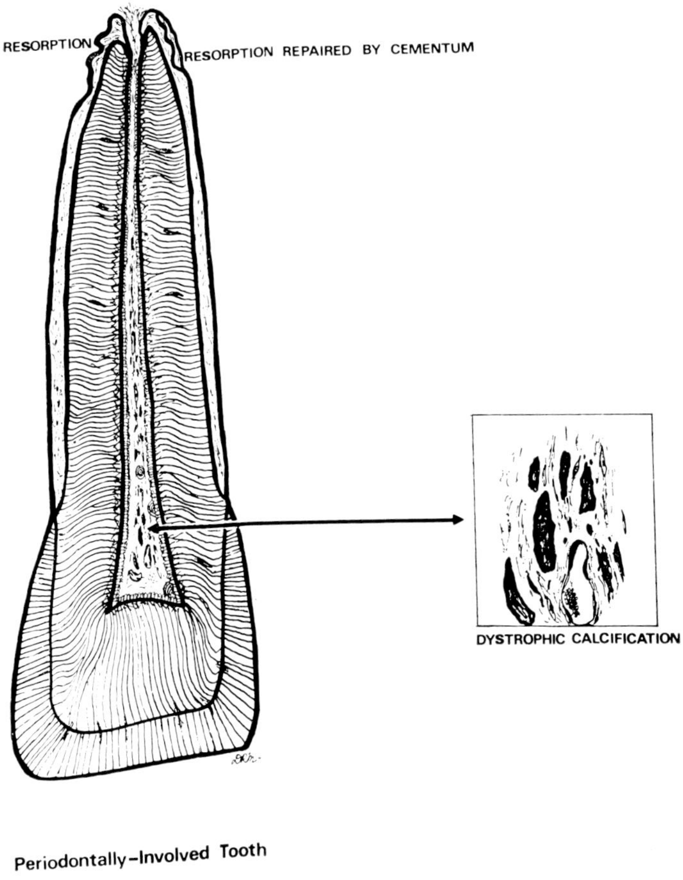

Figure 164. Periodontally-involved tooth, low power view and a higher power view showing dystrophic calcification.

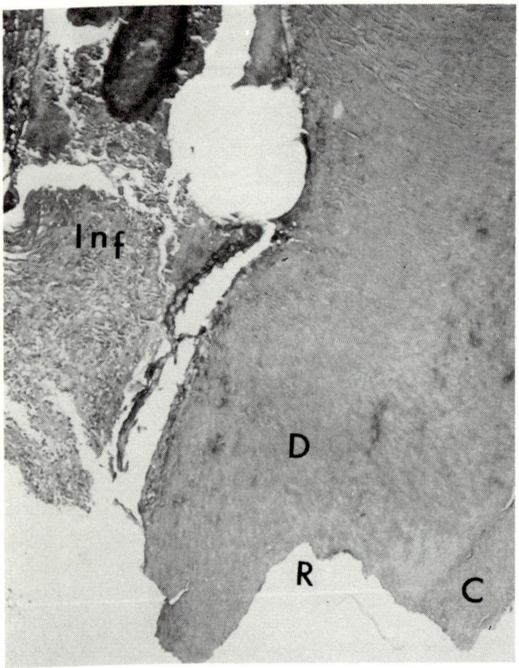

Figure 165. Root resorptions not repaired; Inf = inflammation, D = dentin, R = resorption, C = cementum (×96). (From S. Seltzer et al, "The Interrelationship of Pulp and Periodontal Disease," *Oral Surgery, Oral Medicine and Oral Pathology,* 16:1474, 1963.)

disease, periodontal disease, occlusal traumatism, cyst pressure, tumor pressure, and pressure from embedded or erupting teeth. It can occur following transplantation, replantation, luxation, radiation therapy, and orthodontic therapy. External root resorption may also be found in systemic disorders such as hypothyroidism, calcinosis, Gaucher's disease, hyperparathyroidism, Turner's syndrome, and Paget's disease. In the pulpally-induced external root resorption, it is believed that the rapid destruction of the root occurs as a result of osteoclastic stimulation from products released from highly virulent root canal microbes. There may be an associated periapical area of rarefaction, but this does not have to be present. Resorptions from periodontal disease are generally shallow and repaired by cementum (Fig. 164). However, sometimes they are deeper and are not repaired (Fig. 165). The root resorption resulting from cysts, tumors, embedded teeth, tooth eruption and orthodontic therapy is probably due to pressure. The resorption that results from replantation and transplantation procedures is apparently a manifestation of a rejection phenomenon. The etiology

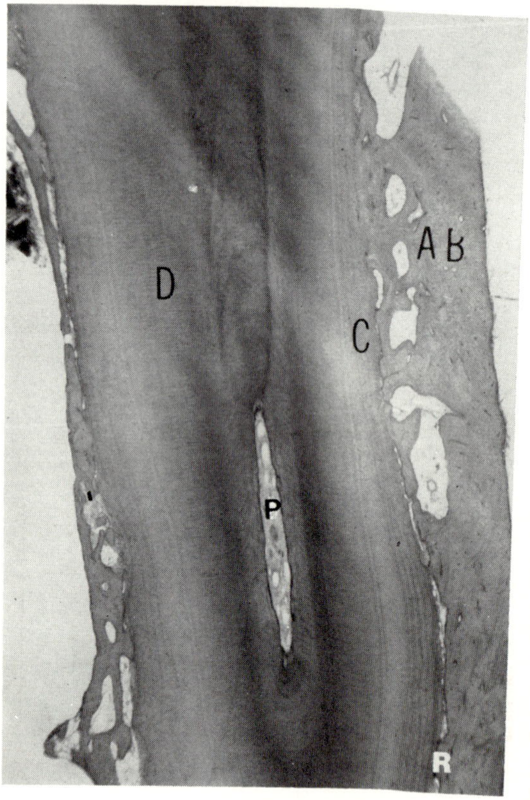

Figure 166. External resorption, ankylosis, and pulposis; D = dentin, C = cementum, AB = alveolar bone, R = resorption, P = pulposis (×8.6). (Courtesy of Dr. S. Seltzer, Philadelphia, Pa.)

of resorption resulting from systemic disorders is unknown but may be related to release of the hormone, parathormone at the local site. Ankylosis (union of bone to root) may occur in any form of external root resorption, probably as a result of destruction of portions of the periodontal ligament (Fig. 166). However, it is found most often along with external root resorption resulting from replantation and transplantation procedures. Resorption symptoms are related to the underlying condition. If pulpal in origin, the pulpal condition may be chronic pulpitis or necrosis. Manifestations of expanding cysts are tooth mobility, and change in the position of the involved teeth. Pain, both locally and referred, can result from tooth eruption. Tumor growth usually causes no symptoms. Root resorption from systemic causes is usually symptomless, as is root resorption resulting from transplantation, replantation, orthodontic movement, and periodontal disease.

The results of clinical tests for pulpally-induced external root resorption depends upon the underlying pulpal condition. In all other cases, except replantation and transplantation procedures, the pulps are vital and should give a normal response to pulp testing. The radiographic appearance of these type external root resorptions, as well as resorption related to orthodontic therapy, show an unevenly appearing root apex that has been shortened by several millimeters (Fig. 30). It may be possible to see the outline of the original length of the root on the radiograph for pulpally-induced cases (Fig. 80). External resorption resulting from cyst expansion, tumor growth, embedded teeth, tooth eruption and periodontal disease, shows various concavities in

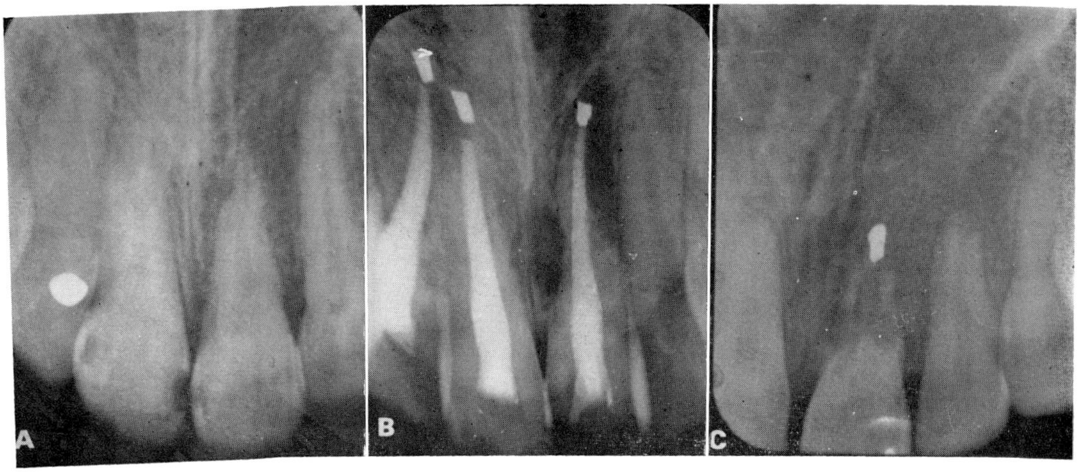

Figure 167. External root resorption in replanted teeth. A. No endodontics was performed, slight resorption is evident. B. Gutta-percha filling and a retrograde seal was placed; severe resorption. C. Only a retrograde was placed; extensive resorption. (From D. R. Morse, "The Significance of Endodontics in Plantation Procedures," *JDA South Africa*, 26:263, 1971)

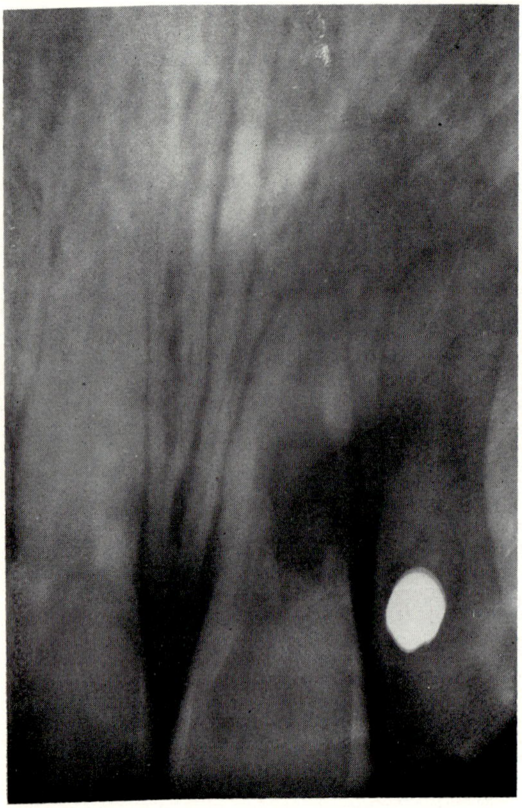

Figure 168. External or internal resorption; it is not possible to distinguish the two possibilities on this radiograph. (From S. Seltzer, *Endodontology,* McGraw-Hill, Inc., 1971. Used with permission of the McGraw-Hill Book Company.)

the surface of the root that is in proximity to the cyst, tumor, erupting tooth, or periodontal pocket (Fig. 81). The resorption resulting from transplantation and replantation appears on many external surfaces of the root and is often found close to the crown of the tooth (Fig. 167). The root resorption occurring in systemic disturbances usually occurs at the apex of several teeth and is bilateral (Fig. 79). Occasionally resorption is of unknown etiology (Fig. 83). When laterally occurring external resorption causes a pulp exposure, it is difficult to distinguish it from internal resorption that has perforated the root (Fig. 168). Vitality tests are not helpful as the pulp may respond vital in both conditions. If the cause of the external resorption can be seen on the radiograph (e.g. embedded tooth, deep pocket), then the two conditions may be differentiated.

The histologic appearance of external resorption shows osteoclastic destruction of the cementum and dentin. Osteoclasts, macrophages and lacunae are found (Fig. 169). In ankylosis, a direct union of the cementum to the alveolar bone is observed. No periodontal ligament is present in the region (Fig. 170).

The prognosis depends upon the underlying cause. Pulpally-induced external resorption usually ceases after successful endodontic therapy is performed (Fig. 80). External resorption due to other local causes is often repaired by amalgam insertion into a prepared cavity made in the resorption defect. The prognosis for this treatment is doubtful. A similar type treatment has been attempted for external resorption resulting from transplantation and replantation procedures. The results of this treatment have only been fair (Fig. 171). Other treatments for transplant and replant cases are fluorides, calcium hydroxide, and cell culture coating. One or all of these may prove to be helpful in inhibiting resorption. In external resorption occurring from systemic causes, treatment of the underlying sys-

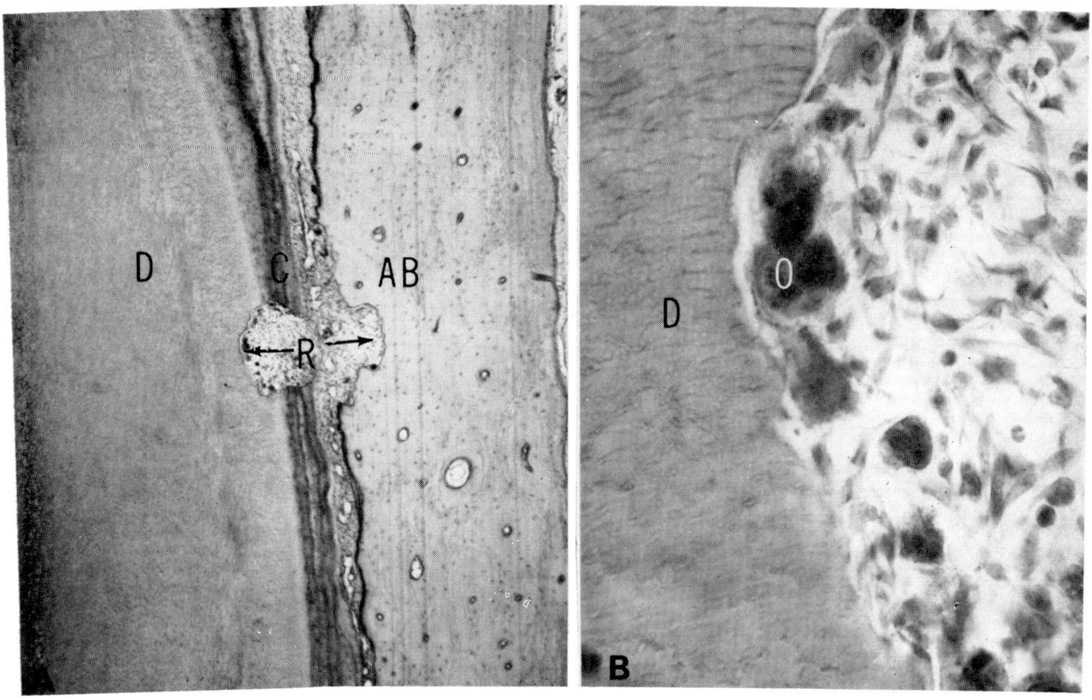

Figure 169. External resorption; histological section. A. D = dentin, C = cementum, R = resorption, AB = alveolar bone (×43.5). B. Higher magnification of area near left arrow; Howship's lacunae showing osteoclast resorbing dentin; D = dentin, O = osteoclast (×370). (From S. Seltzer, *Endodontology*, McGraw-Hill, Inc., 1971. Used with permission of McGraw-Hill Book Company.)

temic disease may cause the resorption to cease. With orthodontic therapy, once the treatment is completed, the resorption ceases.

Hypercementosis

This condition is an overgrowth of cementum. It can be caused by pulpal disease, disuse atrophy, systemic diseases such as Paget's disease (Fig. 17), hyperpituitarism, Cooley's anemia, sickle cell anemia, Gardner's syndrome, and for no apparent reason. The pulpally-induced hypercementosis may be present along with a periapical rarefaction. It may also be present concomitantly with condensing osteitis, or with no periapical lesion. Just as pulpally-induced external root resorption is believed to be caused by highly virulent root canal microbes, the reverse is suggested for the development of hypercementosis, as well as for condensing osteitis. For the latter two conditions, the root canal microbes are believed to be of low virulence. Symptoms are related to the underlying pulpal condition or systemic disease. Clinical test results also depend upon the underlying pulpal disease present. Periapical radio-

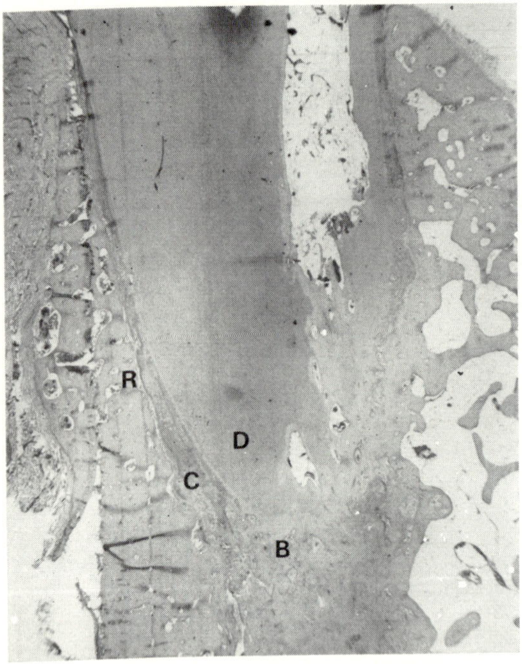

Figure 170. Ankylosis and external resorption; histologic section; D = dentin, B = bone, C = cementum, R = resorption (×8.3). (Courtesy of Dr. S. Seltzer, Philadelphia, Pa.)

graphs show a radiopaque knob-like extension of the root apexes. Condensing osteitis or periapical rarefactions may also be present (Fig. 172A). In systemically caused hypercementosis, the condition is found on many teeth and is bilateral (Fig. 172B). The teeth are all vital and should respond normally to pulp testing. Histological results show a large increase in cementum (either cellular, acellular, or both) in the apical region (Fig. 173). In pulpally-involved cases, prognosis for tooth retention is favorable after successful endodontic therapy. The hypercementosis does not revert to normal (as is the case with condensing osteitis) (Fig. 172). These teeth are very difficult to extract. Therefore, intentional replantation would be contraindicated. In systemically-induced cases of hypercementosis, the condition may stop following treatment of the underlying disease. However one condition, Paget's disease, is incurable.

Endodontic-Periodontic (Pulpodontic-Periodontic) Sydrome

This is a syndrome involving inflammation or degeneration of the pulp

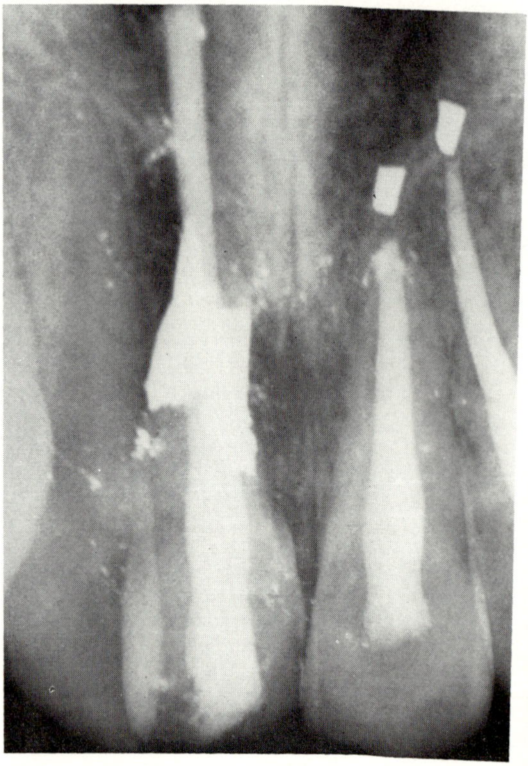

Figure 171. External resorption; attempted repair with amalgam; a replant case in which an endodontic implant was inserted and the resorption defect was sealed with amalgam. (From D. R. Morse, "The Significance of Endodontics in Plantation Procedures," *JDA South Africa*, 26:263, 1971.)

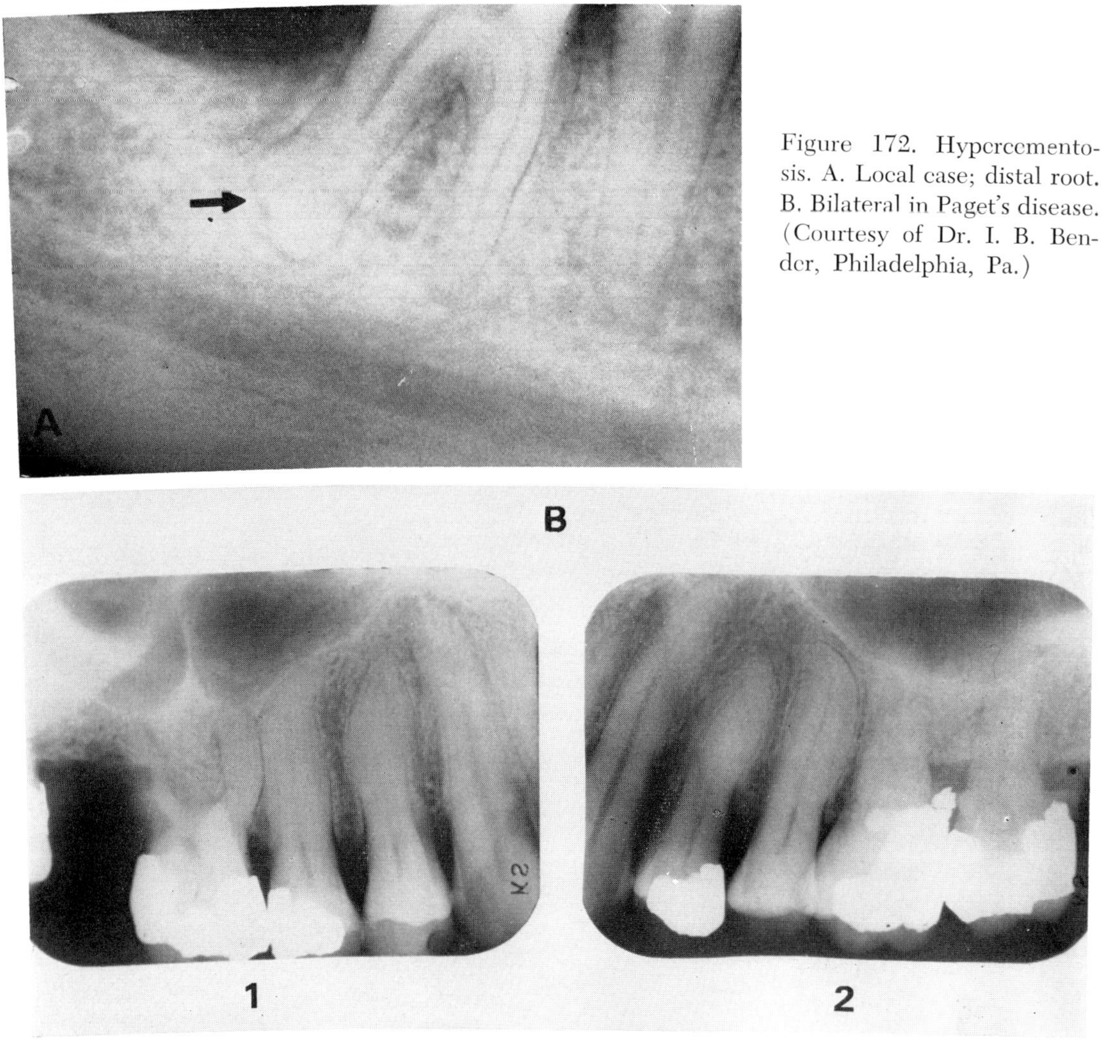

Figure 172. Hypercementosis. A. Local case; distal root. B. Bilateral in Paget's disease. (Courtesy of Dr. I. B. Bender, Philadelphia, Pa.)

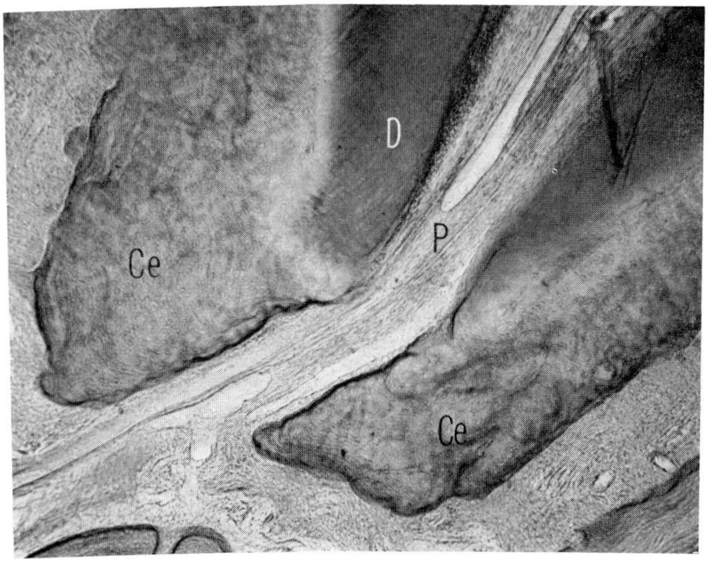

Figure 173. Hypercementosis (Cementum hyperplasia); histologic section; Ce = cementum, D = dentin, P = pulp (×47.5). (From S. Seltzer, *Endodontology*, McGraw-Hill, Inc., 1971. Used with permission of McGraw-Hill Book Company.)

with a clinical pocket on the same tooth. There is a cause and effect relationship between the two disease processes. The syndrome can be initiated by either pulpal or periodontal disease.

Etiology

(1) The interrelationship of the two disease processes is based primarily on the presence of lateral and accessory canals, apically, laterally, and in furcation areas. As there are more of these canals found in molars, this syndrome is more prevalent in molars (Figs. 174, 175). Patients with periodontal disease may have lateral and accessory canals that were previously covered with cementum, become exposed as the result of the inflammatory process. This can lead to microbial and tissue breakdown irritants entering the pulp.

(2) The same outcome can occur as the result of root planing during periodontal treatment.

(3) Also, during periodontal treatment, root desensitizing agents may be used, with resultant chemicals entering the pulp via lateral canals, dentinal tubules, or through the dentin.

(4) The endodontic-periodontic syndrome can also result from an apical inflammatory response progressing toward the crestal and interradicular bone (Fig. 175H).

(5) Other pathways are via sinus tracts opening into the furca or into the gingival sulcus (Fig. 175H). The inflammatory products might then act to cause bone destruction in those regions.

(6) Root perforations, perforating root caries, root fractures, and perforating cases of internal resorption can also lead to pocket and furca formation (Fig. 175).

(7) Also, rapid nonphysiological orthodontic tooth movement can lead to furcation involvements and indirect pulp involvements. Inflammatory products can diffuse pulpally via lateral canals and dentinal tubules (Fig. 175D).

(8) Long standing occlusal traumatism may also contribute to pulpal degeneration (Fig. 175N).

Various possible causes of the endodontic-periodontic syndrome and other endodontic-periodontic interrelationships are shown in Figure 175.

Clinical Manifestations

The signs, symptoms, and test results depend upon the initiating factors.

(1) *Pain*—The presence of pain is generally indicative of endodontic disease. Mild to moderate pain can occur in periodontal disease, but severe pain is almost invariably indicative of endodontic disease. Pain caused by destructive occlusal forces usually occurs when contact is made between opposing teeth, or soon after. The pain may be severe, but usually not as severe as the pain associated with pulpal or periapical inflammation. The pain is usually short-lived. Pain experienced on awakening or during tense

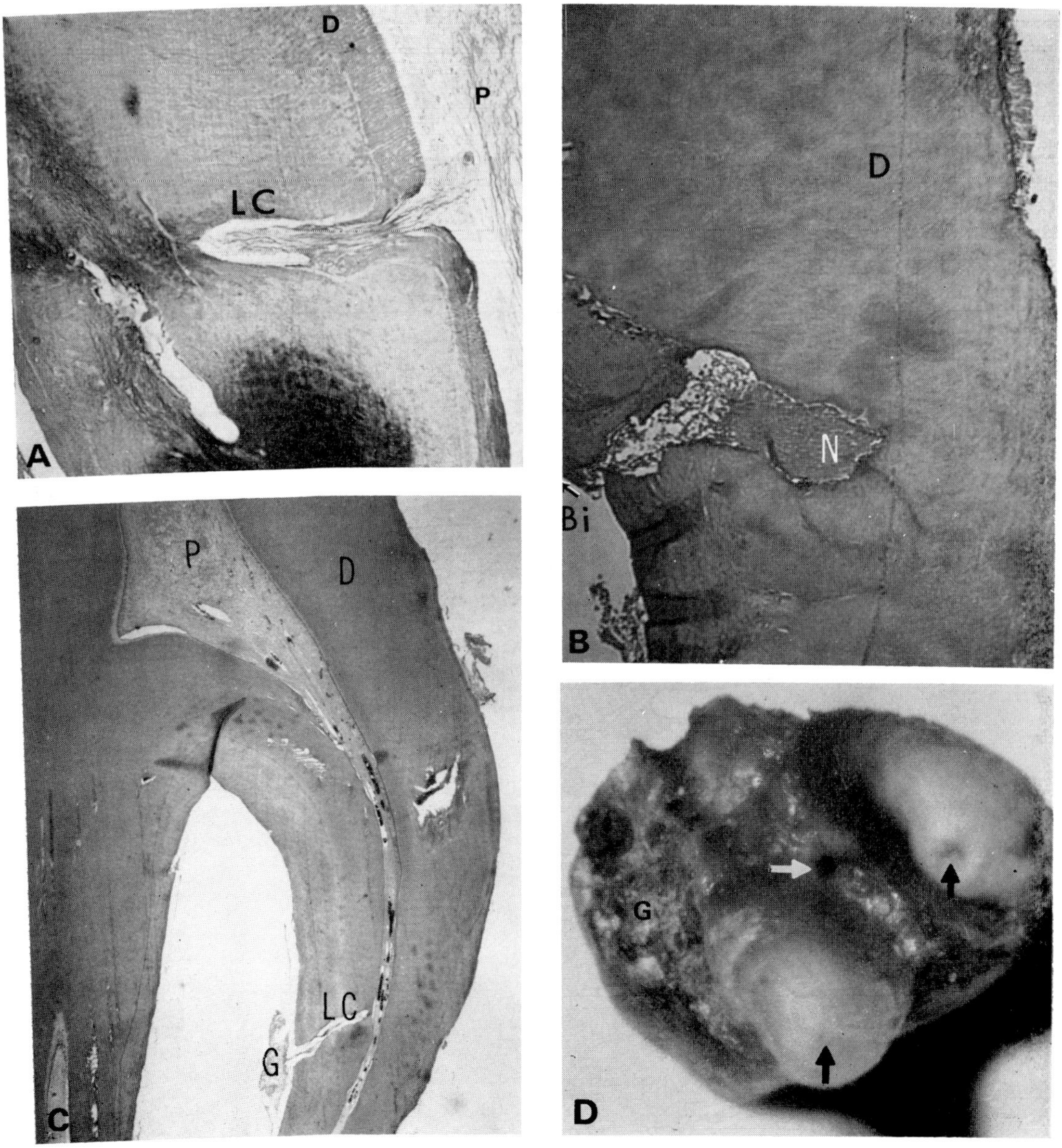

Figure 174. Lateral canals; histologic sections. A. Lateral canal with vital tissue; LC = lateral canal, D = dentin, P = pulp (×96). B. Lateral canal with necrotic tissue; D = dentin, Bi = bifurcation area, N = necrosis, D = dentin (×96). (From S. Seltzer et al, "The Interrelationship of Pulp and Periodontal Disease," *Oral Surgery, Oral Medicine and Oral Pathology,* 16:1474, 1963). C. Lateral canal with attached furcation granuloma; P = pulp, D = dentin, LC = lateral canal, G = granulomatous tissue (×8.4). (From S. Seltzer, *Endodontology,* McGraw-Hill, Inc., 1971. Used with permission of McGraw-Hill Book Company.) D. Extracted lower molar with the roots facing the reader showing a furcation lateral canal (white arrow); black arrows point to apical foramina; G = granuloma. (Courtesy of Dr. L. Muldorf, Philadelphia, Pa.)

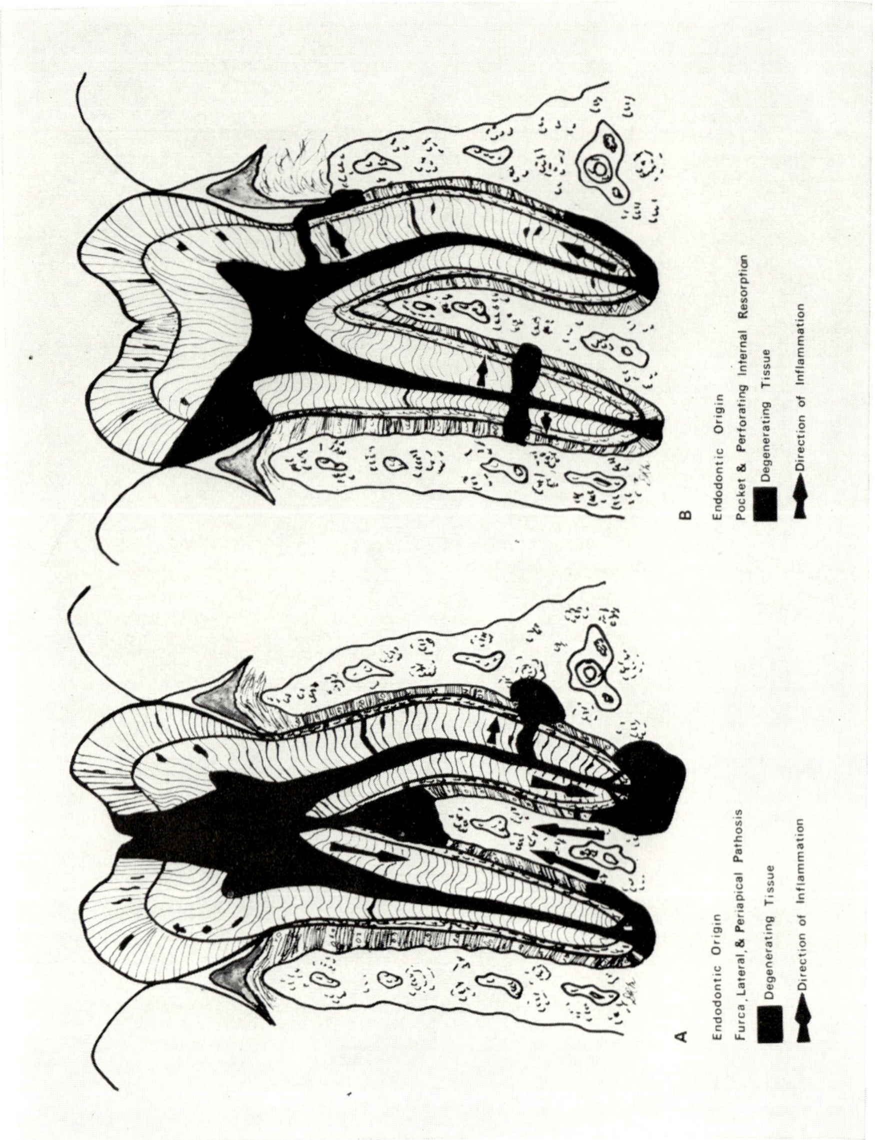

Figure 175 A-N. Various possible causes of the endodontic-periodontic syndrome and other endodontic-periodontic interrelationships.

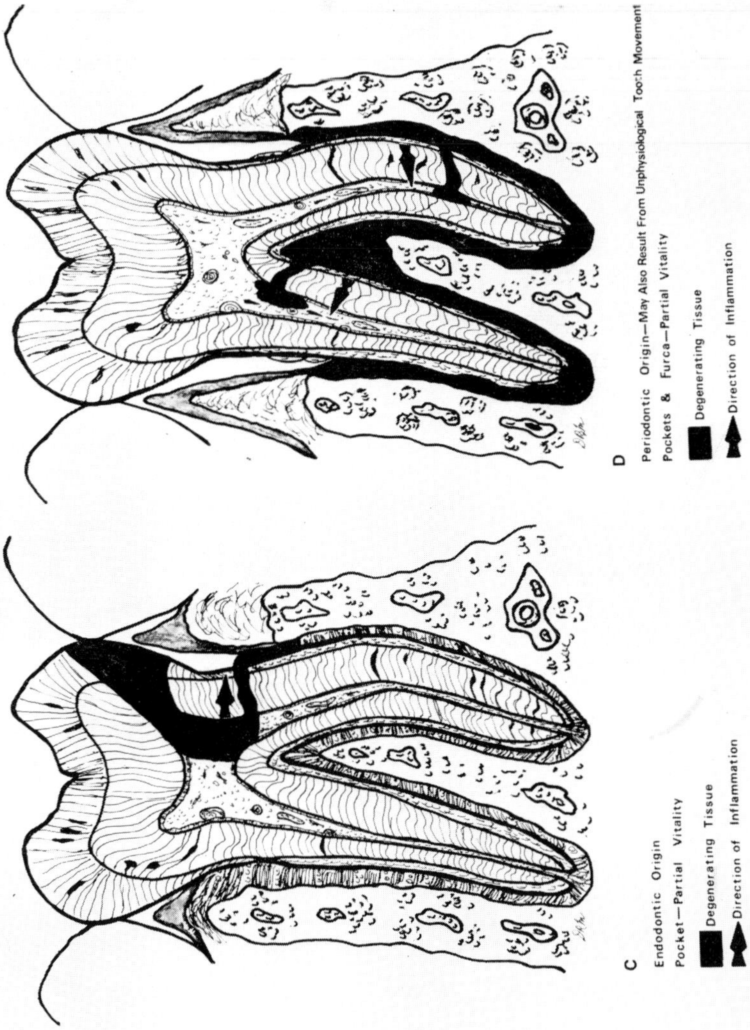
C
Endodontic Origin
Pocket—Partial Vitality
Degenerating Tissue
Direction of Inflammation
D
Periodontic Origin—May Also Result From Unphysiological Tooth Movement
Pockets & Furca—Partial Vitality
Degenerating Tissue
Direction of Inflammation

Figure 175

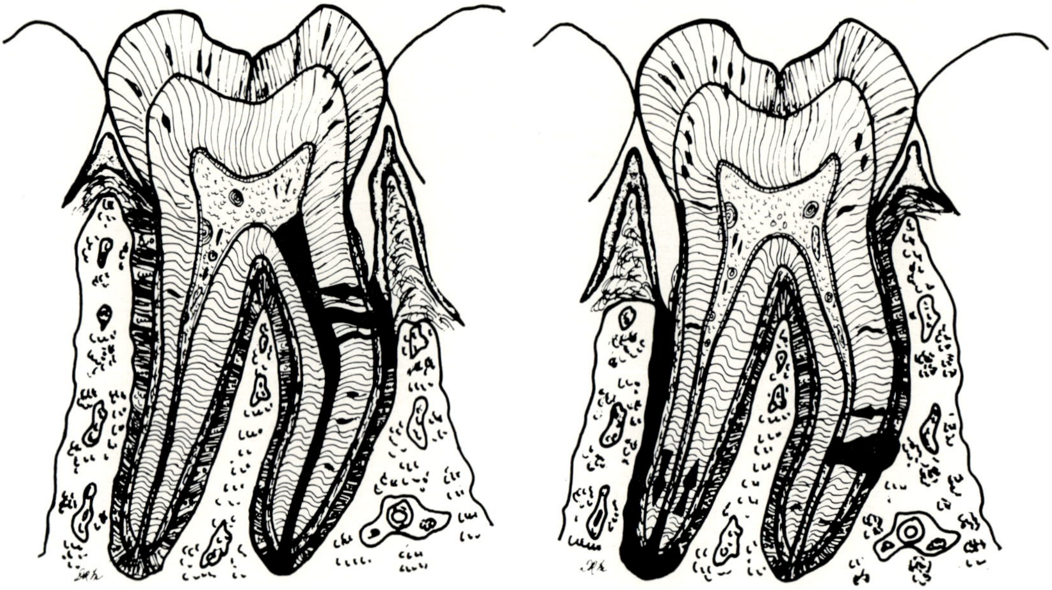

E

Periodontic Origin— Disease or Treatment (Root Planing, Hypersensivity) (Treatment)

Pocket— Partial Vitality

Degenerating Tissue

Direction of Inflammation

F

Periodontic Origin

Pocket, Perforating External Resorption—Partial Vitality

Degenerating Tissue

Direction of Inflammation

Figure 175

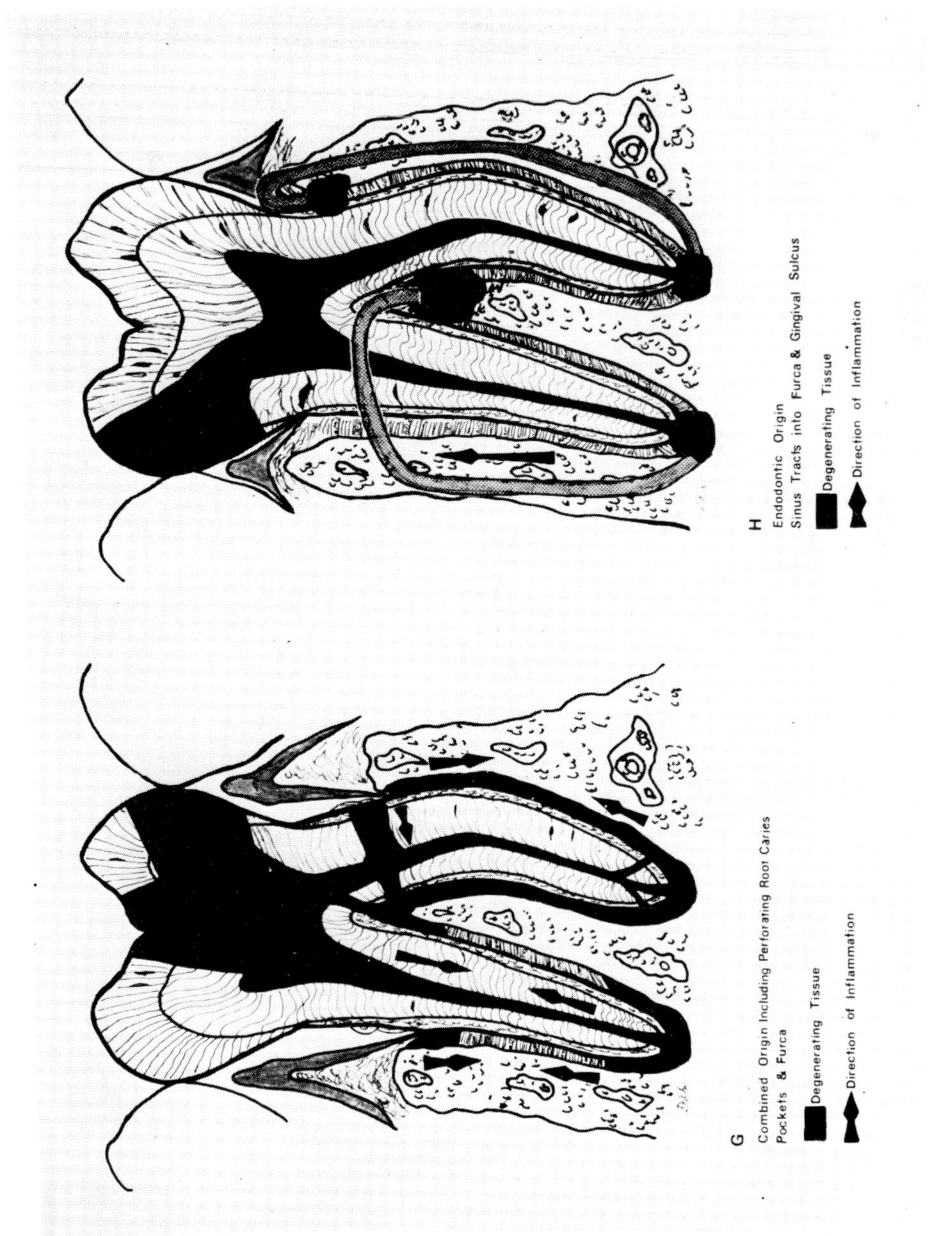
G
Combined Origin Including Perforating Root Caries
Pockets & Furca
Degenerating Tissue
Direction of Inflammation
H
Endodontic Origin
Sinus Tracts into Furca & Gingival Sulcus
Degenerating Tissue
Direction of Inflammation

Figure 175

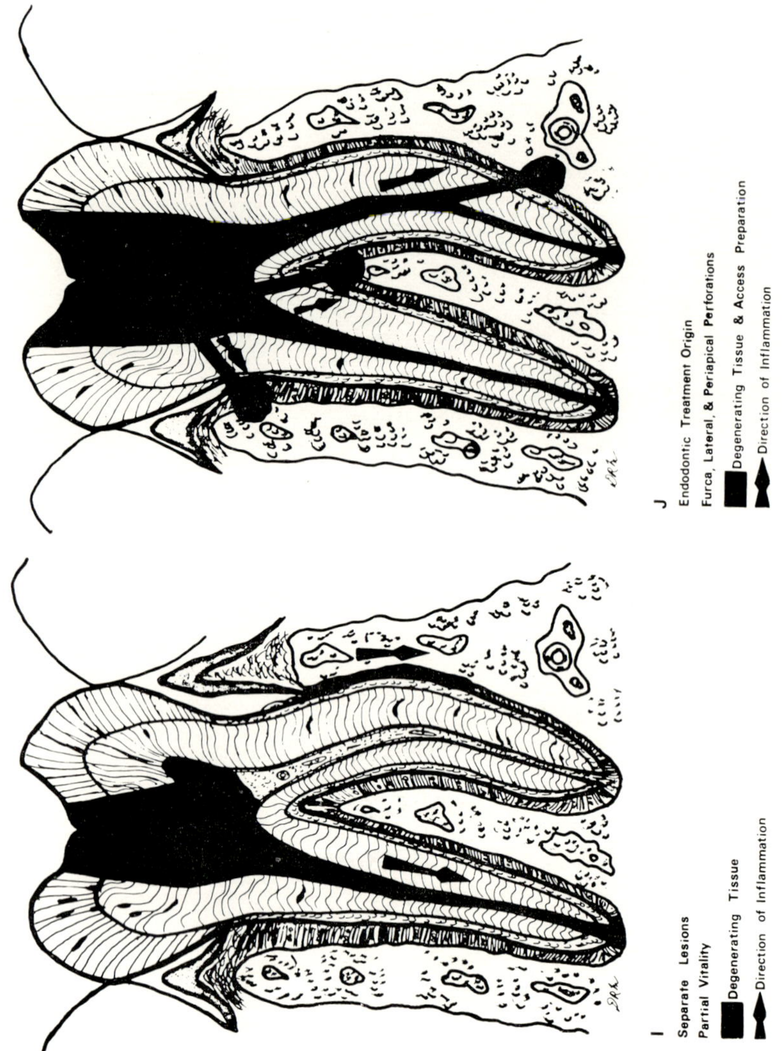
I
Separate Lesions
Partial Vitality
Degenerating Tissue
Direction of Inflammation
J
Endodontic Treatment Origin
Furca, Lateral, & Periapical Perforations
Degenerating Tissue & Access Preparation
Direction of Inflammation

Figure 175

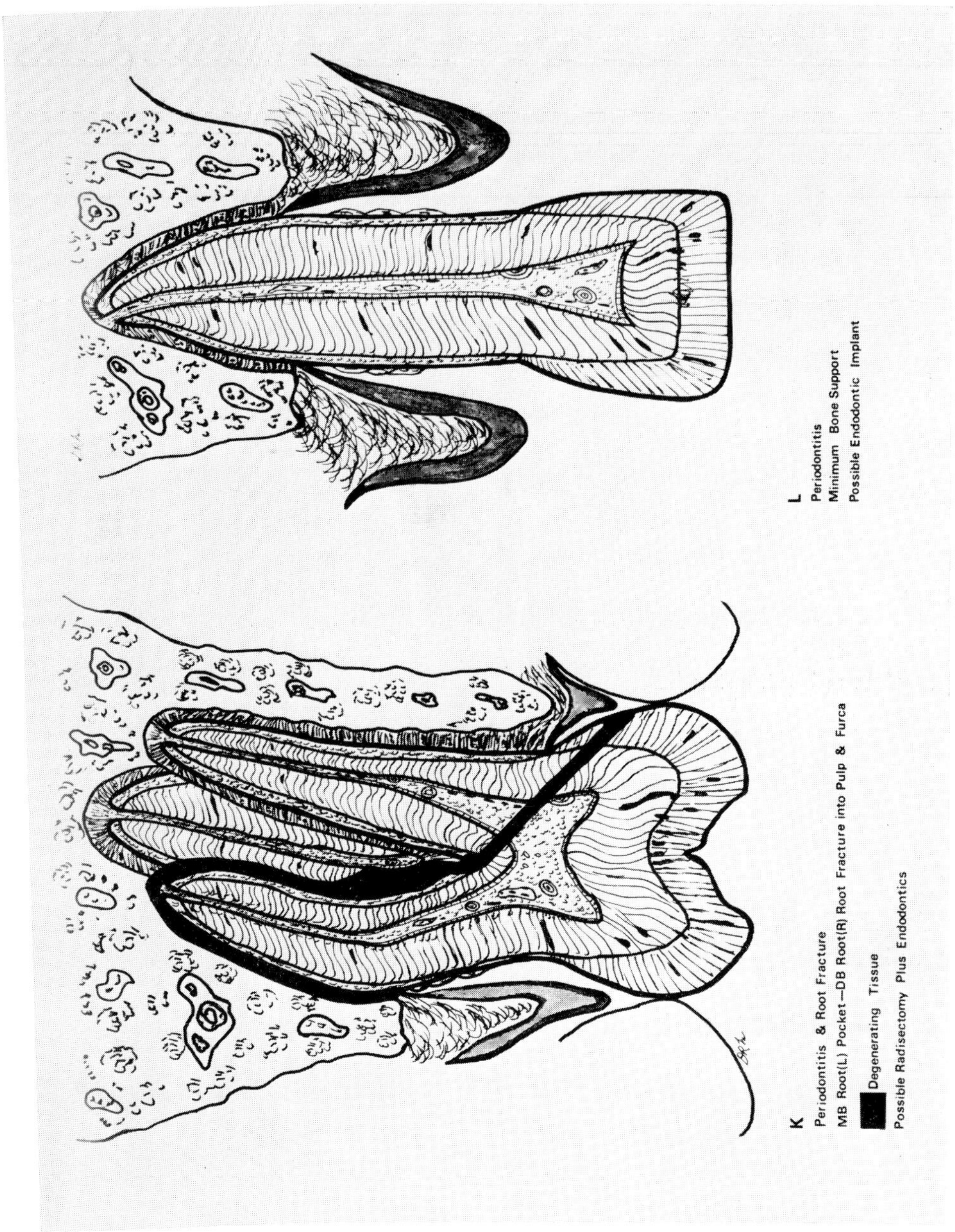
K
Periodontitis & Root Fracture
MB Root(L) Pocket—DB Root(R) Root Fracture into Pulp & Furca
Degenerating Tissue
Possible Radisectomy Plus Endodontics
L
Periodontitis
Minimum Bone Support
Possible Endodontic Implant

Figure 175

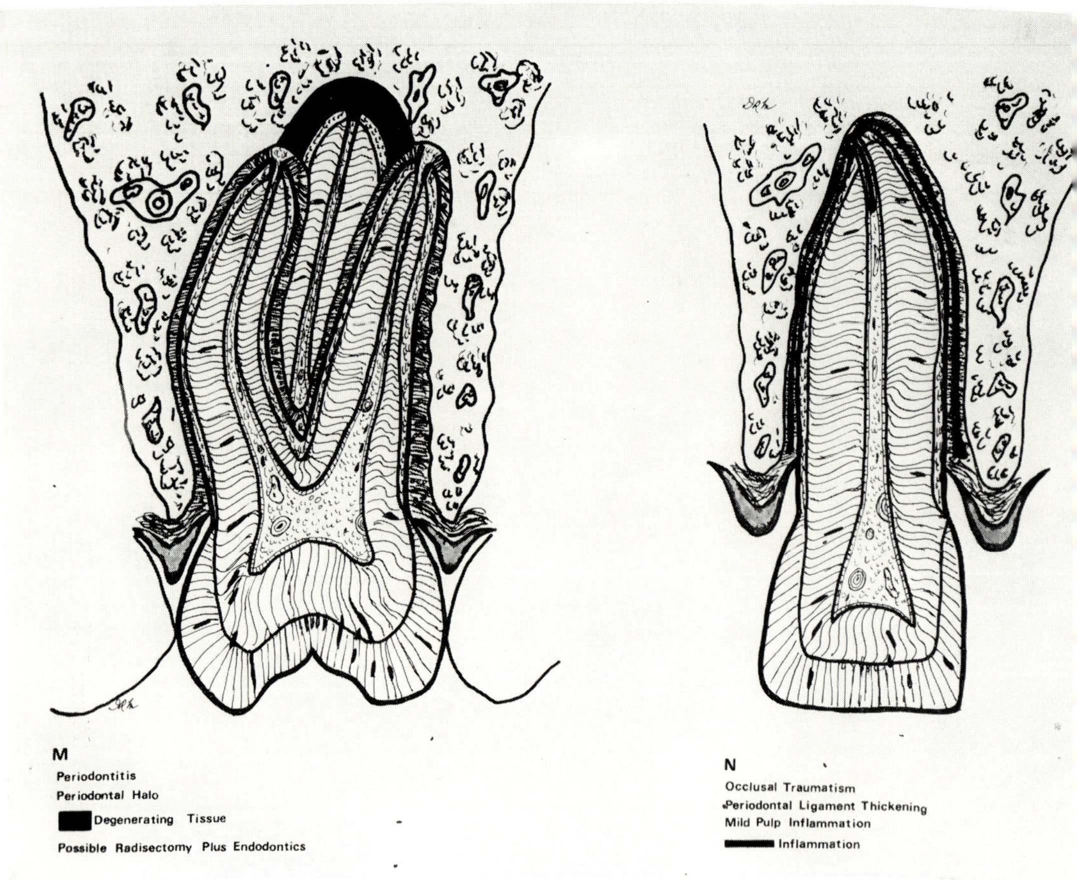

Figure 175

periods is usually related to bruxism.

(2) *Swelling*—Swelling resulting from pulpal-periapical disease occurs in the mucobuccal fold (Fig. 149) and/or in one of the superficial or deep spaces, such as the canine, buccal, submaxillary, or sublingual spaces (Figs. 46, 47, 130). In periodontal disease, the swelling is usually limited to the labial (buccal) or lingual (palatal) gingiva or alveolar mucosa (Figs. 222-225). The onset of pain and swelling is usually rapid in cases of endodontic origin. In cases of periodontal origin, the manifestations are generally chronic.

Diagnostic Tests and Visual Examination Results

(1) *Pulp Tests*—With periodontal disease, pulp test findings are usually normal. With endodontic disease, if the pulp is necrotic,

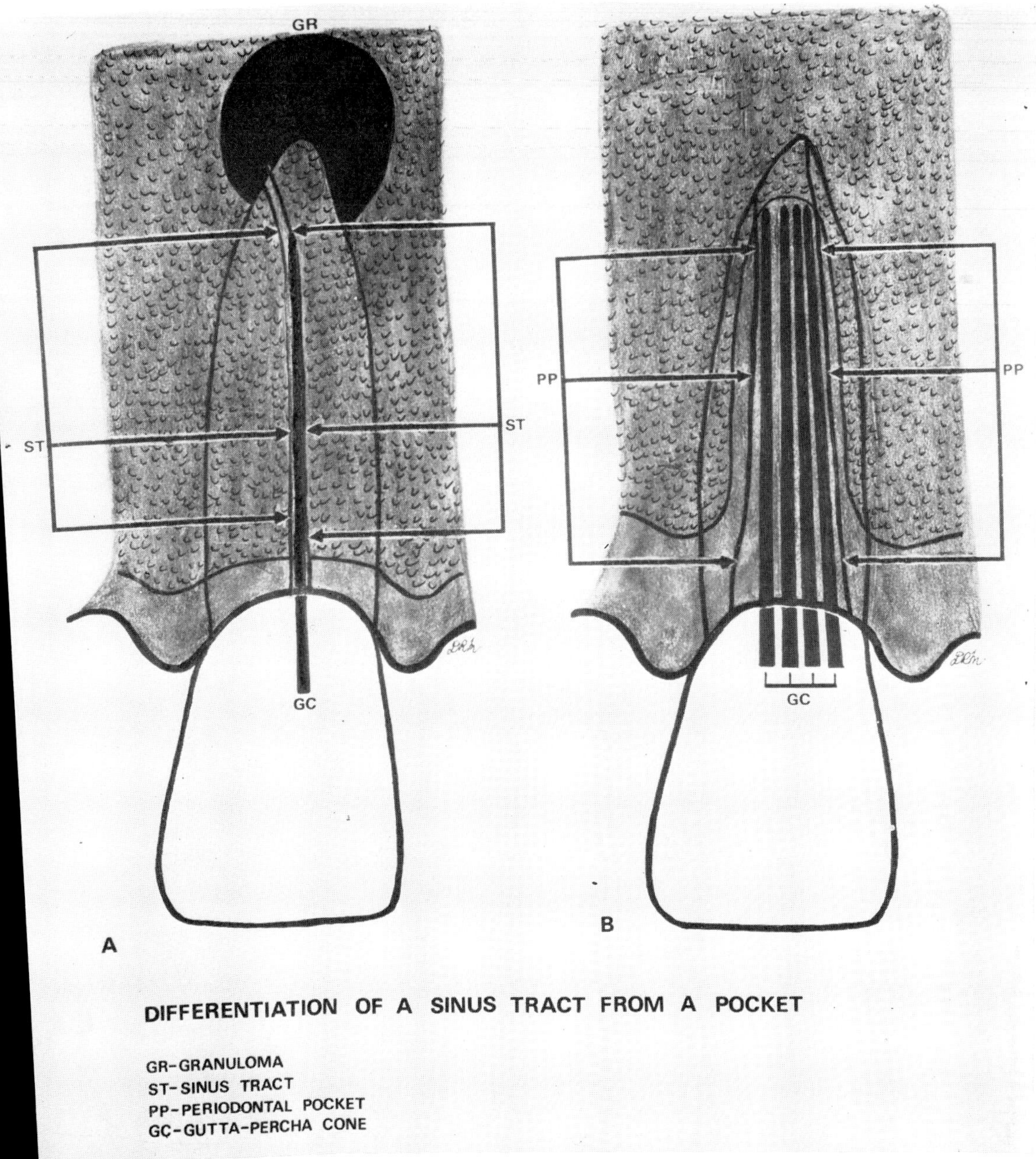

Figure 176. Differentiation of a sinus tract from a pocket. A. Sinus tract. B. Pocket.

there will be no response to the electric pulp tester, thermal tests or test drilling.

(2) *Visual Examination*

(a) When there is no sign of caries, shallow caries, shallow restorations, or normal appearing crowns, then periodontal disease is the usual initiating factor.

(b) In pockets and furca involvement of endodontic origin, calculus is usually absent, unless the lesions are long standing (not usual as these cases are generally acute). In periodontally originating pockets, furca and calculus is often present (these cases are usually chronic).

(3) *Probing*—Probing of sinus tracts and pockets also helps to distinguish the initiating factors. Presence of a sinus tract indicates endodontic disease, while pocket presence indicates periodontal disease, although it is possible for a sinus tract to lead into a furcation or other periodontal defect. If a sinus tract opens into the gingival sulcus, then usually only one diagnostic wire can be inserted into it. If several wires or probes can be inserted, then the lesion is a periodontal pocket (Fig. 176).

(4) *Radiographic Findings*—In the case of periodontal disease, the radiographic findings usually show that several teeth have bone loss, with or without furca involvement (Figs. 88, 177). If a furcation involvement is isolated

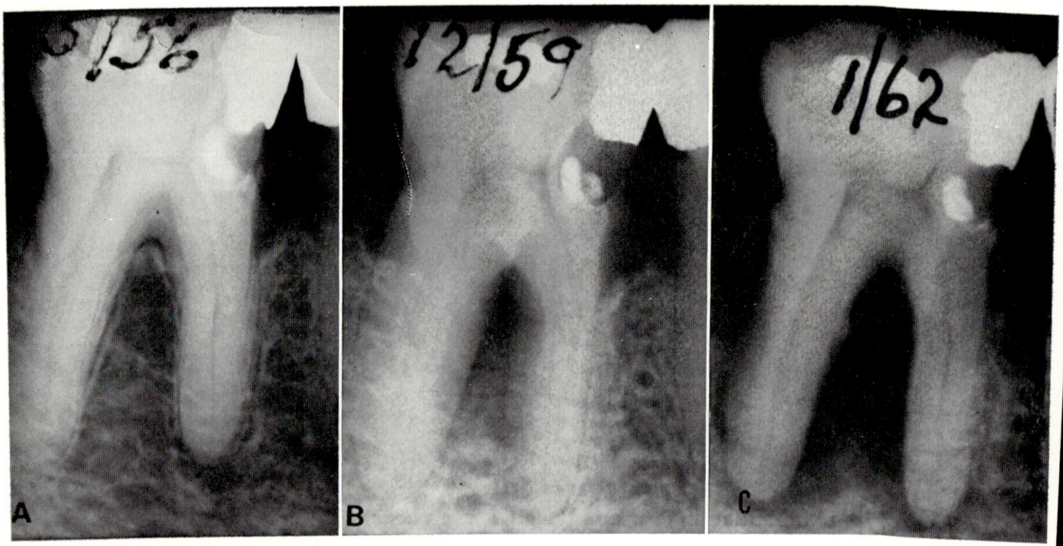

Figure 177. Endodontic-periodontic syndrome, periodontic origin; 6-year progression (Courtesy of Dr. W. Updegrave, Philadelphia, Pa.). A. Slight furcation involvement. B. Three years later; deeper furca is present; slight alveolar *bone loss*. C. Three years later; severe periodontal bone destruction in furca region and around distal root.

to one tooth, and the alveolar crest bone is normal, then the case is probably of endodontic origin (Figs. 178, 179). With a lateral *area* and no pocket (probing fails to reach the area), the case is usually of endodontic origin (Fig. 180). It has been shown by histological examination that it is possible to have an intact epithelial attachment (no clinical pocket) and still have periodontal fiber and bone destruction at a more apical level. Therefore, a sinus tract and a lateral *area* can develop from a periodontitis, even though there is no detectable pocket. It has been postulated that the cause of the periodontal fiber and bone breakdown with the intact attachment, is the release of microbial products through the epithelium into the periodontal fibers and alveolar bone. This type case would present a diagnostic problem because there would be a sinus tract and lateral *area;* the tooth would test vital; and pocket probing would reveal no abnormality. A radiolucent halo around the palatal root of an upper molar often occurs in a tooth affected with chronic periodontitis and occlusal traumatism. The tooth usually tests vital, although the apical pulp may be necrotic (Figs. 175M, 181). Also, periodontally involved teeth often have extensive root resorption and root canal calcifications (Figs. 164, 182).

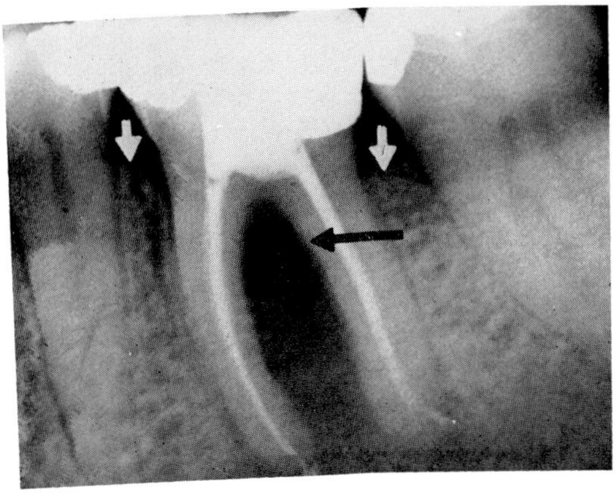

Figure 178. Endodontic-periodontic syndrome, endodontic origin, furca involvement. Black arrow; normal level of interproximal bone. (From D. R. Morse, "The Management of Endodontic Problem Cases," *JDA South Africa*, 27:387, 1972)

(5) *Histologic Results*—Histologic findings show granulomatous tissue in the apical, lateral and furcation regions. If the furcation lesion is of endodontic origin, there is usually no epithelial lining (Fig. 183). However, if it is of periodontal origin, epithelial migration usually has occurred, and an epithelial lining can be found (Fig. 184).

Prognosis

The prognosis depends upon the etiological factors. Cases of endodontic origin have a much better prognosis than cases of periodontic or combined origin.

Treatment Planning

Treatment also depends upon the initiating factors. If the case is of endodontic origin, then nonsurgical endodontic therapy is often all that is necessary for complete regeneration of lateral, apical, and furcation areas of rare-

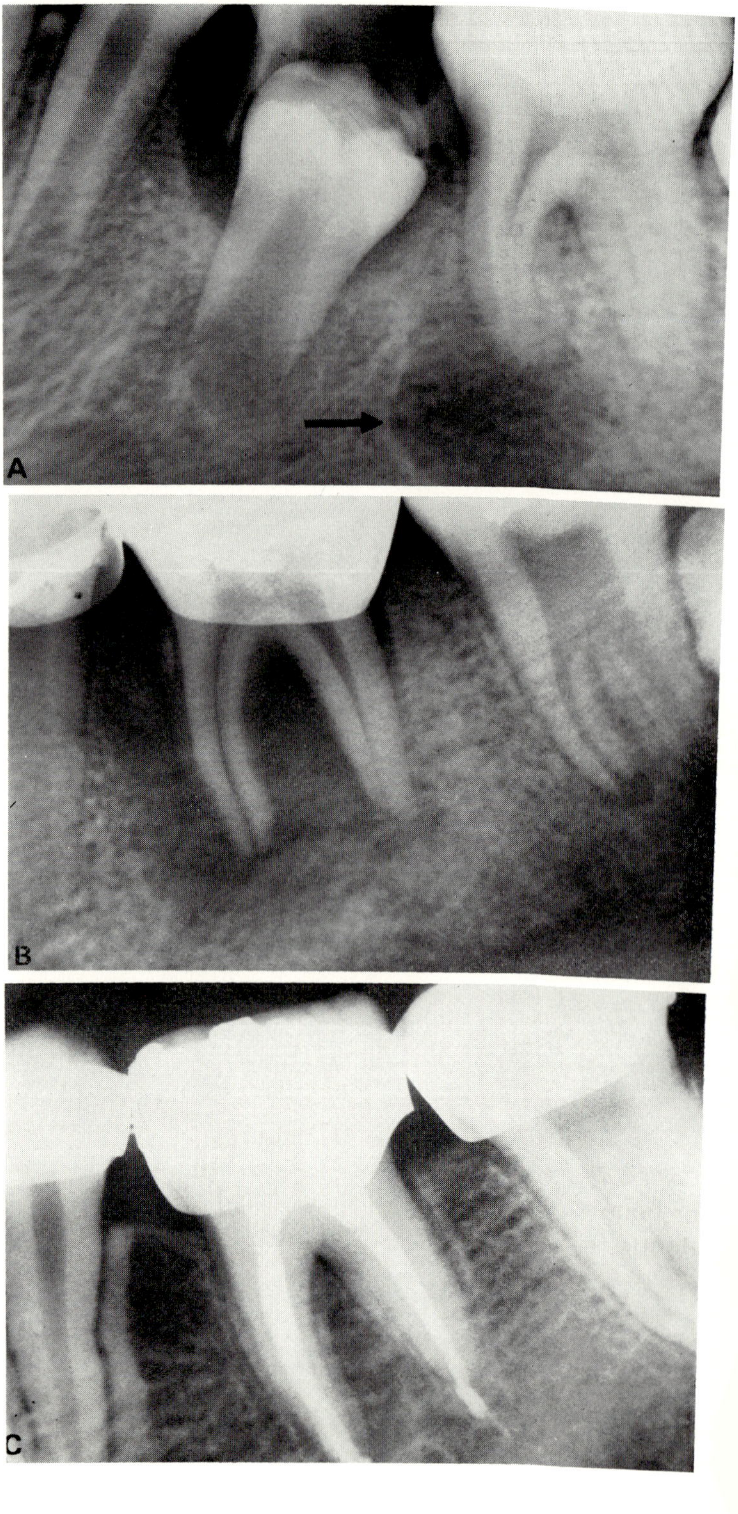

Figure 179. Endodontic-periodontic syndrome; endodontic origin. A. Periapical *area* present on mesial root of lower first molar; tooth was not treated because patient failed to show up for appointments. B. One year later; extensive destruction of furca, apical, and mesial regions. C. Two years after completion of endodontic therapy (gutta-percha-chloropercha obturation), bone repair is evident.

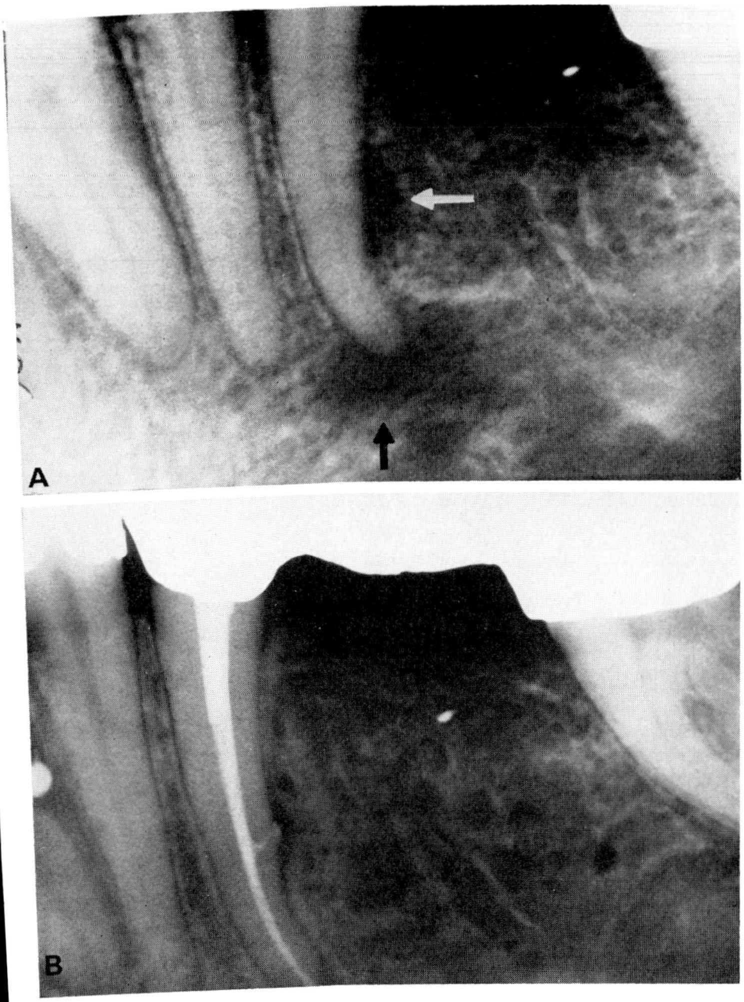

Figure 180. Lateral *area;* endodontic origin. A. Before treatment; lateral *area*—white arrow; periapical *area*—black arrow. B. One year after completion of endodontic therapy, lateral canal sealed; canals filled with gutta-percha-chloropercha; *areas* are healing.

faction. When the case is of periodontic origin, periodontal treatments must be instituted first. If a case does not resolve (e.g. pain or swelling doesn't decrease, pocket depth doesn't diminish or bone doesn't regenerate), then endodontic therapy should be performed. At times, root resection, hemisection, or endodontic implantation may be necessary for cases requiring combined endodontic and periodontic treatment. For treatment of these various categories, see Chapters 9 through 12.

Oral Pathways of Infection

Once an infectious process has reached the periapical region, there are several possible pathways of infection (Fig. 185). The paths and possible results of a typical exudate are the following:

(1) Root canal into the *apical periodontal ligament;* where an *acute* or *chronic apical periodontitis* may develop, may also go into the *lateral periodontal*

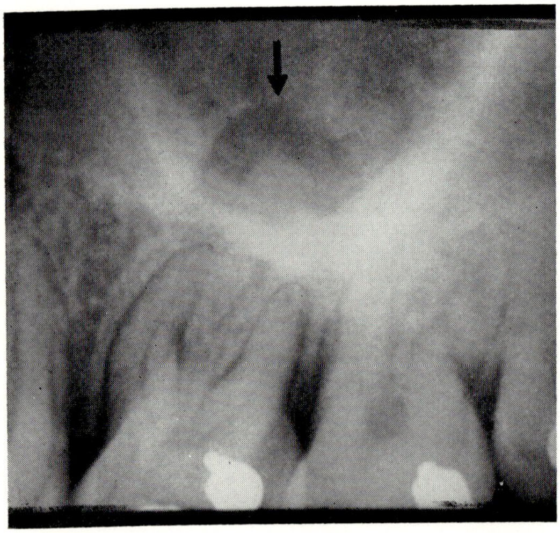

Figure 181. Palatal *halo*, this is indicative of periodontal disease on the palatal root; the pulp is usually vital.

ligament and form a *periodontitis,* then through the

(2) *lamina dura.* When the irritant is of low grade and the host resistance is high, a proliferative reaction of the alveolar bone can occur resulting in a *condensing osteitis;* in other cases directly into the

(3) *marrow spaces,* where depending upon the microbial virulence and the host's resistance the following entities can develop: *acute apical abscess, granuloma, cyst,* or an *osteomyelitis.* The exudate can then bore through the

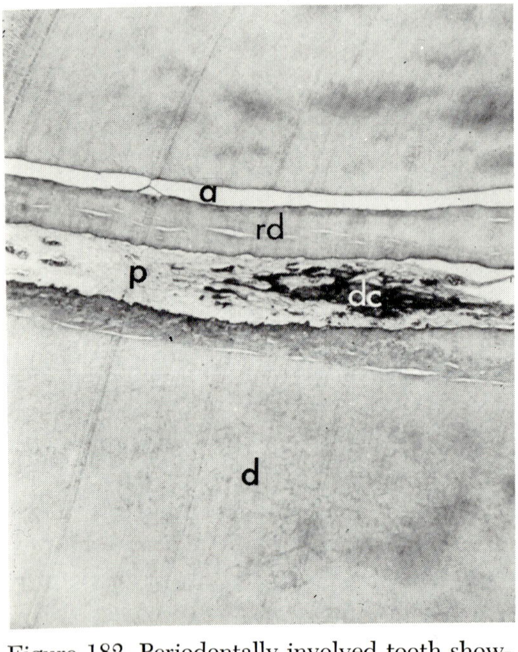

Figure 182. Periodontally involved tooth showing dystrophic calcification of the pulp; a = artifact, rd = reparative dentin, p = pulp, dc = dystrophic calcification, d = dentin. (From S. Seltzer et al, "The Dynamics of Pulp Inflammation: Correlation Between Diagnostic Data and Actual Histologic Findings in the Pulp," *Oral Surgery, Oral Medicine, and Oral Pathology,* 16:846, 1963.)

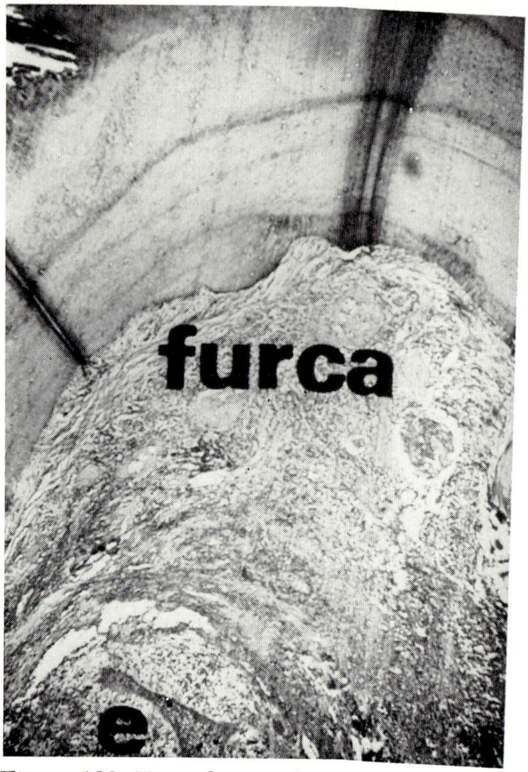

Figure 183. Furca lesion of endodontic origin; granulomatous tissue is evident with scattered epithelium (e) present (×35). (Courtesy of Dr. S. Seltzer, Philadelphia, Pa.)

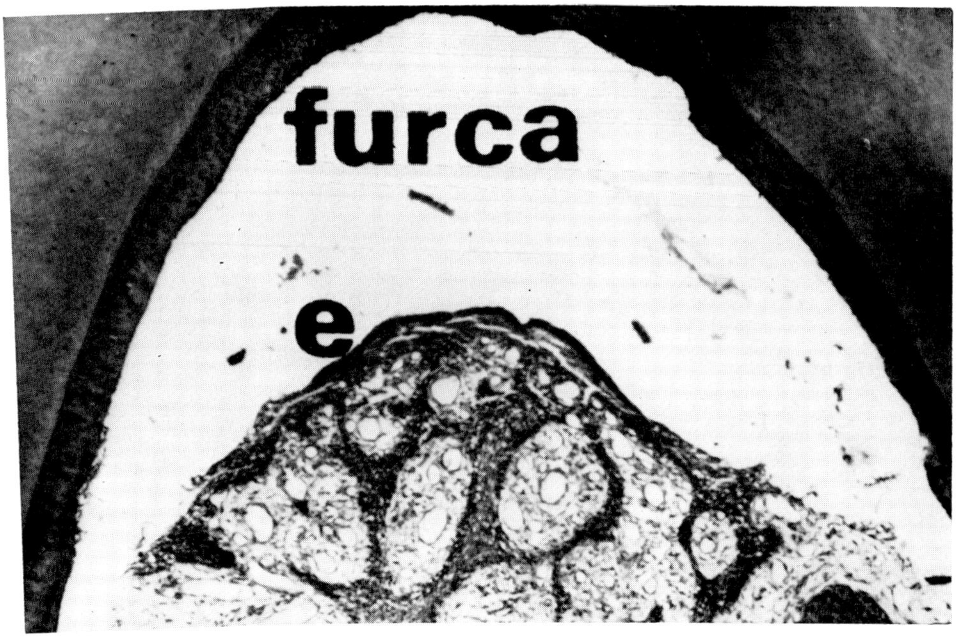

Figure 184. Furca lesion of periodontic origin; an epithelial lining is evident (e) (×35). (Courtesy of Dr. S. Seltzer, Philadelphia, Pa.)

(4) *cortex.* When the cortex is penetrated, then radiographic visualization of an *acute apical abscess, granuloma,* or *radicular cyst* occurs. If bone destruction continues, penetration can occur into either the region of the *nasal fossa* producing a *nasal abscess, maxillary sinus,* producing a *maxillary sinusitis* (which may produce in a radiograph a radiopaque thickening at base of sinus), or *inferior alveolar canal* (or mental foramen) producing an inflammation of the inferior alveolar nerve with a resultant *paresthesia.* The fluid can next reach the

(5) *mucoperiosteum.* When the exudate reaches this point, it is temporarily checked by the dense tissue, and a *subperiosteal abscess* can develop. When enough fluid accumulates, a swelling occurs and this is manifested clinically as a *parulis* (stoma, gum boil) (Fig. 149). From this region, several alternative pathways are possible. The subperiosteal abscess can perforate the labial (buccal) or lingual (palatal) mucosa and drain into the

(6) oral vestibule, producing an *oral vestibule abscess.*

(7) A *sinus tract* can form from the subperiosteal abscess and create a path somewhere along the alveolar mucosa (not necessarily close to the involved tooth) and drain into the oral vestible forming an *oral vesti-*

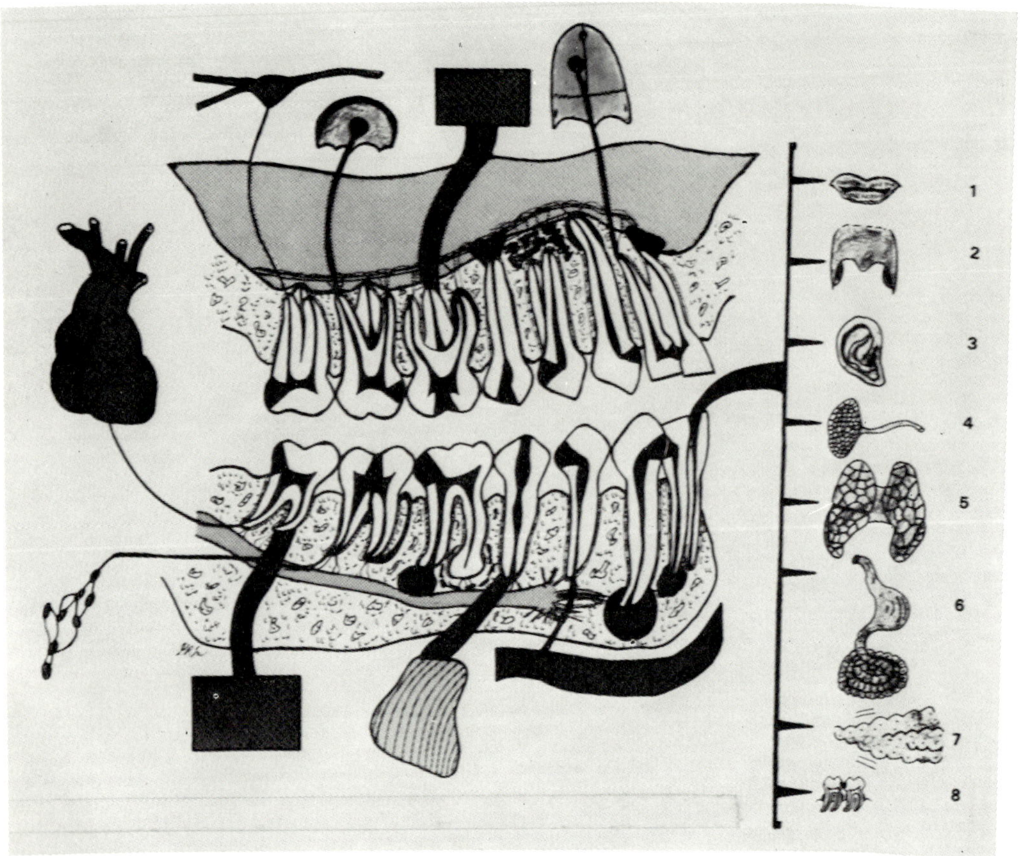

UC—Into Nasal Fossa
UL—Into Palate
UCa—Apical Periodontitis &/or Acute Apical Abscess
U1P—Osteomyelitis
U2P—Into Maxillary Sinus
U1M MB—Into Periodontal Ligament
U1M P—Superficial Cellulitis
U2M—Into Vestibule
U3M—To Cavernous Sinus
L3M D—To Heart
L3M M—Deep Cellulitis
L2M D—To Lymph Nodes
L2M M—Into Sulcus
L1M D—Paresthesia
L1M M—Hypercementosis & Condensing Osteitis
L2P—To Muscle
L1P—Into Skin
LCa—Cyst
LL—Granuloma
LC—Into Oral Cavity
1 Lips
2 Tonsils
3 Ear
4 Parotid
5 Lungs
6 GI Tract
7 Air Pollution
8 Caries & Periodontal Disease

Figure 185. General paths of endodontic infection.

bule abscess.

(8) The sinus tract can also drain through the gingival sulcus or a periodontal pocket creating a *gingival sinus tract.*

(9) At times the tract can be through the cheeks and drainage occurs via the skin resulting in a *skin sinus tract.* Most common sites are chin (lower anteriors—Fig. 53), angle of mandible (lower posteriors—Fig. 416), cheek (upper posteriors), nasal-labial area (upper anteriors).

(10) Rather than draining from the

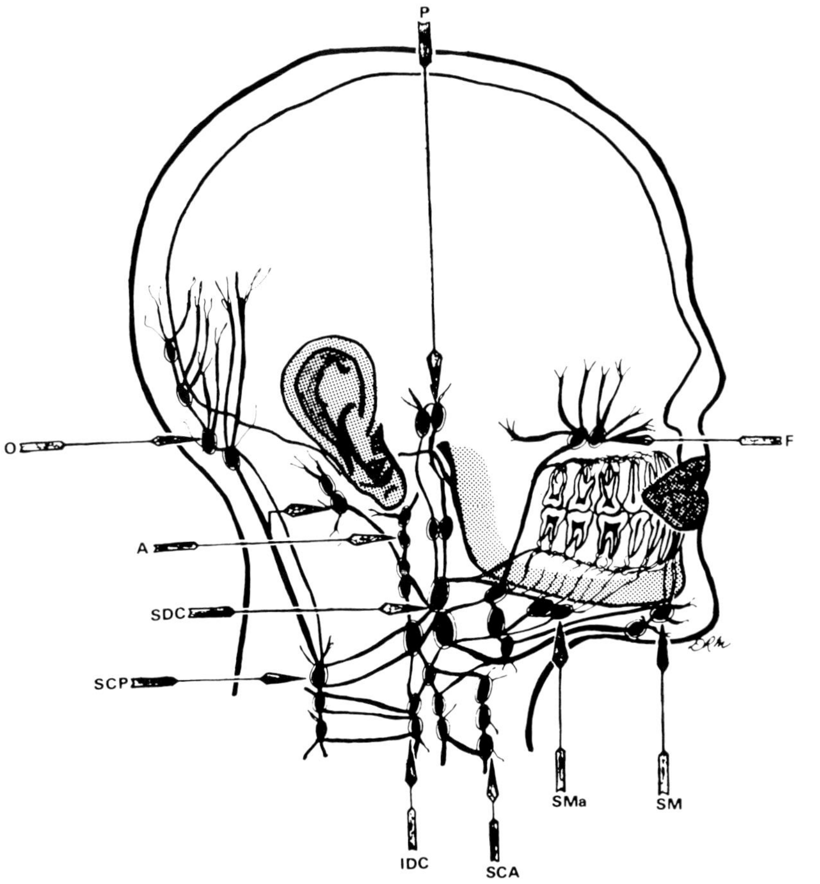

LYMPHATIC DRAINAGE OF HEAD AND NECK

VARIOUS LYMPH NODES
P—Parotid
O—Occipital
A—Auricular
SDC—Superior Deep Cervical
SCP—Superficial Cervical-Posterior
IDC—Inferior Deep Cervical
SCA—Superficial Cervical—Anterior
SMa—Submaxillary
SM—Submental
F—Facial

Figure 186

apical end, the exudate can travel through a coronal opening and pass into the oral cavity, forming an *oral cavity abscess.* From the oral cavity, the exudate can be swallowed and may contribute to *gastrointestinal disease,* it may be aspirated and contribute to *pulmonary disease,* it may initiate a *cheilitis,* it may cause the exacerbation of a *tonsillitis,* it may ascend via the salivary gland ducts and contribute to salivary gland infections, such as a *sialadenitis,* it may remain in the oral cavity and contribute to the oral flora's most prominent diseases, *caries* and *periodontal diseases,* or it may be expectorated and contribute to *air pollution.*

(11) The exudate from the subperiosteal abscess can also drain backwards into the circulatory system. It can drain via the

(12) *lymphatics,* travel to the regional lymph nodes and cause a *regional lymphadenopathy.* Lower anterior teeth drain into the submental nodes. The remaining teeth drain into the submaxillary nodes (except that lower third molars can drain directly to the cervical nodes) and both sets of nodes drain into the deep cervical nodes (Fig. 186). Drainage can also occur into the

(13) *venous system* with possibilities of focal infections, such as *subacute bacterial endocarditis* and serious diseases such as *cavernous sinus thrombosis* (cavernous sinus thrombophlebitis) (Fig. 187). However, after successful endodontic therapy, drainage can occur vis the circulatory system without any mal-effects to the patient.*

(14) Finally, the exudate from the subperiosteal abscess can penetrate into the *soft tissues* of the cheek or floor of the mouth and form a *cellulitis.* A cellulitis is an acute inflammation of the alveolar and loose connective tissues. It is a diffuse spreading type of inflammation that is often caused by streptococci. The cellulitis can be superficial or deep. In the superficial cellulitis, the exudate courses between the superficial fascia and the superficial layer of the deep cervical fascia. Examples of *superficial cellulitis* are involvements of the *canine space,* the *buccal space* (Fig. 46) and the *mental space.* In the deep cellulitis, the exudate travels beneath the superficial layer of the deep cervical fascia, below muscle attachments, and between fascial sheets (Fig. 188). Examples of *deep cellulitis* are involvements of the *submental space, sublingual space, submaxillary space* (Figs. 47, 130), and *masticator spaces.* With severe in-

---

* It has been shown in animal experiments that the principal pathway taken by microbes from a primary focus is via the lymphatics and then later into the blood stream. It is not known whether this also occurs in the periapical region.

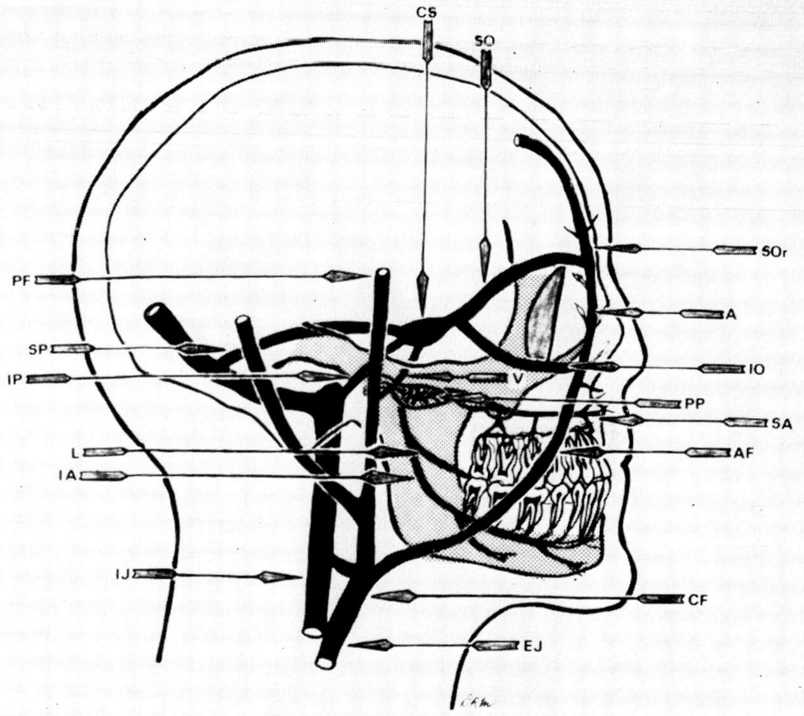

CAVERNOUS SINUS WITH ITS VENOUS CONNECTIONS

CS–Cavernous Sinus
PF–Posterior Facial
SP–Superior Petrosal Sinus
IP–Inferior Petrosal Sinus
L–Lingual
IA–Inferior Alveolar
IJ–Internal Jugular
EJ–External Jugular
CF–Common Facial
AF–Anterior Facial
SA–Superior Alveolar
PP–Pterygoid Plexus
IO–Inferior Opthalmic
V–Vesalian
A–Angular
SOr–Supraorbital
SO–Superior Opthalmic

Figure 187

fectious disease, more posterior spaces become involved including the *lateral pharyngeal* and *retropharyngeal spaces*. When many of the deep spaces are affected, a condition known as *Ludwig's angina* can occur (Fig. 49). It is even possible for *mediastinitis* and a *brain abscess* to develop. The infectious process from a cellulitis may rarely spread directly into the regional *muscles* forming an *acute suppurative myositis*.

The outcome of periapical inflammation is related to certain factors. These

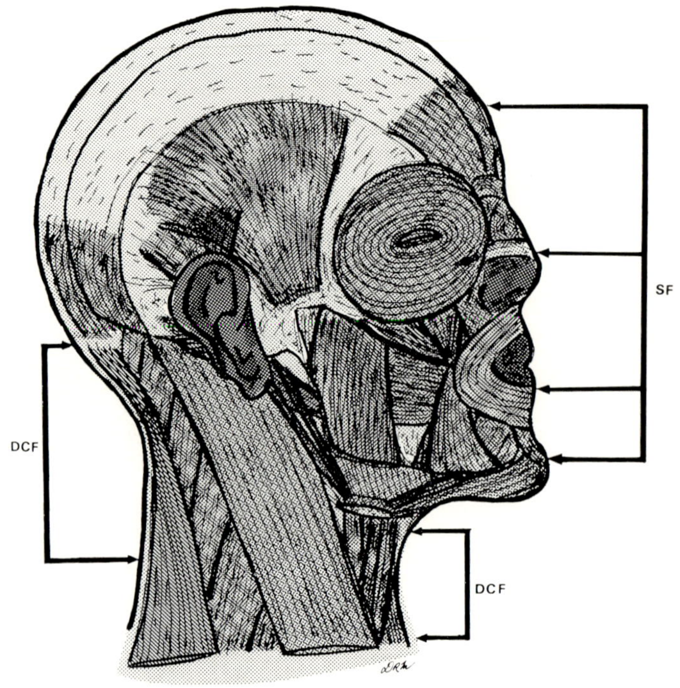

MUSCLES OF THE HEAD AND NECK WITH THEIR OVERLYING FASCIAL SHEATHS
SF—Superficial Fascia—Contains Platysma & Muscles of Facial Expression
DCF—Deep Cervical Fascia—Consists of (3) Connecting Layers &(2) Special Sheaths
(1)—Superficial—Structures Invested Include: Trapezius; Sternocleidomastoid; Masseter; Temporalis; Hyoid; Zygoma; Styloid P.; Mandible
(2)—Middle—Invests Infrahyoids & Neck Viscera (not shown)
(3)—Deep—Invests Deep Posterior Neck Muscles & Cervical Vertebrae (not shown)
Special Sheaths (not shown)
(1)—Carotid—Contains Carotid Arteries, Internal Jugular Veins, & the Vagus Nerves
(2)—Axillary—Contains Brachial Plexus & Subclavian Vessels

Figure 188

are the general resistance of the host, the local resistance of the host, and the population and virulence of the microbes. The general resistance is determined by heredity, nutritional factors, (adequate nutrients in the diet), systemic diseases, drug intake, and amount of sleep, among other factors. The local resistance is determined by muscle attachments, fascial planes, tooth and bone anatomy, salivary flow, type of microbial flora, etc. Actively multiplying virulent organisms, or even actively multiplying avirulent organisms may cause breakdown of tissue resistance. It is the interplay of host and parasite that determines the type of disease that results from periapical breakdown. The various disease entities are now to be discussed.

Space Involvements

Where a specific exudate will localize is determined by muscles and their bony attachments, bony surfaces (maxilla, mandible, zygoma, hyoid), and fascial sheaths. For each tooth there are certain possible infectious pathways, which are discussed below.

The Upper Central Incisor. The

root is often close to the labial surface, with the swelling limited by the attachment of the orbicularis oris muscle and the dense subcutaneous tissue at the base of the nose. A subperiosteal abscess may form with the subsequent development of a parulis (stoma or gum boil). When the lesion bursts, it drains into the oral vestibule (Fig. 189A).

The Upper Lateral Incisor. The root is close to the labial surface 50 per cent of the time and the outcome is similar to that described for the central incisor (Fig. 189A). For the other cases, the root is close to the palatal surface, where the swelling is limited by the attachment of the dense palatal mucosa. Perforation then yields a palatal abscess (Fig. 189B).

The Upper Canine. The root is generally close to the labial surface, with the swelling being limited by the attach-

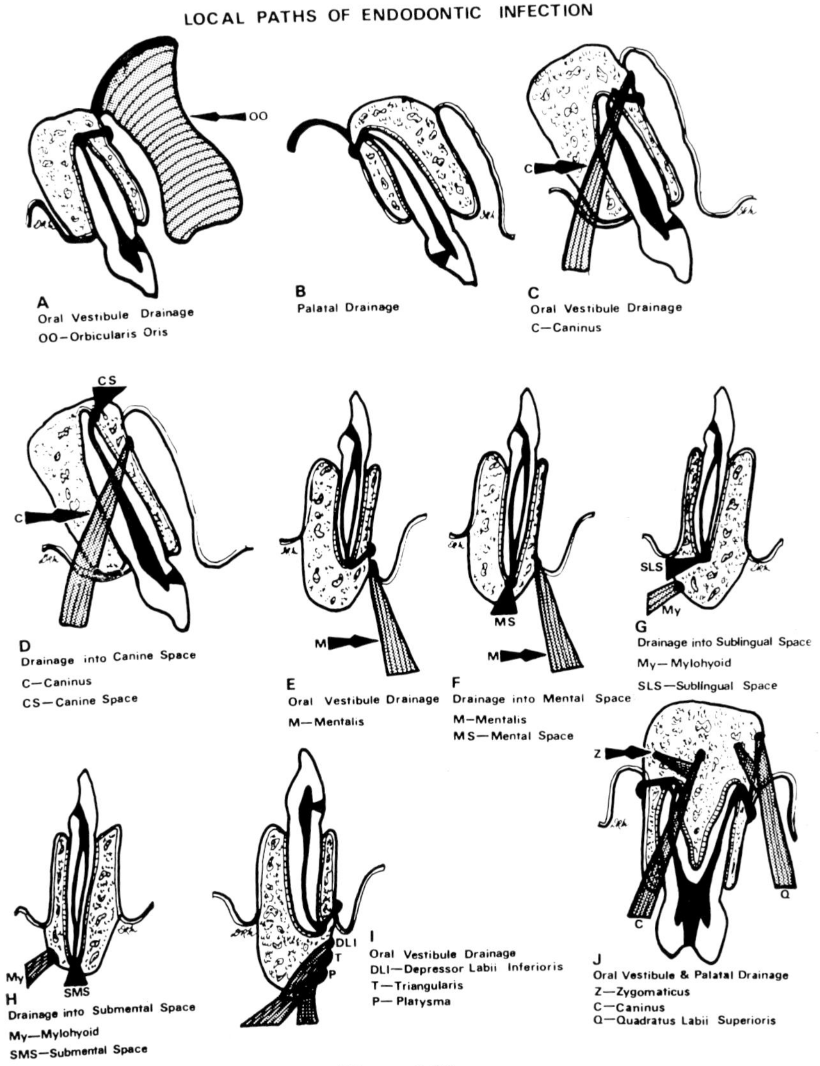

Figure 189

ment of the levator anguli oris muscle (caninus). With the canine, there are two possibilities: (1) with perforation occurring below the origin of the caninus, infection can go into the oral vestibule (Fig. 189C) and (2) with perforation occurring above the origin of the caninus, the exudate can go into the canine space (Fig. 189D). Infection of the canine space produces a superficial cellulitis. This space contains connective tissue and fat, and occupies the area between the anterior surface of the maxilla and the levator muscles of the upper lip (Fig. 190B). The upper canine is the principal tooth involved in this space involvement. Occasionally, the upper centrals, laterals, and premolars may be the precipitating teeth. Clinically, one notes a facial swelling that tends to obliterate the nasolabial fold, and an edema of the eyelids, that closes the eye. Swelling of the upper lip and drooping of the corner of the mouth may be observed. The side of the face is tender and painful to touch, and the skin is taut and red (Fig. 191C). Rare complications include skin perforation, abscess at the inner canthus of the eye, orbital cellulitis, optic neuritis, and retrobulbar neuritis.

THE LOWER CENTRAL AND LATERAL INCISORS. The roots often are close to the labial surface, at times they approach the lingual surface. There are four possible sites of perforation:

(1) With the perforation on the labial surface, the attachment of the mentalis muscle becomes the determinant of the path of infection.

(a) If the site of perforation is above the origin of the mentalis muscle, then exudation goes into the oral vestibule (Fig. 189E).

(b) If the site of perforation is below the origin of the mentalis, then the inflammatory exudate travels into the mental space (Fig. 189F). The mental space (submentalis space) is another site of a superficial cellulitis. It occupies the area between the anterior surface of the mandible, and the skin and superficial fascia overlaying the lower lip depressor muscles (Fig. 190A, P). Clinical observation reveals a firm, red, ovoid swelling of the chin that is painful to touch (Fig. 191B). The pain results from pressure of the exudate against the depressor labi inferiorus and mentalis muscles. The teeth are often mobile and painful to touch.

(2) With perforation occurring on the lingual surface, the attachment of the mylohyoid muscle determines the path of infection.

(a) If the site of perforation is above the mylohyoid origin, infection goes into the sublingual space (Fig. 189G). The sublingual space (paralingual) is a site for a deep cellulitis. It contains the sublingual gland, Wharton's duct, the lingual and hypoglossal nerves, and the sublingual artery. This space occupies the area between the oral mucosa (above) and the mylohyoid muscle (below) (Fig. 190 P, Q). The lower molars are the teeth most often involved, but any lower tooth can be etiologically implicated in this cellulitis. The clinical picture reveals a swelling that raises the floor of the mouth on the affected side. Displacement of the tongue occurs, both superiorly and medially, and the sublingual glands are elevated (Fig. 191G). There is pain and difficulty in swallowing. Infections of this space are potentially dangerous because of connections between it and the submaxillary and lateral pharyngeal spaces (discussed below).

(b) With the site of perforation below the origin of the mylohyoid, infection goes into the submental space (Fig. 189H). The submental space (superficial sublingual space) is another site for a deep cellulitis. It contains the anterior digastric muscle. It is found between the mylohyoid muscle (above) and the platysma muscle (below) (Fig. 189P). Clinically, a firm, definite swelling of the submental region is observed (Fig. 191F). The swelling is board-like in early stages, and the skin is painful and taut. This space connects with the posterior, submaxillary space.

THE LOWER CANINE. Often, the canine root is close to the labial surface, but it may approach the lingual surface. There are four possible sites of perforation:

(1) If the perforation is on the labial surface, there are two possibilities.
   (a) In rare cases, the site of perforation is below the mentalis origin, and mental space infection results (Fig. 189F).
   (b) In the usual situation, the origins of the lower lip depressor muscles are below the apex of the canine, and perforation results in an oral vestibule abscess (Fig. 189I).

(2) With perforation on the lingual surface, again there are two possible results.
   (a) If the site is above the origin of the mylohyoid muscle, then a sublingual space involvement results (Fig. 189G).
   (b) With the perforation site below the mylohyoid attachment, a submental cellulitis is the outcome (Fig. 189H).

THE UPPER PREMOLARS. The roots are usually close to the buccal surface but the palatal root may be closer to the palatal surface. As a result, there are three possible sites of perforation:

(1) When the perforation occurs on the buccal surface, there are two possibilities.

  (a) In rare cases, the perforation is above the caninus origin and a canine space involvement occurs (Fig. 189D).

  (b) In the usual situation, the origins of the upper lip levator muscles are located well above the apexes of the upper premolars, and perforation results in an oral vestibule abscess (Fig. 189J).

(2) If a palatal perforation occurs, a palatal abscess develops (Fig. 189J).

THE LOWER PREMOLARS. Generally, the roots are close to the buccal surface; rarely, they are closer to the lingual cortical plate. There are three possible perforating sites:

(1) In the usual buccal perforation, the origins of the lower lip depressor muscles are located well below the lower premolar apexes with a resulting oral vestibule penetration (Fig. 189K).

(2) Rarely a lingual perforation occurs.

  (a) If the site of perforation is above the mylohyoid attachment then a sublingual space infection occurs (Fig. 189G).

  (b) If the perforating site is below the mylohyoid origin, then a submaxillary space involvement occurs (Fig. 189L). The submaxillary space (submandibular) is another area where a deep cellulitis occurs. It contains the submaxillary gland and its associated lymph nodes. This space lies between the mylohyoid muscle (superior) and the digastric muscle (inferior) (Figs. 189Q, 190C, E). Teeth involved include the lower molars, the primary molars, and occasionally the lower premolars. The clinical picture reveals a facial swelling of the submaxillary region that covers the line of the mandibular border (Figs. 47, 191E). The patient has both pain and tenderness to palpation, and may have pain with swallowing. The overlying skin of the area is red, shiny, and taut. The submaxillary, sublingual, and submental spaces are contiguous with each other. Some authorities consider the entire complex as the submandibular space. The submaxillary space readily connects with the lateral pharyngeal and retropharyngeal spaces (discussed below). In debilitated patients, dangerous complications can occur with involvement of all these spaces in the clinical entity known as Ludwig's angina. This con-

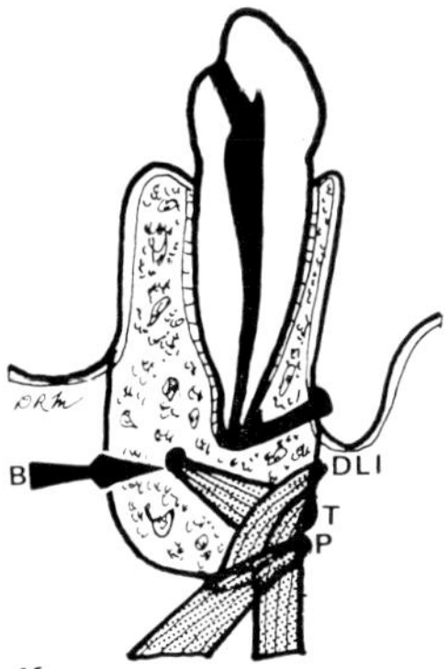

K
Oral Vestibule Drainage
B—Buccinator
DLI—Depressor Labii Inferioris
T—Triangularis
P—Platysma

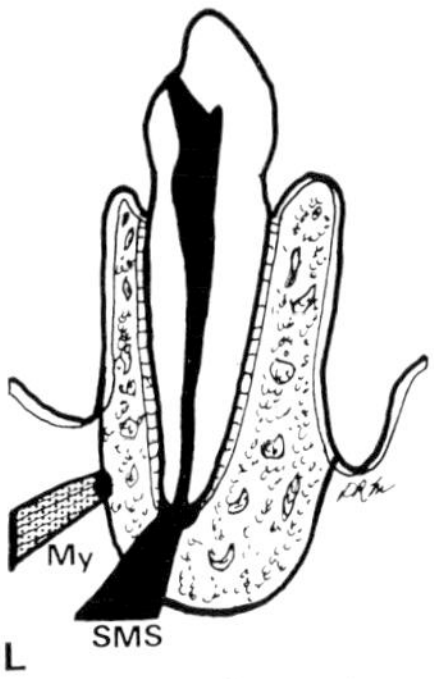

L
Drainage into Submaxillary Space
My—Mylohyoid
SMS—Submaxillary Space

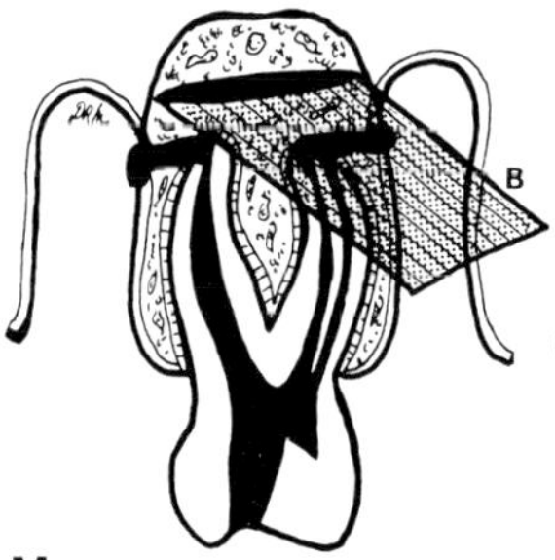

M
Oral Vestibule Drainage
B—Buccinator

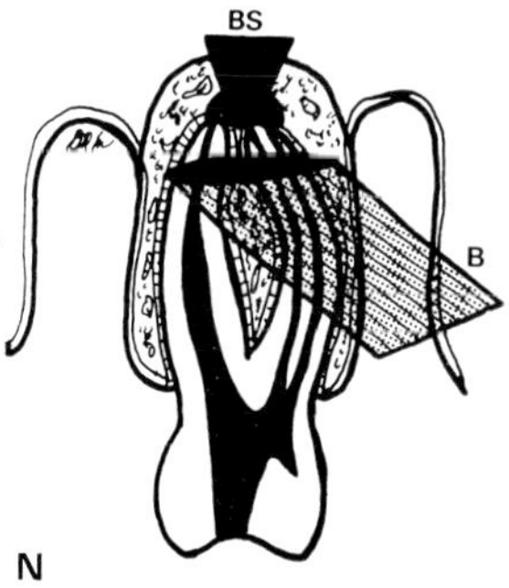

N
Drainage into Buccal Space
B—Buccinator
BS—Buccal Space

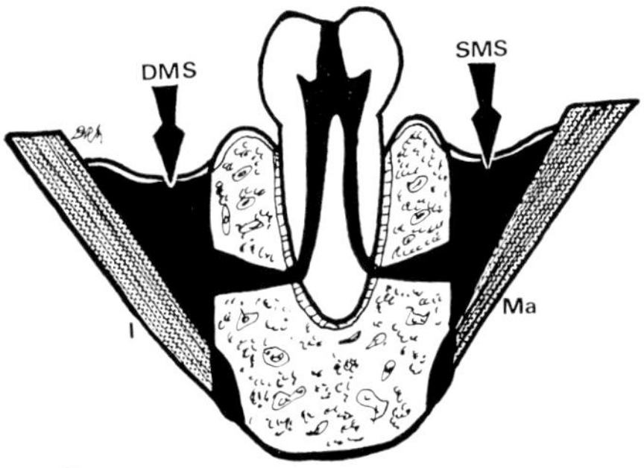

O
Drainage into Masticator Spaces
I—Internal Pterygoid
Ma—Masseter
DMS—Deep Masticator Space
SMS—Superficial Masticator Space

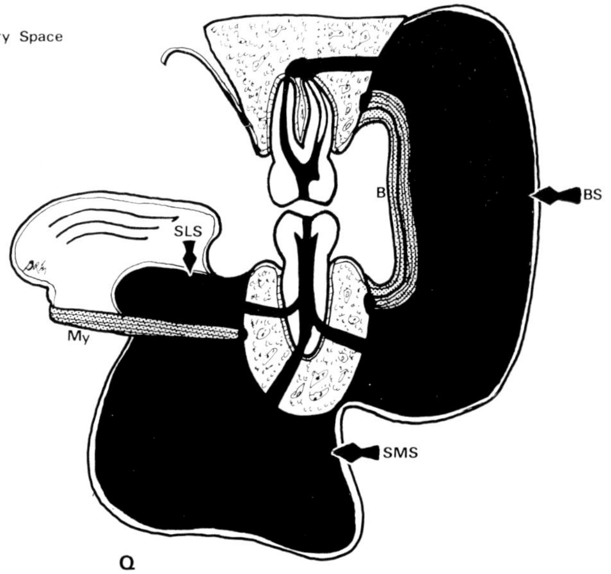

Q
Combined Spaces—Posterior
B—Buccinator
My—Mylohyoid
SLS—Sublingual Space
SMS—Submaxillary Space
BS—Buccal Space

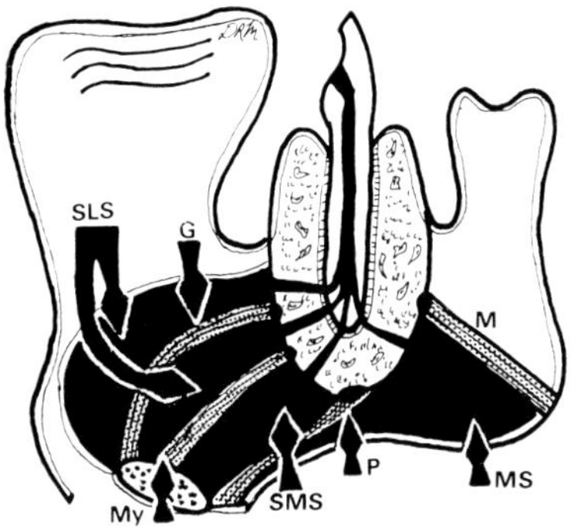

P
Combined Spaces—Lower Anterior
G—Geniohyoid
My—Mylohyoid
P—Platysma
M—Mentalis
MS—Mental Space
SMS—Submental Space
SLS—Sublingual Space

Figure 189

dition shows a massive cellulitis that is bilateral in scope (Figs. 49, 191H). The tongue is enlarged, and is displaced superiorly and posteriorly against the soft palate. This leads to difficulty in respiration. The floor of the mouth tissues have a board-like consistency. Even with antibiotics and drainage, this is a difficult condition to control, fortunately, it is rare.

THE UPPER MOLARS. The buccal roots approximate the buccal surface, and the palatal root is often closer to the palatal surface. There are four sites of penetration (three usual, one rare).

(1) On the buccal surface, the path of infection is limited by the buccinator origin.

(a) If the site of perforation is below the buccinator origin, then an oral vestibule abscess results (Fig. 189M).

(b) If the site of penetration is above the origin of the buccinator, then a buccal space infection occurs (Fig. 189N). The buccal space is a superficial space containing the buccal fat pad. It lies between the buccinator muscle (medially) and the skin and superficial fascia of the cheek (laterally, Figs. 189Q, S, 190D). Teeth involved are both the maxillary and mandibular molars. Clinically, one detects a facial swelling ovoid in shape and confined to the cheek. The swelling begins at the lower border of the mandible and extends upward to the zygomatic arch. It develops rapidly and is easy to palpate. Periorbital involvement usually occurs (Figs. 46, 191D). Although this is a superficial cellulitis, it is potentially dangerous as it communicates with the submaxillary, the temporal and masticator (discussed below) spaces.

(2) Palatal perforation is revealed by a palatal abscess (Fig. 189M).

(3) In extremely rare cases, the infection courses superiorly and posteriorly to the infratemporal space. The infratemporal space (fossa) is another site of a deep cellulitis. It contains the pterygoid plexus of veins and the internal maxillary artery. It lies beneath the sphenoid bone, and between the maxillary tuberosity (anteriorly) and the mandibular fossa (posteriorly, Fig. 189R). Infections have occurred following maxillary molar extractions, after tuberosity and inferior alveolar nerve injections, as a complication of pericoronitis of the lower third molar, and as a rare complication of maxillary sinusitis. Clinical manifestations are swelling above the zygoma and beneath the temporal muscle, trismus, pain, fever, dysphagia, and deviation of the mandible to the affected side upon opening. This space is contiguous with the lateral pharyngeal and temporal

spaces. Severe complications include intracranial abscesses, orbital cellulitis, cavernous sinus thrombosis, and mediastinitis.

THE LOWER FIRST MOLAR. Most often the roots lie close to the buccal surface. In other instances, they are lingually inclined; rarely they are distally directed. As a result, there are six possible exits of infection.

(1) On the buccal, the buccinator origin is the determining factor.

  (a) If the site of the perforation is above the buccinator origin, then an oral vestibule abscess results (Fig. 189K).

  (b) If the perforating site is below the origin of the buccinator, then a buccal space infection develops (Fig. 189Q).

(2) The origin of the mylohyoid is the limiting factor on the lingual.

  (a) If the site of the perforation is above the mylohyoid origin, then a sublingual space involvement occurs (Fig. 189Q).

  (b) With the site of perforation below the origin of the mylohyoid, a submaxillary space infection results (Fig. 189Q).

(3) Rarely, the course of infection

S Various Spaces

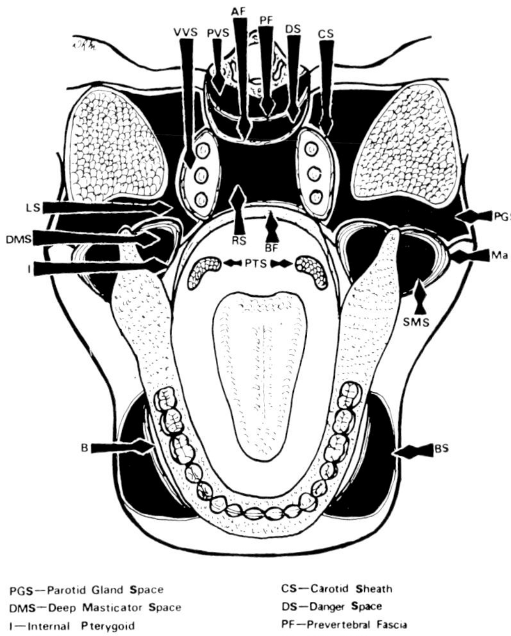

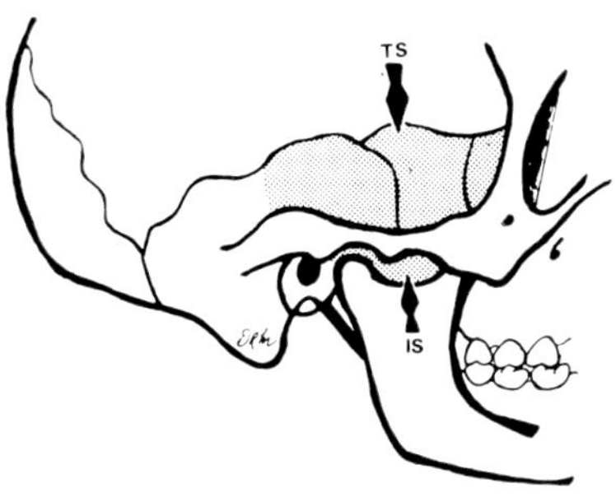

R
Temporal Area
TS—Temporal Space
IS—Infratemporal Space

PGS—Parotid Gland Space
DMS—Deep Masticator Space
I—Internal Pterygoid
B—Buccinator
BS—Buccal Space
SMS—Superficial Masticator Space
Ma—Masseter
LS—Lateral Pharyngeal Space
CS—Carotid Sheath
DS—Danger Space
PF—Prevertebral Fascia
AF—Alar Fascia
PVS—Prevertebral Space
VVS—Visceral Vascular Space
RS—Retropharyngeal Space
BF—Buccopharyngeal Fascia
PTS—Palatine Tonsils & Peritonsillar Space

Figure 189

is distally inclined, and the mandibular ramus is penetrated.

(a) With a buccal exit, infection enters the superficial masticator space (Fig. 189O). The superficial masticator space (lateral) is a deep space that is found between the lateral aspect of the ramus and the medial surface of the masseter muscle (Fig. 189S). Any of the lower molars may be involved but the third molar is most often involved. Clinical examination reveals a large, brawny, facial swelling involving the masseter muscle. There is a boring, prolonged type of pain over the ascending ramus along with severe trismus and high fever. The tissues are tense and shiny. This space communicates with the superficial temporal space.

(b) If the infection exits on the lingual, it enters the deep masticator space (Fig. 189O). The deep masticator space (medial, pterygomandibular) lies between the medial aspect of the ramus and the lateral surface of the internal pterygoid muscle (Fig. 189S). The same teeth are involved as in the superficial infection. An inferior alveolar injection penetrates this space. Clinically, no external swelling is evident. There is an anterior deviation of both the soft palate and the anterior tonsillar pillar and the uvula is displaced to the unaffected side. Other manifestations are sore throat, fever, trismus, dysphagia, intoxication, and possible septicemia. This space interconnects with the deep temporal and lateral pharyngeal spaces. Some authorities combine the masticator and temporal spaces into the masseteric space.

THE LOWER SECOND MOLAR. The possible sites of perforation are the same as for the first molar. The only difference is in frequency; 50 percent of the time the roots are close to the buccal surface, and 50 percent of the time they approach the lingual surface.

THE LOWER THIRD MOLAR. The perforating sites include the six seen in the other lower molars. Most perforations are on the lingual, with the submaxillary space infection being the most frequent. There are two other possible paths of penetration for this tooth:

(1) With mesioangularly inclined or horizontally positioned third molars, the infection can go beyond the mylohyoid muscle directly into the deep masticator space (Fig. 189S).

(2) The exudate can also spread directly into the lateral pharyngeal space, by passing medially to the internal pterygoid muscle (Fig. 189S). The lateral pharyngeal space (parapharyngeal, peripharyngeal, pharyngomaxillary) is a deep space that lies between the lateral wall of the pharynx

(medially) and the fascia covering the internal pterygoid muscle (laterally). Its superior-inferior extent is from the sphenoid to the hyoid bones (Fig. 190E). There are two compartments that are separated by the styloid process; these are the anterior and the posterior. The anterior (muscular, prestyloid) is in close relationship with the tonsillar fossa and the internal pterygoid muscle. The posterior (neurovascular, retrostyloid) contains the carotid sheath and the cranial nerves. The potential space located within the carotid sheath is the visceral vascular space (Fig. 189S). Aside from lower third molar infection, involvement can occur via a misplaced inferior alveolar injection that penetrates the space. The lateral pharyngeal space communicates with several spaces including the sublingual, the submaxillary, the retropharyngeal, the parotid, the deep masticator, the infratemporal, and the palatal muscle spaces. Clinical manifestations are a small, firm, tender external swelling (when present) beneath the angle of the mandible, dysphagia, sore throat, high fever, intoxication, severe trismus, and swelling of the lateral wall of the pharynx and medial displacement of the tonsils, tonsillar pillars, and the uvula. These manifestations simulate a peritonsillar abscess. If the carotid sheath is involved, marked septicemia and hemorrhage can occur. Thrombosis may involve the internal jugular vein or the cavernous sinus. Rarely, spread of the infection can travel down the sheath into the superior and posterior mediastina. From the lateral pharyngeal space, infection can pass readily into the retropharyngeal space. The retropharyngeal space (posterior visceral, retrovisceral, retroesophageal) is a deep space that lies between the middle layer of the deep cervical fascia surrounding the pharynx and esophagus, and the alar layer of the deep cervical fascia (Fig. 189S). It extends from the base of the skull to the superior mediastinum (Fig. 190E). It communicates with the lateral pharyngeal space and the superior mediastinum. The thin alar fascia can easily be destroyed, and then the *danger space* is involved (discussed below). Clinical symptoms are pain, dyspnea, dysphagia, anorexia, snoring, and swelling of the glands of the neck. Complications include rupture into the airway, septicemia, thrombosis of the internal jugular vein, hemorrhage, bronchial erosion, laryngospasm, and mediastinitis. Extension can go into various other spaces. Involvement of the *danger space* is a most serious complication. This space contains loose areolar tissue, and it is located between the alar and prevertebral layers of the deep cervical fascia (Fig. 189S). It extends from the base of the skull to the

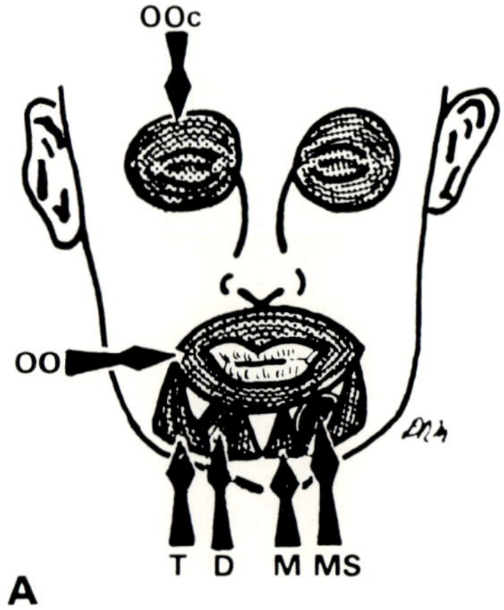

A

MENTAL
OOc—Orbicularis Oculi
OO—Orbicularis Oris
T—Triangularis
D—Depressor Labii Inferioris
M—Mentalis
MS—Mental Space

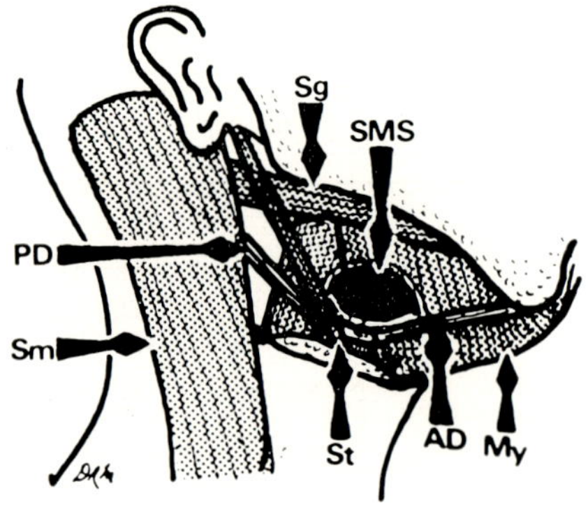

C

SUBMAXILLARY
Sg—Styloglossis
PD—Posterior Digastric
Sm—Sternocleidomastoid
St—Stylohyoid
AD—Anterior Digastric
My—Mylohyoid
SMS—Submaxillary Space

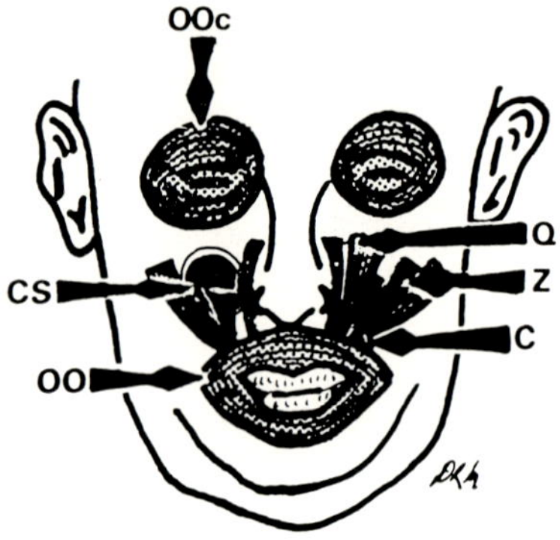

B

CANINE
OOc—Orbicularis Oculi
Q—Quadratus Labii Superioris
Z—Zygomaticus
C—Caninus
OO—Orbicularis Oris
CS—Canine Space

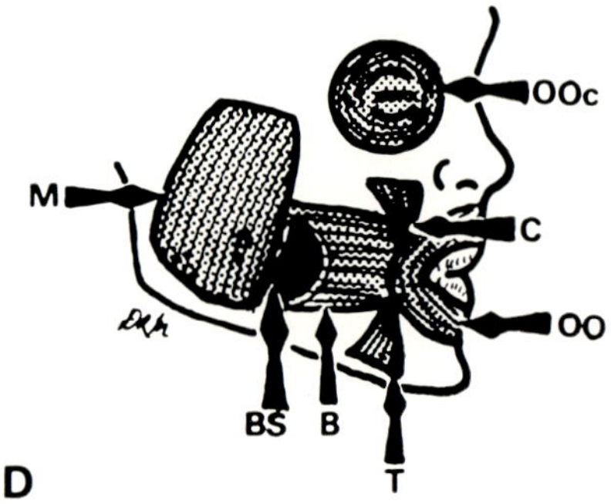

D

BUCCAL
M—Masseter
OOc—Orbicularis Oculi
C—Caninus
OO—Orbicularis Oris
T—Triangularis
B—Buccinator
BS—Buccal Space

Figure 190

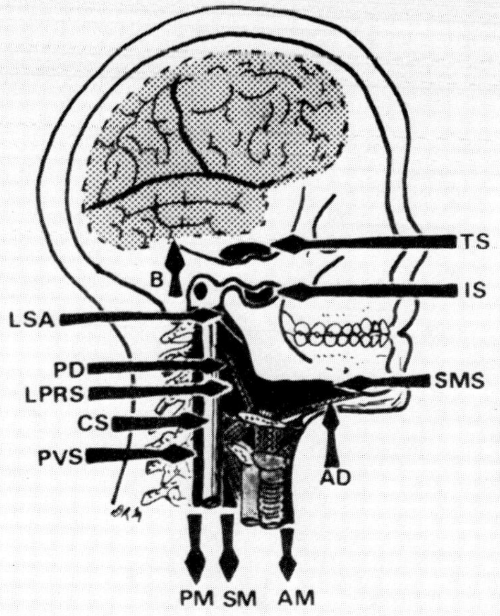

E

POSTERIOR
B— To Brain
LSA—Lateral Pharyngeal Space—Anterior
PD—Posterior Digastric
LPRS—Lateral Pharyngeal Posterior & Retropharyngeal Spaces
CS—Carotid Sheath
PVS—Prevertebral Space
PM—To Posterior Mediastinum
SM—To Superior Mediastinum
AM—To Anterior Mediastinum
AD—Anterior Digastric
SMS—Submaxillary Space
IS—Infratemporal Space
TS—Temporal Space

Figure 190 A-E. Various spaces—Muscle and bony attachments.

posterior mediastinum. Infection can rapidly travel to the mediastinum. Clinically, the symptoms are similar to those in retropharyngeal space involvement. With mediastinitis, the symptoms are chest pain, persistant fever, dyspnea, and roentgenographic evidence of a widened mediastinum. Other spaces, such as the parotid, temporal, peritonsillar, prevertebral and pterygopalatine can be involved in severe infections (Figs. 189S, 190E). Potential interconnections of the various spaces are shown in Plate One. Microbial assay and antibiotic sensitivity testing (anaerobically as well as aerobically) are important measures to help in the treatment of the space infectious diseases. Treatment includes adequate dosage of correct antibiotics and incision and drainage procedures when indicated. The prognosis depends upon the resistance of the patient and whether adequate drainage can be established without extraction of the involved teeth. Generally speaking, the deep cellulitis cases are more dangerous than the superficial cellulitis cases, and the poorest prognosis is for space involvements resulting from lower third molar infections. In the latter cases, in debilitated individuals, life-threatening situations can arise. Fortunately, this is quite rare, but the dental practitioners must never lose sight of the possibilities of dissemination of periapical infection.

Osteomyelitis

This is an inflammation of bone that begins in the marrow spaces, then involves the associated periosteum, and finally becomes established in the cortical plates. Ischemia occurs and various portions of the calcified tissues become necrotic and are sequestered. Osteomyelitis can occur as the result of direct medul-

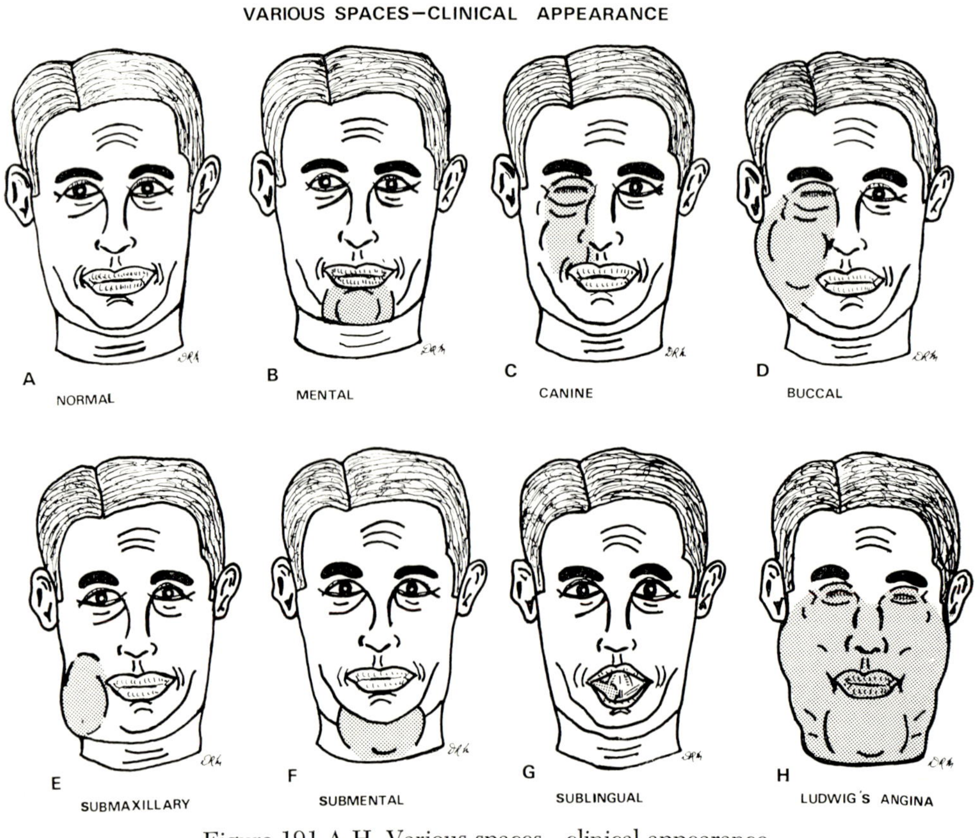

Figure 191 A-H. Various spaces—clinical appearance.

lary spread from the apex of an acute or chronically infected tooth. The mandible is affected much more commonly than the maxilla, presumably because of the poorer blood supply of the former. A precipitating factor in the development of the disease is thrombosis of the inferior alveolar artery. Considering the common occurrence of pulpally-induced periapical pathosis, it is fortunate that osteomyelitis is a rare complication. Too early surgical intervention and application of external heat have been considered as factors stimulating the development of osteomyelitis. Also poor general resistance of the host, impaired vascularity, and extreme virulence of the microbes are important etiologic factors. Staphylococcus aureus is one of the principal microbes implicated, but Staphylococcus albus, streptococci, pneumococci, Salmonella typhosa, and bacteroides species can also be responsible. There are several types of osteomyelitis: acute, chronic, Garre's, chemical, and radiation. Only acute, chronic, and Garre's can result from periapical pathosis. Osteomyelitis can also occur in diseases such as syphilis (Fig. 7), tuberculosis, and Paget's disease.

ACUTE OSTEOMYELITIS. In this disease, patients usually have severe, boring type pain. A firm swelling appears over the affected region of the mandible, and the overlying cheek, and lip paresthesia may occur. Teeth in the involved area become mobile, and are painful to percussion. A purulent exudate often drains either through the gingival sulcus or a sinus tract. The submaxillary lymph nodes are swollen and tender, and a temperature of about 100°F is usual. Pathologic fracture of the mandible can occur. Possible outcomes are chronic osteomyelitis, and in debilitated individuals, septicemia, pneumonia, meningitis, and cavernous sinus thrombosis. Radiographic changes are not evident for the first three weeks. The first change seen is an irregular type of radiolucency. Later on a characteristic *motheaten* bony appearance is seen. This results from sequestrum formation (Fig. 192A-C). Histologic examination reveals a massive infiltration of the marrow spaces by polymorph leucocytes. The lacunae are empty and there are lymphocytes and plasma cells in the peripheral areas. There is a connective tissue attempt at walling off the necrotic bone. The prognosis depends upon the resistance of the host, the destruction by the disease process, and the susceptibility of the microbes to antibiotics. Often the involved teeth have to be extracted. However, with early use of large doses of effective antibiotics and establishment of good drainage, osteomyelitis can be controlled. It is possible to effect a complete cure and even save the teeth after complete endodontic therapy has been performed. If incomplete antibiotic therapy had been given, a possible result would be the conversion of an acute case into a chronic one.

CHRONIC OSTEOMYELITIS. A chronic osteomyelitis can occur directly from a periapical pathosis, if the bone is invaded by microbes of low virulence. It can also occur secondarily to an acute osteomyelitis, bony diseases such as Paget's disease and osteopetrosis, and other systemic diseases such as syphilis, tuberculosis and actinomycosis. The patient's symptoms are not severe. Pain is mild

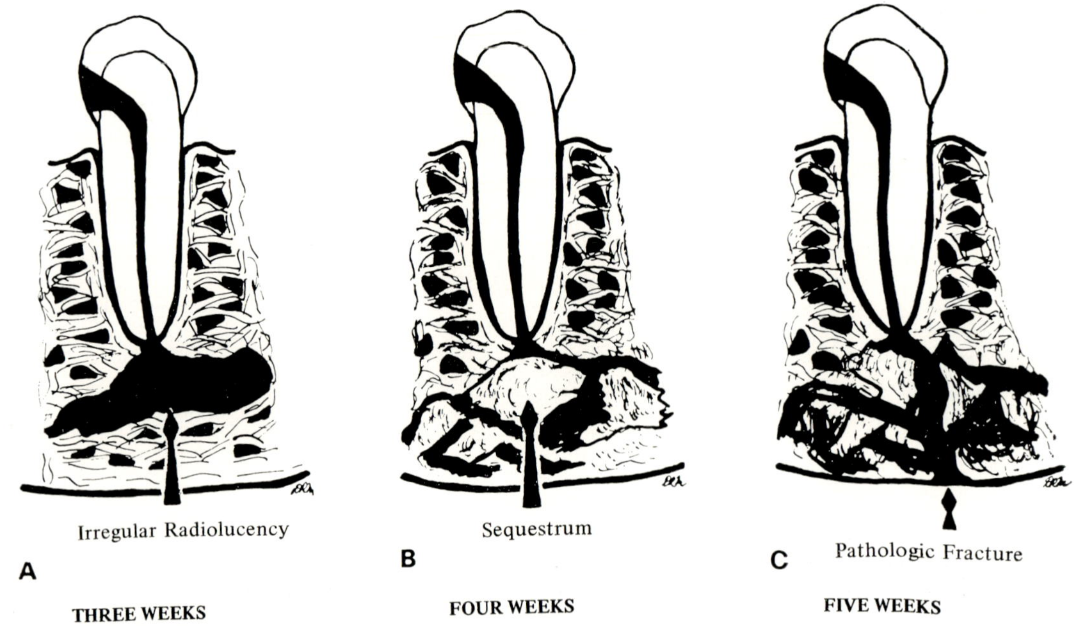

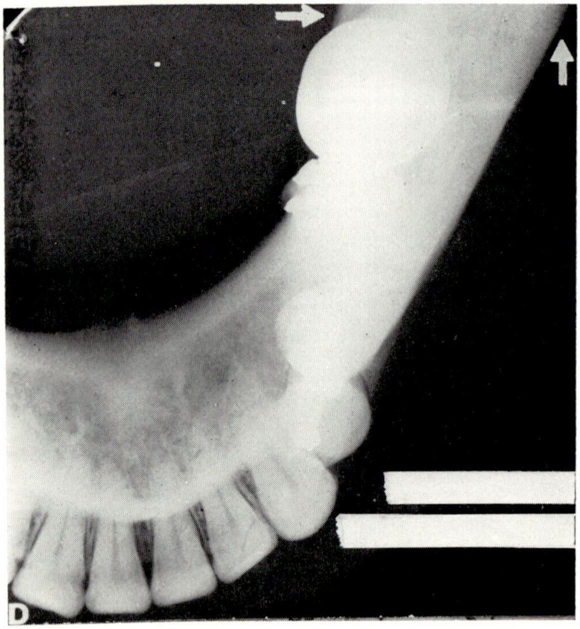

Figure 192 A-C. Three stages of acute osteomyelitis. D. Garre's Osteomyelitis. (Courtesy of Dr. E. Wolfson, Philadelphia, Pa.)

and of infrequent occurrence. Temperature is normal. However, there may be acute flare-ups and then the symptomology is like that of the acute disease. The chronic disease can persist for years.

Histologically, there are usually large sequestra involved, with areas of bone formation and bone destruction present. Chronic inflammatory cells are found in the marrow spaces, and there are areas where polymorph leucocytes

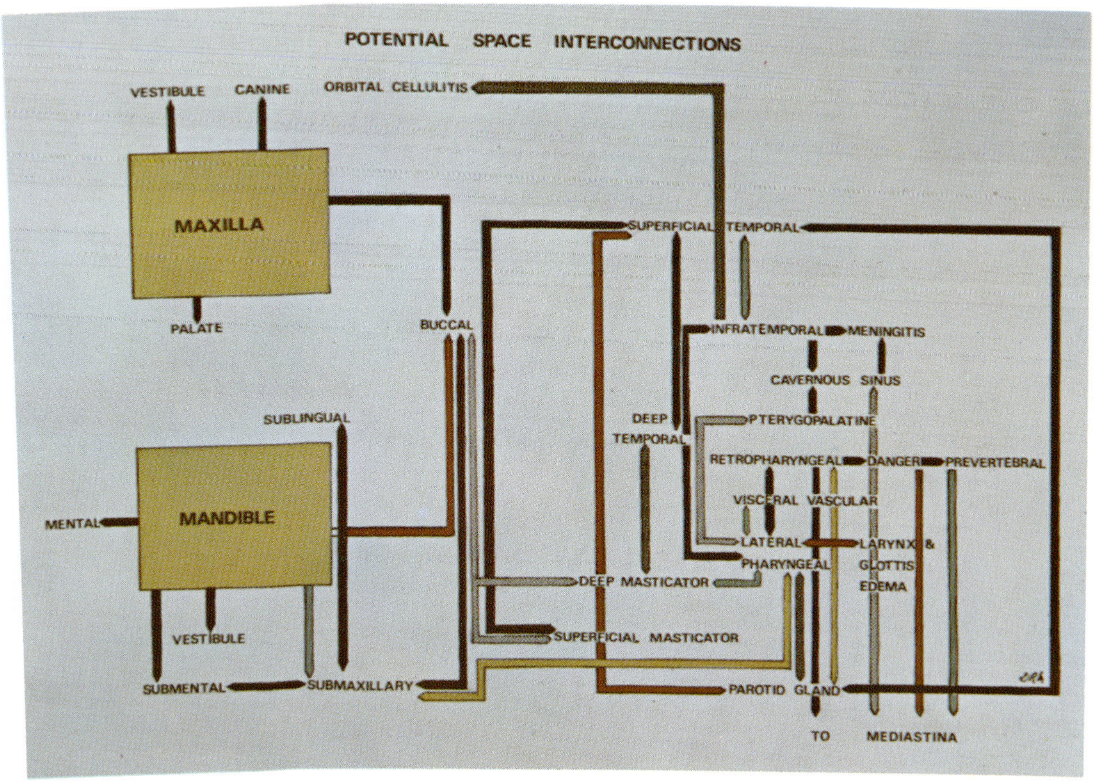
POTENTIAL SPACE INTERCONNECTIONS
VESTIBULE
CANINE
ORBITAL CELLULITIS
MAXILLA
PALATE
BUCCAL
SUPERFICIAL TEMPORAL
INFRATEMPORAL
MENINGITIS
CAVERNOUS SINUS
SUBLINGUAL
DEEP TEMPORAL
PTERYGOPALATINE
RETROPHARYNGEAL
DANGER
PREVERTEBRAL
MENTAL
MANDIBLE
VISCERAL VASCULAR
LATERAL PHARYNGEAL
LARYNX & GLOTTIS EDEMA
DEEP MASTICATOR
VESTIBULE
SUPERFICIAL MASTICATOR
SUBMENTAL
SUBMAXILLARY
PAROTID GLAND
TO MEDIASTINA

Plate One

predominate. Necrotic bone is readily seen. The lamina dura around the involved teeth may be lost.

If the necrotic bone can be removed without damage to the teeth, then the teeth are treatable. Usually, the extent of bone destruction is so great that the involved teeth have to be extracted.

Garre's Osteomyelitis. This condition is a nonsuppurative osteosclerosis that results from the stimulating effect of a relatively avirulent infection. It appears to be a reaction to a mild chronic osteomyelitis and may follow pulpally-induced periapical disease. It resembles condensing osteitis, but the degree of bony proliferation is of a much greater magnitude. This disease occurs primarily in younger individuals. The organisms may be located subperiosteally and can stimulate bone building by the periosteum. The affected bone becomes thickened and is clinically palpable as a hard mass over the involved site. Pain is usually present in the affected region of the mandible. Radiographic findings show a dense radiopaque mass in the involved region of the mandible, which may have isolated areas of radiolucency (Fig. 192D). The histologic findings show many regions of bone formation surrounding fibrous marrow spaces containing an infiltration of plasma cells and lymphocytes. Prognosis is good provided complete endodontic therapy can be performed and the bony involvement is not too great. However, if the lesion is extensive and removal causes extreme damage to the teeth, extraction has to be performed. The lesion must be removed surgically as there are malignant neoplasms, such as Ewing's sarcoma which can have a similar radiographic appearance. After endodontics or extraction and partial bony removal, the remaining mass of bone often undergoes resolution. However, in certain cases, complete recontouring does not occur and the bone remains thickened. Chemical and radiation osteomyelitis will be discussed in a later section.

Cavernous Sinus Thrombosis (Cavernous Sinus Thrombophlebitis)

This is a thrombophlebitis of the cavernous sinus that can result from direct extension of infectious processes from adjoining veins such as the facial, the internal jugular and the pterygoid plexus. The most common dental route is from maxillary and mandibular third molars via the pterygoid plexus (Fig. 187). Other possible routes are from visceral vascular or pterygopalatine space infections (Fig. 190E, Plate 1) and from infected upper anterior teeth via the angular and/or orbital veins to the superior ophthalmic vein and thence to the cavernous sinus (Fig. 187). This disease is a dangerous condition that causes impairment of cerebral vascular drainage. Although it is of much less frequent occurrence since the advent of antibiotics, it can still follow severe periapical pathosis in debilitated individuals. Manifestations include headache, pain in the orbital regions (which may be referred to upper teeth), swelling of the eyes and eyelids on the involved side, high fever, and severe nausea and vomiting. Septic emboli can occur from the breaking off of the thrombi and their passage through the blood stream. This can result in lung abscesses

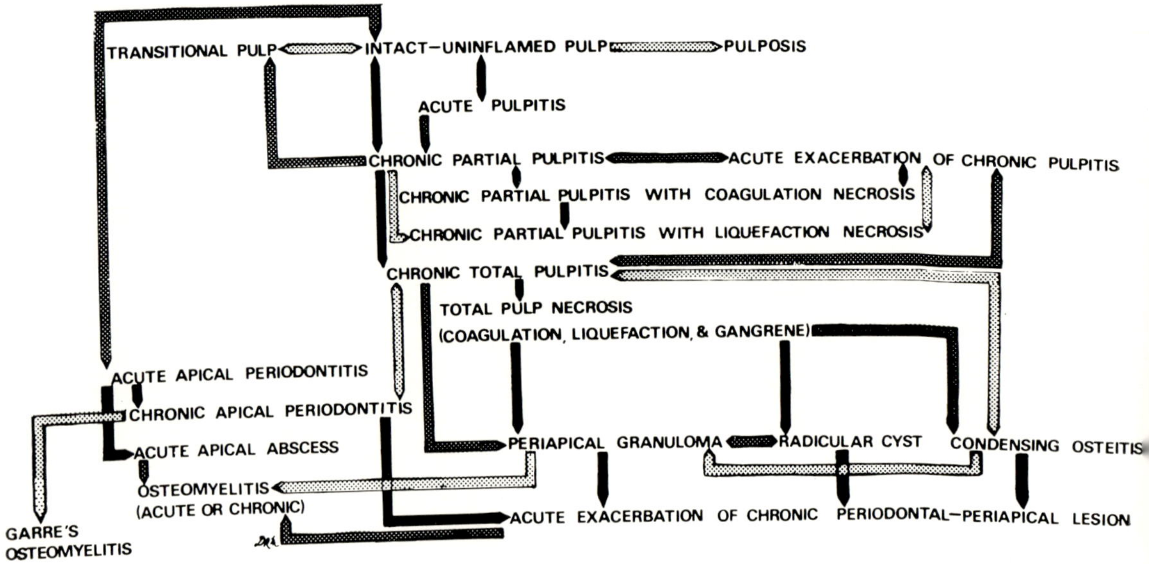

Figure 193. Interrelationship of histologically-classified endodontic diseases.

and cerebral abscesses, among other possibilities.

Histological examination reveals a massive concentration of polymorph leucocytes, microorganisms, and necrotic tissue. Formerly, prognosis was extremely bad. Even today, it is a very serious condition, and recovery can still result in residual brain damage. Treatment consists of massive antibiotic therapy and surgical drainage.

Focal Diseases

As discussed in Chapter 1, the focal infection theory as related to dental abscesses is questionable except for the development of subacute bacterial endocarditis. Eye, ear, and nasal infections can occur as the result of direct extension of severe periapical pathosis and conceivably also as a result of hematogenous spread of microbes and/or their products. If a patient has periapical disease and symptoms persist in the eye, ear, or nasal region, after the return to normalcy of the dental condition, then the patient should be referred to the appropriate physician for consultation.

A histologic classification of endodontic diseases (pulpal and periapical) is shown in Figure 193.

NORMAL ANATOMIC LANDMARKS

Radiographic Landmarks

For each landmark is given the definition, the radiographic appearance, the endodontic lesions that the landmark simulates, and the means to differentiate the two types of conditions.

Anterior Palatine Foramen (Incisive Foramen)

This is the palatine orifice of the anterior palatine canal and it contains palatine blood vessels and nerves. It appears as a radiolucent area of varying size (contingent upon size, shape, thickness of the maxilla, and the inclination of the palate). It is normally seen on periapical radiographs between and above the upper central incisors. Many times the image of the anterior palatine foramen is superimposed over the apex of one of the central incisors, when radiographs are taken of the upper lateral incisors. The foramen appears as a radicular cyst or a periapical granuloma. A second radiograph is taken directly between the central incisors, to differentiate the normal from the pathologic. If the radiolucency is the anterior palatine foramen, the image will appear between the central incisors or

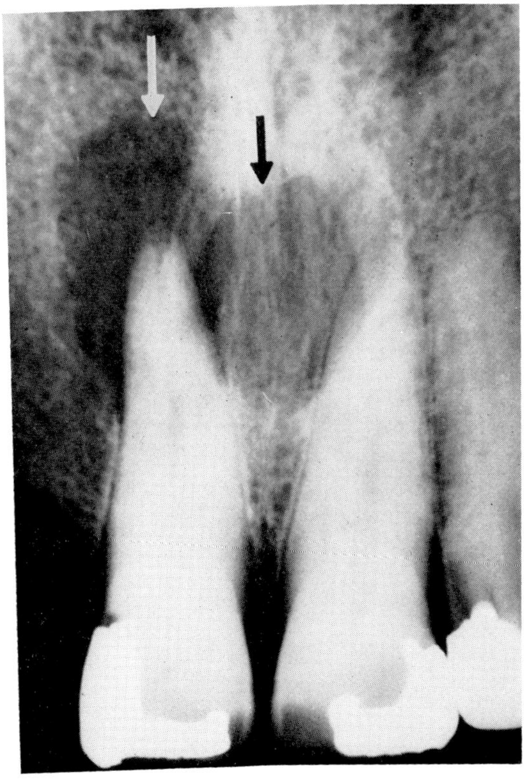

Figure 194. Nasopalatine foramen and periapical area of pathosis; white arrow indicates periapical area of pathosis; black arrow indicates large nasopalatine foramen. (Courtesy of Dr. W. Updegrave, Philadelphia, Pa.)

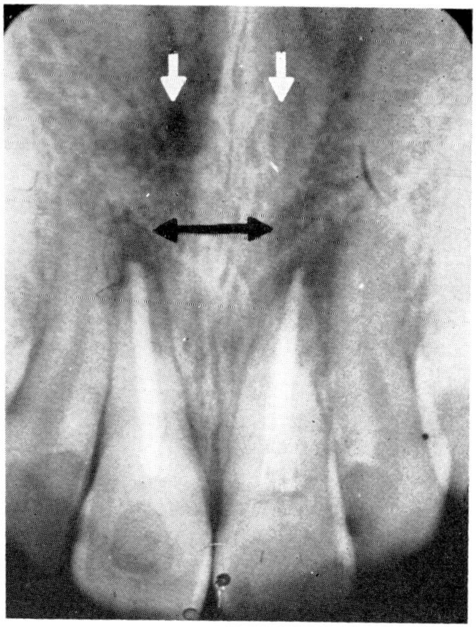

Figure 195. Nasal fossae and periapical areas of pathosis; black arrows indicate periapical areas of pathosis; white arrows indicate the nasal fossae. (From D. R. Morse, "The Significance of Endodontics in Plantation Procedures," *JDA South Africa,* 26:263, 1971.)

away from the apex of the tooth that it had been superimposed over. The condition is related to the tooth, if the image remains over the apex (Fig. 194). Also if the radiolucency is the result of pulpally induced-periapical pathosis, then the lamina dura should not be continuous around the apex. A normal continuous lamina dura should be visible, if the image is created by the foramen. Pulp testing further differentiates the pathosis from the normal landmark. The response from the landmark is a vital one, and the periapical pathosis response usually is a nonvital one.

Nasal Fossae

These are the bony cavities of the nares. They appear as two large radio-

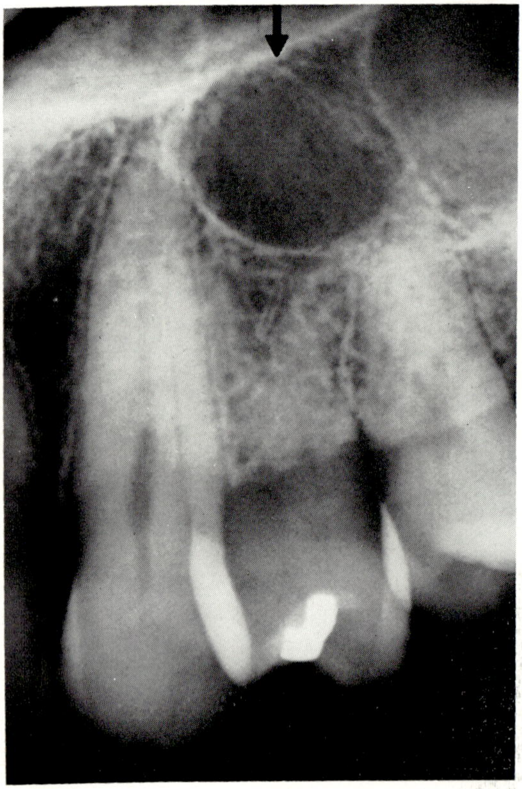

Figure 196. Maxillary sinus extension simulating a radicular cyst. (Courtesy of Dr. W. Updegrave, Philadelphia, Pa.)

lucent images above the roots of the central incisors (Figs. 195, 248). In rare cases when there are large fossae present along with long rooted central incisors, the images of these landmarks may simulate pulpally-induced periapical lesions. The means of differentation are the same as those described for the anterior palatine foramen.

Maxillary Sinus

This is a cavity of varying dimensions (depends upon age, function, loss of teeth and particular individuals). It occurs in the maxilla and is visible in periapical radiographs of upper canines, premolars and molars. The sinus appears as a large radiolucent area with a radiopaque border. It appears above the apexes of the upper posterior teeth, but may appear below the apex in certain views. The sinus often appears as an inverted "Y" shaped structure. It may be misinterpreted as a large radicular cyst, as the image may appear above the apex of any of the upper posterior teeth (Fig. 196). Differentiation between the sinus and a pulpally-induced

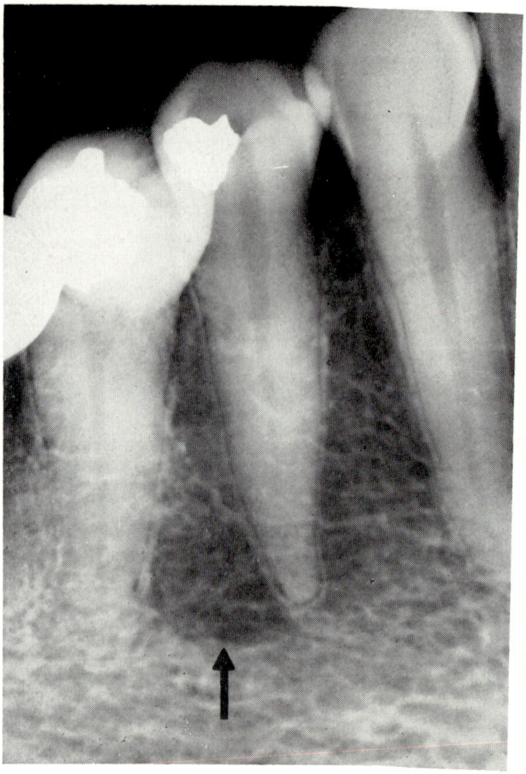

Figure 197. Mental foramen located near the apex of a lower premolar; lamina dura and periodontal ligament space is visible around the entire root of the first premolar. (Courtesy of Dr. W. Updegrave, Philadelphia, Pa.)

periapical lesion is made by the means described for the anterior palatine foramen (Fig. 68). Also, if a periapical area of pathosis has a radiopaque border, it is generally more definite and with a straighter outline than is the case for the sinus border.

Mental Foramen

This foramen contains the branches of the inferior alveolar nerve and blood vessels that exit to the gingiva and alveolar mucosa. It lies between and beneath the lower premolar apexes. The radiographic image shows a round radiolucent area that may appear directly below the apex of one of the premolars (Fig. 197). The foramen then simulates a periapical cyst or granuloma. A change in angulation changes the location of the image of the foramen relative to the premolar apex. The other considerations for differentiation are the same as has been described for the anterior palatine foramen. Another means of differentation is that often the image of the mental foramen can be found to be continuous with the image of the inferior alveolar canal (Figs. 198, 300).

Inferior Alveolar Canal (Mandibular Canal)

This canal houses the inferior alveolar nerves and blood vessels. It appears on the radiograph as a radiolucent line, often with a radiopaque border. The canal is generally seen in lower molar periapical radiographs. It may appear toward the lower border of the mandible, but at other times it can appear to be superimposed over the apexes of the molars, particularly the third molars. In the latter case with an isolated periapical radiograph it may be misinterpreted as a periapical granuloma or

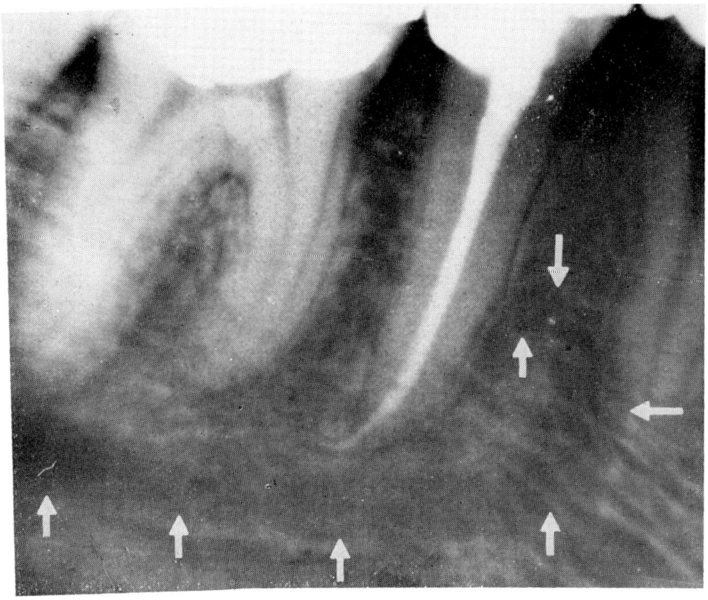

Figure 198. Inferior alveolar canal joins the mental foramen; arrows point to the outline of the canal and mental foramen.

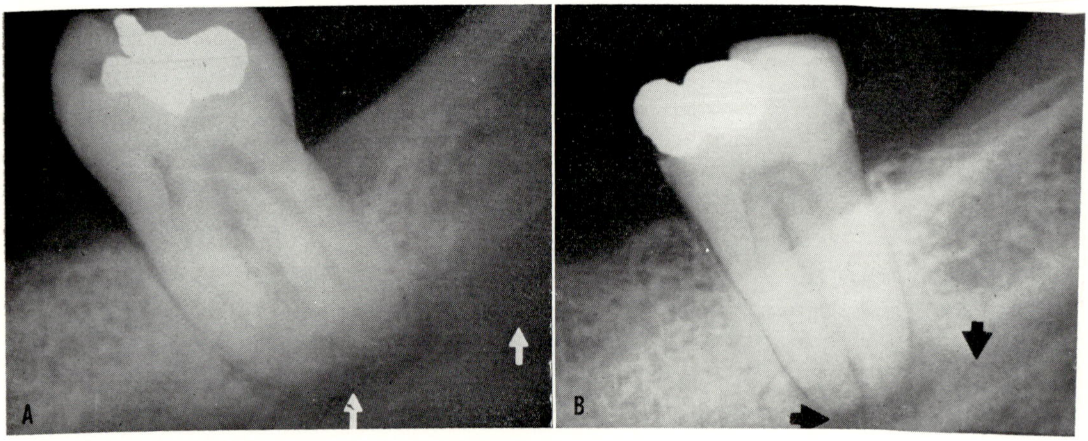

Figure 199. Inferior alveolar canal or periapical area of pathosis? A. Inferior alveolar canal; arrows point to canal; lamina dura and periodontal ligament space is visible around the roots. (Courtesy of Dr. W. Updegrave, Philadelphia, Pa.) B. Inferior alveolar canal and periapical pathosis; right arrow points to canal; left arrow points to periapical pathosis. There is loss in continuity of the apical lamina dura.

cyst (Fig. 199). The canal may be differentiated as described in the section on the anterior palatine foramen. However, instead of changing the horizontal angulation of the second radiograph, the vertical angulation is changed. If the canal is the cause of the radiolucency, it will appear to move up or down on the second radiograph as compared to the original. The image will also move away from the root apex (Fig. 109). With the use of a panograph radiograph, the complete continuity of the canal can be seen and this differentiates the canal from a lesion.

Nutrient Canals and Foramina

These canals house smaller branches of nerves or blood vessels that supply the alveolar bones and the teeth. They appear radiographically as small radiolucent lines and circumferential areas. At times they can be superimposed over root apexes and simulate small pulpally-induced periapical lesions (Fig. 200). Differentiation is as described previously for the other landmarks.

The Lingual Foramen

This is a small radiolucent area that represents the space between the genial tubercles of the mandibular symphysis. The radiographic appearance shows a small radiolucent area that is usually found between the lower central incisors (Fig. 84A). In occasional cases, it may be superimposed over the apex of an incisor root and then appear as if it were a small granuloma. Differentiation is as described previously.

Normal Radiolucent Area

In individuals with a relatively thin cortex, the alveolar bone in the lower incisor or premolar regions may appear radiolucent. The radiolucency may be

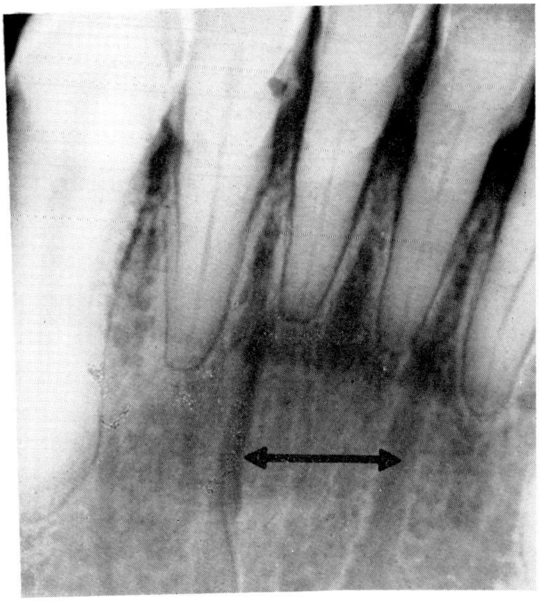

Figure 200. Large nutrient canals that simulate pathoses or fractures. (Courtesy of Dr. T. Simpson, Philadelphia, Pa.)

confined to one area and then simulate periapical pathosis. To differentiate these conditions, it is necessary to look carefully at the radiolucency. It should be possible to see evidence of bony trabeculation in the area and the presence of an intact lamina dura around the roots (Fig. 201). The teeth in the area should all test vital.

Stafne Bone Cyst

This is the superimposition of the submaxillary glands on a radiograph. The radiographic image shows a large radiolucent image near the border of the posterior part of the mandible. It is rarely confused with a periapical lesion as it is usually close to the border of the mandible. However, it is possible that in a thin mandible and with molars with long roots it can appear to be related to root apexes (Fig. 202). Differential between this landmark and periapical lesions is the same as for the anterior palatine foramen.

Teeth with Incomplete Root Formation and Tooth Buds

Developing teeth with incomplete apexes may appear as teeth with periapical areas of rarefaction (Fig. 203). As immature teeth can give a negative response to the electric pulp tester, this

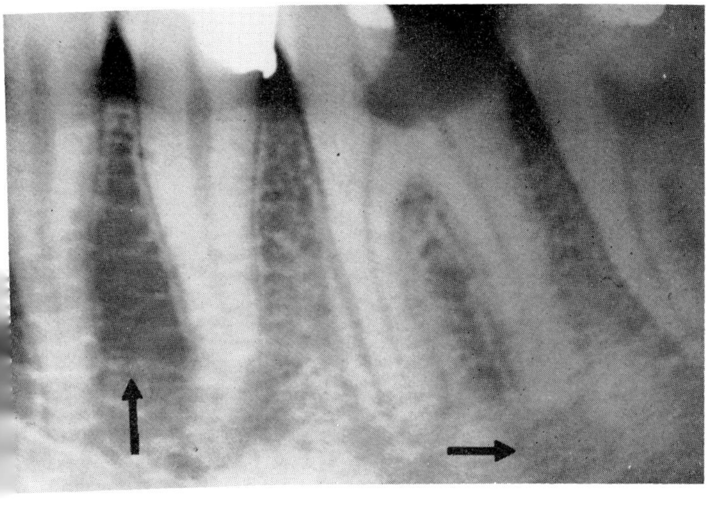

Figure 201. Normal radiolucencies that may simulate pathosis. (Courtesy of Dr. W. Updegrave, Philadelphia, Pa.)

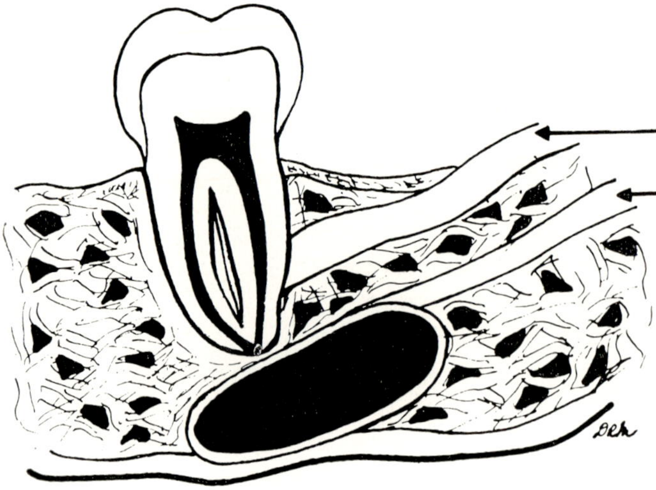

Figure 202. Stafne bone cyst.

cannot be used to differentiate the conditions. If the teeth cause no symptoms, no treatment should be done. If the roots do not continue to develop, then it can be assumed that pathosis is present and endodontic therapy should be performed. A permanent tooth bud can be superimposed over the apex of a primary molar, thereby simulating a periapical lesion (Fig. 204).

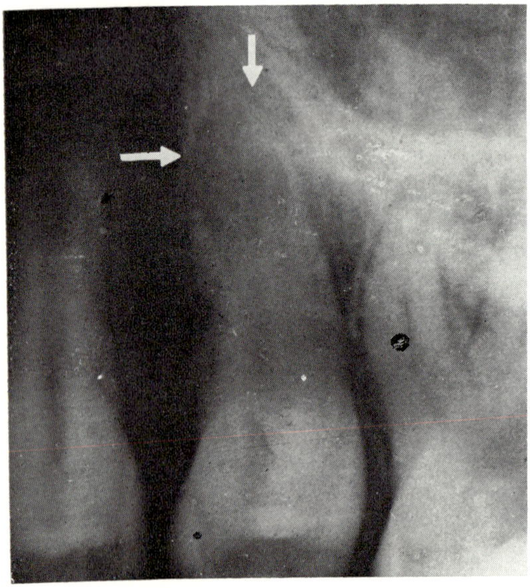

Figure 203. Tooth with wide open apex that simulates a periapical area of pathosis.

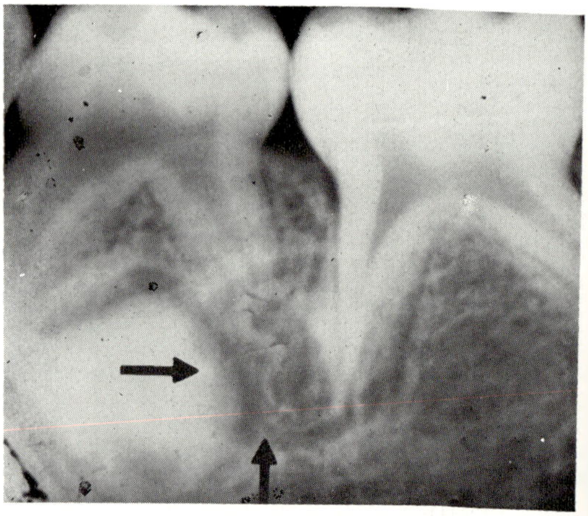

Figure 204. Tooth bud of lower first premolar located over the apex of lower first primary molar simulates a peripical area of pathosis. (Courtesy of Dr. W. Updegrave, Philadelphia, Pa.)

The Maxillary Tuberosity

This is found in the upper posterior region distal to the third molar. It appears as a radiolucent area that may be in proximity to the third molar root apexes (Fig. 205). Differentiation is by use of radiographs from different angles and vitality testing of the teeth in the area.

Radiopaque Landmarks

There are certain radiopaque landmarks that may simulate the appearance of condensing osteitis. They can be differentiated from this lesion by the following means. The teeth related to the landmarks are all vital. The landmarks appear over more than one tooth and this can be readily observed by the use of an occlusal or panograph film. If the landmark appears to be superimposed over the apex, a second film is taken from a different horizontal direction. This should show that the image has moved away from the root apex. In the maxilla, the radiopaque landmarks are the following.

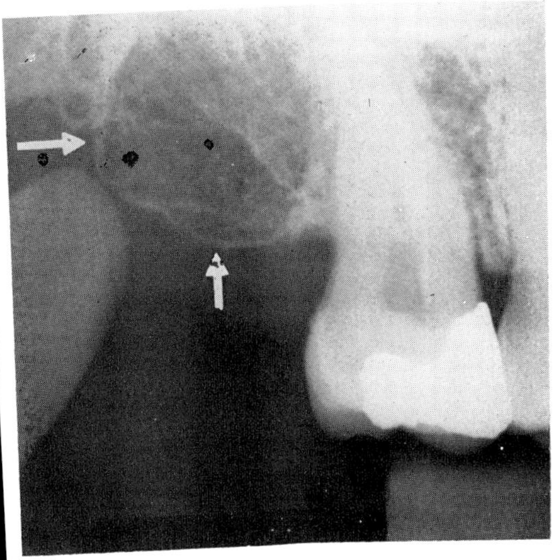

Figure 205. Maxillary tuberosity; shows up as a slight radiolucency (arrows). (Courtesy of Dr. W. Updegrave, Philadelphia, Pa.)

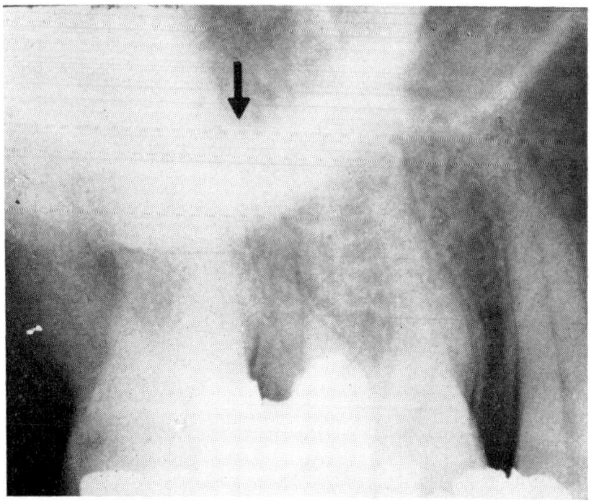

Figure 206. Zygoma.

THE ZYGOMA. This forms the zygomatic arch and it appears as a broad radiopaque mass on upper molar periapical radiographs (Fig. 206).

NASAL SEPTUM AND SPINE. The septum is between the nasal fossa and the spine is between the central incisors (Fig. 207).

TORUS PALATINUS. This is a bony prominence that is found in the midline of the hard palate in some individuals. On periapical radiographs, it may be superimposed over premolar and molar roots.

In the mandible, the radiopaque landmarks are the following:

THE MENTAL RIDGE. This is a dense radiopaque appearing bony septum that extends from the mandibular symphysis to the premolar region (Figs. 208, 209).

GENIAL TUBERCLES. These are four radiopaque-appearing rounded ring-like structures, that are found between and below the central incisors (Fig. 209).

THE EXTERNAL OBLIQUE RIDGE

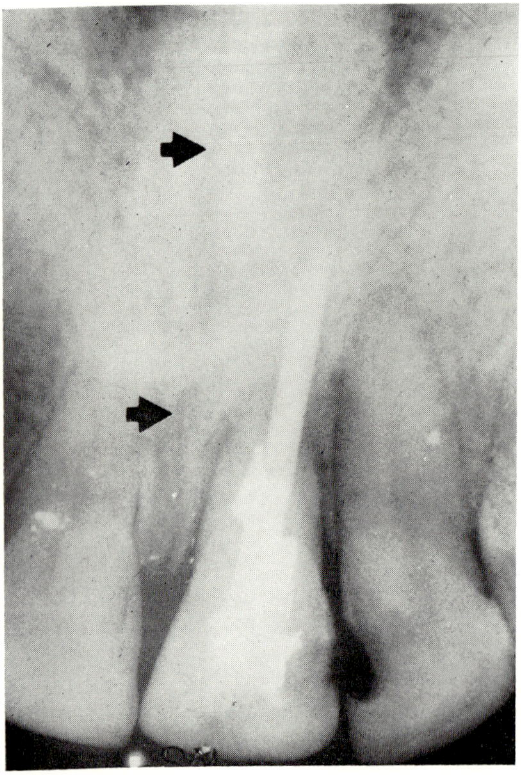

Figure 207. Nasal septum and spine; upper arrow indicates septum; lower arrow indicates spine. (From D. R. Morse, "The Significance of Endodontics in Plantation Procedures," *JDA South Africa,* 26:263, 1971.)

(LINE). This is a thick bony ridge that goes from the mental process up to the anterior border of the ramus. It can appear on lower molar films as a radiopaque band around the apexes (Figs. 210, 211).

THE INTERNAL OBLIQUE RIDGE (MYLOHYOID RIDGE). This ridge is found on the inner aspect of the mandible from the symphysis to the ramus. It may also appear in lower molar radiographs beneath the image of the external oblique ridge (Fig. 211).

TORUS MANDIBULARIS. These are bony exostoses that are found in some individuals on the lingual aspect of the lower posterior avelolar bone. They can be superimposed over the roots of lower posterior teeth (Fig. 212).

EXOSTOSIS. Occasionally there is a normal exostosis of bone that can appear in the vicinity of root apexes (Fig. 213).

Soft Tissue Landmarks

For each landmark is given the definition, the clinical appearance, the endodontic lesions it simulates, and the means of differentiation of the two types of conditions.

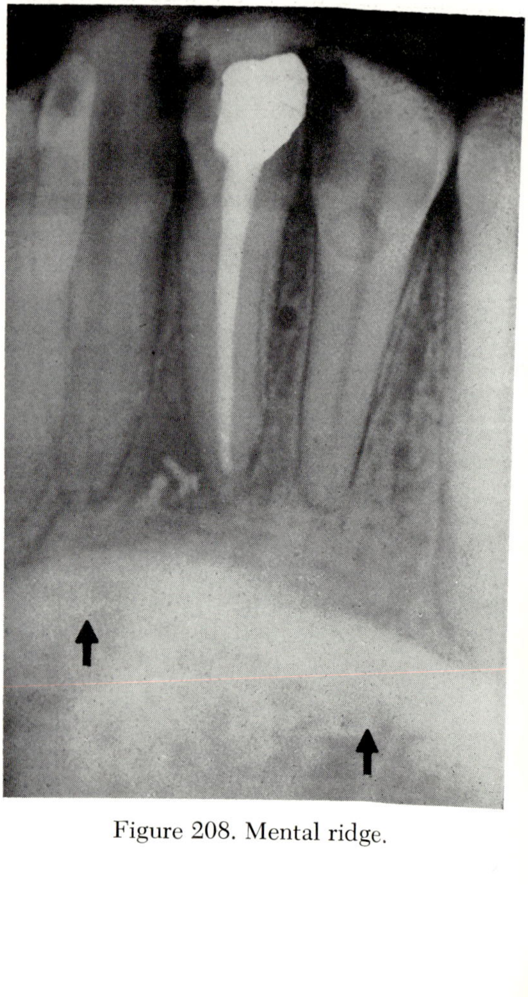

Figure 208. Mental ridge.

Fordyce's Granules

These are ectopically placed sebaceous glands. They are usually found in the buccal mucosa, especially around the internal aspect of the commissure of the lips. Rarely, isolated Fordyce granules can occur in the mucobuccal fold and simulate sinus tracts (Fig. 214). Differential diagnosis is by probing and histologic examination of the excised tissue.

Macroglossia

An enlarged tongue, especially on the inferior border, can simulate a swelling of the floor of the mouth. This must be differentiated from a lingual swelling originating from an abscessed lower molar. Macroglossia would show bilateral swelling and there would be no associated abnormality of the lower posterior teeth (Fig. 215).

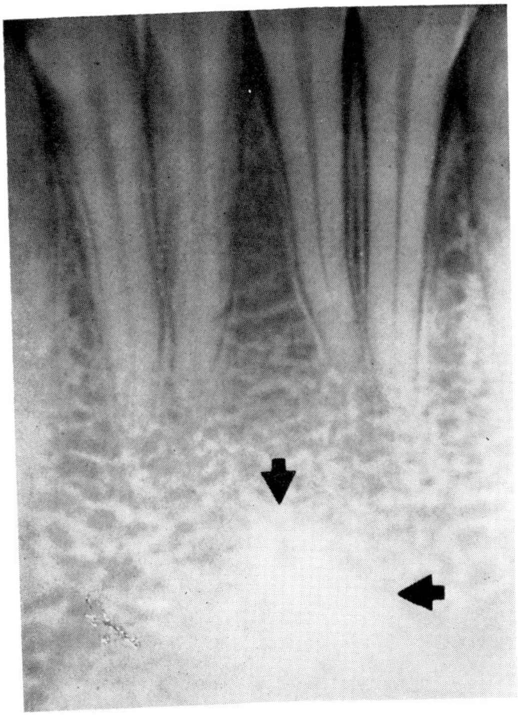

Figure 209. Genial tubercles and mental ridge; left arrow indicates genial tubercles; right arrow indicates mental ridge. (Courtesy of Dr. T. Simpson, Philadelphia, Pa.)

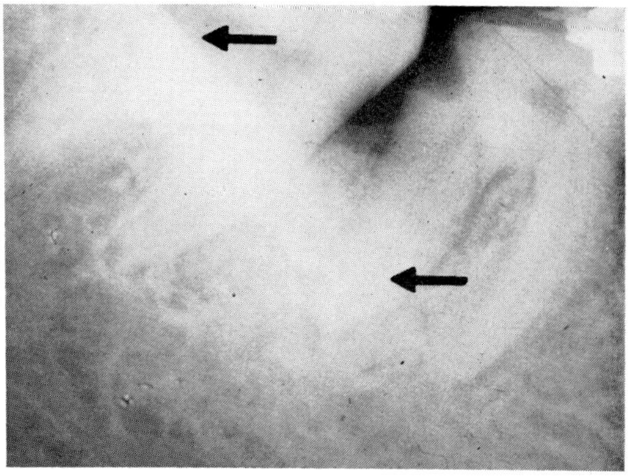

Figure 210. External oblique ridge. (From D. R. Morse, "The Management of Endodontic Problem Cases," *JDA South Africa*, 27:387, 1972.)

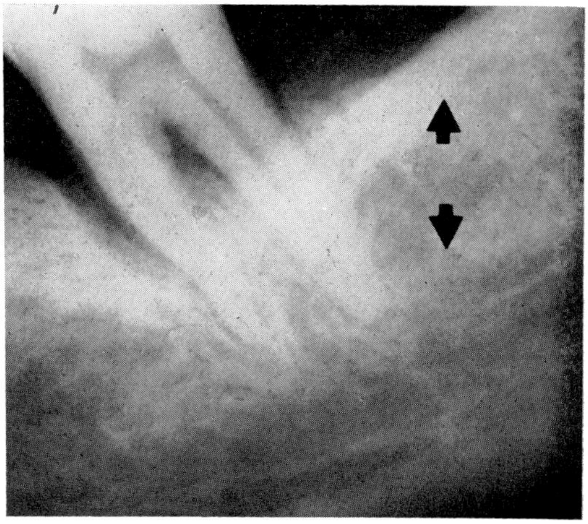

Figure 211. Oblique ridges; upper arrow indicates external ridge; lower arrow indicates internal ridge. (From D. R. Morse, "The Significance of Endodontics in Plantation Procedures," *JDA South Africa*, 26:263, 1971.)

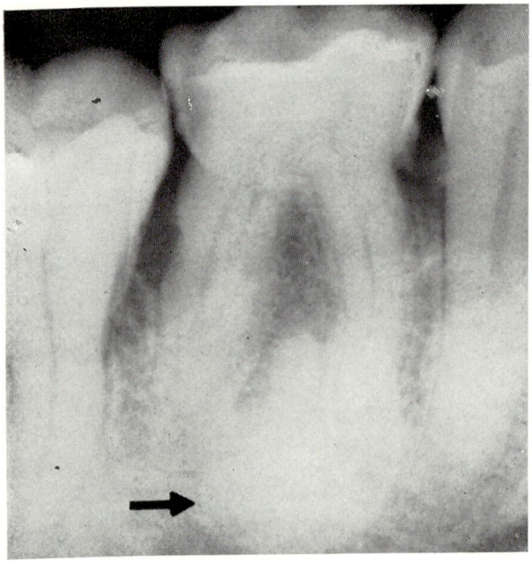

Figure 212. Torus mandibularis superimposed over the apexes of a lower molar. (Courtesy of Dr. T. Simpson, Philadelphia, Pa.)

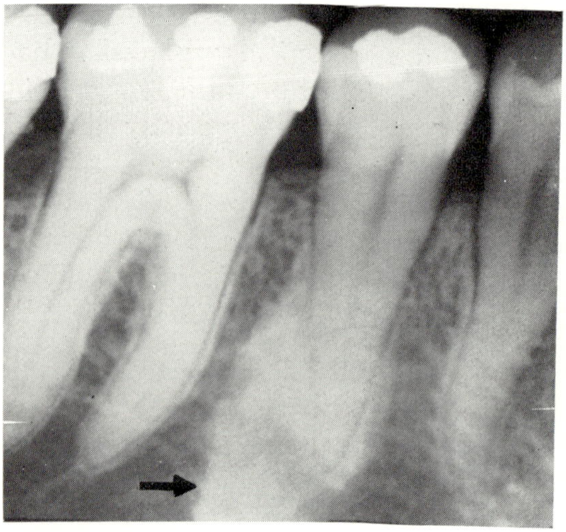

Figure 213. Exostosis. (Courtesy of Dr. W. Updegrave, Philadelphia, Pa.)

Salivary Duct Orifices

The orifice of the parotid duct (Stenssen's) is on the buccal mucosa opposite the upper second molar (Fig. 216). The orifices of the submaxillary and sublingual ducts are found in the anterior floor of the mouth in the vicinity of the lingual frenum (Fig. 215). These orifices can simulate sinus tracts. They are differentiated from the latter by their specific locations and by the vital responses of associated teeth.

Frenums and Papilla

The labial and lingual frenums and the incisive papilla (anterior palatine) (Fig. 215) may simulate a parulis (gum boil). Their specific location, and nor-

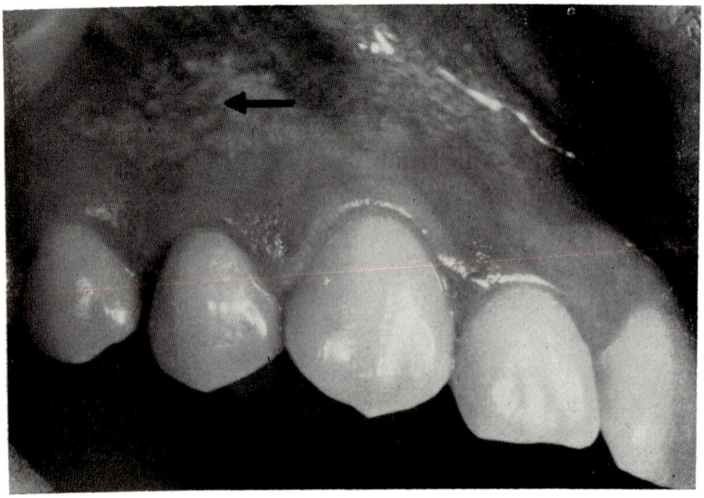

Figure 214. Fordyce granules in the muco-buccal fold. (Courtesy of Dr. T. Simpson, Philadelphia, Pa.)

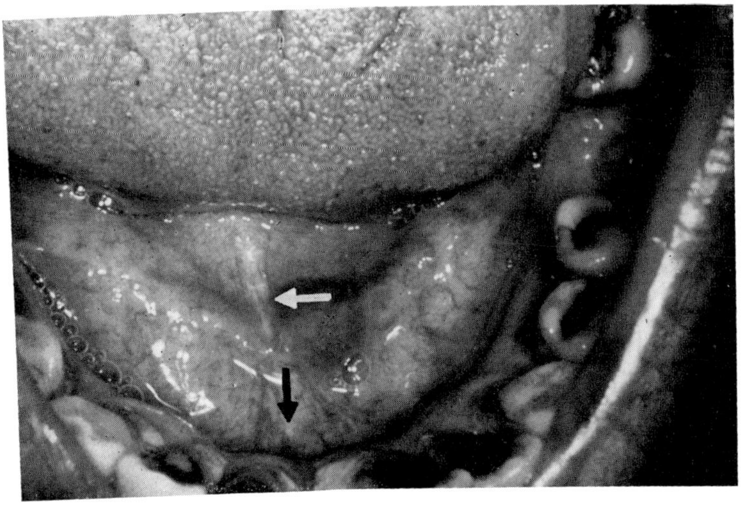

Figure 215. Macroglossia, orifices of the submaxillary and sublingual ducts (black arrow), and lingual frenum (white arrow). Courtesy of Dr. T. Simpson, Philadelphia, Pa.)

mal vitality of associated teeth serves to differentiate the conditions.

Palatal Opening of the Nasopalatine Duct

There have been cases of palatal openings of the nasopalatine duct in the anterior palate. These openings can simulate a sinus tract originating from an upper incisor. Differential diagnosis of the two conditions is obtained by means of probing and pulp testing. With the nasopalatine duct opening, the probe would not penetrate into the region of a tooth apex (determined by a radiograph) and the associated teeth would test vital.

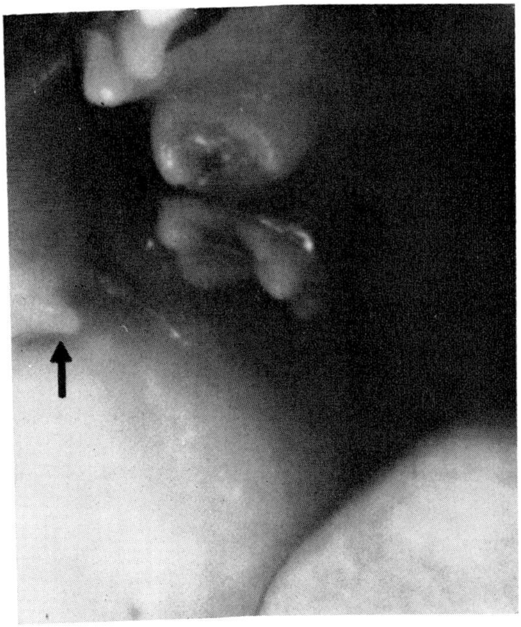

Figure 216. Orifice of Stenssen's duct. (Courtesy of Dr. K. Bomze, Cherry Hill, N. J.)

Benign Masseteric Hypertrophy

This is an enlargement of the masseter muscle of unknown etiology, that can simulate a facial swelling. It may occasionally be unilateral and then appear similar to an endodontically-involved swelling. However, all tests would be normal.

NORMAL PHYSIOLOGIC CONDITIONS

Each of these conditions has one or more pulpal or periapical signs or symptoms that are not related to pulpal or periapical disease.

Menstruation and Pregnancy

During these periods, women can have oral signs and symptoms. Herpetic lesions and gingivitis may occur. Symptoms of apical periodontitis and odontalgia may occur in apparently sound teeth. These manifestations may localize to one or several teeth. Symptoms related to menstruation or pregnancy and not pulpal or periapical disease, terminate at the end of the menstrual period or pregnancy. The symptoms may then recur with the onset of the following menses or pregnancy. As the teeth test vital, the apical periodontitis and odontalgia appear to be related to the hyperemia and capillary dilation present during menstruation and pregnancy. The blood vessel alterations may be triggered by hormonal changes.

Tooth Eruptions

An erupting third molar can cause referred pain to teeth anterior to it. Radiographs and vitality tests of adjoining teeth aid in the diagnosis. As described previously, an erupting tooth may cause external root resorption of an adjoining tooth.

Aging

Pulp calcification and fibrosis may occur with aging of teeth. Tooth age is not necessarily related to chronological age, although generally as one gets older, pulpal calcification and fibrosis increase. These teeth may give little or no response to pulp testing. As teeth with pulposis are difficult to differentiate from teeth with symptomless necrosis (without any periapical rarefactions), the best treatment is a watch and wait attitude.

TREATMENT COMPLICATIONS RESULTING IN ORAL FACIAL SWELLINGS OR RADIOGRAPHIC RAREFACTIONS

Swellings

Included in this section are hematoma, ecchymoses, buccal fat pad swelling, angioneurotic edema, and surgical emphysema.

Hematoma and Ecchymosis

A hematoma is a tumor-like collection of effused blood. A local anesthetic injection into a blood vessel can cause its production (Fig. 42). It may also occur following periapical surgery, when a large pool of blood accumulates. A hematoma may result from a facial accident. Only in the latter case should there be any problem with differential diagnosis, and then the history should help in the diagnosis. The swelling of the hematoma is usually dark in appearance due to the pooled blood in the subsurface tissues. It may take several days to weeks to completely resolve. Treatment is discussed in Chapter 16. An ecchymosis is a large and blotchy area *(black & blue)* resulting from hemorrhage. Etiology and prognosis is the same as for hematoma.

Buccal Fat Pad Swelling

A local anesthetic injection into the buccal fat pad, in the region of the upper molars, can cause this rapidly produced swelling. As in the case with the hematoma, several days may be necessary for the swelling to disappear. If the swelling comes up slowly, it may be confused with a swelling arising from an infection. However, with a fat pad injection, the patient usually states that the swelling was noticeable soon after he (or she) left the dental office (see Chapter 16).

Angioneurotic Edema

This is an allergic-type response that is characterized by a sudden, transient, circumscribed, edematous swelling. It may involve the lips, the skin around the eyes and the chin, the tongue, and the oral mucous membranes or the glottis. Angioneurotic edema is believed to occur as a result of small blood vessel dilation with subsequent transudation of fluid through capillary walls into the adjoining subcutaneous or submucosal tissue. It can be hereditary, a response to drugs, including antibiotics, or it may result from a food allergy. Angioneurotic edema may be precipitated by trauma of dental surgery. The history should help in the differentiation of this swelling from a pulpal-periapical disease swelling. The swelling of angioneurotic edema usually lasts only one day. Treatment is discussed in Chapter 16.

Surgical Emphysema

This is the introduction of air into the subcutaneous tissues, resulting in a noticeable swelling. It can occur following a clinical procedure. In dentistry, it usually appears following the use of the air turbine handpiece during oral surgery or following the introduction of forced air directed into the pulp cavity. The latter procedure should never be performed during endodontic therapy. Most cases of surgical emphysema follow surgical procedures on lower molars. Air can be forced into the submaxillary space and then into the deeper spaces and finally into the mediastinum. If emphysema occurs during endodontics, air could get into other spaces and produce swellings mimicking cellulitis cases. There should be no problem in differentiating this condition from periapical pathosis by a knowledge of the history. Other diagnostic signs are sudden swelling of the involved region and a characteristic crepitus or crackling sound heard upon palpation of the swollen mass. Depending upon where the air masses are, it is possible to visualize them as radiolucent areas on radiographs. For treatment see Chapter 16.

Fibrous Scar

This consists of normal fibrous connective tissue in a periapical area that formerly contained granulomatous tissue or a radicular cyst (Fig. 217C). It usually occurs after periapical surgery had been performed for a lesion that had destroyed both cortical plates of bone (labial and lingual). Rarely, it occurs after nonsurgical endodontic therapy. The radiographic appearance reveals an extremely radiolucent area at a distance from the root apex, although it may be continuous with the apex (Figs. 73C, 217B). In the latter instance, the scar may be confused with a pulpally-induced periapical lesion.

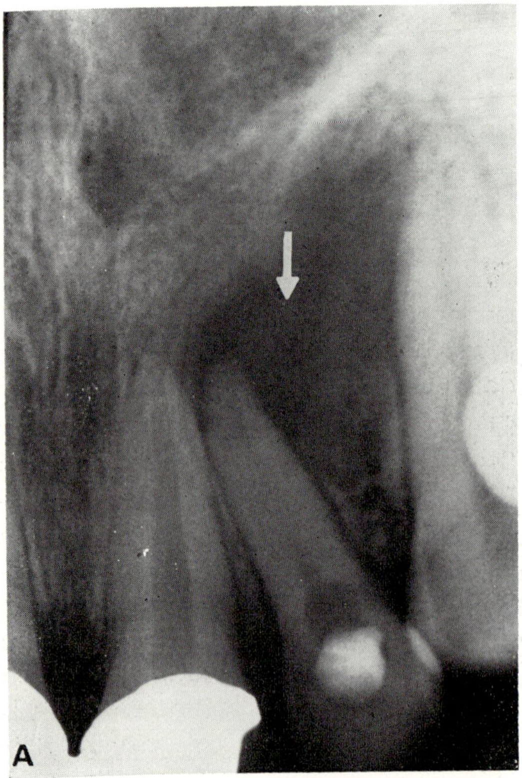

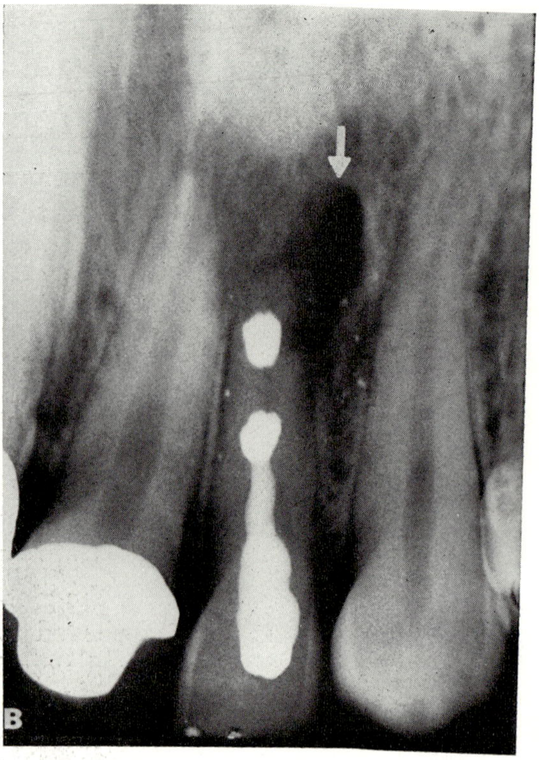

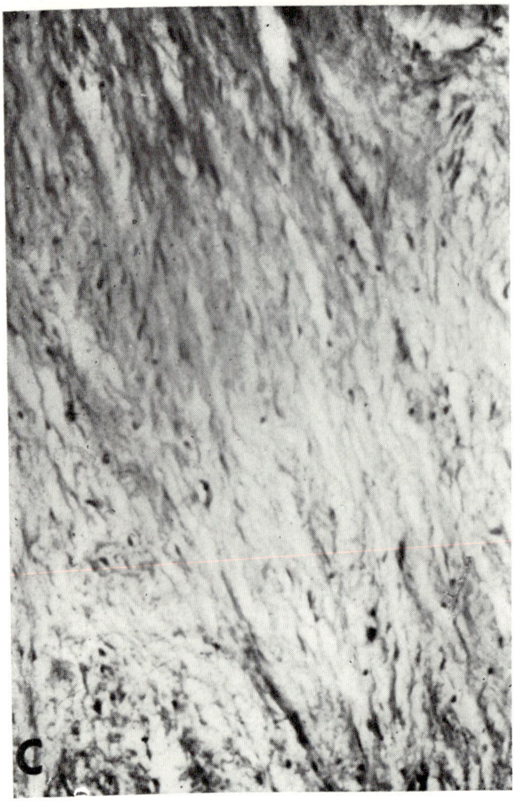

Figure 217. Globulomaxillary cyst, pulp necrosis, perforation, and development of fibrous scar. A. Globulomaxillary cyst was present and removed; pulp of lateral incisor subsequently became pulpless; root was perforated during access preparation. B. Three years after endodontic therapy, periapical curettage (bone was destroyed on both labial and palatal plates of bone), and amalgam seal of the apex and perforation, tooth has uprighted; periapical area of pathosis has healed and a fibrous scar remains. C. Histologic section of tissue (arrow in B) revealed fibrous connective tissue.

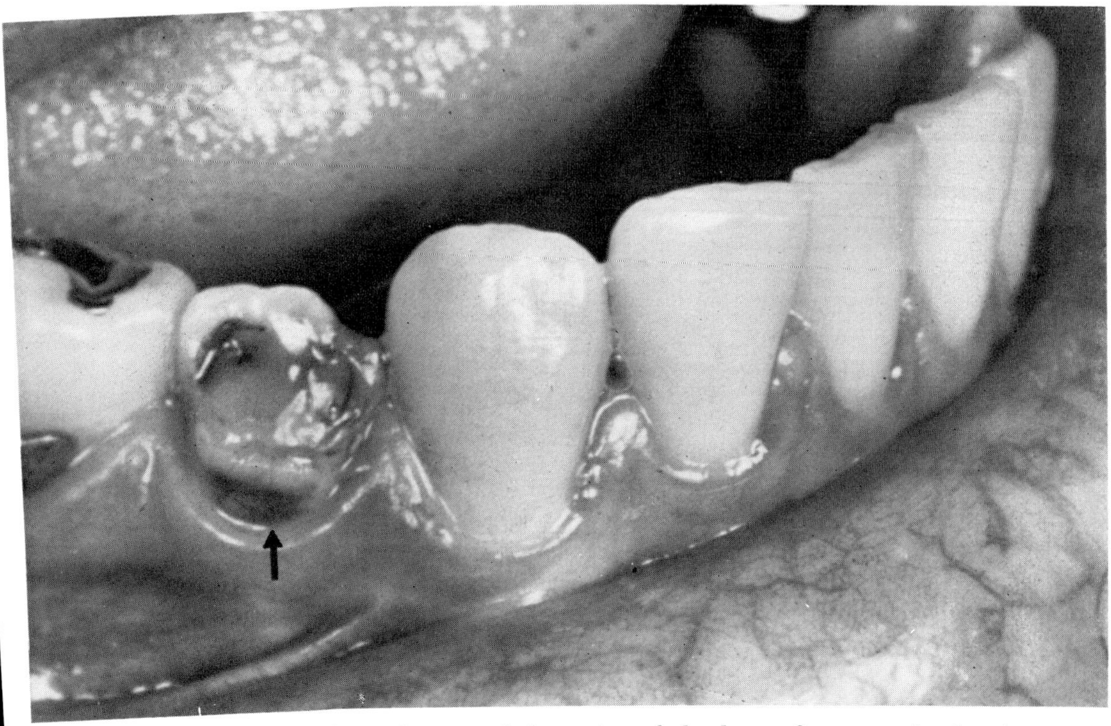

Figure 218. A Turner's tooth; enamel formation of the lower first premolar has been impeded because of inflammation of its predecessor, the primary first molar. (From S. Seltzer and I. B. Bender, *The Dental Pulp*, J. P. Lippincott Co., 1965. Used with permission of J. P. Lippincott Company.)

The principal means of differential diagnosis is by the history and an examination of pre- and post-treatment radiographs.

NON-ENDODONTIC DENTAL, PERIODONTAL, OR TEMPOROMANDIBULAR LESIONS, DISEASES AND CONDITIONS

These entities can show certain manifestations that may simulate endodontic disease symptoms or signs. The manifestations include pain, swelling, tooth discolorations, pulp canal enlargements, pulp canal calcifications, periapical areas of pathosis, and root resorption. The involved teeth should test vital.

Turner's Tooth

A local cause of enamel hypoplasia is injury to the permanent tooth germ, resulting from an infection of the overlying primary molar. The involved tooth is called a Turner's tooth (Fig. 218). If the only alteration is hypoplasia, the tooth should test vital.

Hereditary Opalescent Dentin

In this genetic disease, the pulp cavities are abnormally large in early stages and then become almost calcified with aging (Fig. 142). The dentin appears opalescent, the enamel flakes away

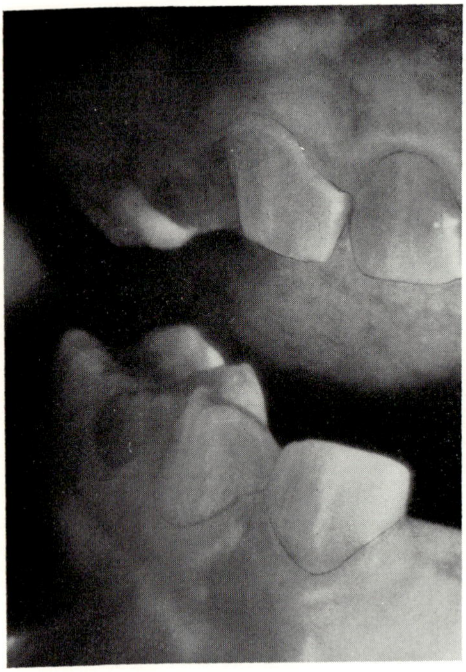

Figure 219. Hereditary opalescent dentin; dentin appears opalescent. (Courtesy of Dr. K. Bomze, Cherry Hill, N. J.)

readily (Fig. 219), and the roots are usually short and pointed (Fig. 142).

Dens Invaginatus (Dens in Dente)

In this genetically-induced lesion, there is an invagination of the dental organ into the dental papilla, forming a *tooth within a tooth*. The involved tooth is most frequently an upper lateral incisor but it may be a lower lateral incisor (Fig. 220). Usually the pulp becomes necrotic, and treatment is by immediate surgical endodontics (Fig. 221). There is also a somewhat similar developmental anomaly appearing as fissure-like channels in the lingual aspect of upper central and lateral incisors. These grooves continue apically for varying lengths and act as a nidus for progressive inflammation. The grooves are usually associated with an infrabony pocket. Reports have stated that these cases are untreatable, and even combined endodontic and periodontic treatment is to no avail. If the groove extends only partially down the root surface, the tooth may be retained, but occasional exacerbations may occur.

Taurodontism

In this genetic manifestation, the teeth have large crowns, short roots and very large pulp chambers that can easily be exposed by caries or dental procedures (Fig. 147). Taurodontism is more common in relatively primitive people like Eskimos, American Indians, and aborigines.

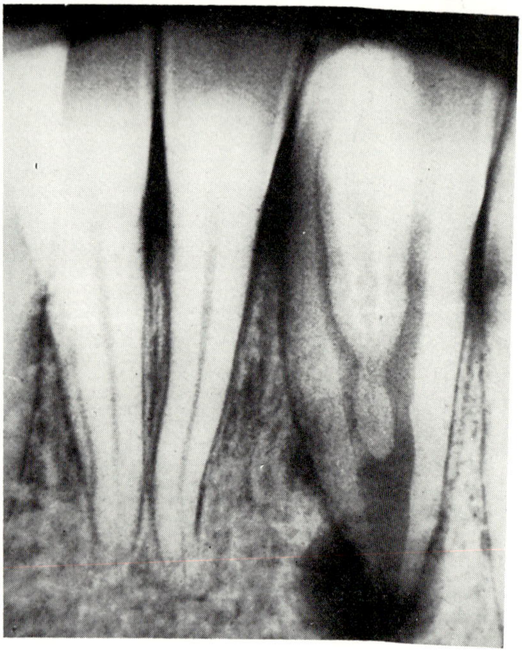

Figure 220. Dens invaginatus (dens in dente) in a lower lateral incisor. (Courtesy of Dr. T. Simpson, Philadelphia, Pa.)

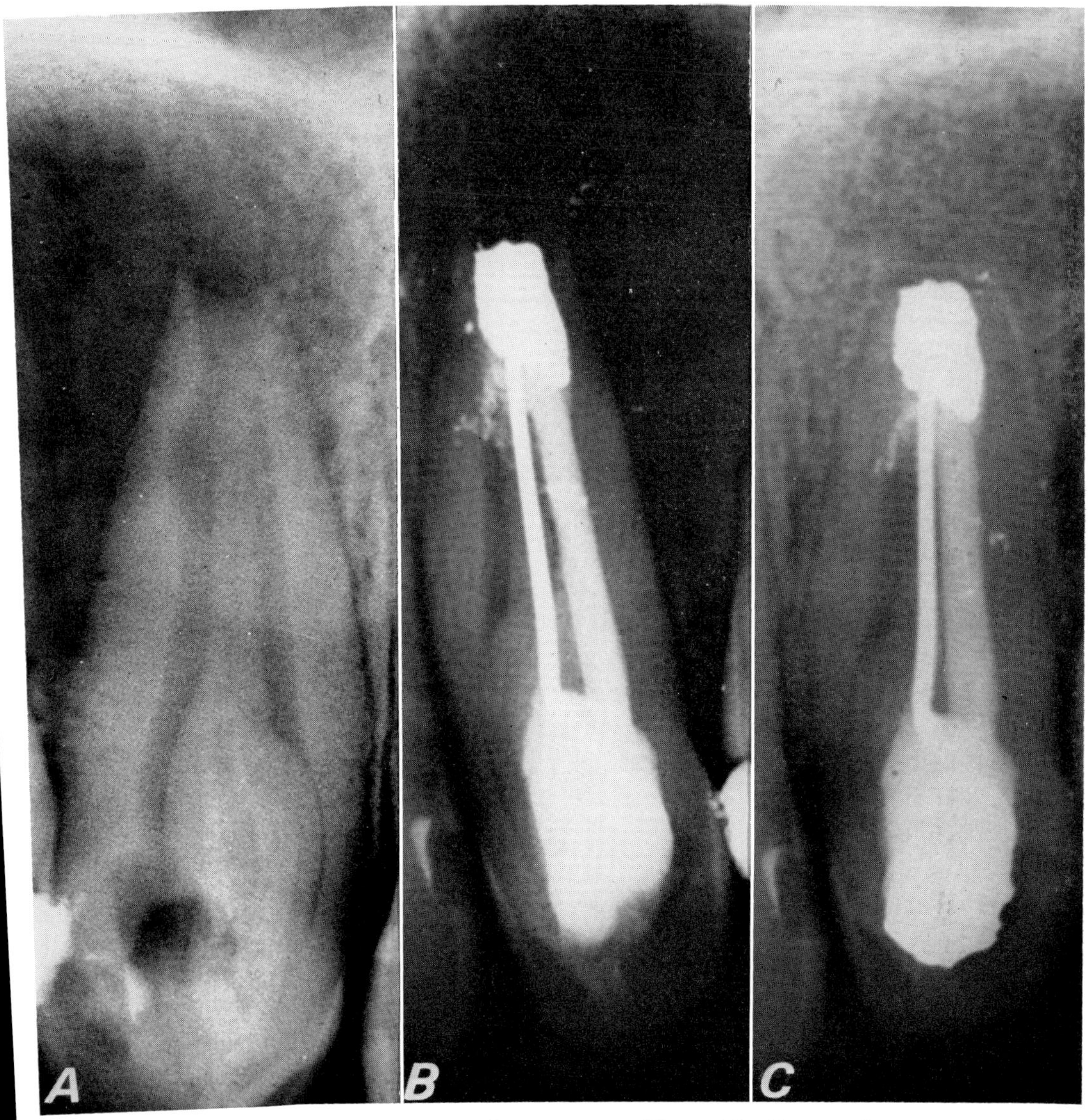

Figure 221. Dens in dente; surgical treatment. (From N. Chivian "Surgical Endodontics—A Conservative Approach," *J N J Dent Assoc,* 40:234, 1969.) A. Before treatment. B. After obturation with a combination of gutta-percha, silver cone, and a periapical curettage and retrograde amalgam seal. C. A. post-operative radiograph showing periapical repair.

Odontodysplasia

In this condition, possibly caused by a somatic mutation, all elements of the dental organ are affected. The teeth have large pulp chambers and hypoplasia of enamel, dentin, and cementum. Pulp exposure is common. The condition usually affects several adjacent teeth, and is very rare.

Pulpal Dysplasia

This is another genetic condition, in which the pulp chambers of all the teeth are usually ovoid or flame-shaped. The pulp canals contain multiple pulp stones, and calcification occurs with aging. Blood tests are normal in this rare condition.

Dentin Dysplasia

This is a rare genetic disease involving the dentin. The roots are short and there is almost complete pulp calcification. Pulp chambers have a radiographic semi-lunar appearance. There are often large periapical areas of rarefaction present which probably result from minute pulpal exposures.

Atypical Dentin Dysplasia with Typical Facies

This is another rare genetic disease in which there is complete obliteration of the pulp cavities in adults, along with a typical facial appearance.

Periodontal Diseases

In most of the periodontal diseases, the lesions are not isolated to single teeth, as usually is the case with endodontic disease. However, occasionally isolated infra-bony pockets may be found (Fig. 175I). Pain is often less severe than in endodontic disease. Swelling, when present, is not at the mucobuccal fold, but is in the region of the alveolar mucosa or gingiva.

Gingivitis

There are various types of gingivitises including marginal, desquamative, acute herpetic gingivostomatitis, and acute necrotizing ulcerative gingivitis (ANUG) (Fig. 222). Gingivitis may accompany systemic diseases and conditions such as vitamin C deficiency (scurvy), vitamin B deficiencies, anemias, leukemias (Fig. 11), polycythemia, agranulocytosis, cystic fibrosis, puberty, pregnancy, post-menopause, rickets, exanthematous diseases, diphtheria, kidney diseases, lung diseases, gastrointestinal diseases, acromegaly, diabetes (Fig. 223), Hand-Schüller-Christian disease, and acatalasemia. In the latter genetic disease, in which there is a deficiency of the enzyme catalase, necrotic ulcerative gingivitis usually occurs. This may be followed by recession and alveolar bone loss. The teeth may eventually loosen and exfoliate. Blood tests show a deficiency in the enzyme catalase, which normally degrades hydrogen peroxide. Generally, there is no problem in differential diagnosis between these conditions and endodontic diseases. In ANUG and herpetic stomatitis, the patients may have extreme pain and a submaxillary lymphadenopathy. In these conditions, the patients also complain of a fetid odor and a foul taste. These manifestations might be confused with

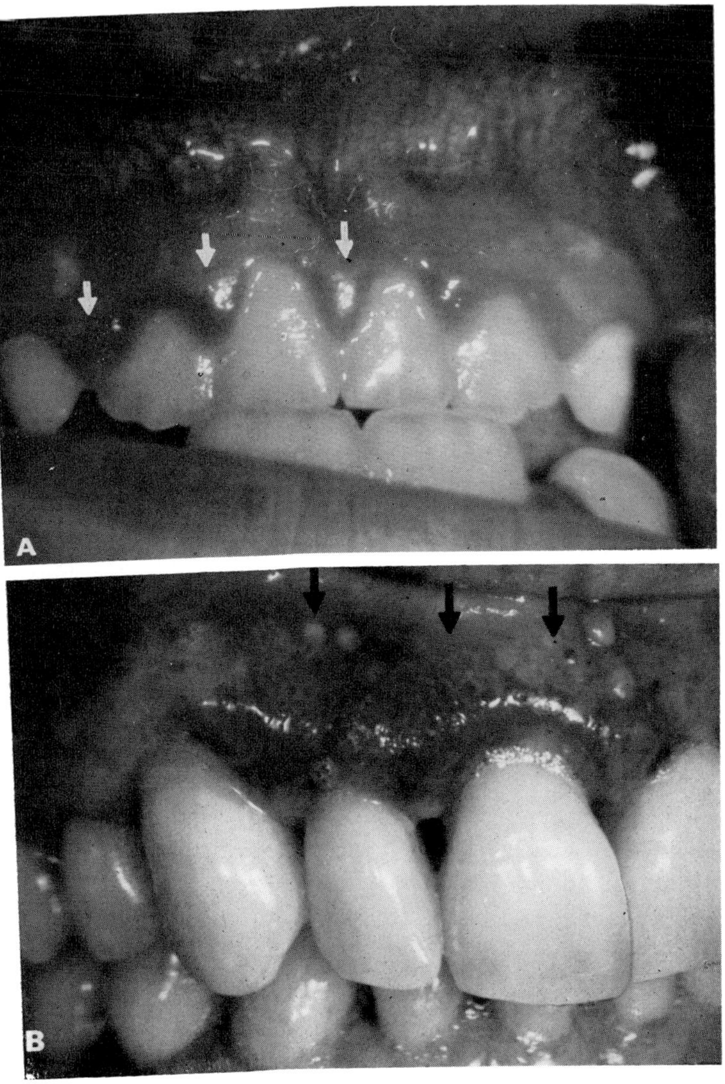

Figure 222. Two types of gingivitis: A. Localized marginal gingivitis. (Courtesy of Dr. K. Bomze, Cherry Hill, N. J.) B. Desquamative gingivitis around an upper central and lateral incisor. (Courtesy of Dr. T. Simpson, Philadelphia, Pa.)

the odor and taste originating from a gangrenous dental abscess. However, examination of the mouth would reveal the marked widespread gingival inflammation, and the possibility of endodontic disease would be dismissed. Also, microbial examination of the involved tissues would show the characteristic fuso-spirochetes of ANUG and the herpes simplex virus of herpetic stomatitis.

Gingival Hyperplasia

This may result from local conditions or systemic alterations. Hyperplasia can result from these possible systemic involvements: Dilantin therapy (Fig. 224), hypothyroidism, amyloidosis, Sturge-

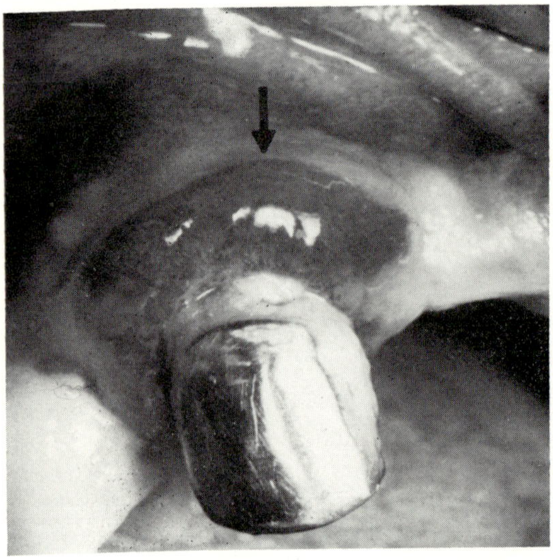

Figure 223. Gingivitis in an uncontrolled diabetic. (Courtesy of Dr. T. Simpson, Philadelphia, Pa.)

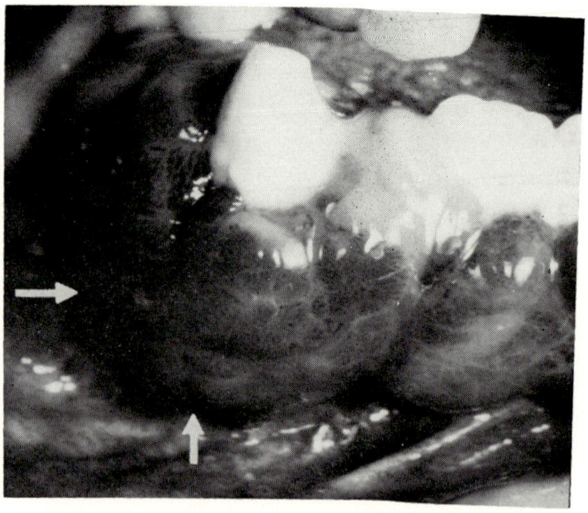

Figure 224. Gingival hyperplasia resulting from Dilantin therapy. (Courtesy of Dr. T. Simpson, Philadelphia, Pa.)

Weber's disease, Wegener's granulomatosis, Crohn's disease, infectious mononucleosis, hypopituitarism, and polycythemia. Local causes are calculus and mouthbreathing. The gingival swelling is rarely limited to one area; hence differential diagnosis is not usually a problem (Fig. 225).

Acute Papillitis

Inflammation and swelling of the interdental papilla may be caused by trauma, such as that initiated by food packing, toothbrush bristle, toothpick, etc. In this condition, manifestations may simulate those of pulpal or periapical disease. The patient may have severe pain that appears to be coming from

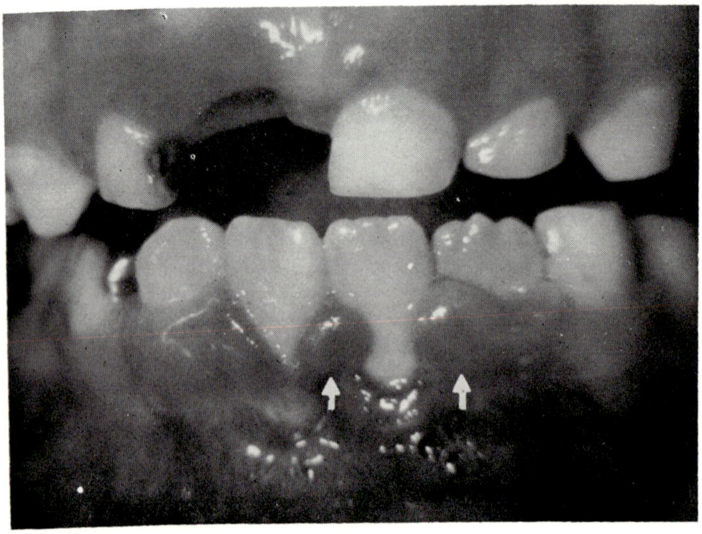

Figure 225. Gingival hyperplasia; local etiology, limited to lower anterior teeth. (Courtesy of Dr. K. Bomze, Cherry Hill, N. J.)

the pulp. The swelling is not in the mucobuccal fold but is in the interdental papilla. The adjoining teeth should test vital and probing of the papilla should allow for the recovery of the culpable object.

Lateral Periodontal Abscess or Cyst

In this case, there also can be pain and/or swelling. The radiograph usually reveals a radiolucency in the lateral or furca aspect of the root (Fig. 226). In the case of the abscess, the tooth tests vital and there is usually a pocket that communicates with the lesion. The exudate often drains through the pocket. After periodontal curettage, the symptoms should cease, if only a perio-

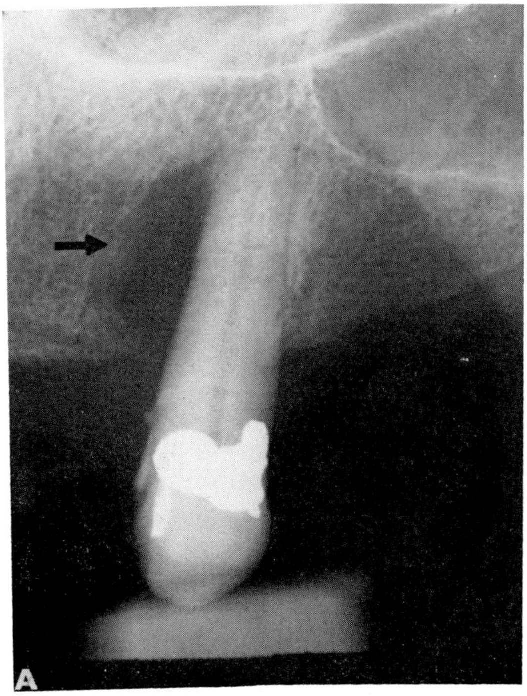

Figure 226. Lateral periodontal abscesses and cysts. A. Lateral abscess. B. Furcation cyst. C. Lateral cyst. (A and B, courtesy of Dr. W. Updegrave, Philadelphia, Pa., C, Courtesy of Dr. T. Simpson, Philadelphia, Pa.)

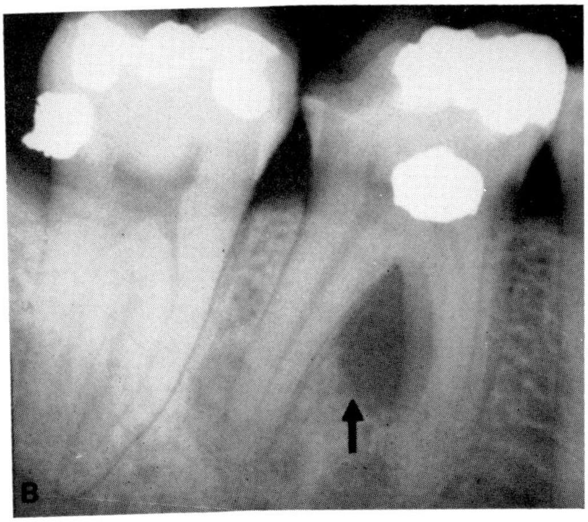

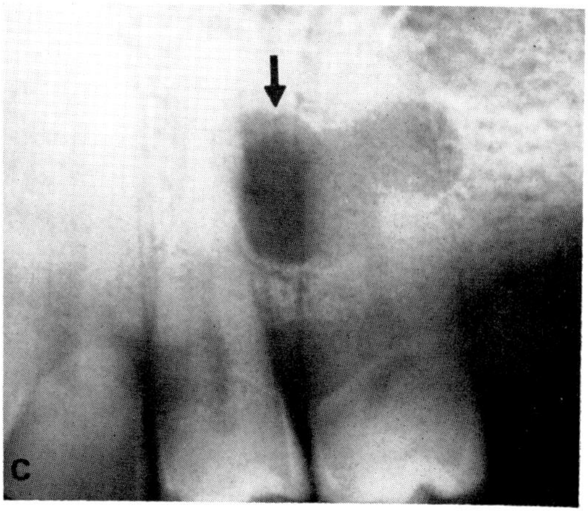

dontal condition is present. The lateral cyst is also involved with a vital tooth. It is often found along the lateral aspect of the root of lower canines and premolars. It does not communicate with the oral cavity as does a lateral abscess. It may result from trauma. The histopathological result shows a cyst lined by either a thin, keratinizing, stratified squamous epithelium, or a non-keratinizing cuboidal epithelium.

Acute Pericoronitis

This is an inflammation of the operculum or flap that partially covers an erupting tooth (usually a lower third molar). It can cause referred pain to the ear, angle of the jaw and to teeth anterior to it. Also a submaxillary lymphadenopathy may occur. Differential diagnosis would be abetted by examination of the inflamed tissues and pulp testing of the teeth in the area (they should test vital).

Periodontitis

Inflammation of the periodontal ligament with subsequent loss of alveolar bone may simulate endodontic diseases. Radiographic examination usually is helpful (Fig. 86). In periodontal disease, the alveolar bone loss is usually not limited to the one tooth (Fig. 88). In palatal root lesions, there may be a halo-like radiolucency around the apex of this root (Fig. 181). This is indicative of periodontal disease rather than endodontic disease. Pocket probing and detection of calculus also aid in the differentiation. At times a parulis or sinus tract may be present. However, probing would show that it usually does not go to the root apex. At times, there may be bone loss to the apex, and then the probe would reach that point. The teeth should test vital if the lesion is periodontal. Following periodontal treatment, if periapical healing does not take place, then it is probably a combined lesion (see endodontic-periodontic syndrome). Alveolar bone loss is widespread in periodontosis and may also occur in uncontrolled diabetes, Addison's disease, and in Hand-Schüller-Christian disease. In leprosy, the anterior nasal spine is missing and there is excessive bone loss in the anterior maxillary region.

Embedded Teeth (Impacted Teeth)

These teeth can occasionally cause pressure on adjacent teeth that results in pain and root resorption (Fig. 81). Embedded teeth may also communicate with the oral cavity via a sinus tract. The removal of these embedded teeth can cause injury to the adjoining teeth.

Temporo-Mandibular Joint Pain Dysfunction Syndrome (TMJPDS) or Myofascial Pain Dysfunction Syndrome (MFPDS)

These conditions are probably the same syndrome. The patients complain of pain over the joints usually elicited by jaw movement, clicking of the joints, limitation of movement, pain on chewing, and stiffness of the joints. Other symptoms include pain in the nasopharyngeal, preauricular and auricular areas, and referred pain to the posterior teeth (temporal muscle to upper teeth, masseter muscle to lower teeth). Symptoms are usually unilateral. The syndrome is known as TMJPDS when the joint and occlusal relationships are stressed. The name MFPDS stresses the importance of spasms of the muscles of mastication. Undoubtedly the temporomandibular joint, the dentition, and the muscles of mastication are all involved. The pain referred to teeth is the only symptom that can simulate pulpal or periapical disease. A careful history, and examination of the occlusion, joints, and muscles should confirm the diagnosis. There are other temporomandibular joint diseases including traumatic arthritis, rheumatoid arthritis and osteoarthritis. In these conditions, odontalgia is usually not present.

NON-ENDODONTIC ORAL-PHARYNGEAL-FACIAL-CERVICAL-CRANIAL LESIONS, DISEASES AND CONDITIONS

These clinical entities can also show manifestations simulating those of pulpal or periapical disease.

Eye Diseases Such as Iritis, Conjunctivitis and Keratitis

Pain can be referred to upper teeth with these conditions. Orbital swelling may occur with orbital cellulitis and lachrymal abscess. However, the patient would have eye manifestations, and the teeth should test vital.

Ear Diseases Such as Tinnitis, Toxic Neuritis, Otitis Media and Mastoiditis

Pain can be referred to posterior teeth and a submaxillary lymphadenopathy can occur. The patient would have ear manifestations and the teeth should test vital.

Nasal Diseases Such as Nasal Abscesses and Common Cold, and Nasal Tumors

Pain may be referred to upper anterior teeth but the patient would have nasal manifestations and the teeth should test vital.

Frontal and Maxillary Sinusitis and Other Sinus Conditions

If the frontal sinus is involved, the patient may have pain referred to the upper anterior teeth. However, the teeth should test vital. Pressure on the frontal region usually elicits pain. In maxillary sinusitis, the upper posterior teeth are sensitive to percussion and palpation (apical region). They may also have a tinny sound upon percussion. Pain may occur in these teeth during the acute stages of the sinus condition. The pain increases when the patient bends forward. In chronic maxillary sinusitis, neoplasms, polyps and cysts of the sinus, the periapical radiograph may show a cloudy, variably radiopaque appearance of the maxillary sinus (Fig. 227). However, this appearance is only suggestive. The involved teeth should test vital to pulp testing. Other means for aiding in the diagnosis of a chronic sinusitis are the following:

(1) The use of transillumination using fiber optics (Fig. 129) or a Welch-Allen transilluminator. The room must be completely dark. The instrument is placed under the zygoma in the region of the maxillary sinus and the palate region on the same side is examined. With a normal sinus,

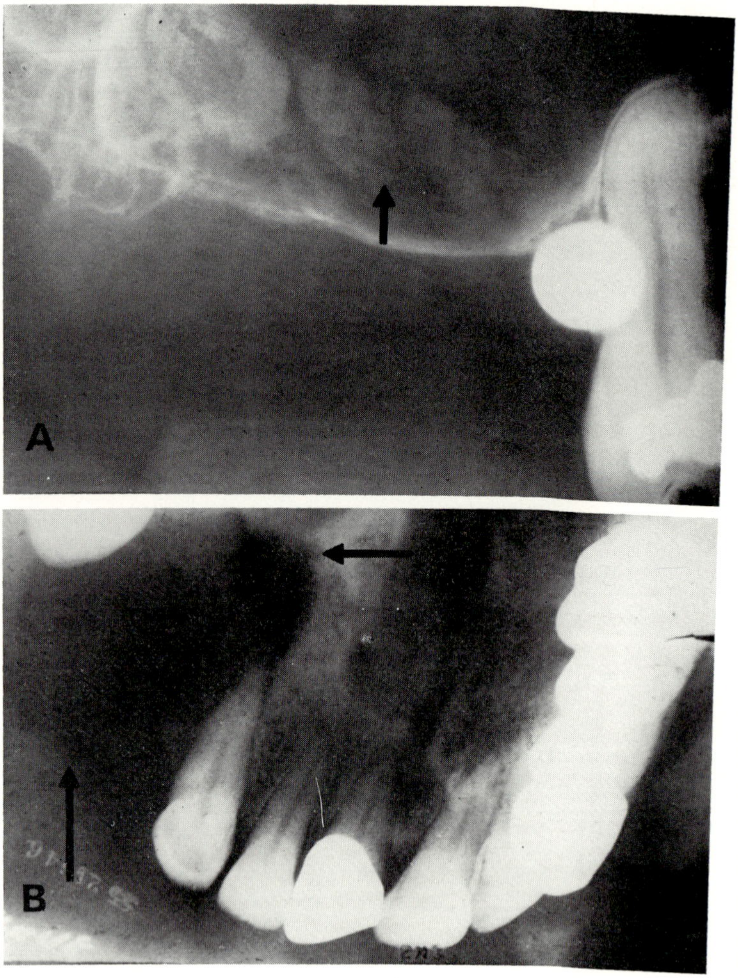

Figure 227. Sinus disorders. A. Radiopaque areas on floor of maxillary sinus are suggestive of polyps (arrow); definite diagnosis requires histopathologic examination. (Courtesy of Dr. T. Simpson, Philadelphia, Pa.) B. Anaplastic carcinoma of the maxillary sinus. (Courtesy of Dr. D. Litwack, Philadelphia, Pa.)

a red glow is visible on the roof of the mouth on that side. When there is an obstruction in the sinus or a sinusitis present, then the light either only penetrates partially or is not transmitted at all and nothing would be visible on the palate. Both sides should be examined for comparative purposes.

(2) The patient is asked to close his (or her) mouth. One nostril is closed with a finger, and the patient is then told to blow through the other nostril. If there is a sinusitis present, the ostium will probably be partially or completely clogged and the patient will have great difficulty in forcing air through that nostril. This is then an indication that sinus on the same side as the clogged nostril is affected by a sinusitis. The same procedure is then used for the other nostril.

(3) A topical anesthetic is sprayed into the nostril on the side that apparently has the sinusitis.

Within a few minutes, the symptoms should be alleviated if a sinusitis is present.

In pulpal and periapical disease, it is rare for more than one tooth to be involved at once, and this helps differentiate sinus disease from endodontic disease.

Throat Conditions

Patients with acute follicular tonsillitis and streptococcal sore throat may have a submaxillary lymphadenopathy and rarely pain may be referred to posterior teeth. As the patients are toxic, and have inflamed throats and/or tonsils, there should be no problem with differential diagnosis. Patients with pharyngeal tumors may also have pain referred to posterior teeth. A peritonsillar abscess simulates a lateral pharyngeal space swelling. However, with the abscess there are no teeth involved, and the tonsils are infected.

Erysipelas

This condition is a bacterial infectious disease that causes extreme redness and swelling of the face and head. Erysipelas is caused by hemolytic streptococci or hemolytic staphylococci. The submaxillary lymph nodes may enlarge and become painful. However, the lymphadenopathy is bilateral and visual examination should serve to differentiate this condition from endodontic diseases.

Facial Boils, Carbuncles, and Insect Stings

Facial swelling can result from these conditions. The history would help in the differential diagnosis.

Major Neuralgias

These neuralgias include trigeminal neuralgia (tic douloureux), geniculate neuralgia, glossopharyngeal neuralgia, post-herpetic neuralgia, and superior laryngeal neuralgia. The pain involved in these syndromes is one of the most severe types that can afflict a person. The pain is usually initiated by a trigger zone somewhere in the oral-pharyngeal-facial-cranial region. The stimulus may be touch, air, talking, smiling, or eating. Onset is sudden and duration is short (usually less than a minute). The pain is limited to part of the pathway of the involved nerve. A diagnostic aid is that pain relief is obtained by injection of a local anesthetic into the trigger area. There is usually no known anatomical or physiological defect of the involved nerves. Remissions and exacerbations are common and unpredictable.

Trigeminal Neuralgia (Tic Douloureux)

This condition is the principal neuralgia. It usually affects the second and third divisions of the trigeminal nerve unilaterally and is more common on the right side. Pain may be interpreted as if it was coming from one or more teeth. However, these teeth are vital, and the history of the condition should be sufficient for the diagnosis. Rarely, pain from undetected pulpal disease, such as in the cracked tooth syndrome or in pulpitis with referred pain, may simulate a neuralgia, but the pain is not as severe. There is usually no trigger zone, and the symptoms often localize to the involved tooth after a period of time. Treatment of trigeminal neuralgia includes surgery, alcohol injections, vitamin B-12 injections, and the use of the antiepileptic drug, carbamazepine (Tegretol®). Trigeminal neuralgia symptoms can occur in patients taking digoxin (a digitalis drug) and in patients with multiple sclerosis.

Other Major Neuralgias

These neuralgias are rare. In geniculate neuralgia, pain is felt within the ear and this should help differentiate it from dental conditions. In glossopharyngeal neuralgia, pain may be felt in the ear, tonsils, larynx or tongue. The pain on occasion can be bilateral. As a result of the history, differentiation of this condition from pain arising from dental disease should not be a problem. In superior laryngeal neuralgia, the pain occurs in the larynx, which should aid in the differential diagnosis. Postherpetic neuralgia follows herpes zoster. The herpetic lesions cover the skin and mucous membranes of the involved cranial nerve branches. The trigeminal nerve may be involved, with the ophthalmic division being the usual site. Other nerves that are occasionally involved are the facial, glossopharyngeal, and vagus nerves. Pain may continue after the disease manifestations have abated and may last for months or years. It probably results from damage to the involved nerve ganglia. Patients have a burning, boring type of pain which is often combined with paresthesia. There is usually no problem with differential diagnosis, unless the mandibular or maxillary branches of the fifth nerve are involved. In this case an adequate history should serve to confirm the diagnosis.

Abnormal Vasodilation Neuralgias (Atypical)

These neuralgias have been given different names by various authors including Sluder's neuralgia, sphenopalatine neuralgia, vidian neuralgia, histaminic cephalgia of Horton, petrosal neuralgia, and *classic* migraine. They all have in common the fact that they are painful conditions that arise from abnormal vasodilation. There is a wide spectrum of symptoms evident.

The histaminic cephalgia of Horton starts on one side of the head in the orbital region and it may spread to the occipital region, neck, or jaws. It has a rapid onset, becomes intense and lasts for 15 minutes to two hours. The pain is steady and severe. A similar type of vasodilating facial pain can occur in the lower face. A good differential diagnosis method is to inject ergotamine tartrate. There is also a sublingual form available. The result of the drug's action stops the vasodilating type of facial pain.

Migraine is usually preceded by a visual aura. The pain is on one side of the head for a particular attack, but it can shift to the other side for a subsequent attack. The painful episodes may last for several hours. Nausea and vomiting may also occur. The history of these conditions should serve to differentiate them from pulpal and periapical disease.

Minor Neuralgias of the Atypical Facial Pain Variety

The pain localizes in the distribution of either of these nerves, the second and third cervical, the glossopharyngeal, or the trigeminal. However, the patterns are not according to the true distribution of the nerves and the pain can cross the mid line. The pain is of a constant, persistent type. It has been described as burning, boring, pulling, etc. The pain often occurs in post-menopausal women. The pain may be localized to a particular jaw or even a particular tooth. However, all tests would show the teeth to be normal. Some other symptoms are burning tongue, palate, lips, or oral mucous membranes. The cause of this syndrome is usually psychogenic. These patients may have underlying neuroses or even psychoses.

Neuritis

In rare cases, a neuritis of some portion of the trigeminal nerve may refer pain to the teeth. This can occur from trauma to the face, dental extractions, or severe bites. A paresthesia is usually present along with the pain. The history should help in the differential diagnosis. In vitamin B deficiencies, there may be a neuritis of the tongue, but this should cause no confusion with dental pain. In Bell's palsy there is a facial nerve inflammation with a flaccid paralysis present on the affected side. Pain is not usually referred to the teeth and the typical appearance should simplify the diagnosis.

Temporal Arteritis

This condition is an inflammation of the temporal arteries. Occasionally, the internal and external maxillary arteries may be involved. Temporal arteritis is considered to be a form of periarteritis nodosa. The affected patients may have pain referred to the upper teeth, the jaws, the zygoma, and the temporo-mandibular joint. The pain may be intensified during eating. Signs of the disease are redness and swelling of the skin overlying the temporal arteries. The region is painful to palpation. Diagnosis is helped by pulp testing, the teeth should test vital. Absolute confirmation of the diagnosis necessitates tissue examination.

Cranial Lesions, Diseases or Conditions

These include thalamic *central pain* syndromes, brain stem tumors and infarcts, cerebellopontine angle tumors, trigeminal neuropathy, tumors of the middle cranial fossa and gasserian ganglion, petrositis, and trigeminal neuralgia resulting from multiple sclerosis. Patients with these entities may have headaches, dizziness, double vision and other eye disturbances, paralysis, and balancing problems. Rarely, pain may be referred to the teeth. A central lesion can cause bilateral symptoms including bilateral pain. Diagnosis usually presents no problem because of the presence of the other manifestations.

Acute Suppurative Myositis

This is an acute inflammation of muscles caused by microorganisms. Aside from the direct spread of infection from a cellulitis as previously discussed, a suppurative myositis can occur from unsterile anesthetic injections, surgical procedures, or traumatic injuries. Depending upon which muscles are involved, facial swelling may develop in different areas. Facial pain and referred pain to the teeth may also occur.

Arthritis of the Neck

In this condition, pain may be referred to the teeth. Pain in the cervical regions is present which should aid in the diagnosis.

Whiplash Injury to the Neck

This condition may also cause pain to be referred to the jaws. The history should aid in the diagnosis.

Benign Thyroid Tumor

There have been reports in the literature of patients having pain referred to the mandible from a benign thyroid tumor.

Branchial Fistulas

These are fistulas that are present along the site of the branchial clefts. They are congenital defects that result from a failure of closure of the branchial clefts. The sites may be anywhere along a line from the bottom of the ear, along the angle of the mandible, to the larynx (Fig. 55). Usually, only one fistula occurs and when it drains, it discharges a mucoid material. A branchial fistula may simulate a sinus tract from a lower molar infection. Differential diagnosis is aided by sinus tract probing with a periapical radiograph, for localization. Histopathological examination reveals that branchial fistulas are lined by stratified squamous or columnar epithelium, while sinus tracts from infected teeth are usually lined with granulomatous tissue.

Hemihypertrophy of the Face (Hemifacial Hyperplasia)

This condition is a congenital malformation in which one half of the face appears swollen. It usually involves the muscles and bone as well as the superficial soft tissues. History is an important diagnostic criterion in this case.

Soft Tissue Local Oral and Cervical Lesions

These lesions include disease manifestations, allergic reactions, traumatic lesions, inflamed soft tissue landmarks, foreign body reactions, and cysts and tumors. They may occur singly or in patches. The cysts and tumors usually occur isolated, while the disease manifestations generally have multiple locations. When any of these lesions are isolated to the mucobuccal fold, they may simulate a parulis (gum boil) or sinus tract. Swelling may occur in salivary glands, in lymph nodes, and in other areas of the neck. Usually the swelling is bilateral, but may occasionally be unilateral. Differential diagnosis is helped by the use of the following:

(1) *Pulp Testing.* The teeth should test vital in these conditions.

(2) *Probing.* If a sinus tract leads from the lesion to a root apex, then a pulpally-induced periapical condition is suspected.

(3) *Biopsy.* This method gives the histopathologic diagnosis.

(4) *History of the Lesion.*

Various Non-Cystic and Non-Tumorous Lesions

These lesions include recurrent herpes, apthous ulcers, traumatic ulcers, stomatitis venenata, herpes zoster, herpangina, white patches, inflamed soft tissue landmarks, foreign body granulomas, and actinomycosis.

Recurrent Herpes. Primary herpes is caused by a virus and is manifested by multiple herpetic vesicles, followed by ulcers, appearing throughout the oral mucous membrane. Therefore, it should not be confused with endodontic diseases. Recurrent herpes (fever blisters) lesions may be isolated. They may occur following trauma, stress, dental appointments, menstruation, or upper respiratory infections. The lesions may occur anywhere on the oral mucous membrane. When located at the mucobuccal fold, they may be confused with sinus tracts. However, the appearance is usually more ulcerated than is the case with a sinus tract. Probing of a herpetic lesion does not allow tissue penetration.

Apthous Ulcers. These lesions are similar in appearance to recurrent herpetic lesions but they are not caused by a virus (Fig. 33). Differential diagnosis is the same as described for recurrent herpes.

Traumatic Ulcers. These may result from burns or drug reactions. These reactions usually result from eating something sharp (Fig. 34), having a foreign object placed into the tissues (Fig. 228), eating hot food (Fig. 36), or placing aspirin or some other chemical (e.g. formocresol, chloroform) into the mucobuccal fold (Fig. 38). These lesions

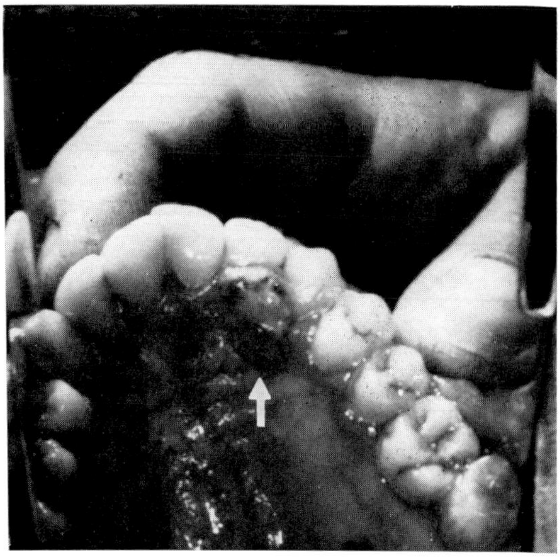

Figure 228. A traumatic ulcer. (Courtesy of Dr. T. Simpson, Philadelphia, Pa.)

also have the same appearance as recurrent herpes (ulcer stage), and diagnosis would be arrived at in the same manner, as described for herpes, plus an evaluation of the history.

Stomatitis Venenata. This is an allergic contact-type reaction, in which vesicles or bullae can occur singly or in multiples. It can occur in the mucobuccal fold, and almost any type of foreign substance can elicit it. Certain patients are very allergic to zinc oxide-eugenol paste, topical antibiotics, sulfonamides, and mercury. The diagnosis is arrived at after examination of the tissue, testing of the teeth in the area (they should test vital), and a history of the drug usage.

Herpes Zoster. This disease is a neurogenic infection caused by a virus. It affects the area of the skin and mucous membrane supplied by the involved sensory nerve. If the mandibular nerve is involved, vesicles and ulcers can appear

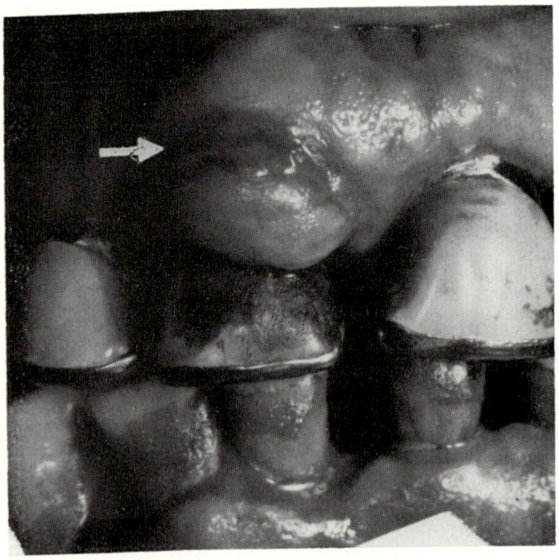

Figure 229. Foreign body granuloma caused by irritating material placed subgingivally. (Courtesy of Dr. T. Simpson, Philadelphia, Pa.)

on the oral mucous membranes. The lesions are rarely isolated to the mucobuccal fold. Differential diagnosis would be arrived at after a consideration of the history, clinical appearance, and probing.

HERPANGINA. This is another virus-induced disease in which oral mucous membrane vesicles and ulcers may occur. The lesions invariably are multiple, and therefore there should be no confusion with endodontic diseases.

WHITE PATCHES. Lesions such as leukoplakia, lichen planus, and pachyderma oris, even if they are isolated to the mucobuccal fold should not present problems in differential diagnosis. They are characteristically white, raised, or flat lesions and this appearance is not similar to paruli or sinus tracts (Fig. 35). In thrush, the white lesions are multiple.

INFLAMED SOFT TISSUE LANDMARKS. The orifices of the salivary gland ducts, the frenums, and the incisive papilla have been described previously. When these landmarks become inflamed, they can more easily be confused with paruli and sinus tracts. However the location and pulp testing (teeth in this area should test vital) should serve to differentiate these entities from endodontic conditions. However, an acutely inflamed frenum may cause a severe pericementitis and an odontalgia. In this instance, a vital pulp response and discovery of a foreign body (e.g. toothpick, piece of food) in the frenum would confirm the diagnosis.

FOREIGN BODY GRANULOMAS. These are granulomatous inflammations of the oral mucous membrane, including the mucobuccal fold, that may appear as localized swellings (Fig. 229). These lesions result from foreign objects, such as toothpicks, food debris, and gutta-percha (overfilled gutta-percha in the mucobuccal fold or alveolar mucosa) lodging in the soft tissues. Differential diagnosis is aided by inspection, palpation, surgical enucleation and examination, and vitality testing. The teeth should test vital except for the overfilled root canal cases. Histopathological examination reveals typical granulomatous tissue with the foreign body surrounded by giant cells.

ACTINOMYCOSIS. This is a suppurative infectious disease caused by Actinomyces israeli (Gram positive microaerophilic filament). Trauma is thought to be a precondition for the onset of the disease. It can occur in the jaws (primarily the mandible), salivary glands, and the lungs. In the cervico-

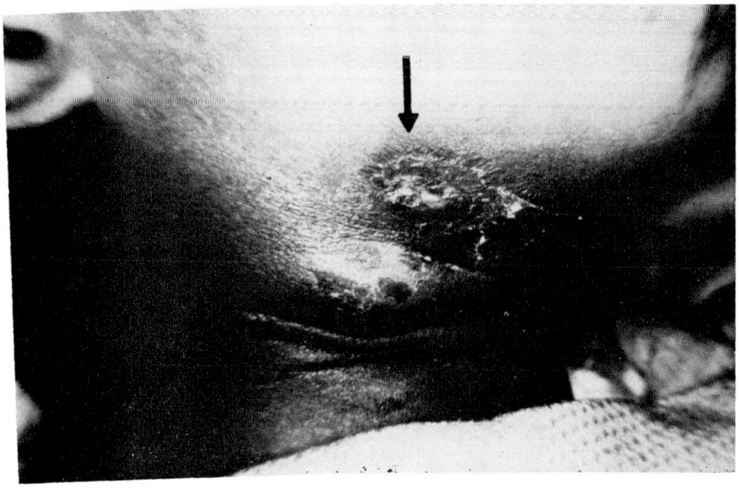

Figure 230. Draining sinus tracts in cervico facial actinomycosis. (Courtesy of Dr. M. Gross, Philadelphia, Pa.)

facial form there may be external sinus tracts draining in the skin (Figs. 54, 230). These can be differentiated from sinus tracts derived from pulpally-induced periapical disease by histopathologic examination and the finding of sulfur granules (Fig. 231). Also, the sinus tracts are usually multiple, unlike the case in endodontic disease. With actinomycosis, there may also be associated periapical destruction and occasionally the pulps can become infected with actinomyces microbes. Clinically, with actinomycosis, there is usually swelling of the neck and the mucous membrane overlying the mandible.

Salivary Gland Diseases and Lesions

The major salivary glands, the parotids and the submaxillaries, are closely associated with the parotid and submaxillary lymph nodes, respectively. Disease processes of the glands usually are manifested by swellings of the glands and the associated nodes. In many of the disease entities, the involvement is bilateral, although this is not always the case. Parotid gland involvement is more common than submaxillary gland involvement. Unilateral swelling might be confused with a lymphadenopathy resulting from a periapical abscess. How-

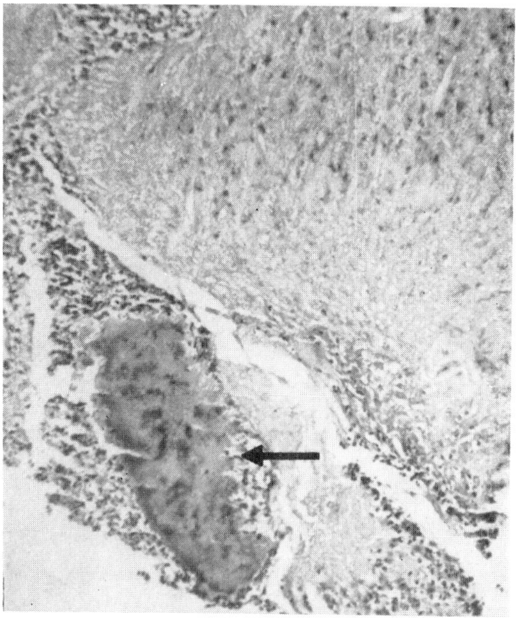

Figure 231. Sulfur granules (arrow) in cervico-facial actinomycosis; histologic section (×96). (Courtesy of Dr. S. Seltzer, Philadelphia, Pa.)

ever, in the case of parotid gland disease, the swelling is above the angle of the jaw and goes up to the ear. In the case of submaxillary gland involvement, the clinical appearance reveals a swelling below the angle of the jaw, including the associated area of the neck. Differential diagnosis of the latter condition from periapically induced lymphadenopathy depends upon history, vitality testing (if the condition is a salivary gland disease, the regional teeth should test vital), periapical radiography (in salivary gland conditions there usually is no periapical rarefactions) and biopsy, for definite determination of the histopathological nature of the lesion. Occasionally salivary gland diseases may refer pain to teeth.

INFECTIOUS OR EPIDEMIC PAROTITIS (MUMPS). This is the most common salivary gland disease. It is an infectious viral disease. The parotid glands are usually involved and occasionally it is a unilateral condition (Fig. 48). Mumps occurs primarily in children. The disease is rapid in onset; it is accompanied by high fever and malaise; and the patients often have a bad taste in their mouths, along with facial pain.

ACUTE SIALADENITIS. This acute infection of the salivary glands usually affects the parotid glands and causes facial pain and swelling. Pus often is discharged from the ducts of the affected glands. Acute sialadenitis is a rare condition and the swelling is not associated with sialoliths (stones, calculi) or eating. It occurs primarily in debilitated individuals.

CHRONIC SIALADENITIS. This chronic infection of the salivary glands usually affects the submaxillary glands. The swelling generally occurs immediately before, during, and immediately after meals. At other times, swelling is minimal. There are usually salivary calculi associated with the condition (sialolithiasis) (Fig. 232). The calculi occur primarily in the major ducts and rarely in the glands themselves. Clinical examination, including palpation and probing, often aids in the detection of stones. The major ducts are often inflamed

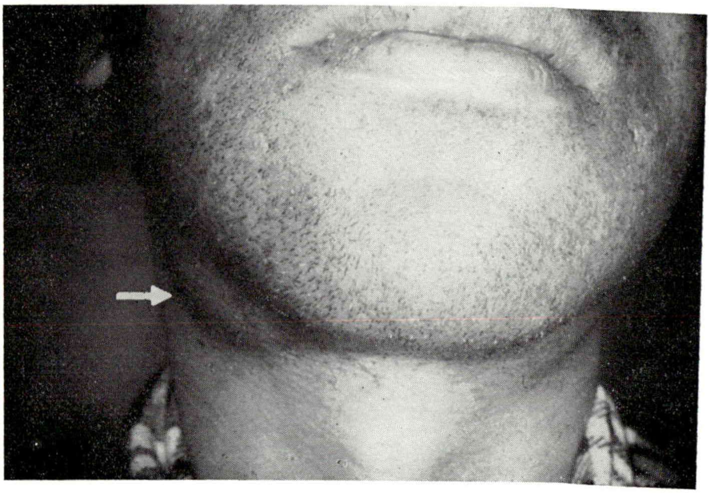

Figure 232. Submaxillary swelling in chronic sialadenitis associated with sialolithiasis. (Courtesy of Dr. T. Simpson, Philadelphia, Pa.)

(sialadochitis). Radiographs are important aids to reveal the presence of stones. Occasionally stones can appear superimposed around the apexes of lower anterior teeth, where they can simulate condensing osteitis. However, the associated teeth are vital. Injections of radiopaque substances such as Lipiodol, followed by lateral jaw or panograph radiography (x-ray sialography) often reveals the presence of numerous constrictions and dilatations in the ducts (sialectasis).

VARIOUS NON-NEOPLASTIC PAROTID GLAND SWELLINGS. These conditions principally involve the parotid glands. They are generally of slow onset and may have been present for several years before they first became noticed. Definite diagnosis entails histopathologic examination of excised tissues. The conditions include lymphoepithelial cyst, hypertrophy, fatty infiltration, Sjögren's syndrome, Mikulicz's disease (benign lymphoepithelial lesion), uveoparotitis, cytomegalic virus inclusion disease, sarcoidosis, tuberculosis of the salivary glands, and various other granulomatous diseases of the salivary glands. In rare cases, tuberculosis cervical adenitis can cause a draining skin sinus tract.

ANIMAL SCRATCH DISEASE (CAT-SCRATCH DISEASE). This is a virally-induced disease, often transmitted by the scratch of a cat and usually found in children. As the face is involved most often, either the parotid or submaxillary lymph nodes enlarge and become painful. This condition is included with the salivary gland diseases as it is not possible to differentiate it from salivary gland diseases by visual or digital examination. The history is the best diagnostic aid.

MUCOCOELES AND RANULAS. These are mucous-containing cysts that are usually lined with granulation tissue. They occur in the ducts of the salivary glands and in the overlying mucous membrane. The mucocoeles are small, circumscribed, usually elevated, and may occur in the floor of the mouth or lip. They result from the traumatic rupture of an excretory duct of a minor salivary gland. This allows for saliva accumulation in the contingent tissues. Mucous retention cysts are larger and are found in the same locations. Occasionally, they are found on the alveolar mucosa and may be lined with epithelium (Fig. 233). Ranulas are much larger than mucocoeles and are found in the floor of the mouth (Fig. 45). They result from trauma to the submaxillary (Wharton's) or one of the major sublingual (Bartholin's) ducts. It is possible to confuse these swellings with those resulting from periapical abscesses draining toward the lingual. However, in the salivary conditions, the teeth in the region test vital.

SALIVARY GLAND TUMORS. These can be either benign or malignant. Generally benign tumors are slow growing, often of long duration, and are not fixed to the underlying tissues. Benign tumors in approximate order of decreasing frequency include pleomorphic adenoma (mixed tumor with cartilage-like tissue and epithelium), Warthin's tumor (with epithelially-lined cystic spaces), adenoma (with duct-like gland-

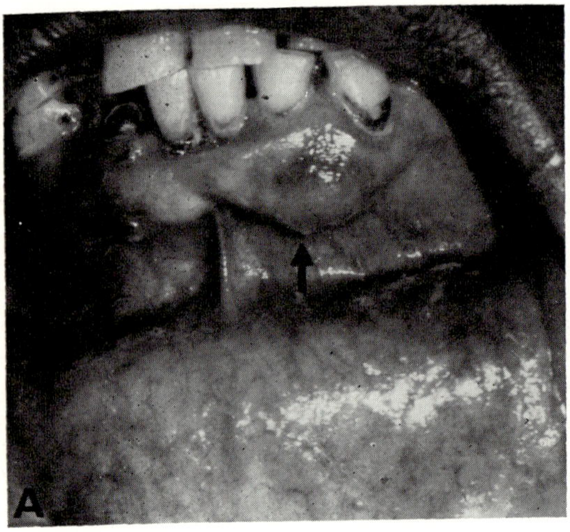

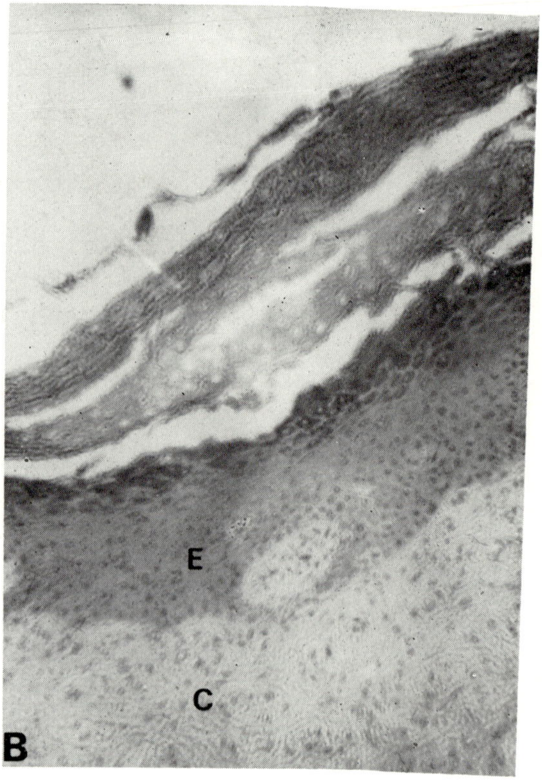

Figure 233. Mucous retention cyst. A. A rare occurrence in the alveolar mucosa. (Courtesy of Dr. T. Simpson, Philadelphia, Pa.) B. Histologic section; E = stratified squamous epithelium, C = connective tissue (×540). (Courtesy of Dr. T. Simpson, Philadelphia, Pa.)

ular tissue), and oncocytoma (with sheets of eosinophilic cells). Malignant tumors in approximate order of decreasing frequency include adenocarcinoma (various types with anaplastic tissue), adenocystic carcinoma or cylindroma (contains small, dark, epithelial cells surrounded by a homogenous material), mucoepidermoid tumor (contains mucous cells, epidermoid cells, dark intermediate cells, and clear cells), and acinic cell carcinoma (contains cells that resemble serous acinar cells). Definite diagnosis necessitates histological examination of excised tissues.

Soft Tissue Tumors and Cysts

These lesions can occur in the mucobuccal fold, alveolar mucosa, gingiva, floor of the mouth, tongue, in other areas of the oral mucous membrane, and the neck. The tumors are either benign or malignant. Included with the benign tumors are the inflammatory lesions of granulation and connective tissue.

The benign tumors, if isolated to the mucobuccal fold or alveolar mucosa, may simulate a parulis. The benign lesions generally are slow growing, of long duration, painless, and are not attached to the underlying tissues. Benign lesions usually are smooth and round in appearance.

The malignant lesions are usually fast growing, of short duration, may be painful, and are fixed to the underlying tissues. They may, on occasion, invade the underlying bone, and they often cause a regional lymphadenopathy. Malignant lesions can appear ulcerated, warty-like, cauliflower-like, or pigmented.

Differential diagnosis depends upon probing of the lesions, radiographs, pulp testing, histologic examination of sections from the biopsied tissue, and the history. In the case of tumors and cysts the lesions cannot be probed (a lesion that is suspicious of being malignant should not be probed), radiographs would not show a periapical rarefaction unless a malignant tumor invaded bone in the neighborhood of the root apex, and the teeth in the area should test vital.

The Soft Tissue Cysts. The mucocoele and ranula have been included with the salivary gland lesions. The other cysts to be discussed are the gingival, epidermoid, nasoalveolar, branchial cleft, thyroglossal duct, cyst of the palatine papilla, and oral cyst with intestinal epithelium.

Gingival Cyst. This is a rare circumferential swelling, usually limited to blacks and principally found in the lower canine and premolar areas. The lesion can erode the bone and then produce a radiolucency similar in appearance to a lateral periodontal cyst. The associated teeth are vital, and there is no pocket present (unless periodontal disease is superimposed). The cyst lining is stratified squamous.

Epidermoid Cyst (Including Dermoid, Epidermal, and Dermal Cysts). The epidermoid cyst is usually seen in the floor of the mouth, where it can cause tongue elevation. It is a roundish, freely movable lesion. The histopathologic picture shows a keratinized stratified squamous epithelial lining. The surrounding connective tissue wall may contain sweat and sebaceous glands, and hair follicles. True dermoid cysts are neoplastic teratoid lesions and are very rare.

Nasoalveolar Cyst. This is a fissural cyst that is usually limited to blacks, especially women. It produces a swelling at the base of the nostrils that is palpable under the upper lip and nose. The lesion can erode through the alveolar bone and produce a radiolucency between the upper central incisors. The radiolucency may appear to be superimposed over the apex of one of the incisors, if the radiograph is not taken directly perpendicular to the long axis of the teeth. Pain may occur in the floor of the nose, but the associated teeth are vital. The cyst lining is of either stratified squamous or respiratory-type epithelium (pseudostratified columnar).

Branchial Cleft Cyst (Lymphoepithelial Cyst). This swelling can occur in the lateral aspect of the neck, the floor of the mouth or the angle of the mandible. It originates from epithelial inclusions found within cervical lymph nodes. The cyst is lined by stratified squamous epithelium, which is surrounded by lymphoid tissue.

Thyroglossal Duct Cyst. This cyst is derived from epithelial remnants of the embryonic thyroglossal duct. The latter, in an early developmental state, connects the tongue with the thyroid gland. The swelling occurs beneath the tongue or in the submental area. It may resemble a submental space infection.

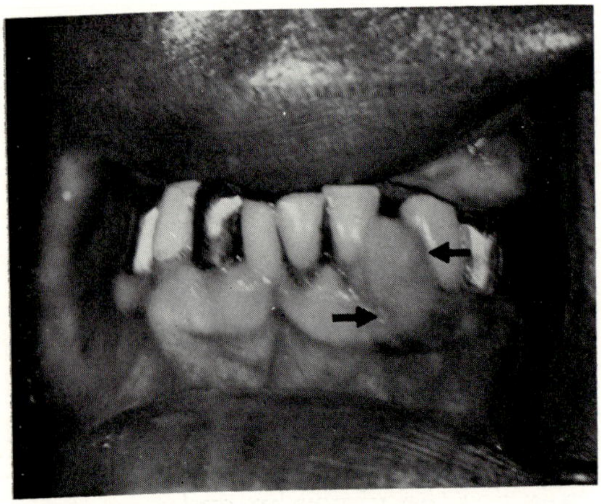

Figure 234. An irritation fibroma (fibrous epulis) located on the interdental papilla. (Courtesy of Dr. T. Simpson, Philadelphia, Pa.)

However, the associated teeth should test vital. The cyst lining is of either ciliated or nonciliated columnar, stratified squamous, or transitional epithelium.

Cyst of the Palatine Papilla. This is a nasopalatine cyst that involves only the incisive (anterior palatine) papilla. It appears as a round, soft swelling that may be found along the midline of the palate. The incisive papilla is elevated by the cyst. This lesion must be differentiated from an inflamed incisive papilla as well as a palatal abscess. With this cyst, the associated teeth should test vital. The cyst lining is of respiratory, cuboidal, or stratified squamous epithelium. The connective tissue wall contains mucous glands, nerves, lymphocytes, and plasma cells.

Oral Cyst with Gastric or Intestinal Epithelium. These rare cysts are lined by gastric or intestinal mucosa. They can be found in the tongue or floor of the mouth.

SOFT TISSUE TUMORS. The tumors included are benign tumors and tumor-like proliferations, and malignant tumors.

Benign Tumors and Tumor-Like Proliferations. These lesions include verruca vulgaris, papilloma, irritation fibroma, fibroma, pyogenic granuloma, pregnancy tumor, peripheral giant cell reparative granuloma, plasma cell granuloma, soft tissue plasmacytoma, hemangiomas, eosinophilic granuloma, cystic hygroma, lymphangioma, benign symmetrical lipomatosis, neurofibromas, lipoma, granular cell myoblastoma, neuroma, and carotid body tumor.

Verruca Vulgaris and Papilloma. Both of these lesions are cauliflower-like white growths. They rarely occur in the alveolar mucosa. The verruca is caused by a virus. The epithelium may show hyperkeratosis or parakeratosis in both conditions.

Irritation Fibroma (Fibrous Epulis). This lesion is an overgrowth of fibrous connective tissue covered by pale-looking epithelium. It occurs in response to local irritation. It can appear clinically as a smooth elevation, a sessile-type growth, a pedunculated-type growth, a hyperkeratinized lesion, or an ulcerated lesion. The epulis may occur on the gingiva, the alveolar mucosa, or in the mucobuccal fold (Fig. 234). Histologically, it consists of few fibroblasts, dense collagen, few blood vessels, varying number of inflammatory cells, and a covering of stratified squamous epithelium.

Fibroma. This lesion is also an overgrowth of fibrous connective tissue. It is much less common than an irritation fibroma, and is a true tumor. The fibroma usually occurs in the region of the interdental papilla, or attached gingiva but may occur in the alveolar mucosa (Fig. 235). The lesion can appear pale or red, and may be elevated, pedunculated, or sessile. Histologically, it contains fibrous connective tissue but with many more fibroblasts than is the case with the irritation fibroma. The fibroma may contain areas of myxomatous and/or calcific degeneration. It is covered by a thin layer of stratified squamous epithelium, which may have ulcerated areas.

Pyogenic Granuloma. This lesion is a tumor-like proliferation of vascular granulation tissue. It occurs probably as an exaggerated response to trauma. The most common site is the interdental papilla, occasionally it is found on the attached gingiva, and rarely it may occur on the alveolar mucosa (Fig. 44).

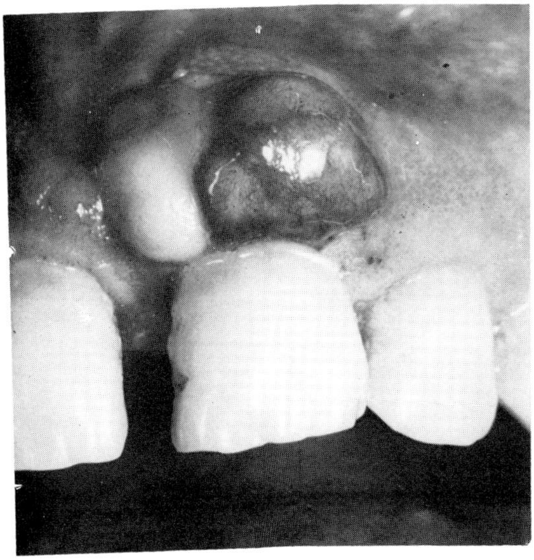

Figure 235. A fibroma located on the attached gingiva and alveolar mucosa. (Courtesy of Dr. T. Simpson, Philadelphia, Pa.)

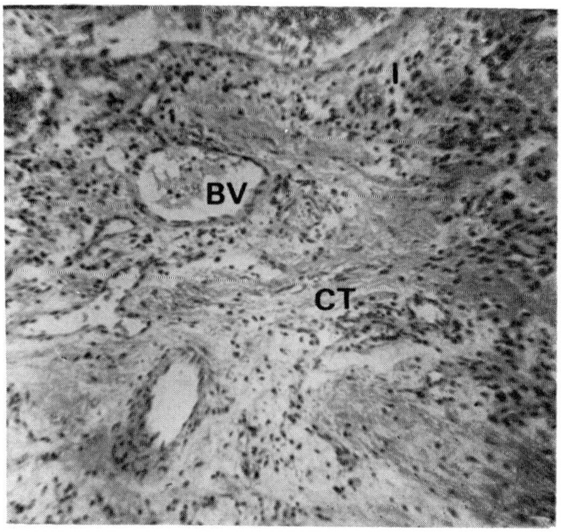

Figure 236. Pregnancy tumor; histologic section; BV = blood vessels, I = inflammation, CT = fibrous connective tissue (×240). (Courtesy of Dr. T. Simpson, Philadelphia, Pa.)

The pyogenic granuloma has a smooth red surface and it may be sessile or pedunculated. It grows rapidly, bleeds easily, and may be ulcerated. The histologic appearance shows granulation tissue with numerous islands of capillaries, plasma cells, lymphocytes, and polymorph leucocytes.

Pregnancy Tumor (Granuloma Gravidarum). This is a localized manifestation of pregnancy gingivitis. It is the same type lesion, both clinically and microscopically, as the pyogenic granuloma (Fig. 236). The pregnancy tumor is also found in the interdental papilla. It usually appears toward the end of the first trimester and often regresses after delivery (Fig. 43).

Peripheral Giant Cell Reparative Granuloma (Giant Cell Epulis). This is another tumor-like lesion composed of granulation tissue. It also may occur as a response to trauma. The giant cell

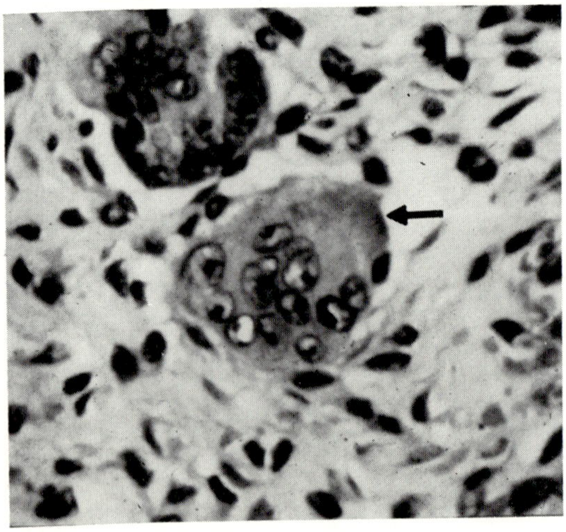

Figure 237. Giant cell reparative granuloma; histologic section; arrow points to a multinucleated giant cell (×960). (Courtesy of Dr. D. Litwack, Philadelphia, Pa.)

epulis occurs primarily on the gingiva, and is usually reddish-blue or dark brown, and smooth in appearance. It can be sessile or pedunculated, and bleeds readily. The histopathologic appearance reveals highly cellular granulation tissue with multinucleated giant cells, and deposits of hemosiderin (Fig. 237). The lining is composed of stratified squamous epithelium and it may be ulcerated.

Plasma Cell Granuloma and Soft Tissue Plasmacytoma. The plasma cell granuloma is also an inflammatory tumor-like growth that occurs principally on the gingiva. The histologic appearance shows a large accumulation of plasma cells, but there are also other inflammatory cells present including lymphocytes, polymorph leucocytes, and eosinophiles. The true tumor, the soft tissue plasmacytoma, consists entirely of plasma cells and is potentially dangerous as it usually is an early stage of multiple myeloma. It has been reported to occur occasionally on the maxillary alveolar mucosa. Definitive diagnosis requires histologic examination.

Hemangiomas. These are tumors of blood vessels. The two principal types are the capillary, with numerous blood filled capillaries, and the cavernous, with large endothelially-lined blood filled spaces. The hemangiomas may appear on the tongue, lip, cheek, or occasionally, the alveolar mucosa. Hemangiomas appear as smooth, reddish or bluish lesions. The lesions can be elevated or nonelevated, circumscribed, or flattened (Fig. 238). The cavernous type often contains phleboliths (calcified thrombi). The latter appear radiopaque in a radiograph, and occasionally they appear superimposed over root apexes. If the hemangioma invades bone, the radiograph may show a radiolucent appearance. Sometimes the lesion causes bony expansion and the patient experiences pain. Teeth in the area should all test vital.

Eosinophilic Granuloma. This is one

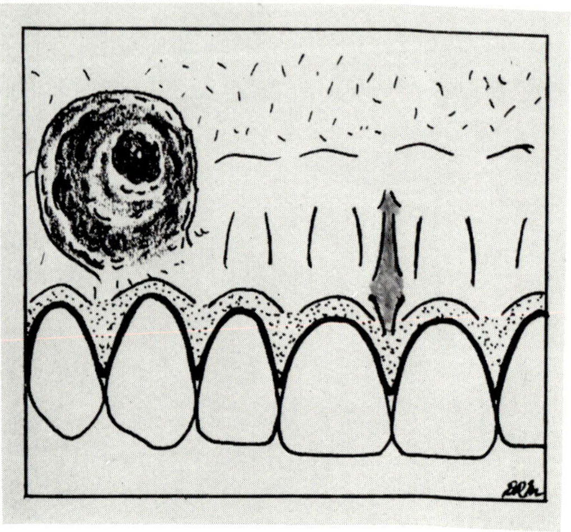

Figure 238. Hemangioma.

of three diseases encompassed in the term histiocytosis X. It can occur as a solitary lesion in the gingiva, but is usually a bony lesion and will be discussed with the bony lesions.

Cystic Hygroma. This is a congenital malformation that consists of large lymph-filled spaces. There are massive unilateral or bilateral swellings of the neck. It occurs in infants and young children.

Lymphangioma. This is a tumor of lymph- or serous-filled endothelially-lined spaces. It occurs principally on the tongue where it can cause a massive enlargement.

Benign Symmetrical Lipomatosis. This rare condition is seen clinically as a bilateral neck swelling. The lesion is composed of a massive accumulation of fatty tissue in the cervical and supraclavicular regions.

Neurofibromas. These lesions of nerve sheath origin can be found in the oral mucous membrane but practically never on the alveolar mucosa.

Lipoma. This is a tumor of fat cells that is rarely found in the oral cavity. When present, it is primarily seen in the cheek and rarely observed on the alveolar mucosa (Fig. 239).

Granular Cell Myoblastoma. This is another rare oral lesion. It occurs principally on the dorsum of the tongue, but may appear elsewhere on the oral mucous membrane. It consists of large granular cells with small, dark round nuclei, covered by hyperplastic epithelium.

Neuroma (Traumatic or Amputation Neuroma). This lesion results from an overgrowth of fibroblasts, Schwann cells, and axis cylinders, after trauma to or severance of a peripheral nerve. It can occur in the oral cavity after a fracture or oral surgical procedure. The neuroma is frequently found in the region of the mental foramen. The overlying alveolar mucosa usually contains movable nodules that may be painful to palpation.

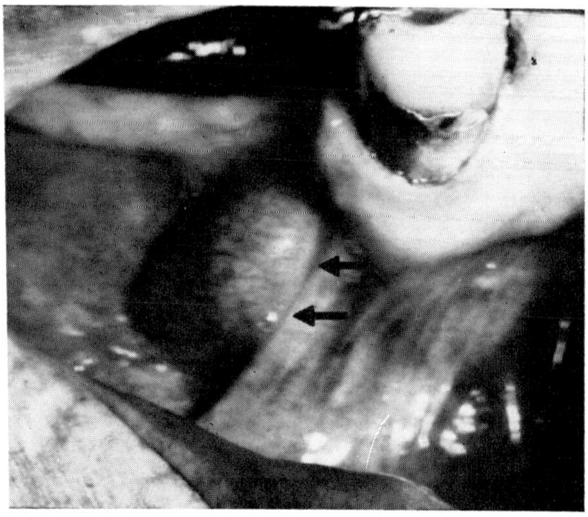

Figure 239. A lipoma located on the alveolar mucosa. (Courtesy of Dr. T. Simpson, Philadelphia, Pa.)

Carotid Body Tumor, Aneurysms of the Carotid Artery, Carotidynia and Carotid Sinus Enlargement Resulting from Extreme Hypertension. The carotid sinus is the enlarged part of the internal carotid artery and it is found just inferior to the angle of the mandible. Any of the above conditions can cause a swelling of the sinus which could simulate a submaxillary lymphadenopathy. However, upon palpation of the sinus a pulsation should be felt.

Malignant Tumors. In most of these lesions, the regional lymph nodes are involved, and at times are the first sign of the disease. Conditions covered are squa-

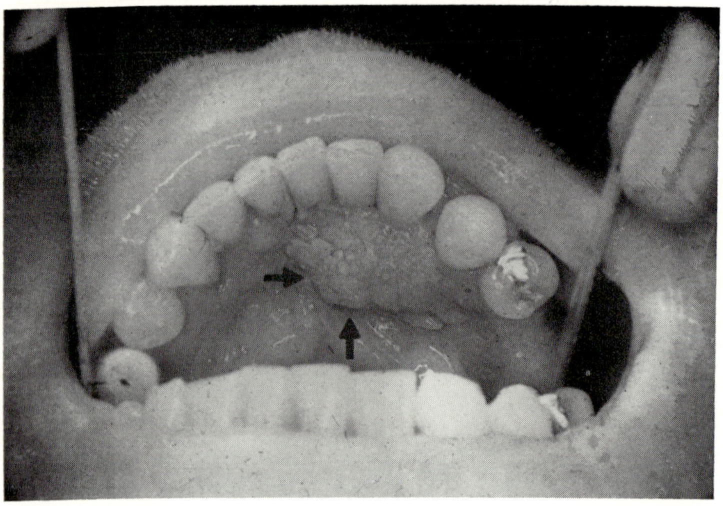

Figure 240. Squamous cell carcinoma located on the anterior portion of the palate. (Courtesy of Dr. T. Simpson, Philadelphia, Pa.)

mous cell carcinoma, verrucous carcinoma, transitional cell carcinoma, lymphoepithelioma, melanoma, lymphosarcoma, reticulum cell sarcoma, fibrosarcoma, liposarcoma, osteogenic sarcoma, and chondrosarcoma.

Squamous Cell Carcinoma (Epidermoid Carcinoma). This is the most common oral malignancy. It is generally found on the lips, less frequently on the tongue, occasionally on the floor of the mouth, and infrequently on the alveolar mucosa, palate, and cheek. The squamous cell carcinoma rarely invades bone. It can occur as an ulcer, a flat erythematous lesion, a warty growth, or a white lesion (Fig. 240). The submaxillary and deep cervical lymph nodes may become involved. The histological appearance depends upon the grade of malignancy. The more malignant the lesion, the greater the anaplastic (more embryonic) appearance. Stratified squamous epithelium with invasion of the underlying mucosa, dyskeratotic appearance, and presence of epithelial and keratin pearls is characteristic of Grade I (less malignant) lesions (Fig. 241). In Grade IV, the tissue is hardly recognizable as stratified squamous epithelium and there are many mitoses present.

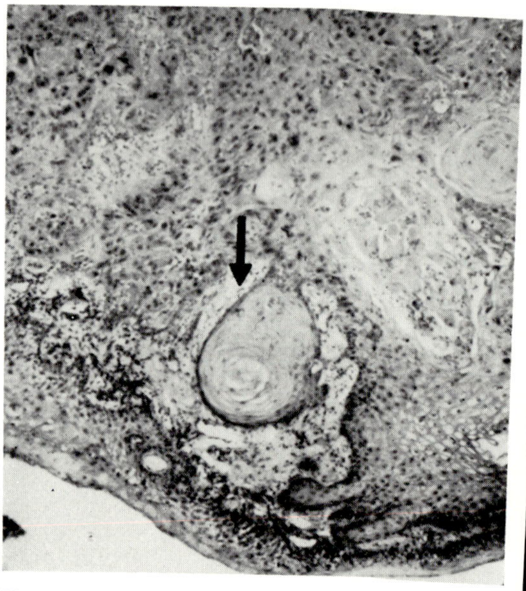

Figure 241. Squamous cell carcinoma; histologic section of Grade I; arrow points to a keratin pearl (×240). (Courtesy of Dr. D. Litwack, Philadelphia, Pa.)

Verrucous Carcinoma. This tumor occurs in older patients. It has a cauliflower-like appearance (papillary folds) and is often found in the alveolar ridge. It is much less malignant than the typical squamous cell carcinoma.

Transitional Cell Carcinoma. This very rare anaplastic tumor occurs at the base of the tongue and in the oral pharynx. Often this primary lesion is hard to find and the first sign is an enlarged regional lymph node. The tumor is composed of sheets and islands of anaplastic epithelial cells.

Lymphoepithelioma. This lesion is often first noticed by a swelling of a regional lymph node. The small primary lesion is found in the tonsillar area or the nasal pharynx. Histologically, the appearance is that of anaplastic epithelial islands, surrounded by a dense collection of lymphocytes.

Melanoma. This is an extremely malignant melanin-containing tumor. It is very rare in the oral cavity, but when present can occur on the maxillary alveolar mucosa, gingiva or hard palate. The melanoma can arise from a nevus, lentigo or form spontaneously, and it metastasizes early. It originates as a pigmented or nonpigmented lesion that later becomes ulcerated and more pigmented. The histologic appearance can vary but the typical formation shows spindle shaped, melanin-containing, anaplastic epithelial cells.

Malignant Lymphomas. These are malignant tumors of lymphoid tissue. In the oral cavity they are quite rare, but may occur on the gingiva. The lymphomas may appear as a tumorous growth or as a gingival hyperplasia. The microscopic appearance for the lymphosarcoma shows masses of lymphocytes, many of which are immature in appearance. There are no other associated cells of the chronic inflammatory series, such as plasma cells or macrophages. The histologic appearance of the reticulum cell sarcoma shows a dense infiltration of pale-staining cells intertwined with reticular fibers. This lesion can also be found in bone, and clinical features of this type are discussed in the section on bone diseases. Two other malignant lymphomas are follicular lymphoma and Hodgkin's disease. These are rarely found in the oral cavity. When present orally, Hodgkin's disease can result in a cervical and submaxillary lymphadenopathy. Occasionally, a gingival hyperplasia is found (Fig. 242).

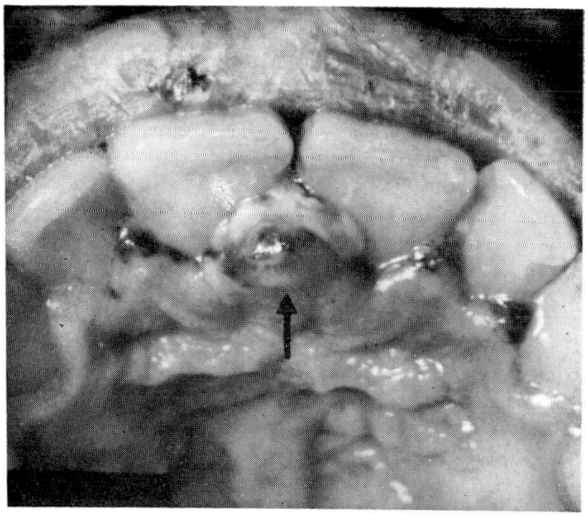

Figure 242. Hyperplasia of the incisive papilla in a case of Hodgkin's disease; histologic section of the excised tissue showed cells typical of this disease. (Courtesy of Dr. T. Simpson, Philadelphia, Pa.)

Fibrosarcoma. This is another rare tumor which occasionally can be found on the alveolar mucosa as a swelling. The histologic appearance varies with the degree of malignancy. It consists of fibroblasts and collagen fibers that appear in a stream-like configuration. The cells vary from spindle-shaped in the less malignant lesions, to hyperchromatic appearing, with many mitoses, in the more malignant lesions.

Liposarcoma. This is a malignant tumor of fat which is very rare in the oral cavity. The tissue consists of bizarre lipoblasts in a myxomatous matrix.

Osteogenic Sarcoma and Chondrosarcoma. The alveolar mucosa may appear swollen with these tumors, but these are tumors of bone and are discussed under bony lesions.

ENDODONTIC MANIFESTATIONS OF SYSTEMIC DISEASES

In these diseases, there may occur signs and symptoms that simulate endodontic diseases. These manifestations are odontalgia, paresthesia, pulposis, pulp canal enlargements, tooth discoloration, bone changes (radiolucency or radiopacity), hypercementosis, oral lesions, regional lymphadenopathy, malodors and tastes, bleeding, loss of lamina dura, widening of periodontal ligament space, gingival changes, external root resorption, and facial swelling. Systemic diseases that cause external root resorption, hypercementosis, and gingivitis have already been discussed under those respective categories. Systemic diseases that cause bone changes will be discussed under bony lesions. For oral manifestations of systemic diseases, in most cases, more than one tooth is involved and the condition is bilateral. Tests which help in differential diagnosis include pulp testing of teeth in area (they should test vital); blood and urine tests, to aid in the detection of certain systemic diseases; cardiac function tests; liver function tests; kidney function tests; gastrointestinal analysis; microbiological analyses; biopsy; visual examination; palpation; and history.

Diseases Causing Odontalgia as the Predominant Oral Manifestation

These include coronary artery diseases, diabetes, leukemias, sickle cell anemia, and miscellaneous diseases.

Coronary Artery Diseases and Pericarditis

In cases of pericarditis, angina pectoris, coronary thrombosis, myocardial infarction, and rheumatic fever, there can be referred pain to the jaws and teeth during an acute episode. Usually the patient has concurrent painful symptoms that radiate down the left shoulder and arm. However, there have been reported cases where the patient only experienced pain in the jaws.

Diabetes Mellitus

Diabetic patients can experience toothaches which are probably related to pulpal arteritis or atherosclerosis. Diabetics, in an advanced stage of the disease, may have a distinctive sweet *acetone breath* (results from ketones being released into the saliva).

Leukemias

Leukemic patients may develop toothaches in clinically sound teeth. Blood smears from leukemic pulps show the presence of abnormal immature leucocytes. These patients can also have a cervical lymphadenopathy, and ulcerative gingivitis (Fig. 11). Rarely, the disease may invade bone (Fig. 12).

Miscellaneous Diseases

There have been reports in the literature (not thoroughly documented) of patients experiencing toothaches apparently as reflex referred pain from systemic conditions such as malaria, aspergillus, gastrointestinal disturbances (constipation, hunger and stomachache), urogenital disturbances (distended bladder and uterine disturbances), gout, influenza, hypoparathyroidism, and exanthematous diseases (diphtheria, measles, chicken pox, scarlet fever). There is also the possibility of anachoresis (blood borne bacteria localizing and fixing in an area of inflammation) resulting in an odontalgia. Although it is difficult to prove, microbes from a remote site (e.g. infected tonsils) could localize in an inflamed pulp and lead to pulpal necrosis and odontalgia.

Diseases Causing Paresthesia as the Predominant Oral Manifestation

These include syphilis and multiple sclerosis.

Syphilis

In tabes dorsalis, a late stage of syphilis, patients may experience loss of pulpal sensation.

Multiple Sclerosis

Some of these patients experience loss of pulpal sensation as well as trigeminal neuralgia symptoms. Systemic signs of nerve degeneration are readily observable.

Diseases Causing Pulp Calcification and Fibrosis as the Predominant Endodontic Manifestation

These include progeria, osteogenesis imperfecta, hypervitaminosis D, and miscellaneous diseases.

Progeria

This is a genetic disease in which there is premature aging of all body tissues and organs. The pulps also may show signs of aging as evidenced by pulpal calcification and fibrosis.

Osteogenesis Imperfecta with Dentinogenesis Imperfecta

In this genetic disease, dentinogenesis imperfecta has been reported to accompany the bony changes in about 15 per cent of the cases. The dental manifestations are the same as has been described for hereditary opalescent dentin (Figs. 146, 243). However, the two diseases are caused by different genetic changes. The bones are very brittle, fracture readily, and show osteoporosis.

Hypervitaminosis D

One of the manifestations of excessive vitamin D has been shown to be calcifications of the pulp (calcinosis).

Miscellaneous Diseases

Other diseases that have been reported as causing pulp calcifications are ar-

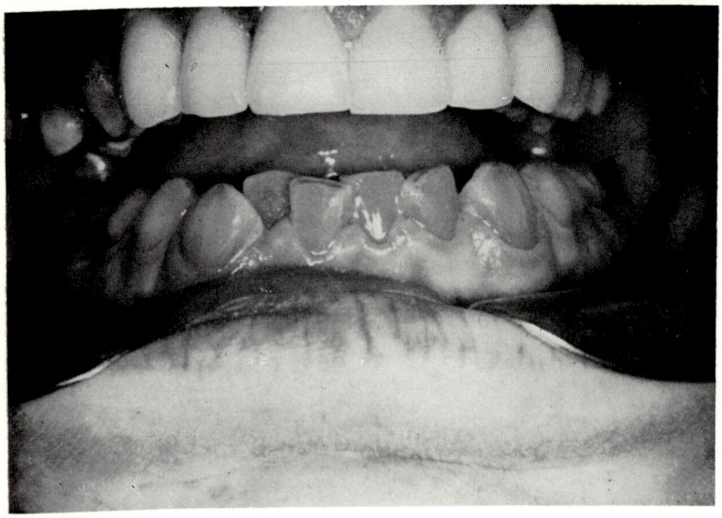

Figure 243. Dentinogenesis imperfecta; the upper anteriors have been crowned. (Courtesy of Dr. T. Simpson, Philadelphia, Pa.)

teriosclerosis, renal lithiasis, gout, Paget's disease, hypercalcemia, and dermatomyositis with calcinosis.

Diseases Causing Pulp Canal Enlargements as the Predominant Endodontic Manifestation

Included in this section are hypophosphatemic vitamin D-resistant rickets, Fanconi's syndrome, osteogenesis imperfecta, and hypophosphatasia.

Hypophosphatemic Vitamin D-Resistant Rickets

This disease is discussed under bony lesions, however, there are large pulp chambers present.

Fanconi's Syndrome

This genetic syndrome has the same dental changes as hypophosphatemic rickets.

Osteogenesis Imperfecta with Dentinogenesis Imperfecta

In this previously discussed disease, the pulp chambers are very wide in early years (Fig. 146A and B).

Hypophosphatasia

This is a genetic disease characterized by low serum alkaline phosphatase, phosphoethanolamine in plasma and urine, and skeletal abnormalities. The oral manifestations are spontaneous or early loss of teeth, often extremely large pulp chambers, and deficiencies of cementum.

Diseases Causing Oral Lesions as the Predominant Oral Manifestation

In these diseases, the lesions are generally not limited to the oral cavity but may be found on the skin and elsewhere. In the mouth, they usually have more than one location. Diseases included are typhoid fever, lupus erythematosus, pemphigus, erythema multiforme, epidermolysis bullosae, syphilis, and gonorrhea.

Typhoid Fever

Typhoid fever patients may have oral involvements, including ulceration of the palate and alveolar mucosa. Pulpal abscesses have been reported, as well as periapical breakdown, including osteomyelitis. Submaxillary lymphadenopathy can also occur. Salmonella typhosa has been isolated from infected pulps and periapical areas.

Lupus Erythematosus

In this disease, irregularly shaped reddish lesions can be found in the oral mucosa, and ulcers may be present. The lesions may also be found on the skin, especially of the nose, ears and forehead. A positive L-E test is diagnostic.

Pemphigus

In this disease, ulcers can also be found both within the oral mucosa and on the skin (Fig. 19). Blood tests show a positive Pels Macht test.

Erythema Multiforme

This is a skin disease in which there may be bullae and ulcerations of the oral mucous membranes.

Epidermolysis Bullosae

This is a genetic skin disease that may show oral erythematous lesions, bullae, ulcerations, and hypoplastic teeth.

Syphilis and Gonorrhea

In these venereal diseases, oral lesions may occur in different stages of the diseases.

Diseases Causing Regional Lymphadenopathy as a Predominant Head and Neck Manifestation

The lymphadenopathy is usually bilateral. Diseases considered are granulomatous diseases and miscellaneous diseases.

The Various Granulomatous Diseases

These diseases can have oral or salivary gland lesions, but they often show lymphadenopathy of the parotid, submaxillary, and deep cervical lymph nodes. The primary lesions are usually in the lungs. These diseases can be detected by various tests, including radiography, delayed hypersensitivity tests, microbial examinations, histologic examinations, and complement fixation tests. The diseases in the category include syphilis, yaws, bejel, lymphogranuloma venereum, tuberculosis, sarcoidosis, histoplasmosis, actinomycosis, South American blastomycosis, thrush, and infectious mononucleosis. In the latter disease, gingival hyperplasia may occur, and detection is aided by a positive reaction with the heterophile agglutination test.

Miscellaneous Diseases That Cause Regional Lymphadenopathy

These include throat infections and scarlet fever.

ACUTE FOLLICULAR TONSILLITIS, TANGIER DISEASE, AND STREPTOCOCCAL PHARYNGITIS. In these throat infections, it is relatively easy to differentiate the infections from endodontic diseases. Examination of the throat reveals the characteristic inflamed and purulent lesions. The patient also has a high fever with the streptococcal diseases.

SCARLET FEVER. These patients also have a high fever, along with skin eruptions. Ulcers and a yellowish membrane may be found on the oral mucous membranes. The disease process can penetrate the alveolar process and cause an osteomyelitis. A positive Dick test is diagnostic.

Other Exanthematous Diseases. In diseases such as measles, chicken pox and diphtheria, a submaxillary lymphadenopathy can also occur.

Iodism. In this manifestation of chronic iodine poisoning, a submaxillary lymphadenopathy can occur.

Diseases Causing Malodors and Bad Tastes as Predominant Oral Manifestations

Agranulocytosis, which mimics acute necrotizing ulcerative gingivitis, can cause a malodor and foul taste. These manifestations can simulate those from an abscessed tooth. Blood tests would help in differential diagnosis, by showing the relative paucity of polymorph leucocytes. Also the gingivitis is widespread. Other diseases causing oral malodors and tastes are lung infections, eosinophilic granuloma, and gastrointestinal diseases. A salty taste has been reported in hypertensive patients, and patients with neurologic disturbances and neuroses may have a sweet taste. Sweet *acetone breath* can occur in patients with advanced diabetes.

Diseases Causing Facial Swelling as a Predominant Oral Manifestation

These diseases include hypothyroidism, Cushing's disease, Cooley's anemia, myositis ossificans, and dermatomyositis.

Hypothyroidism

In this disease of sluggish thyroid activity, facial swelling caused by facial edema may occur. However, it can be differentiated from a cellulitis by the fact that it is bilateral. Blood tests and tests for thyroid metabolism would help in the diagnosis of the condition.

Cushing's Disease

As a result of the high level of circulating corticosteroids, one of the clinical manifestations of this disease is a bilateral facial swelling, resulting in the typical *moon faced* appearance (Fig. 5). The bilateral aspect of the swelling should differentiate it from endodontic disease. Blood, urinary, radiographic, and other medical tests should help in the diagnosis of this systemic disease.

Cooley's Anemia

This disease is discussed under bone lesions. However, there is a characteristic facial appearance related to hyperplasia of bone marrow of the facial bones. The appearance simulates a facial swelling, but the bilateral nature helps in the differential diagnosis (Fig. 10).

Myositis Ossificans

When this debilitating muscle disease involves the temporal muscle, a facial swelling can occur.

Dermatomyositis with Calcinosis

This is a rare collagen-type disease in which there may be bilateral facial swelling. Cutaneous lesions and generalized soft tissue calcifications are found. Root resorptions and pulpal calcifications may also occur.

Diseases Causing Bleeding as a Predominant Oral Manifestation

Oral bleeding can occur in leukemias, polycythemia, vascular diseases, coagulation disorders such as classical hemophilia, Von Willebrand's disease, Christmas disease, and platelet disorders. In all of these diseases, systemic manifestations and blood tests help in the evaluation.

Diseases Causing Loss of Lamina Dura as a Predominant Endodontic Manifestation

Loss of lamina dura can occur in hyperparathyroidism (Fig. 16), Paget's disease, and fibrous dysplasia.

Diseases Causing Widening of Periodontal Ligament Space as a Predominant Endodontic Manifestation

Widening of the periodontal ligament space has been reported for diffuse scleroderma (Fig. 20) and osteopetrosis. In hypoparathyroidism, there may be incomplete root formation with wide open apexes. In these cases, the teeth should test normal.

Diseases Causing Tooth Discoloration as a Principal Oral Manifestation

Teeth may be discolored as the result of stains, enamel hypoplasia, or hypocalcification. Usually in all of these cases of tooth discoloration, the signs are seen on several teeth. The involved teeth are vital. In the case of tooth discoloration resulting from endodontic disease, one tooth is usually involved (Fig. 52). However, in cases in which trauma is the etiologic agent, several teeth may be discolored. In this instance, the teeth should not respond to the electric pulp tester, and the negative response would aid in differential diagnosis.

Teeth can become stained as the result of tetracycline ingestion (Fig. 51), chromogenic microbes, foods (Fig. 50), tobacco, ingestion of chemicals such as arsenic, mercury, bismuth, phosphorus, fluoride, copper, iron, chromium, silver, lead and iodine, use of silver nitrate on floors of cavities and margins of crowns, and systemic diseases and conditions such as jaundice, congenital porphyria, sickle cell anemia, osteogenesis imperfecta with dentinogenesis imperfecta (Fig. 243), erythroblastosis fetalis, leprosy (blue or purplish hue), dermatomyositis with calcinosis, cystic

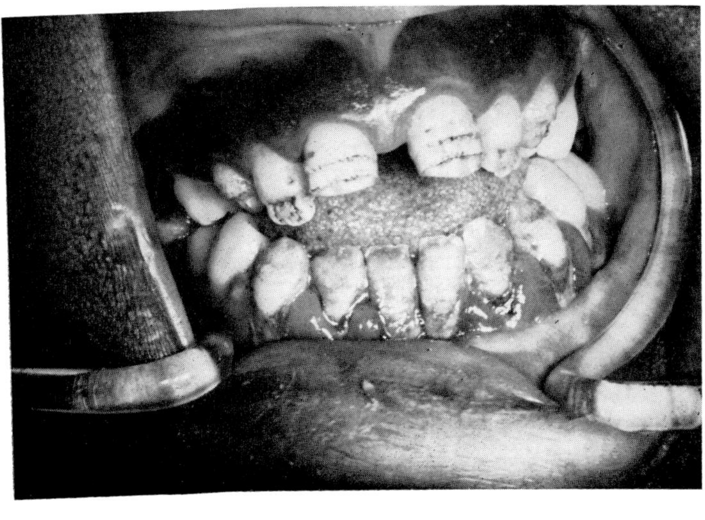

Figure 244. Severe enamel hypoplasia resulting from rickets in early childhood. (Courtesy of Dr. T. Simpson, Philadelphia, Pa.)

TABLE III

PERIAPICAL OR LATERAL RADIOLUCENCIES AND RADIOPACITIES

The possible etiologies of periapical or lateral radiolucencies and radiopacities are listed in order of decreasing frequency. Normal radiographic landmarks are not included. As there have been no complete reports of frequency, this order is an approximation based on clinical experience and a review of the literature.

Condition	*Causative Factors*	*Local or Systemic*
	Radiolucencies	
Periapical granuloma	Pulpal disease; microbes	Local
Radicular cyst	Pulpal disease; microbes	Local
Fibrous scar	Post-surgical; perforation through labial (buccal) and palatal (lingual) plates of bone	Local
Periodontal bone loss (especially on palatal roots)	Periodontal disease; microbes	Local
Cholesteatoma	Pulpal disease; microbes	Local
Lateral abscess or cyst	Periodontal disease; microbes	Local
Cementoma (early stages)	Unknown	Local
Dentigerous cyst	Congenital	Local
Primordial cyst	Congenital	Local
Nasopalatine cyst	Congenital	Local
Globulomaxillary cyst	Congenital	Local
Traumatic bone cyst	Trauma	Local
Fibrous dysplasia	Unknown	Local and/or systemic
Giant cell reparative granuloma, single or multiple as in hyperparathyroidism	Unknown for local; for hyperparathyoidism; tumor, kidney disease, or genetic	Local and/or systemic
Foreign body granuloma	Foreign bodies, e.g. cotton, gauze, etc.	Local
Paget's disease (early stages)	Genetic	Systemic
Ameloblastoma	Unknown; may be associated with dentigerous cyst	Local
Osteomyelitis	Pulpal-periapical disease and other microbial diseases	Local
Aneurysmal bone cyst	Trauma?	Local
Disuse atrophy	Lack of function; no occlusion	Local
Osteoporosis related to:		
Senility	Old age	Systemic
Post-menopausal period	Lack of estrogen	Systemic
Hypercortinism	Excess corticosteroids	Systemic
Protein deficiency	Inadequate proteins	Systemic
Vitamin C deficiency	Inadequate vitamin C	Systemic
Thyroid diseases	Excess or deficiency of thyroid hormones	Systemic
Diabetes mellitus	Lack of insulin	Systemic
Acromegaly	Excess growth hormone	Systemic
Ovarian dysgenesis	Lack of female hormones	Systemic
Osteogenesis imperfecta	Genetic	Systemic
Adrenal atrophy	Lack of adrenal hormones	Systemic
Cystic fibrosis	Genetic	Systemic
Median palatine and median alveolar cysts	Congenital	Local

TABLE III—*Continued*

Condition	*Causative Factors*	*Local or Systemic*
Cleft palate	Congenital; genetic	Local
Ameloblastic fibroma	Unknown	Local
Actinomycosis	Microbes	Local or systemic
Ameloblastic odontoma	Unknown	Local
Adenoameloblastoma	Unknown	Local
Acanthomatous ameloblastoma	Unknown	Local
Hemolytic anemias: Sickle Cell and Cooley's	Genetic	Systemic
Burkitt's tumor	Unknown; virus	Systemic
Histiocytosis X: eosinophilic granuloma; Hand-Schüller-Christian disease; Letterer-Siwi disease	Unknown	Systemic
Multiple myeloma	Unknown	Systemic
Osteogenic sarcoma	Unknown	Local
Reticulum cell sarcoma	Unknown	Local
Osteoradionecrosis	Radiation therapy	Local
Metastatic tumors	Some unknown; others have various causes including genetic	Systemic
Cental hemangioma	Unknown	Local
Cherubism	Genetic	Local
Calcifying odontogenic cyst	Unknown	Local
Leukemias	Radiation; genetic; other factors	Systemic
Osteomalacia	Vitamin D deficiency	Systemic
Cementifying fibroma	Unknown	Local
Gingival cyst	Congenital; traumatic	Local
Myxoma	Unknown	Local
Diffuse scleroderma	Unknown	Systemic
Nasalveolar cyst	Congenital	Local
Multilocular cyst	Congenital	Local
Chondroma	Unknown	Local
Odontogenic myxoma	Unknown	Local
Arterio-venous aneurysm	Congenital; trauma	Local
Squamous cell carcinoma	Smoking; other factors; genetic	Local
Hurler's syndrome	Genetic	Systemic
Chondrosarcoma	Unknown	Local
Ewing's tumor	Unknown	Local or systemic
Fibrosarcoma	Unknown	Local
Malignant salivary gland tumors of the palate	Unknown	Local
Neurogenic tumors	Unknown	Local
Gaucher's disease	Genetic	Systemic
Osteoid osteoma	Unknown	Local
Fibroma	Unknown	Local
Odontogenic fibroma	Unknown	Local
Lipoma	Unknown	Local
Liposarcoma	Unknown	Local
Median mandibular cyst	Congenital	Local

TABLE III—*Continued*

Condition	*Causative Factors*	*Local or Systemic*
Benign (true) cementoblastoma	Unknown	Local
Gout	Faulty uric acid metabolism; related to genetic and dietary factors	Systemic
Ameloblastic fibrosarcoma	Unknown	Local
True giant cell tumor	Unknown	Local
	Radiopacities	
Condensing osteitis	Pulpal disease; microbes	Local
Odontomas (compound, complex and cystic)	Unknown	Local
Osteosclerosis related to:		
Trauma	Trauma	Local
Estrogen administration	Excess estrogen; iatrogenic	Systemic
Occlusal relations	Occlusal traumatism	Local
Phosphorous exposure	Environment; excess phosphorus	Systemic
Sclerosteosis	Genetic	Systemic
Generalized cortical hyperostosis	Genetic	Systemic
Pyknodysostosis	Genetic	Systemic
Engleman's disease	Unknown	Systemic
Hyperostosis corticalis deformans juveniles	Genetic	Systemic
Miscellaneous conditions and objects including:		
Foreign bodies (bullets, amalgam, (etc.)	Environmental; dentistogenic	Local
Root fragments	Dentistogenic	Local
Sialoliths	Microbial; foreign bodies; mechanical obstruction	Local
Calcifications of lymph nodes or thrombi	Dietary; genetic?	Local
Calculus (subgingival)	Microbial; dietary; genetic?	Local
Cementoma (late stages)	Unknown	Local
Osteomas	Unknown	Local
Paget's disease (late stages)	Genetic	Systemic
Garre's osteomyelitis	Pulpal-periapical disease; microbes	Local
Osteopetrosis	Genetic	Systemic
Gardner's syndrome	Genetic	Systemic
Leontiasis ossea	Genetic	Systemic
Mucous cyst of the antrum	Unknown	Local
Dentinoma	Unknown	Local

fibrosis (may result from tetracycline ingestion, Fig. 18), and primary hyperoxaluria with oxalosis. In cases of mercury poisoning (acrodynia) the patient may also have a gingivitis, sloughing of the teeth and necrosis of the jaw bones.

Hypocalcification as well as discolorations may result from fluoride ingestion (enamel fluorosis, mottled enamel, Fig. 1), and in the bone disease, osteopetrosis. Hypoplasia may result from certain systemic diseases, such as the exanthematous diseases (measles, chicken pox, rickets, and scarlet fever, Figs. 15, 63), syphilis (peg shaped incisors, mulberry molars, Fig. 6), vitamin A deficiency, vitamin D deficiency (Fig. 244), amelogenesis imperfecta (a genetic disease), epidermolysis bullosa (another genetic disease), hypoparathyroidism, and hypothyroidism.

BONY LESIONS

These lesions produce radiolucencies, radiopacities, or a combination of both, on radiographs (see Table III). The lesions can be local cysts, tumors, and conditions, or oral manifestations of systemic diseases and tumors. Differential diagnosis from endodontic diseases depends upon pulp testing of the regional teeth, blood and urine chemistry (certain diseases have distinctive changes in blood calcium, phosphorus and alkaline phosphatase), radiography (systemic conditions often show bilateral involvement), biopsy, and history.

Primarily Radiolucent Lesions

Odontogenic Cysts

These cysts usually are found in the lower third molar area, but may occur

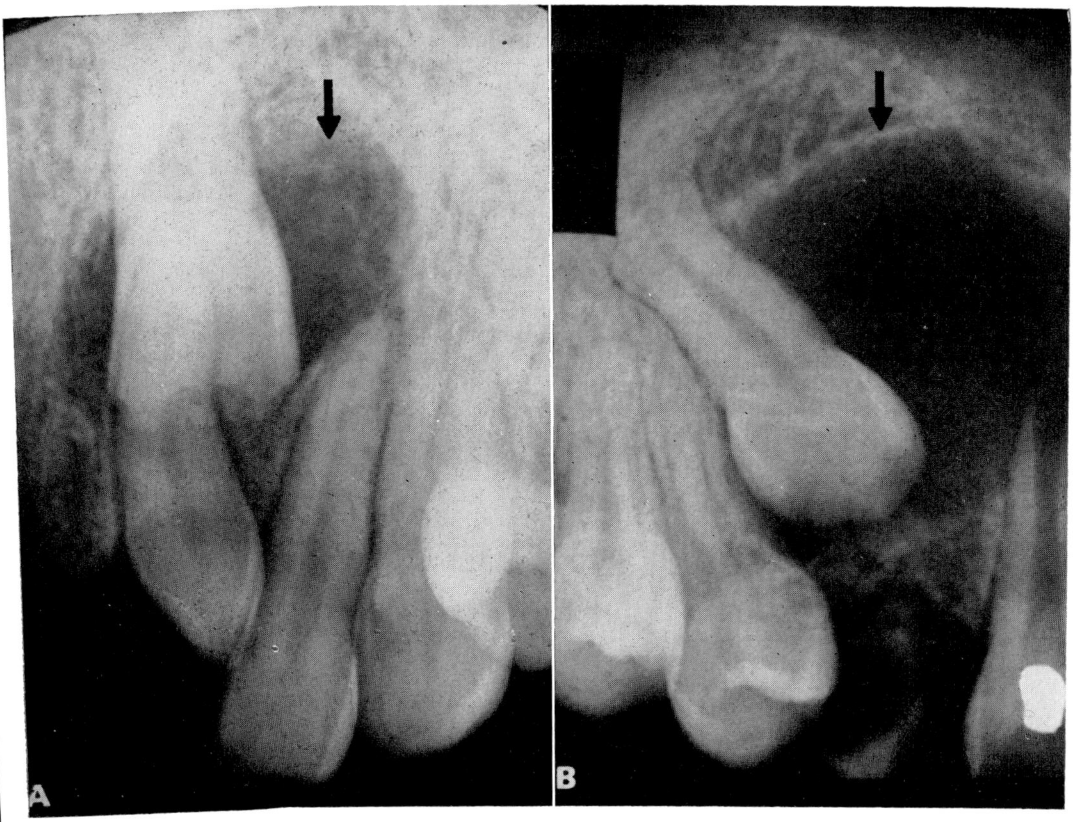

Figure 245. Dentigerous cysts. A. Dentigerous cyst associated with an embedded upper central incisor; the lateral incisor is vital. (Courtesy of Dr. T. Simpson, Philadelphia, Pa.) B. Dentigerous cyst associated with an embedded canine; the central incisor is pulpless and its necrotic products have contributed to the bony destruction. (Courtesy of Dr. W. Updegrave, Philadelphia, Pa.)

elsewhere. The most common odontogenic cysts, the radicular and lateral periodontal, have already been discussed. In rare cases, odontogenic cysts may develop into squamous cell carcinoma. The cysts discussed include primordial, dentigerous, multilocular, and calcifying odontogenic.

PRIMORDIAL (FOLLICULAR) CYST. This cyst develops from a degenerated tooth germ. There may be an associated jaw swelling. The primordial cyst is often found in the lower third molar area, but the tooth is absent. The radiographic image shows a large radiolucent area, not associated with a tooth. This cyst is lined by stratified squamous epithelium which is covered by a thin layer of keratin.

There is a rare genetic syndrome in which there are multiple primordial cysts, multiple cutaneous nevoid basal cell carcinomas, and various skeletal abnormalities.

DENTIGEROUS CYST. This cyst develops around a partially developed crown after degeneration of the dental organ. There is a jaw swelling associated with the lesion. The dentigerous cyst is usually found in the lower third molar area and occasionally in the upper canine region. The radiographic appearance shows a partially developed crown surrounded by a large radiolucent area (Fig. 245). The typical histologic picture shows a stratified squamous epithelially-lined cystic cavity surrounding the crown of a partially developed tooth. The covering connective tissue wall contains a mild chronic inflammatory cell infiltration and it may have foci of odontogenic epithelium. Dentigerous cysts can occasionally give rise to ameloblastomas (Fig. 246). Multiple dentigerous cysts may be found in the genetic diseases, cleidocranial dysostosis (hypoplasia or aplasia of clavicles with large and short skull, Fig. 247), and amelogenesis imperfecta.

MULTILOCULAR CYST. On rare occasions, a multilocular cyst can develop from a degenerating tooth germ. The involved jaw is swollen. The usual site is the lower third molar area. Recently,

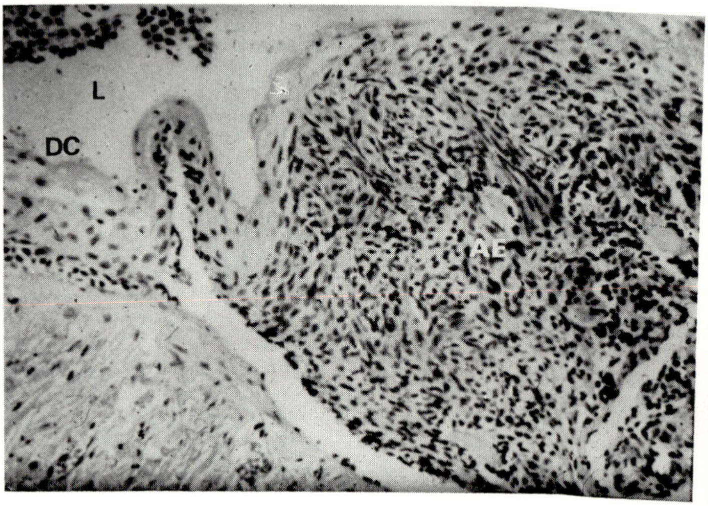

Figure 246. Dentigerous cyst with foci of ameloblastic epithelium; histologic section; L = lumen of cyst, DC = dentigerous cyst epithelium, AE = ameloblastic epithelium (×240). (Courtesy of Dr. D. Litwack, Philadelphia, Pa.)

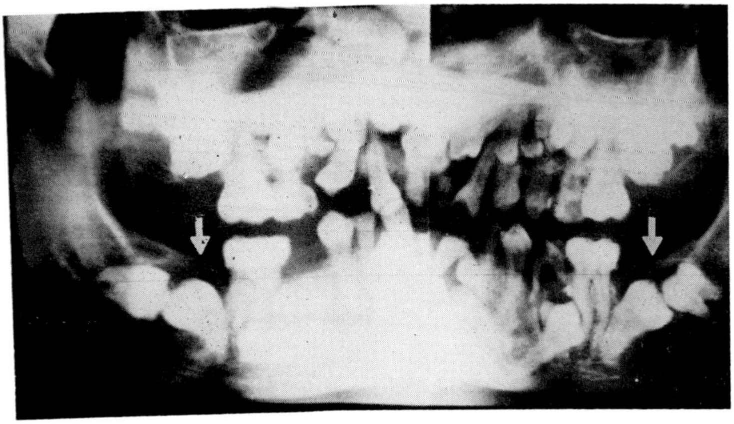

Figure 247. Cleidocranial dysostosis showing multiple embedded and partially erupted teeth, with possible dentigerous cysts (arrows). (Courtesy of Dr. M. Gross, Philadelphia, Pa.)

a multilocular cyst has been described in the lower canine area (botyroid odontogenic cyst). The usual radiographic picture shows a soap-bubble appearance in the area of the missing tooth. The usual histologic appearance shows stratified squamous epithelially-lined intercommunicating cyst-like cavities. The epithelial lining may be keratinized.

CALCIFYING ODONTOGENIC CYST. This lesion is a transition form between a cyst and a neoplasm. It usually occurs within the mandible. The etiology is unknown. The radiographic appearance shows a radiolucent area with several radiopaque foci of calcification. The histopathologic picture shows that there is a low cuboidal basal layer above which are irregular, swollen cells, scattered throughout are pale *ghost* cells, which may be keratinized, and some *ghost* cells are calcified.

Non-Odontogenic Cysts

These include cysts such as globulomaxillary, nasopalatine, median posterior palatine, median alveolar, and median mandibular.

GLOBULOMAXILLARY CYST. This is a fissural cyst located between the upper lateral incisor and canine. The cyst develops from epithelial remnants. There may be an associated swelling of the alveolar mucosa. The radiographic picture shows a pear-shaped radiolucency separating the roots of the involved teeth (Figs. 75, 217). The microscopic appearance shows a cyst lined by stratified squamous epithelium or ciliated columnar epithelium (Fig. 75B).

NASOPALATINE CYST (INCISIVE CANAL, MEDIAN ANTERIOR MAXILLARY). This is a fissural cyst within bone; the soft tissue counterpart, the cyst of the palatine papilla has already been described. It develops from epithelial remnants of the nasopalatine ducts. There may be an enlargement of the anterior midline portion of the hard palate and suppuration may occur. The radiographic appearance shows an oval, circular, or heart-shaped radiolucency above and between the roots of the upper central incisors (Fig. 248). In smaller cysts (less than 0.6 cm), it is difficult to differentiate the lesion from a normal incisive fossa. The microscopic picture shows a

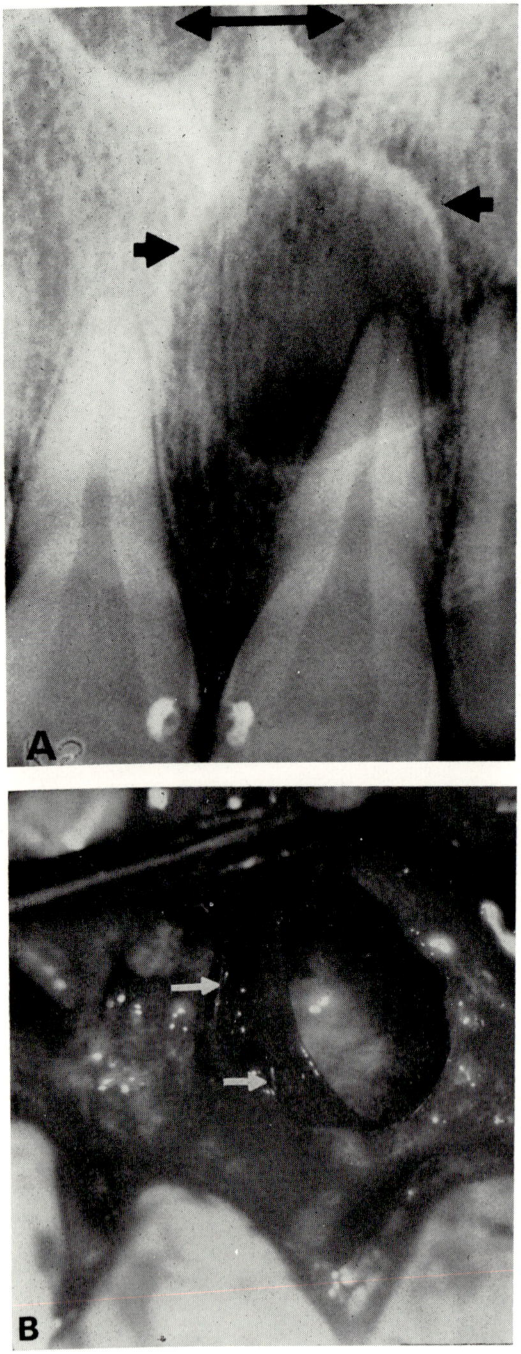

Figure 248. Nasopalatine cyst. (Courtesy of Dr. J. Levy, Philadelphia, Pa.) A. Radiographic; lamina dura and periodontal ligament space can be seen around the upper right central incisor; upper arrows indicate the nasal fossae. B. Clinical picture; arrows point to the thin epithelial lining that was evident when the lesion was uncovered.

cyst lined by stratified squamous, cuboidal, or ciliated columnar epithelium The connective tissue wall usually contains mucous glands, adipose tissue, blood vessels, nerves, and some chronic inflammatory cells.

MEDIAN POSTERIOR PALATINE CYST AND MEDIAN ALVEOLAR CYST. These are fissural cysts that apparently develop from epithelial rests left in the midline of the palate. The alveolar cyst is on the alveolar process behind the central incisors and in the midline of the palate. The palatine cyst is within the palate. Clinically, there is usually a firm swelling in the midline of the palate. The radiographic appearance shows a circumscribed radiolucent area. For the alveolar cyst, the radiolucency is in a lower position than is found with the nasopalatine cyst. The histopathologic appearance shows a cyst lined by stratified squamous epithelium, ciliated columnar epithelium, or both. The connective tissue wall may show slight chronic inflammation.

MEDIAN MANDIBULAR CYST. This is a rare fissural cyst located within the lower jaw and below the apexes of the lower central incisors. It probably forms from epithelial remnants in the midline of the mandible. The radiographic view shows either single or multilocular radiolucent areas. The microscopic picture shows a cystic cavity lined by stratified squamous epithelium or a combination of stratified squamous and ciliated columnar epithelium.

Pseudocysts

There are cyst-like lesions that are not lined by epithelium. The two lesions covered are the *traumatic* bone cyst and the aneurysmal bone cyst.

"TRAUMATIC" BONE CYST (EXTRAVASATION CYST, SIMPLE BONE CYST, HEMORRHAGIC BONE CYST). This cyst-like lesion usually occurs in the mandible, between the canine and the ramus, but it can occur in the lower anterior region. It may be related to traumatically-induced intraosseous hemorrhage, but this has not been definitely proven. The

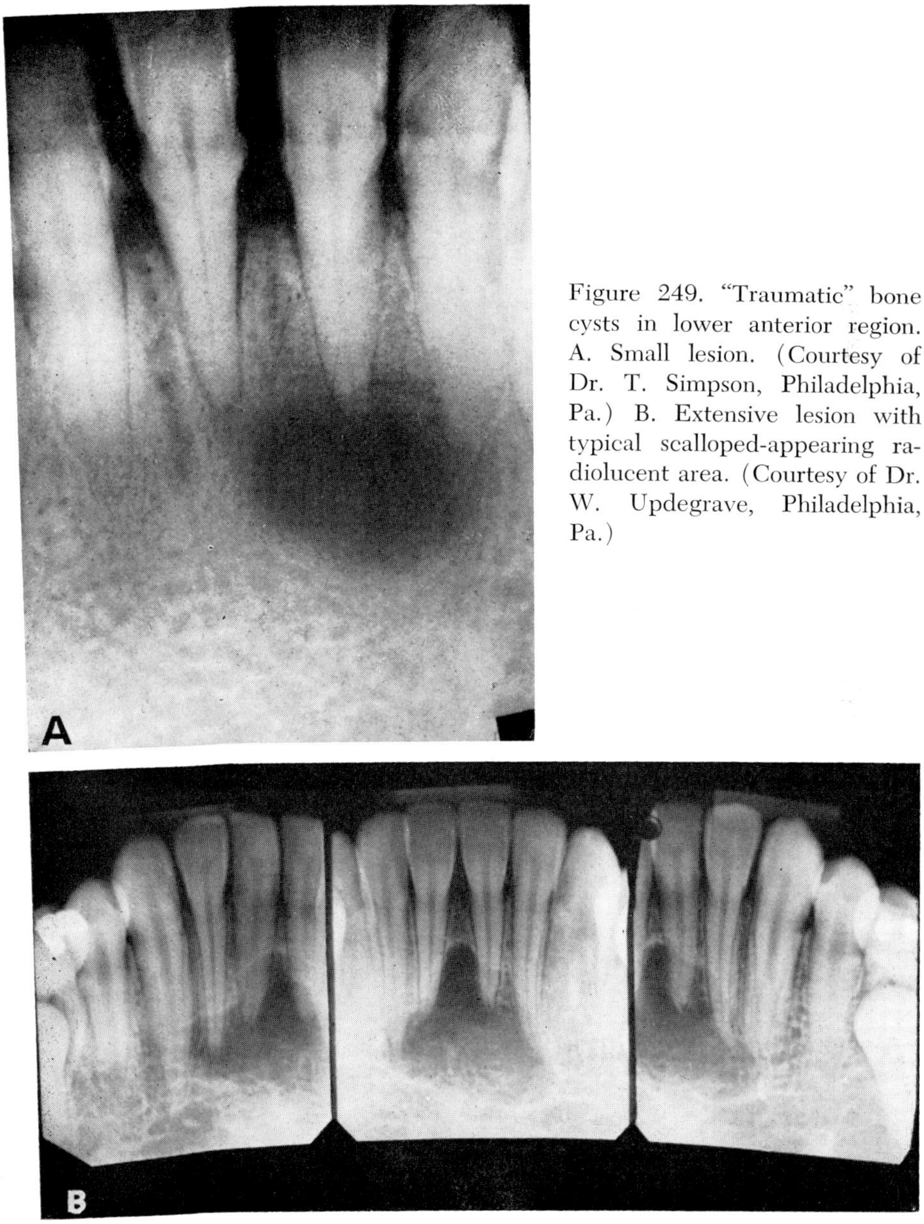

Figure 249. "Traumatic" bone cysts in lower anterior region. A. Small lesion. (Courtesy of Dr. T. Simpson, Philadelphia, Pa.) B. Extensive lesion with typical scalloped-appearing radiolucent area. (Courtesy of Dr. W. Updegrave, Philadelphia, Pa.)

traumatic bone cyst is usually symptomless, but may cause expansion of the involved jaw. The typical radiographic picture shows a scalloped-appearing radiolucent area extending between teeth (Fig. 249). The microscopic view shows a hollow cavity or a cavity filled with small amounts of clear fluid or serum. The cavity is covered by a thin layer of connective tissue.

ANEURYSMAL BONE CYST. This pseudocyst also usually occurs in the mandible, and generally there is a history of trauma. A swelling of the jaw and overlying mucosa is seen. The bony cavity contains blood and reddish-brown tissue. The radiographic appearance shows a unilocular or multilocular radiolucency. Histopathologic features show prominent vascular spaces containing blood, fibroblasts, and collagenous tissue containing many giant cells, hemosiderin, and blood vessels.

Disuse Atrophy

There is generally loss of trabeculation of supporting bone around teeth that do not have opponents in the dental arch. The radiographic appearance usually shows radiolucent spaces that may occur around the roots. The periodontal ligament space is often narrowed and hypercementosis may be found (Fig. 250).

Radiolucent Diseases of the Jaws

Diseases included in this category are fibrous dysplasia, cherubism, giant cell reparative granuloma, hyperparathyroidism, osteoporosis, osteomalacia, rickets, hypophosphatemic vitamin D-resistant rickets, actinomycosis, histiocytosis X, Gaucher's disease, Paget's disease, cleft palate, Hurler's syndrome, gout, diffuse scleroderma, hemolytic anemias, and leukemias.

FIBROUS DYSPLASIA. These are lesions of unknown etiology containing immature fibrous connective tissue and bone. They are not neoplastic. If they involve one bone, the disease is the monostotic variety. Synonyms for this condition are fibroma and ossifying fibroma. If several bones are involved, this is the polyostotic variety. The monostotic variety is much more common and it occurs mainly in females, primarily children and young adults. Reports show that about 10 to 15 per cent of the cases involve the jaws. The maxilla is affected more often then the mandible. The usual site in the maxilla is the posterior region and the maxillary sinus is often involved. In the mandible, the premo-

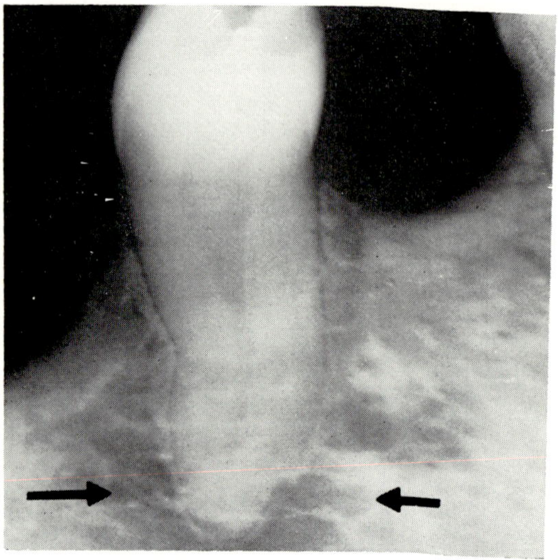

Figure 250. Disuse atrophy; a local form of osteoporosis. (Courtesy of Dr. W. Updegrave, Philadelphia, Pa.)

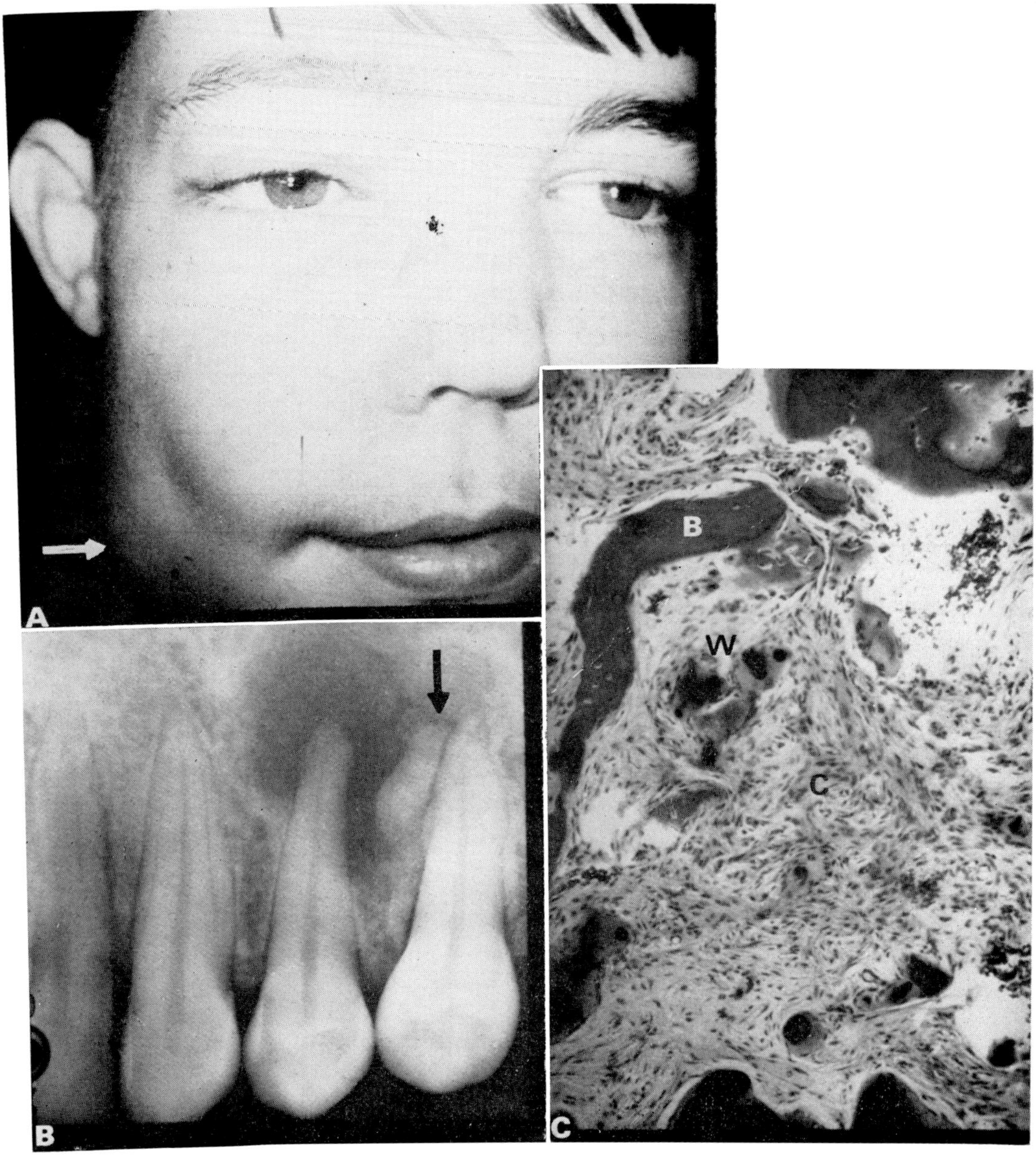

Figure 251. Fibrous dysplasia; monostotic variety. A. Clinical picture of a patient with fibrous dysplasia of the right mandible; showing unilateral swelling. (Courtesy of Dr. M. Gross, Philadelphia, Pa.) B. Radiograph of fibrous dyplasia appearing in the periapical region of an upper right first premolar; note the radiopaque foci in the radiolucent area—arrow. C. Histologic section of the lesion; B = bone, W = woven bone, C = fibrous connective tissue (×240). (B and C, Courtesy of Dr. D. Litwack, Philadelphia, Pa.)

lar-molar area is the usual site. If the polyostotic variety is combined with sexual precocity and areas of abnormal cutaneous pigmentation, the disease is called Albright's syndrome. The bony lesions may be bilateral or unilateral. Clinically, there is usually a painless swelling of the jaw and overlying mucosa (Fig. 251A). Teeth may be displaced and fail to erupt. Usually the blood chemistry is normal. However it has been reported that in 20 percent of the cases, the blood calcium level is elevated to between 11 and 13.8 mg/100 ml. In approximately 40 percent of child patients, the phosphorus level is decreased below 3.5 mg/100 ml. In about 50 percent of the patients, serum alkaline phosphatase levels are elevated. The radiographic appearance may show loss of lamina dura plus radiolucent areas containing sections of radiopaque foci giving a mottled appearance (Fig. 251B).

Histologically, the important features are replacement of normal bone by fibrous connective tissue. Interspaced within the mass of connective tissue are trabeculae of woven or fiber bone along with more mature bone (Fig. 251C). On rare occasions, malignant transformation into sarcomas may take place.

CHERUBISM. This is a genetic disease affecting the jaws. It often begins at ages 2 to 5. Usual clinical features show a bilateral swelling involving the posterior mandible. The regional lymph nodes may be swollen during the acute phase and tooth migration can occur. Jaw growth is rapid for a few years and then ceases. By adulthood, the jaws usually appear normal. During the early years, the radiographs show multiloculated radiolucencies with a few transverse bony septa, giving a *soap bubble* appearance. The histologic appearance often shows mature fibroblasts, pale ground substance, abundant collagen, clusters of giant cells, and bone spicules.

GIANT CELL REPARATIVE GRANULOMA (SOLITARY AND MULTIPLE) AND HYPERPARATHYROIDISM. These are giant cell lesions of bone that are similar histologically to the soft tissue peripheral giant cell reparative granuloma. If they occur along with lesions in other bones plus other systemic manifestations, the disease is called hyperparathyroidism (Von Recklinghausen's disease or osteitis fibrosa cystica generalisata). There is also a genetically-induced form of hyperparathyroidism called familial hyperparathyroidism. Hyperparathyroidism may also be secondary to renal osteodystrophy. It is also possible for giant cell reparative granulomas to be multiple without the condition being part of hyperparathyroidism.

Clinical findings in the localized condition report that it is more common in females, especially under 30 years of age, most lesions occur in the anterior half of the mandible and the involved region is usually swollen, and there is often a history of trauma.

Radiographs usually show a multilocular *soap bubble* appearance. Roots are often displaced (Figs. 252, 253A-D). The microscopic pattern reveals many multinucleated giant cells, hemosiderin, erythrocytes, numerous capillaries, immature fibroblasts, and osteoid or bone formation (Fig. 253E-G).

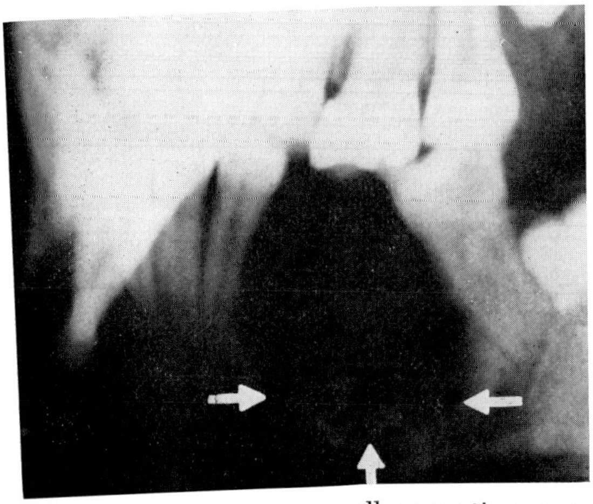

Figure 252. Large giant cell reparative granuloma of the mandible. (Courtesy of Dr. D. Litwack, Philadelphia, Pa.)

Clinically, features of hyperparathyroidism are fatigue, weakness, spontaneous fractures, and constipation. The etiology is often a tumor of the hyperparathyroid glands. Blood chemistry usually shows an increased calcium (11-18 mg/100 ml), a decreased phosphorus (less than 2.5 mg/100 ml), and a slight increase in alkaline phosphatase. There is also an increase in urinary calcium and phosphorus excretion. In the localized condition, the blood and urine chemistry are normal. The jaw radiographic picture in hyperparathyroidism may show, in addition to those changes described for the reparative granuloma, a generalized diffuse rarefaction.

Occasionally a loss of the lamina dura, with a widening of the periodontal ligament space occurs (Fig. 16). The histologic picture is identical to that described for the local condition. Rarely, if ever, a true giant cell tumor is found in the jaws. This lesion is usually found in the long bones and is aggressive and can metastasize. It is indistinguishable histologically from the giant cell reparative granuloma.

Osteoporosis. This is a generalized term that is related to failure of bone matrix formation by osteoblasts. It can occur in the jaws with many diseases and conditions. One form of osteoporosis has already been discussed under disuse atrophy (Fig. 250). The most frequent types are *senile,* which occurs in elderly individuals that have decreased secretion of steroids and possibly higher intake of phosphates (may be related to high meat ingestion) and *postmenopausal,* which occurs in women with decreased estrogen secretion. In these cases, blood chemistry values are normal. Other systemic inducing factors are protein deficiency, in which the blood calcium is often lowered (4-8.5 mg %), vitamin C deficiency, in which there is usually an increased blood calcium and a decreased blood ascorbic acid, a lack of fluoride for a prolonged period, and corticoid excess, which can occur in Cushing's syndrome or as the result of patients being treated with corticosteroids. Some diseases in which corticosteroids are given are asthma, the collagen diseases, nephrosis, leukemias, lymphomas, and transplant cases. There are other systemic diseases in which osteoporosis occurs. These include the following:

Hyperthyroidism. In this disease, there may be an associated alveolar bone loss (Fig. 254), an increased flow of saliva, an increased calcium excretion in feces, a decreased blood cholesterol, an increased iodine, a decreased glucose tolerance, and an increased basal metabolic rate.

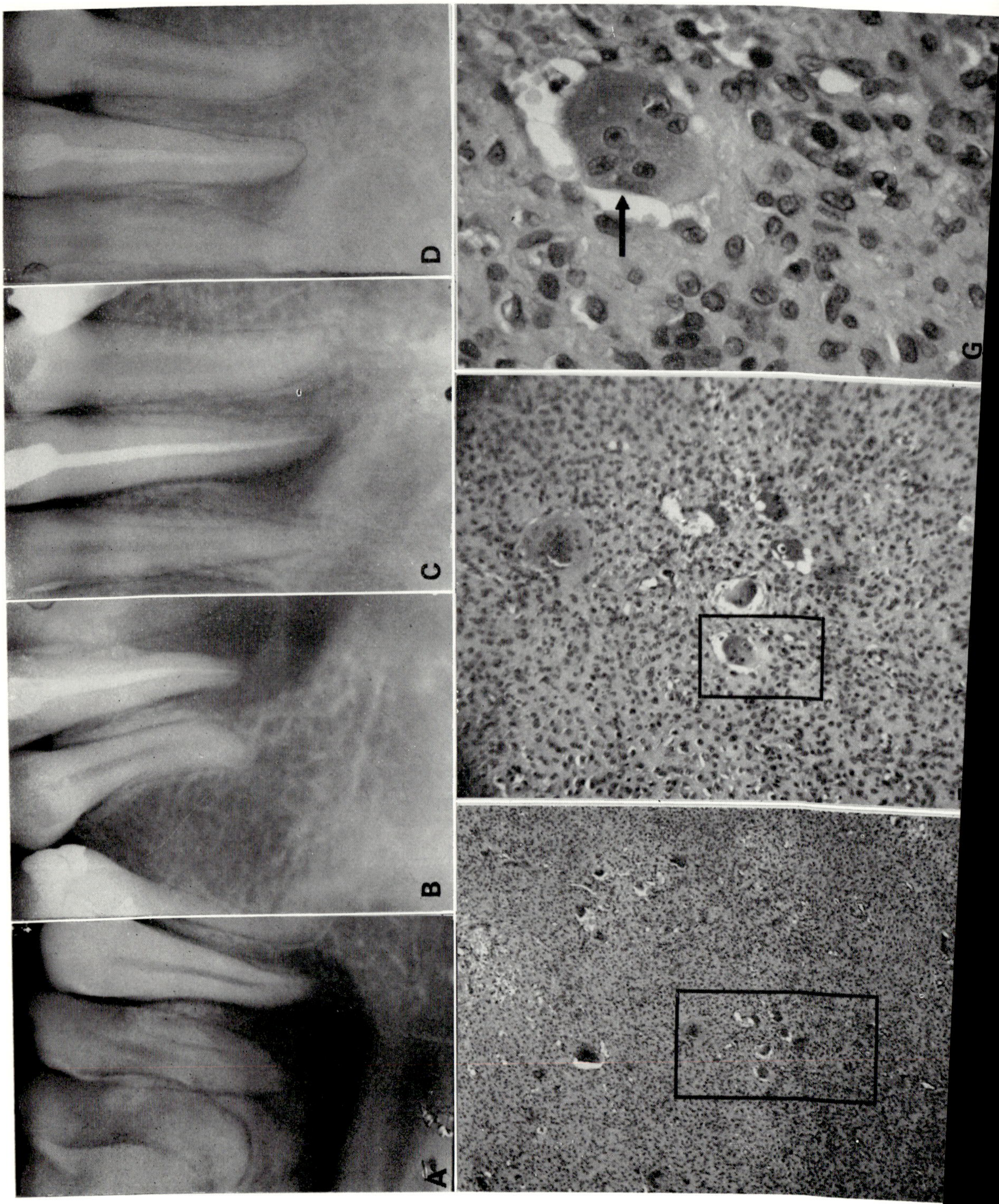
A
B
C
D
G

Hypothyroidism. In this disease, root resorptions and hypoplastic teeth may occur.

Diabetes Mellitus. In this disease, there may also be alveolar bone loss. Tests show a hyperglycemia, an increased glucose tolerance test, and a glucosuria.

Acromegaly (Adult Hyperpituitarism). In this disease, osteoporosis occurs in the mandible and the teeth often show hypercementosis.

Ovarian Dysgenesis. In this condition, there is also a deficiency in female hormones.

Osteogenesis Imperfecta. This is a genetic disease showing osteoporosis, brittle bones, blue sclerae, deafness, and often a dentinogenesis imperfecta (previously described).

Adrenal Atrophy. In this condition, there is a lack of adrenal hormones.

Cystic Fibrosis. This is a wasting disease involving the pancreas. It is found often with celiac disease. Accompanying conditions usually found are anemia, scurvy and rickets. In cystic fibrosis, excess calcium is excreted as insoluble calcium soaps, which result from disturbed fat metabolism.

←

Figure 253. Giant cell reparative granuloma; radiographic and histologic views. (From S. Seltzer, *Endodontology*, McGraw-Hill, Inc., 1971. Used with permission of McGraw-Hill Book Company.) A-D. Radiographic views of the lesion. E-G. Histologic views of the lesion. E. Abundant fibroblastic proliferation (×36). F. Higher magnification through rectangular area in E; giant cells are evident (×90). G. Higher magnification through rectangular area in F; arrow indicates multinucleated giant cell (×306).

The radiographic picture with osteoporosis shows a diffuse radiolucency that may be seen around root apexes. The microscopic view shows that the bone trabeculae are resorbed and replaced with fatty marrow.

Osteomalacia, Rickets, and Hypophosphatemic Vitamin D-Resistant Rickets. The term osteomalacia refers to a failure of osteoid tissue to calcify, while osteoporosis refers to a failure in matrix formation. The radiographic picture of both conditions look identical. Vitamin D deficiency is manifested as rickets in the child and osteomalacia in the adult. Clinical oral manifestations of rickets are retarded tooth eruption, enamel hypoplasia, tooth malposition, and hypoplasia of the mandible. In both rickets and osteomalacia, there are generalized radiolucent lesions of bone. The jaws are rarely involved but can occasionally show osteoporotic looking changes. Blood tests usually show a lowered calcium and phosphorous and an increased alkaline phosphatase. There is a low urine calcium. Renal rickets (secondary hyperparathyroidism) causes a result similar to primary hyperparathyroidism, with bone demineralization and excessive loss of calcium. The disease is caused by chronic renal disease. The jaw manifestations are a combination of rickets, osteomalacia and hyperparathyroidism. The radiographic picture shows marked osteoporosis and absence of lamina dura. Hypophosphatemic vitamin D-resistant rickets is a genetically-induced disease in which the primary defect is either a decreased renal tubular reabsorption of phosphorus, a decreased gastrointestinal

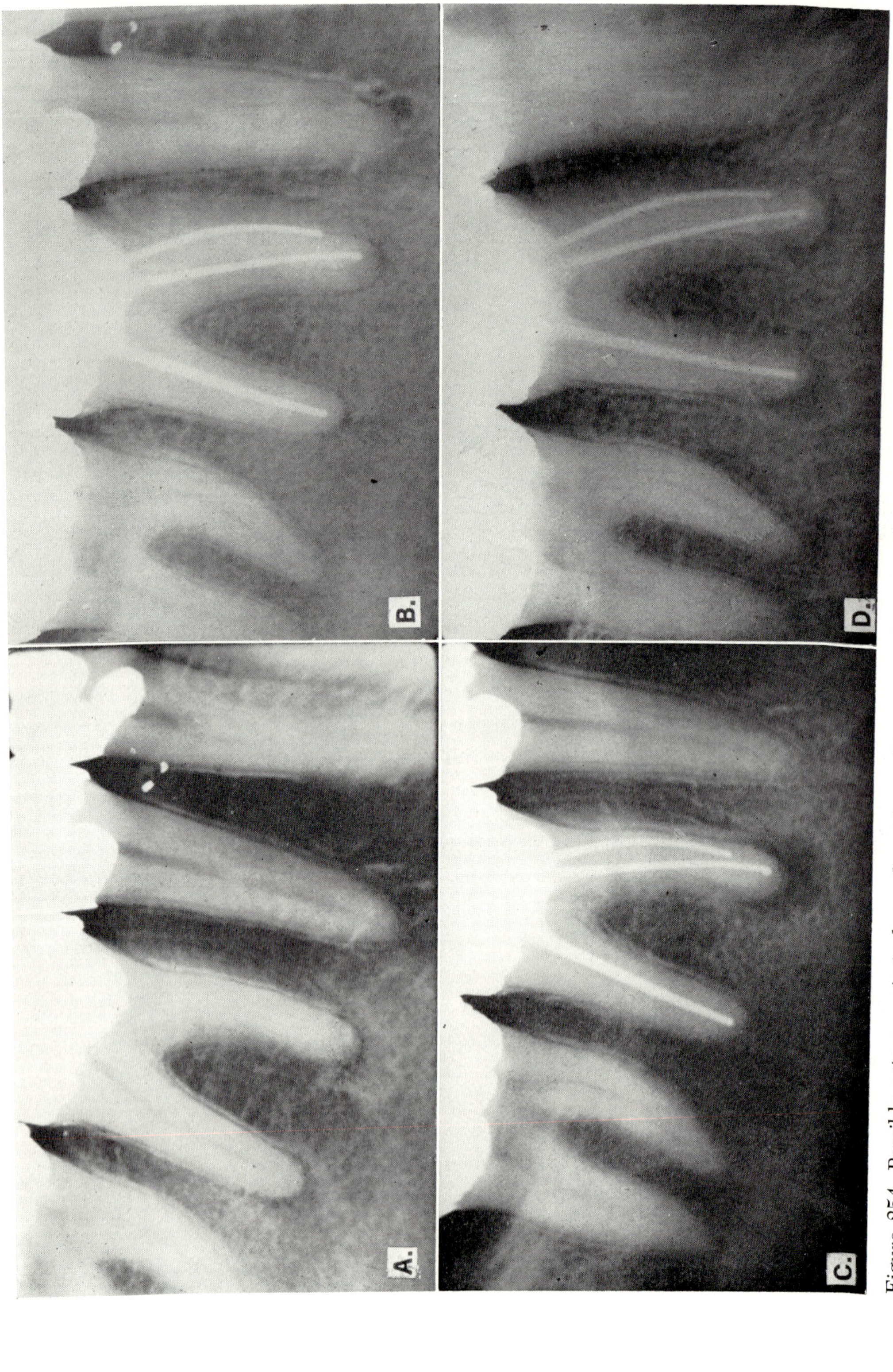

Figure 254. Possible osteoporosis in hyperthyroidism. (From S. Seltzer, *Endodontology*, McGraw-Hill, Inc., 1971. Used with permission of McGraw-Hill Book Company.) A. Preoperative x-ray of lower left first molar, which required endodontic therapy. B. Endodontic therapy completed. C. One year later, rarefaction at apex has developed; shortly afterwards, the thyroid glands were ablated. D. Seven years later; periapical rarefaction reduced, but not completely eliminated.

absorption of phosphorus, or a combination of both. The clinical result is a hypophosphatemia (low blood phosphorus). In this condition, rickets and/or osteomalacia may also be present. An important consideration for differential diagnosis in these patients is the presence of gingival abscesses, sinus tracts, and periapical rarefactions. The involved teeth appear intact but may be hypoplastic, and there is usually no caries or history of trauma. Radiographs often show large pulp chambers with enlarged pulp horns and periapical areas of pathosis. Apparently, microbes gain ingress into the pulp through enamel defects and cause the pulpal and periapical pathoses. Fanconi's syndrome is another genetic syndrome, which is associated with vitamin D-resistant rickets. The patients have the same dental changes as in the latter condition. The blood chemistry shows a low level of phosphorus, glucose and bicarbonate.

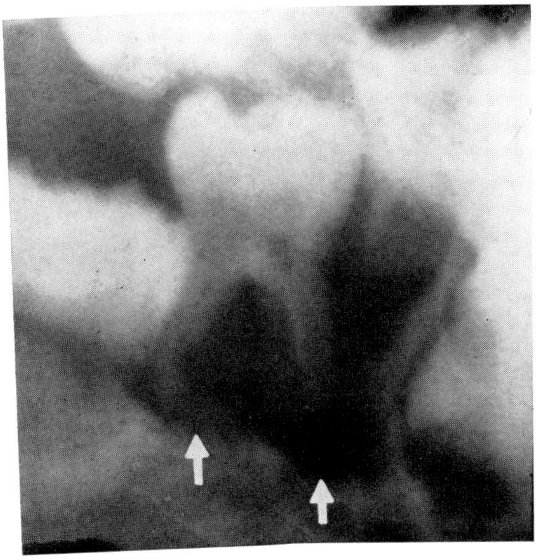

Figure 255. Letterer-Siwe's disease showing involvement around a primary molar; the tooth appears to "hang in space." (Courtesy of Dr. T. Simpson, Philadelphia, Pa.)

Actinomycosis. This disease has been discussed previously as far as the multiple sinus manifestation and regional lymphadenopathy are concerned. It can also occur as a central bony lesion. The radiographic picture shows a radiolucency that may appear around a tooth apex or can involve a large portion of the jaw (usually the mandible). Differential diagnosis depends upon microbial examination of the purulent discharge or tissue to look for sulfur granules and actinomycotic colonies.

Histiocytosis X. This is a descriptive term encompassing three diseases of the reticuloendothelial system (which includes macrophages of connective tissue and reticulum cells of lymph nodes, spleen, liver, and bone marrow). The three diseases, Letterer-Siwe's disease, Hand-Schüller-Christian disease, and eosinophilic granuloma are believed to be different forms of the same disease.

Letterer-Siwe's Disease. This is the most serious form of histiocytosis X. As it occurs almost always in the first year of life, it is usually not a consideration for differential diagnosis of endodontic and non-endodontic bony lesions. The jaws and other bones may have diffuse radiolucencies, but the primary involvement is in the liver, spleen, lymph nodes, lungs, skin and bone marrow. Disseminated histiocytes are found in these organs. In a case seen at Temple University, involvement occurred around a lower first primary molar (Fig. 255).

Hand-Schüller-Christian Disease. This form of histiocytosis X occurs primarily

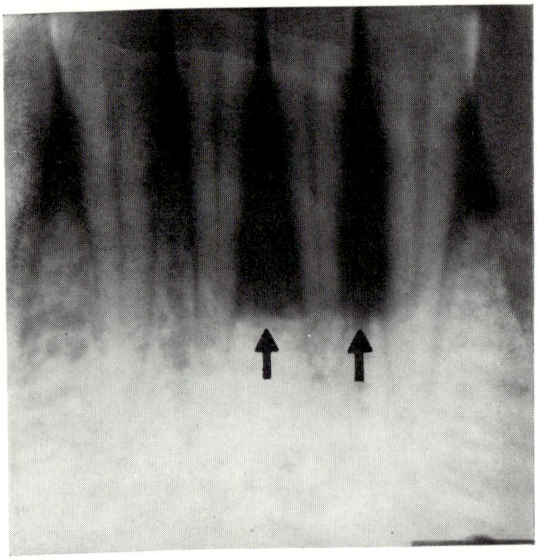

Figure 256. Eosinophilic granuloma of lower anterior teeth; the teeth have minimal bone support. (Courtesy of Dr. T. Simpson, Philadelphia, Pa.)

in children. The bone marrow is the principal organ involved, and numerous macrophages are found. This disease is more chronic than Letterer-Siwe's disease. Other organs that may be involved are the liver, spleen, lymph nodes, and skin. In a certain number of cases, there is a triad composed of bone lesions, exophthalmos, and diabetes insipidus. The disease can affect many bones, but the jaws and skull are often involved. In the oral cavity, there can be a gingivitis, and lesions simulating periodontal and periapical diseases. The bony lesions may look like endodontic-periodontic cases, but they affect many teeth. The radiographic picture reveals that the teeth often appear to have no bone support at all, and there are rarefied areas around the apexes. The histologic characteristics are sheets of histiocytes, some with lipid *(foam cells)*, plus some eosinophiles and increased amounts of collagen in the tissues (may be variable). The same type cells may be found in the dental pulp.

Eosinophilic Granuloma. This form of histiocytosis X occurs mainly in early adulthood, and more commonly in males. It has the most favorable prognosis of the three forms of the disease. The lesions occur primarily in marrow spaces. They are usually solitary, but may be multiple. The jaws are often involved and may be the sole manifestation of the disease. As is the case with Hand-Schüller-Christian disease, the disease can simulate periodontal and periapical disease and the pulp can be involved. The gingiva may be swollen or ulcerated. The involved tooth (or teeth) may be mobile and painful. The premolars and molars are the teeth most frequently involved. The patients may complain of an unpleasant taste and fetid breath. Another clinical manifestation of this disease is an extraction site that fails to heal. The radiographic picture is similar to cases of jaw involvement of Hand-Schüller-Christian disease. The involved tooth (or teeth) seem to be hanging in space with no apparent bone support (Fig. 256). There is usually a dark radiolucency with sharp margins. The histologic picture is characteristic with sheets of histiocytes alternating with collections of eosinophiles.

Gaucher's Disease. This genetic disease is also one of the reticuloendothelial system. In this condition, a lipid (glucosyl cerebroside) is deposited in the reticulum cells of the liver, spleen, bone marrow and lymph nodes. The patient manifestations are weakness, pigmented skin lesions, and bone lesions, which may involve the jaws. The radiographic picture of the jaws shows diffuse radiolucent areas, particularly in the lower molar region. Root resorption can occur (Figs. 257, 261). Serum acid phosphatase is often elevated. The diagnosis is confirmed by the demonstration of Gaucher's cells either in the bone marrow or other involved organs. The cells are large, striated, foamy cells. Frequently, several nuclei are present (Fig. 258). Neiman-Pick's disease is another lipid reticuloendothelial disease that can cause jaw radiolucencies, but as it occurs only in infants, it will not be considered further.

PAGET'S DISEASE (OSTEITIS DEFORMANS). This is a systemic disease of bone that is characterized by concomitant resorption and deposition of bone. In the early stages, the resorption is more prevalent and in the later stages the apposition is more frequent. The typical signs of this disease are enlarged head (Fig. 58) including jaws, in patients usually over 40 years of age, bowed legs, sunken chest, and curved back. Hearing and eyesight are often affected and patients may have headaches. Oral involvement occurs mainly in the maxilla. Radiographically, there is usually a loss of the lamina dura and the teeth often show root resorption and hypercementosis (Figs. 17, 79). The

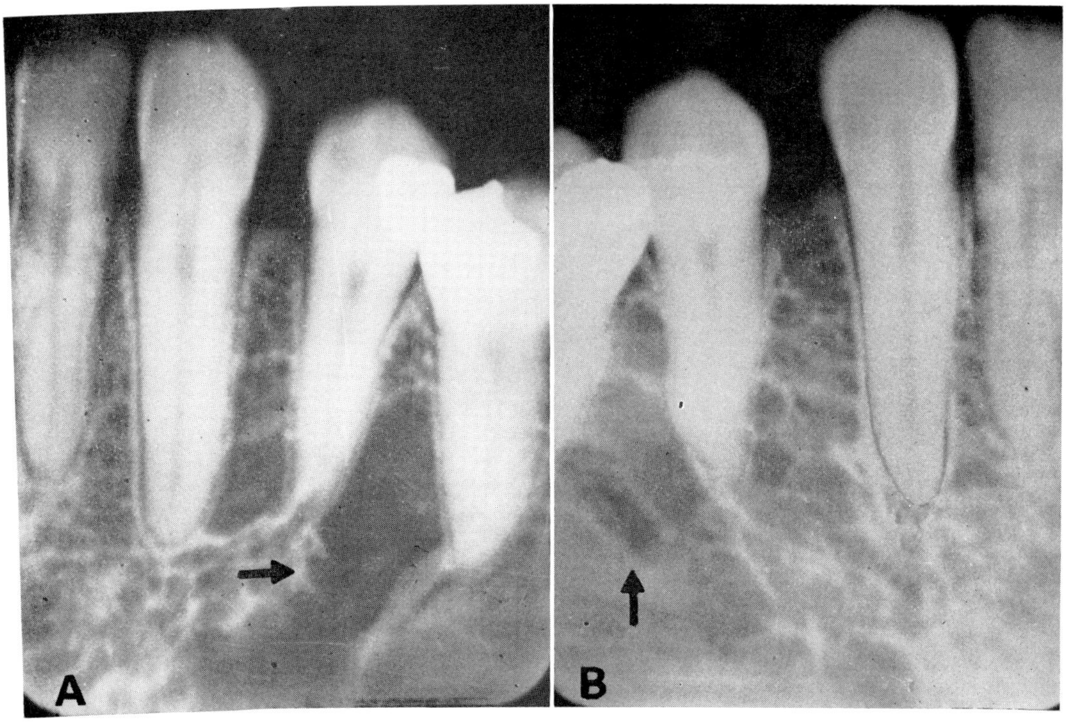

Figure 257 A and B. Gaucher's disease, radiographic views; two sites in an affected patient showing bony rarefactions (arrows). (Courtesy of Dr. I. B. Bender, Philadelphia, Pa.)

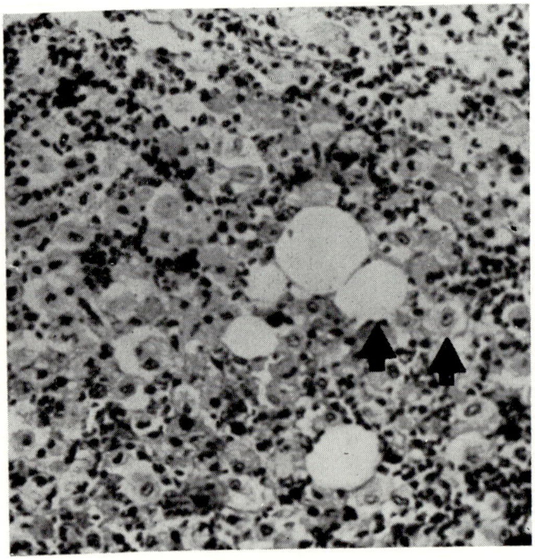

Figure 258. Gaucher's disease; histologic view. Arrows point to foam cells (×450). (Courtesy of Dr. T. Simpson, Philadelphia, Pa.)

alveolar ridge enlarges, teeth migrate, and may loosen. The bony radiographic findings vary with the stage of the disease. In the early stages, irregular radiolucencies are noted, which alternate with patches of radiopacities as the disease progresses. Finally in later stages, *cotton wool* appearing radiopacities are found (Figs. 58, 79). Histologically, there is found alternating patterns of bone formation and bone resorption (Fig. 259). As a result of the disease, bone blood circulation is poor and when infection occurs, osteomyelitis can follow rapidly. It has been reported that osteogenic sarcomas develop in 25 per cent of these patients. An important blood test finding in Paget's disease is a marked increase in blood alkaline phosphatase (usually 15-40 Bodansky units).

Cleft Palate. This genetically-induced defect in the palate occurs as a result of the failure of the palatal processes to fuse with each other and/or with the frontonasal process. These patients can have a periapical radiolucency (as seen on a radiograph) that may be superimposed over the apex of one of the upper central incisors. This can simulate an endodontic involvement. It is important to carefully examine the radiograph to see if the cleft continues between the incisors. This would then show that a cleft is present, rather than a periapical area of pathosis (Fig. 260).

Hurler's Syndrome. This is a genetic disorder of one of the mucopolysaccharides and it affects the skeleton. The symptoms include skeletal deformities, mental retardation, deafness, cardiac

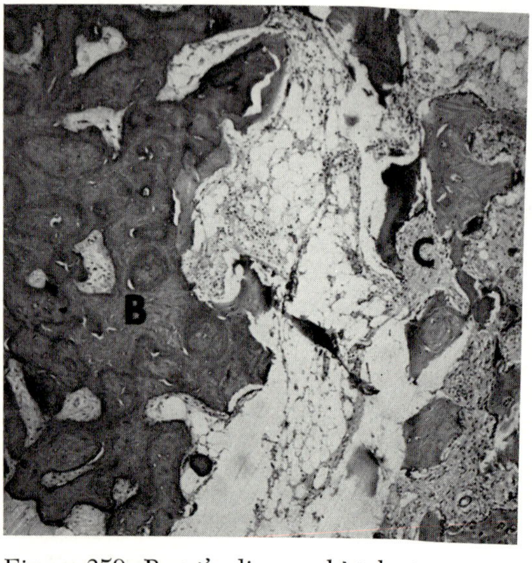

Figure 259. Paget's disease; histologic section; B = bone, C = connective tissue (×103.5). (Courtesy of Dr. A. Miller, Philadelphia, Pa. From S. Seltzer, *Endodontology*, McGraw-Hill, Inc., 1971. Used with permission of McGraw-Hill Book Company.)

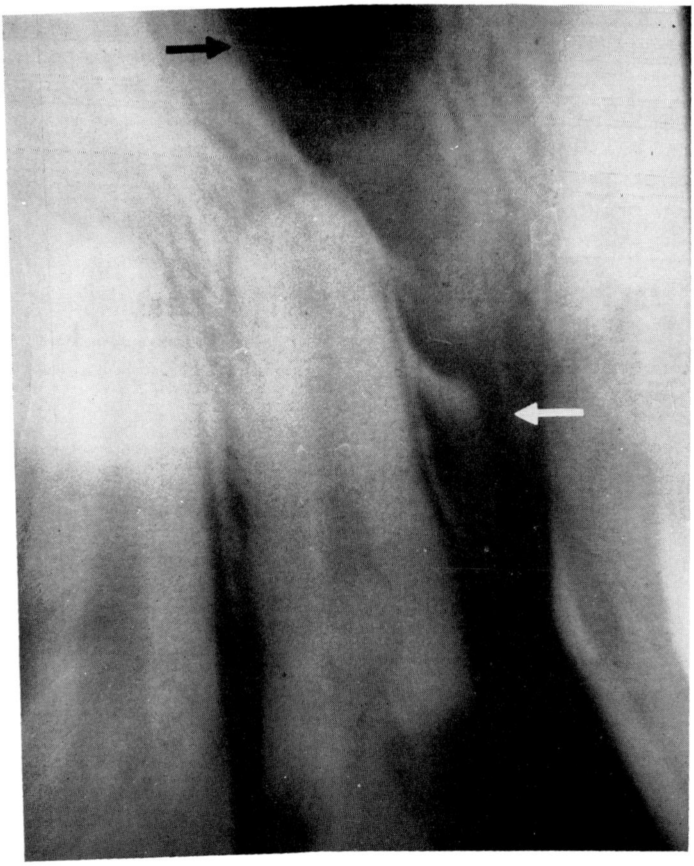

Figure 260. Cleft palate; radiolucency indicated by black arrow could be confused with a periapical area of pathosis; true diagnosis can be confirmed by following the continuity of the radiolucency (white arrow). (Courtesy of Dr. L. Muldorf, Philadelphia, Pa.)

anomalies, and hepatosplenomegaly. The mandible often contains radiolucent areas around crowns of the unerupted first and second molars. These probably represent *pools* of chondroitin sulfate B, rather than dentigerous cysts. Urine tests show large amounts of chondroitin sulfate B and heparin sulfate present.

GOUT. This is a disease of uric acid metabolism. In this condition, various bones in the body, including the jaws (rarely), can show multiple punched out radiolucent areas on radiographs. There have been reports of reflex referred pain to teeth, although these reports are questionable. The diagnosis is aided by urine and blood examination for uric acid.

DIFFUSE SCLERODERMA. This is a skin disease manifested by sclerosis of collagen. The skin becomes hard and fixed to underlying tissues and bones (Fig. 57). Other organs that can be affected are the lungs, kidneys, esophagus, blood vessels, heart, skeletal muscle, and the oral cavity. In the latter instance, the patients can have difficulty in opening their mouths. White or yellow sclerotic oral lesions can occur on the oral mucous membranes. The jaws can be affected with distinct widening of the periodontal ligament space (an estimated 7% of cases) and an associated periodontal and periapical rarefaction (Fig. 20). Histologically, hyalinized collagenation of tissues occur.

HEMOLYTIC ANEMIAS. These anemias are sickle cell and Cooley's (Mediterranean, thallasemia), and homozygous hemoglobin C disease (HHC). These are genetic diseases that predominantly affect blacks (sickle cell and HHC) and Mediterranean-type people (Cooley's). In sickle cell anemia, the red blood cells are sickle shaped and contain an abnormal type of hemoglobin (Hemoglobin S). The cells are readily destroyed in the liver, spleen and bone marrow. The patients usually die young because of insufficient oxygenation of tissues. Blood tests confirm the diagnosis. Possible oral manifestations are pigmentation of teeth, rarefied areas on jaw radiographs, and hypercementosis (in some cases, Figs. 8, 261C). During a *sickling crisis,* patients may have acute joint, abdominal, muscle, and occasionally jaw and/or tooth pain. Fever also occurs. In Cooley's anemia, there are also structurally defective red blood cells that are deficient in normal hemoglobin and contain large amounts of hemoglobin F. Oral signs may show enlargement of the facial bones due to marrow hyperplasia that simulates bilateral facial swelling, protrusion of upper anterior teeth (Fig. 10), short and spiked roots (variable), and similar type radiographic changes as seen in sickle cell anemia (Figs. 9, 261B). Homozygous hemoglobin C deficiency disease is not as serious as the others. Radiographic findings are similar.

LEUKEMIAS. Leukemias can cause bone rarefactions as a result of pressure resorption (Fig. 12). The presence of odontalgia has already been discussed.

Miscellaneous Conditions Causing Radiolucencies

These include foreign body granuloma, arteriovenous aneurysm, and osteoradionecrosis.

FOREIGN BODY GRANULOMA. If a foreign body is left in the periapical tissues, a granuloma, similar in radiographic and histological appearance to a typical periapical granuloma, would form. Some objects that have been found are sutures, sponges, needles, root canal instruments, cotton, root canal filling materials, and amalgam.

ARTERIOVENOUS ANEURYSM (FISTULA)

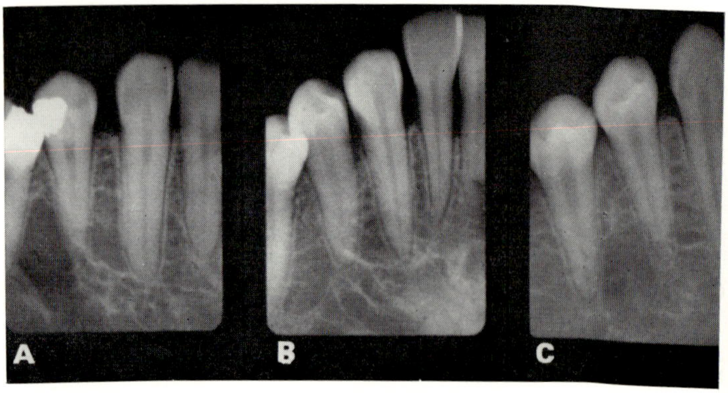

Figure 261. Bone changes seen in sickle cell anemia, Cooley's anemia, and Gaucher's disease. A. Gaucher's disease. B. Cooley's anemia (thalassemia). C. sickle cell anemia. (Courtesy of Dr. I. B. Bender, Philadelphia, Pa. From S. Seltzer, *Endodontology,* McGraw-Hill, Inc., 1971. Used with permission of McGraw-Hill Book Company.)

OF THE JAWBONES. This condition may be congenital or related to trauma. It is an abnormal communication between arterial and venous channels. Clinical manifestations reveal swelling and often discoloration over the involved area of the jaw (usually mandible). There may be extensive bone destruction and loosening of the teeth at the site of the fistula. The radiographic image shows extensive rarefaction, usually in the region of the inferior alveolar canal or retromolar-ramus area. The histologic picture shows several large arteries and veins communicating inside the bony lesion.

OSTEORADIONECROSIS (RADIATION NECROSIS). This is a severe destructive form of osteomyelitis that results from radiation treatment (Fig. 13). It follows by weeks, months or years, radiation therapy to the jaws. It usually occurs when teeth have been left in the jaws, but can occur even without teeth. The bone changes result from the direct effect of the radiation on bone cells and interference with the blood supply of the bone. Secondary effects result from introduction of infection into the pathological bone. If teeth had been left in the jaws, patients could develop toothaches resulting from pulpal arteritis. Other dental manifestations are rapid root caries, tooth discoloration, paresthesia, and pulpal necrosis (Fig. 14). The histologic and radiographic picture of osteoradionecrosis is similar to that previously described for osteomyelitis.

Odontogenic Tumors

These tumors originate from the dental lamina or its derivative structures. They are benign endosteal tumors, except for the ameloblastic fibrosarcoma. They are derived from the epithelium, the mesoderm, or both. Those that have radiolucent appearances are discussed in this section. These include ameloblastomas, calcifying epithelial odontogenic tumor, ameloblastic fibroma, ameloblastic odontoma, cementoma, fibromas, cementoblastoma, odontogenic myxoma, and ameloblastic fibrosarcoma.

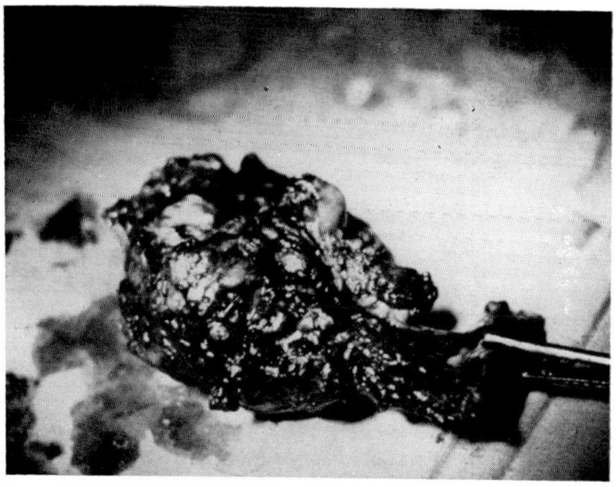

Figure 262. Gross specimen of an ameloblastoma; note the multicystic appearance. (Courtesy of Dr. D. Litwack, Philadelphia, Pa.)

AMELOBLASTOMA. This is the most common and most aggressive epithelial odontogenic tumor. It arises from either the dental lamina, the lining of a dentigerous cyst (Figs. 246, 264), remnants of the dental organ, or the basal layer of the oral mucous membrane. The incidence of the ameloblastoma is approximately 1 percent of the tumors and cysts of the jaws. It occurs primarily in the molar and ramus area of the mandible in the age bracket 20 to 49. Clinically, the involved area often shows swelling and absence of other manifestations. The gross lesion is multicystic in appearance (Fig. 262). The

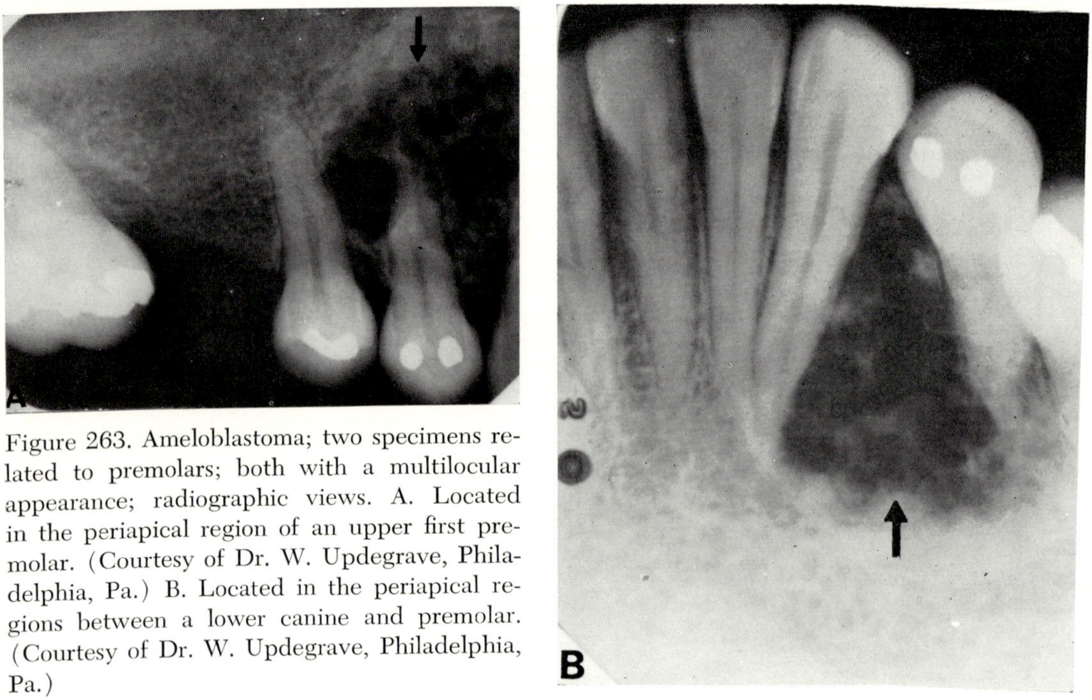

Figure 263. Ameloblastoma; two specimens related to premolars; both with a multilocular appearance; radiographic views. A. Located in the periapical region of an upper first premolar. (Courtesy of Dr. W. Updegrave, Philadelphia, Pa.) B. Located in the periapical regions between a lower canine and premolar. (Courtesy of Dr. W. Updegrave, Philadelphia, Pa.)

usual radiographic appearance shows multilocular (soap bubble-like) radiolucent areas (Figs. 111, 263). Occasionally, the areas are unilocular. The histologic picture shows epithelial islands, strands, cords, or sheets in a collagenous fibrous connective tissue stroma. The peripheral epithelial cells resemble ameloblasts and the central cells resemble stellate reticulum, but in some rare lesions the central cells are granular. There is no encapsulation (Fig. 264).

ACANTHOMATOUS AMELOBLASTOMA. This is a variety of ameloblastoma which differs only in its histological appearance. The tumor consists of epithelial strands of squamous cells which may be keratinized. Also, regular ameloblastic-type epithelium and connective tissue are usually present.

ADENOAMELOBLASTOMA (ADENOMATOID ODONTOGENIC TUMOR). This is another rare epithelial odontogenic tumor. Its origin is unknown, but it may arise from the pre-ameloblast cells. The adenoameloblastoma occurs more often in the anterior maxilla than in other areas, and the usual age affected is approximately 20 years. It may be associated with unerupted teeth and can be located between teeth. Radiographically, the adenoameloblastoma usually appears radiolucent and can be confused with a lateral periodontal cyst or a dentigerous cyst. There may be some areas of radiopacity within the lesion. Microscopically, the tumor is composed of numerous duct-like structures, lined by columnar epithelium. In between the duct-like structures are epithelial cells, and calcified material may be scattered throughout. The lesion is usually en-

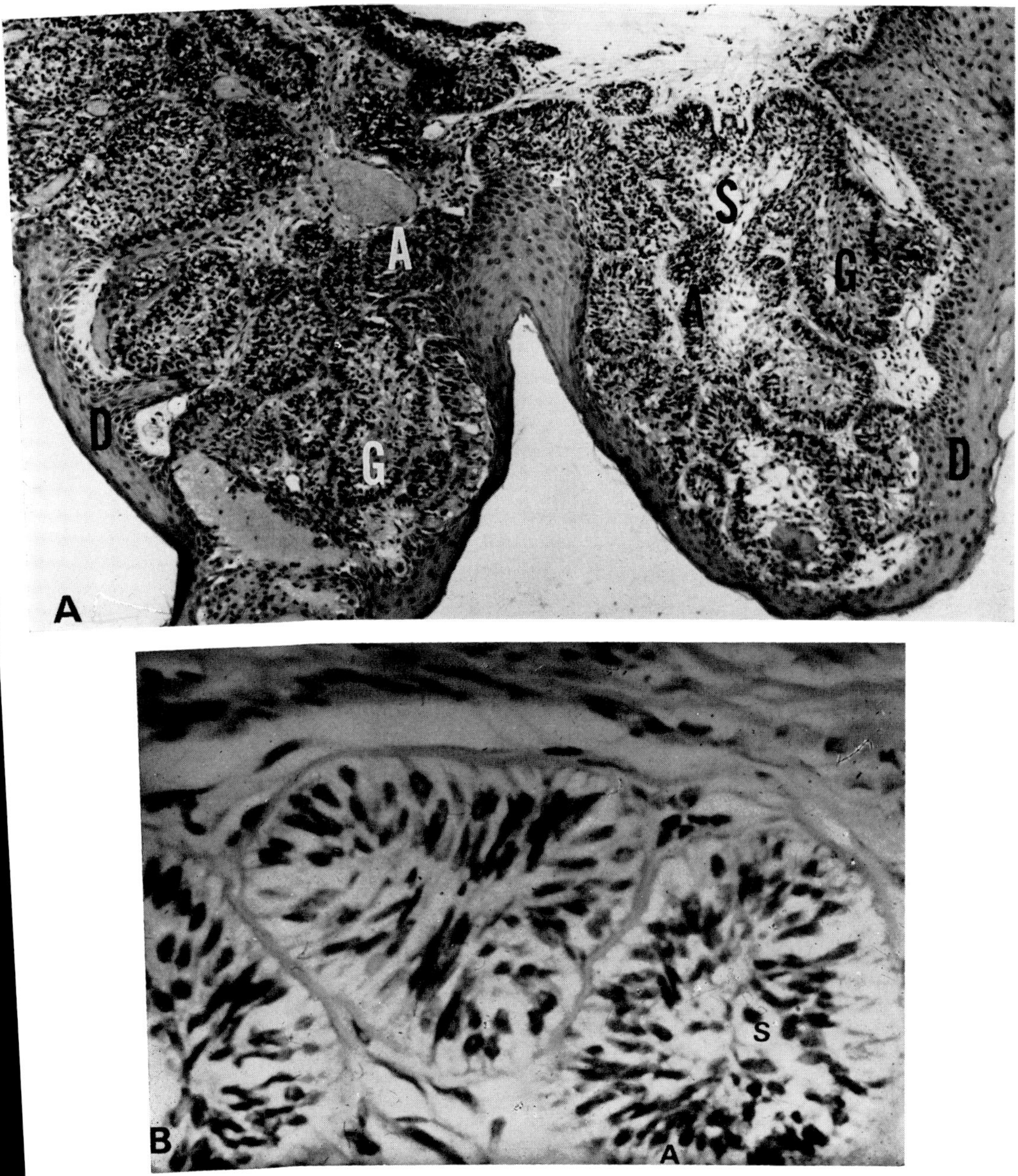

Figure 264. Ameloblastoma; histologic views. A. A granular cell ameloblastoma arising in the wall of a dentigerous cyst; D = dentigerous cyst epithelial lining, G = granular cells, A = ameloblastic epithelium, S = stellate reticulum cells (×100). (Courtesy of Dr. C. Leifer, Philadelphia, Pa.) B. Higher magnification of an ameloblastoma showing ameloblastic epithelium with stellate reticulum cells; A = ameloblastic epithelium, S = stellate reticulum cells (×450). (Courtesy of Dr. D. Litwack, Philadelphia, Pa.)

capsulated by fibrous connective tissue.

MELANOAMELOBLASTOMA. This is a very rare epithelial odontogenic tumor that causes a radiolucent radiographic appearance in periapical films. As the melanoameloblastoma only occurs in children less than one year of age, it will not be considered in differential diagnosis of endodontic and non-endodontic lesions.

CALCIFYING EPITHELIAL ODONTOGENIC TUMOR. This is a rare aggressive epithelial odontogenic tumor that occurs primarily in the premolar-molar area of the mandible. Swelling usually occurs in the involved region. This odontogenic tumor often appears in association with an impacted tooth. The radiographic appearance usually shows a combination of radiolucency and radiopacity. The histologic picture typically shows sheets of polyhedral epithelial cells separated by a slight connective tissue stroma. The epithelial cells may be pleomorphic. There may also be present islands of amyloid-like material.

AMELOBLASTIC FIBROMA. This odontogenic tumor contains epithelial and mesodermal tissue elements. It may be derived partly from Hertwig's epithelial root sheath. The ameloblastic fibroma occurs primarily in the premolar-molar region of the mandible, in patients generally younger than twenty-five years of age. It is usually symptomless, except for swelling of the involved region. Radiographically, it appears as a distinct unilocular, or rarely a multilocular, radiolucency. The histological picture shows a fibrous encapsulated lesion composed of thin strands, cords, and islands of cuboidal epithelium similar to the dental lamina, dispersed in a bed of young mesenchymal connective tissue. The mesenchyme appears similar in appearance to the dental papilla.

AMELOBLASTIC ODONTOMA. This is a rare mixed odontogenic tumor containing odontogenic epithelium, mesenchyme, and calcified dental tissue. It is derived from a later stage of tooth development than the previously described tumors. The ameloblastic odontoma occurs more often in the maxilla and in patients 15 years of age and under. It is asymptomatic except for swelling of the involved area (most frequently the premolar-molar area). Radiographs reveal radiolucencies interspersed with radiopaque areas. The microscopic picture usually shows a random arrangement of odontogenic epithelium embedded in a *sea* of mesenchyme with varying proportions of ameloblasts, stellate reticulum, enamel matrix, enamel, dentin, osteodentin, cementum, bone and pulp.

CEMENTOMA (PERIAPICAL CEMENTAL DYSPLASIA; PERIAPICAL FIBROMA). This mesodermal odontogenic tumor is one of the lesions that is most frequently confused with a pulpally-induced periapical lesion. It may be derived from the apical part of the dental follicle. Cementomas occur primarily in the lower anterior region. There is a higher incidence in females, middle age, and blacks. The lesion is symptomless and may occur singly or multiply. The involved teeth are vital. The radiographic appearance depends upon the stage. In the early stages, there are periapical radiolucencies found that appear radiographically identical to pulpally-in-

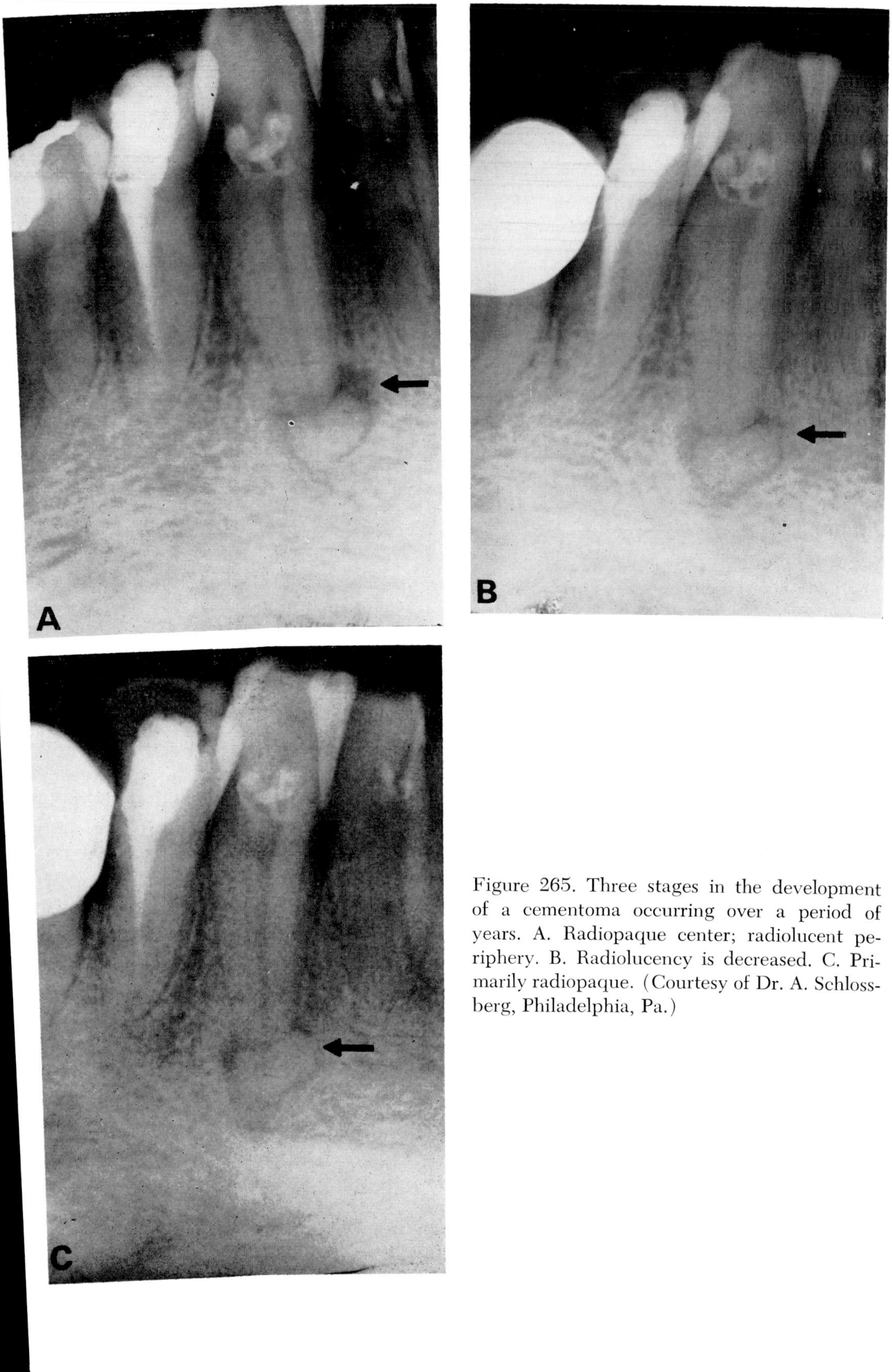

Figure 265. Three stages in the development of a cementoma occurring over a period of years. A. Radiopaque center; radiolucent periphery. B. Radiolucency is decreased. C. Primarily radiopaque. (Courtesy of Dr. A. Schlossberg, Philadelphia, Pa.)

duced periapical rarefactions. In the next stage, there are radiolucencies with specks of radiopacity, and the roots may show hypercementosis. In the final stage, which may occur years later, the appearance is of circumscribed radiopacity (Figs. 74, 265). In the latter stage, the apical periodontal ligament space can usually be seen. The microscopic picture varies with the stage. In the initial stage, young fibroblasts, collagen, and blood vessels are found. In the second stage, in addition to the above description, cementoblasts, osteoblasts, and cementicles can be found. In the final stage, calcified masses are the predominant find, either of osteoid, bone, cementum, or some combination (Fig. 266). There are also some marrow spaces, with a few cells present. No treatment should be performed for these cases.

Cementifying Fibroma. This is a rare mesodermal odontogenic tumor that is unrelated to tooth apexes. It usually occurs singly in the lower premolar-molar region and the patients are often past middle age. There may be swelling of the involved jaw region. The radiographic appearance shows a well limited radiolucency with radiopaque specks. The microscopic view shows a fibrous stroma containing cementicles and/or acellular cementum.

Benign (True) Cementoblastoma. This is a very rare mesodermal odontogenic tumor that is attached to the root apex. The usual site is the lower premolar-molar area. It often occurs in individuals younger than age 25. The involved area may show swelling. Radiographically, there is a radiopaque center with a radiolucent periphery in the periapical region. The microscopic picture shows an encapsulated lesion containing fused cementum-like bodies.

Odontogenic Fibroma. This is also a very rare mesenchymal odontogenic tumor. Some authorities believe it is more common than has been reported, as it can be confused radiographically with a dentigerous cyst. It usually occurs in the mandible in young adults and is generally symptomless. The radiograph-

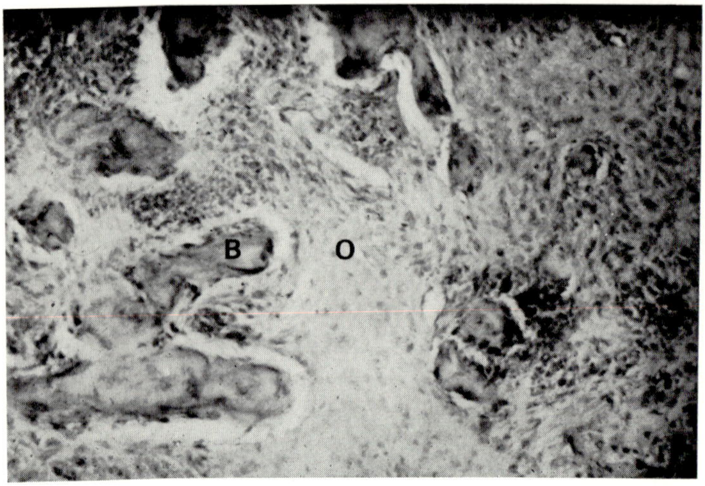

Figure 266. Cementoma; third stage; histologic section; B = bone or cementum, O = osteoid (×100). (Courtesy of Dr. D. Litwack, Philadelphia, Pa.)

ic appearance shows a distinct radiolucent lesion. Histologically, the odontogenic fibroma is characterized by fibrous connective tissue stroma containing strands and islands of nonameloblastic epithelium.

Odontogenic Myxoma. This is another rare mesenchymal odontogenic tumor. It is typically found in the maxilla in patients less than 35 years old. There may be swelling of the involved jaw area with displacement of teeth. The radiographic image shows a definite radiolucency with some radiopaque septa. The histologic picture shows myxomatous tissue with isolated strands of odontogenic epithelium.

Ameloblastic Fibrosarcoma. This is an extremely rare malignant odontogenic tumor, which may arise from an ameloblastic fibroma. The tumor is generally found in the mandible in young-middle aged patients. Pain usually precedes the swelling, which is different than with most odontogenic tumors. The swelling develops rapidly. Radiographically, the lesion shows an irregular, diffuse radiolucency. The microscopic appearance shows ameloblastic epithelium in a stroma of fibrous connective tissue that contains bizarre, spindle shaped, and polyhedral cells with atypical mitoses.

Nonodontogenic Tumors

These tumors can occur in many bones including the jaws. They may be benign or malignant and do not arise from any dental structures.

Benign Tumors. These tumors include myxoma, chondroma, central hemangioma, fibroma, neurogenic tumors, and osteoid osteoma.

Myxoma (Myxofibroma). Some authorities do not differentiate this lesion from the odontogenic myxoma. The true myxoma (if it is different than the odontogenic myxoma) usually occurs in the jaws, although it can occur in other bones. It can occur in either jaw and the age incidence is not specific. The myxoma is a slow growing tumor that may expand the involved jaw, but rarely produces pain. Paresthesia of the lip has been reported in certain cases. The radiographs show either unilocular or multilocular radiolucencies. The roots may be displaced and show root resorption. Microscopically, the tumor is not encapsulated and contains myxomatous tissue and stellate shaped cells with a mucoid stroma.

Chondroma. This cartilagenous tumor is very rarely found in the jaws. It may occur in either jaw, and cause swelling of the involved area. Tooth resorption and displacement of teeth can occur. The roentgenographic picture shows a radiolucent area that may have radiopaque flecks present. The histopathologic view shows typical hyaline cartilage with chondrocytes and often some areas of calcified cartilage. This tumor may become malignant.

Central Hemangioma. This has been mentioned under soft tissue hemangiomas. It occurs primarily in the mandible, in young female adults. The involved jaw area usually shows swelling and pain may occur. The roentgenographic features show multilocular rarefactions giving a *soap bubble* appear-

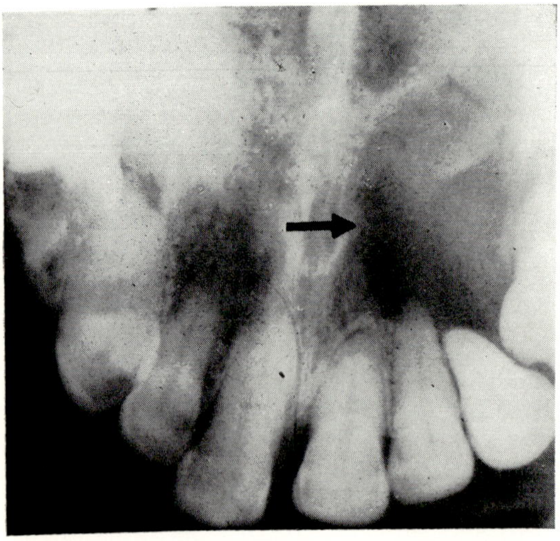

Figure 267. A fibroma of the maxilla; an extremely rare lesion. (Courtesy of Dr. D. Litwack, Philadelphia, Pa.)

ance and root resorption may occur. This histologic picture typically shows a combination of the capillary and cavernous type hemangiomas.

Fibroma. These fibrous tumors are extremely rare in the jaws. They occur primarily in the mandible and show well defined radiolucent rarefactions (Fig. 267). Histologically, the picture is of fibrous connective tissue.

Neurogenic Tumors. The soft tissue neurofibromas and schwannomas rarely can be encased in bone and produce a radiolucent x-ray image (Fig. 268).

Lipomas. These lesions are as described under soft tissue lipomas. Rarely, they occur in the jaws where they

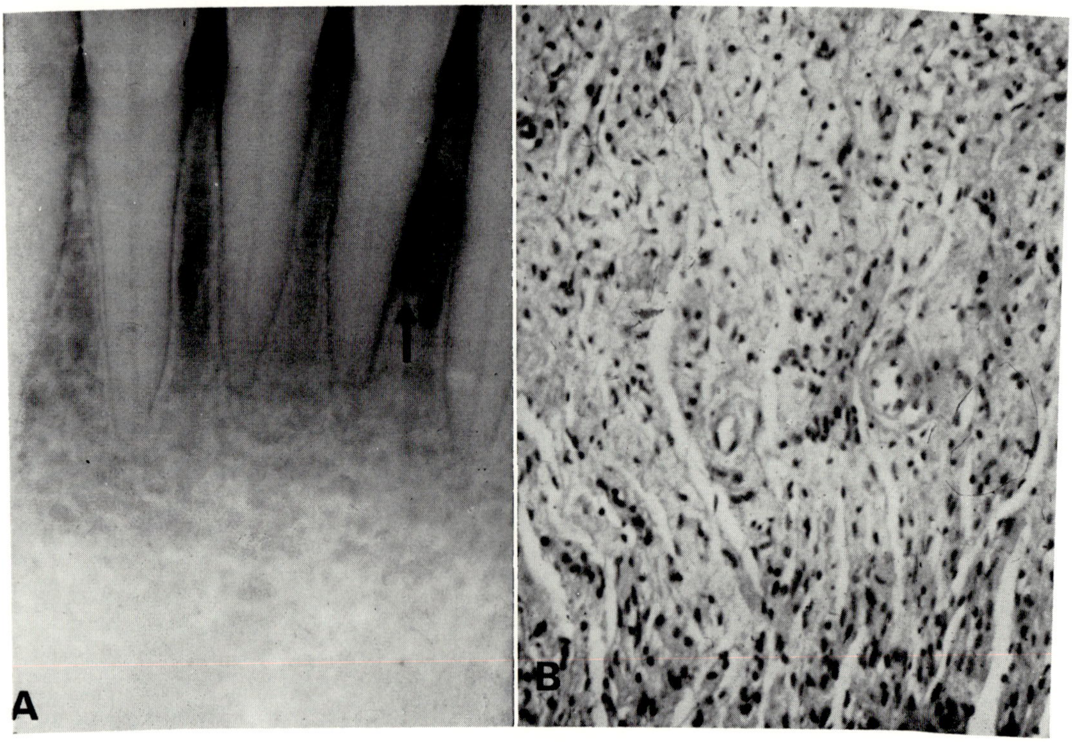

Figure 268. Neurofibroma of the mandible; another very rare lesion. A. Radiographic view. (Courtesy of Dr. T. Simpson, Philadelphia, Pa.) B. Histologic section of a neurofibroma (×240). (Courtesy of Dr. D. Litwack, Philadelphia, Pa.)

produce a radiolucent roentgenographic image.

Osteoid Osteoma. This tumor occurs in long bones and rarely in the jaws. It is composed of osteoid and bone deposited within a substrate of vascular osteogenic connective tissue. The osteoid osteoma occurs in people 20 years of age or less and usually at the lower border of the mandible. Patients often have severe localized pain and swelling. The radiographic picture shows a round radiolucent area covered by an area of dense radiopacity. The inner radiolucent nidus may have some radiopaque flecks within it. Histologically, the radiolucent area contains osteoid and vascular fibrous connective tissue. Areas of radiopacity are dense bone. Another similar lesion is the giant osteoid osteoma (benign osteoblastoma). It grows faster, and is less painful than the osteoid osteoma. It also lacks the surrounding area of dense radiopaque bone, found in the osteoid osteoma.

MALIGNANT TUMORS. These tumors include sarcomas, multiple myeloma, Burkitt's tumor, carcinomas, leukemias, and metastatic tumors.

Osteogenic Sarcoma. This is a malignant tumor of bone that rarely occurs in the jaws. When present, it is more prevalent in the mandible, with the usual age bracket being 10 to 33. It is manifested as a rapidly swelling mass that causes expansion of the involved jaw area. Pain is common, and paresthesia has been reported in about 25 per cent of the mandibular cases. Displacement of teeth, root resorption, mobility, and spontaneous fractures may also occur. The radiographic appearance varies from radiolucency, through a combination of irregular radiolucency and radiopacity, to the typical *sunburst* or *sun ray* effect (results from radiating bone trabecullae). A symmetrical widening of the periodontal ligament space of teeth in the involved area may occur. The histological appearance shows pleomorphic osteoclasts and fibroblasts with hyperchromatic nuclei and numerous mitoses, alternating with atypical bony trabeculae.

Chondrosarcoma. This is another malignant bony tumor that is infrequently found in the jaws. It is slightly more prevalent in the maxilla than in the mandible, and occurs primarily in middle age. The chondrosarcoma also occurs as a rapidly swelling mass that expands the cortex of the involved jaw. It may cause pain, paresthesia, resorption, migration, and mobility of the teeth in the area. The roentgenogram usually shows a radiolucency with flecks of radiopacity interspersed. The microscopic picture shows numerous atypical chondrocytes, in various sizes and stages of differentiation, containing irregular nuclei. Multinucleated cells and bone are usually present.

Fibrosarcoma. This malignant tumor occurs more often in the soft tissues and the histologic features have been described under the section of soft tissue lesions. When it is found in the jaws, it occurs predominantly in the mandible, during middle age. The fibrosarcoma forms a discernible mass. Paresthesia in the involved area can occur. The radiographic picture may show radiolucency and root resorption of teeth in the vicinity of the tumor.

Multiple Myeloma. This is a malignant tumor of bone marrow, specifically of the plasma cells. It occurs in many bones including the jaws, the skull, the vertebrae, pelvis and femur. The mandible is affected more often than the maxilla. The patients generally are in the 40 to 70 year age bracket. Clinical features are bone pain, pathologic fractures, nausea, vomiting, anemia, weakness, weight loss, lethargy, and easy fatiguability. Clinical tests may show multiple punched out radiolucent areas in x-rays of various bones, abnormal plasma cells in bone marrow, elevated gamma globulin level in the blood, Bence-Jones protein in the urine, and a hypercalcemia. Oral features are gingival bleeding, pain, jaw swelling, paresthesia, and tooth mobility. Oral radiographs show many punched out areas of radiolucency and the teeth in the area may show root resorption and loss of the lamina dura. Histologic sections reveal sheets of normal and abnormal plasma cells with frequent mitoses.

Reticulum Cell Sarcoma. This is a malignant tumor which occurs in soft tissue or bone. The histologic aspects have been discussed under the soft tissue lesions. When it occurs in the jaws, the mandible is the usual site. Men are involved more frequently than women, and the age is usually below forty. The tumor can cause tooth mobility, odontalgia, paresthesia, and swelling of the involved region. The radiographic area shows a diffuse radiolucency.

Ewing's Sarcoma (Tumor). This is a malignant tumor of bone marrow (as is multiple myeloma) causing a proliferation of small round cells. It occurs in many bones, and the jaws are volved in approximately 10 per cen thc cases. The mandible is the prefe site and the patients are usually u the age of thirty. The jaws are ra the site of the primary tumor. Clin manifestations include rapidly deve ing swelling of the affected site, p and paresthesia. The radiographic ture usually shows radiolucencies v some areas of radiopacity. The mic scopic appearance reveals sheets or co of closely packed small round cells tertwined with a fibrous, vascular c nective tissue stroma.

Burkitt's Tumor. This is a malign lymphoma that is prevalent in Afric children, although it can occur el where. These are deposits in many gans including the adrenals, thyro kidneys, ovaries, liver, pancreas, vario lymphoid tissues, salivary glands, a the jaws. Clinical manifestations i clude gross swelling of the face ove lying one or more jaw quadrants, faci pain, mobility, and exfoliation of pr mary teeth. Tumor growth is rapid. Ra diographically, a widespread radiolu cency is evident. The microscopic pic ture reveals sheets of lymphoid ster cells with round nuclei, interspersed with clusters of histiocytes.

Squamous Cell Carcinoma, Adenocystic Carcinoma, Liposarcoma, and Leukemias. These malignancies of soft tissue and blood have previously been described. In rare occasions, they can invade bone and cause the visualization of radiolucencies on periapical radiographs (Fig. 227B). In extremely rare cases, dental cysts (usually dentigerous or follicular) can undergo malignant degeneration into squamous cell carcinomas.

Metastatic Tumors. Primary malignancies rarely metastasize to the jaws (principally mandible). The clinical features vary but may show expansion of the involved area, pain, paresthesia, tooth mobility or trismus. The sites of primary tumors in the approximate order of decreasing frequency are breast, large intestine, prostate, kidney, thyroid, testes, ovaries, and liver. The roentgenographic features generally show radiolucencies and root resorptions (Fig. 269). Lesions from breast and prostate can give a radiopaque appearance.

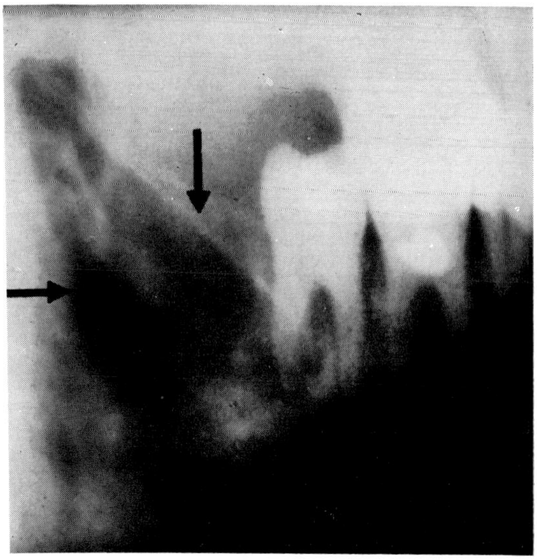

Figure 269. A metastatic carcinoma of the mandible. (Courtesy of Dr. D. Litwack, Philadelphia, Pa.)

Primarily Radiopaque Lesions

The only radiopaque lesions related to endodontic disease are condensing osteitis and Garre's osteomyelitis. Both of these conditions are rarely found, especially the osteomyelitis. Other radiopaque lesions of the jaws are also found less frequently than are the radiolucent jaw lesions. In the former conditions, the radiopacity is not usually limited to the periapical region, but is more widespread and may be bilateral. Therefore, the differential diagnosis between radiopaque endodontic and non-endodontic lesions is usually not that difficult. However pulp testing is not helpful, as a vital response is possible in both the endodontically-induced lesion and in the non-endodontic cases.

Diseases with Radiopaque Jaw Manifestations

These diseases include osteopetrosis, leontiasis ossea, myositis ossificans, and miscellaneous diseases.

OSTEOPETROSIS (ALBERS-SCHÖNBERG DISEASE). This is a genetic disease in which there is increased osseous density leading to *marble bones.* Bone formation is normal, but there is an absence of bone resorption. Clinical signs include anemia, hepatosplenomegaly, deafness, blindness, paralysis, expanding bones, and osteomyelitis. Oral features are nonerupting teeth, incomplete root formation, malformed and hypocalcified teeth, and spontaneous jaw features. Osteomyelitis can readily occur after periapical involvement; apparently because of the deficient blood supply in the jaws (the red marrow is crowded out by the proliferating bone). Usual radiographic findings are dense, widespread radiopacities, unerupted teeth, short-rooted teeth, and an increased width of the periodontal ligament space (Fig. 270). Histologically, there is a

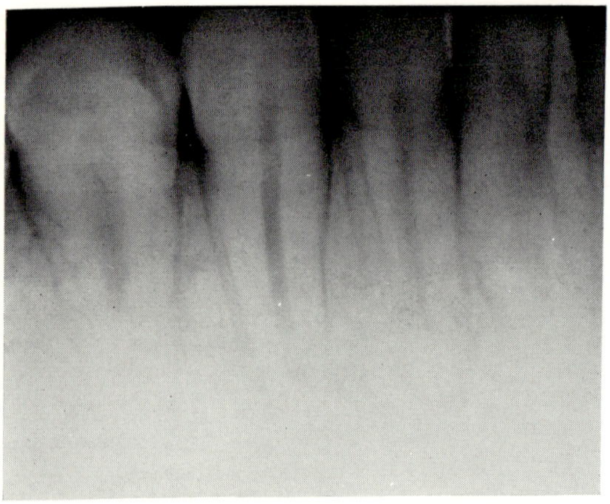

Figure 270. Osteopetrosis (Albers-Schönberg disease); radiograph reveals extreme radiopacity of the mandible. (Courtesy of Dr. T. Simpson, Philadelphia, Pa.)

great increase of trabeculae, and a replacement of the red marrow by fibrous connective tissue.

Leontiasis Ossea. This may or may not be a distinct disease. It has been considered a form of osteopetrosis, fibrous dysplasia, or Paget's disease. Leontiasis ossea is manifested by a hyperostosis that primarily affects the bones of the upper face. Clinical features are large head, open mouth, flat nasal bridge, deafness, blindness, mental retardation, and facial nerve paralysis. As with the other conditions, the roentgenogram reveals dense radiopacities. Blood levels of calcium, phosphorous and alkaline phosphatase are normal.

Myositis Ossificans. When this serious muscle disease occurs in the temporalis muscle, it can produce fan-shaped calcifications which may appear as irregular radiopacities on posterior radiographs.

Miscellaneous Diseases Causing Osteosclerosis. These are generally genetic diseases that cause widespread dense sclerotic changes in bone. The radiographic appearance shows radiopacities. The diseases are sclerosteosis, generalized cortical hyperostosis, pyknodysostosis, Engleman's disease, and hyperostosis corticalis deformans juvenitis (juvenile Paget's disease). Caffey's disease (infantile cortical hyperostosis) occurs primarily in infants.

Miscellaneous Conditions with Radiopaque Jaw Appearance

The following conditions may be found in the region of the root apex. They include foreign bodies, root fragments, sialoliths, calcified thrombi and

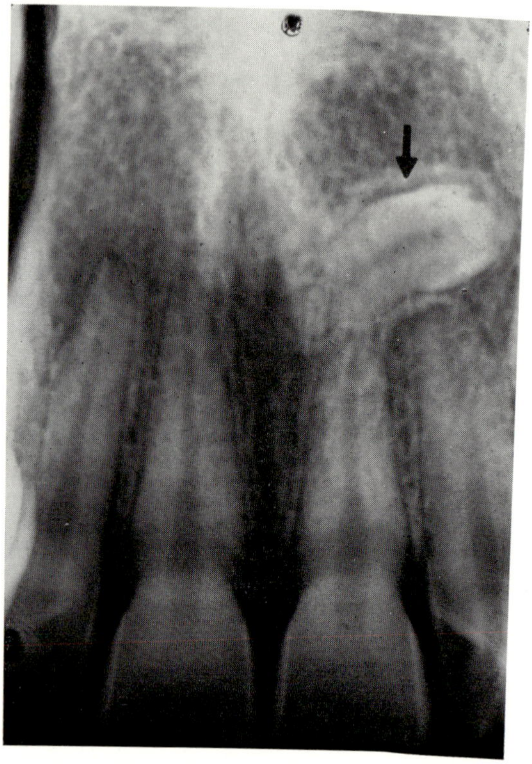

Figure 271. A supernumerary tooth at the apex of an upper central incisor. (Courtesy of Dr. T. Simpson, Philadelphia, Pa.)

nodes, and calculus and osteosclerosis.

FOREIGN BODIES, BULLETS, AMALGAM, ETC. These can be readily differentiated by the extreme radiopacity and the history (Fig. 103).

ROOT FRAGMENTS OR A SUPERNUMERARY TOOTH. These usually can be differentiated by the radiographic evidence of a lamina dura, periodontal ligament space, pulp canal, and by the history of the case (Figs. 91, 271).

SIALOLITHS. Salivary stones can appear in periapical radiographs. X-ray sialography, and probing of salivary gland ducts, helps in the differential diagnosis.

CALCIFICATIONS OF LYMPH NODES OR PHLEBOLITHS (CALCIFIED THROMBI). These can show up as irregularly sized radiopacities, which may appear on periapical radiographs. Lateral jaw radiographs help in the true determination of these conditions.

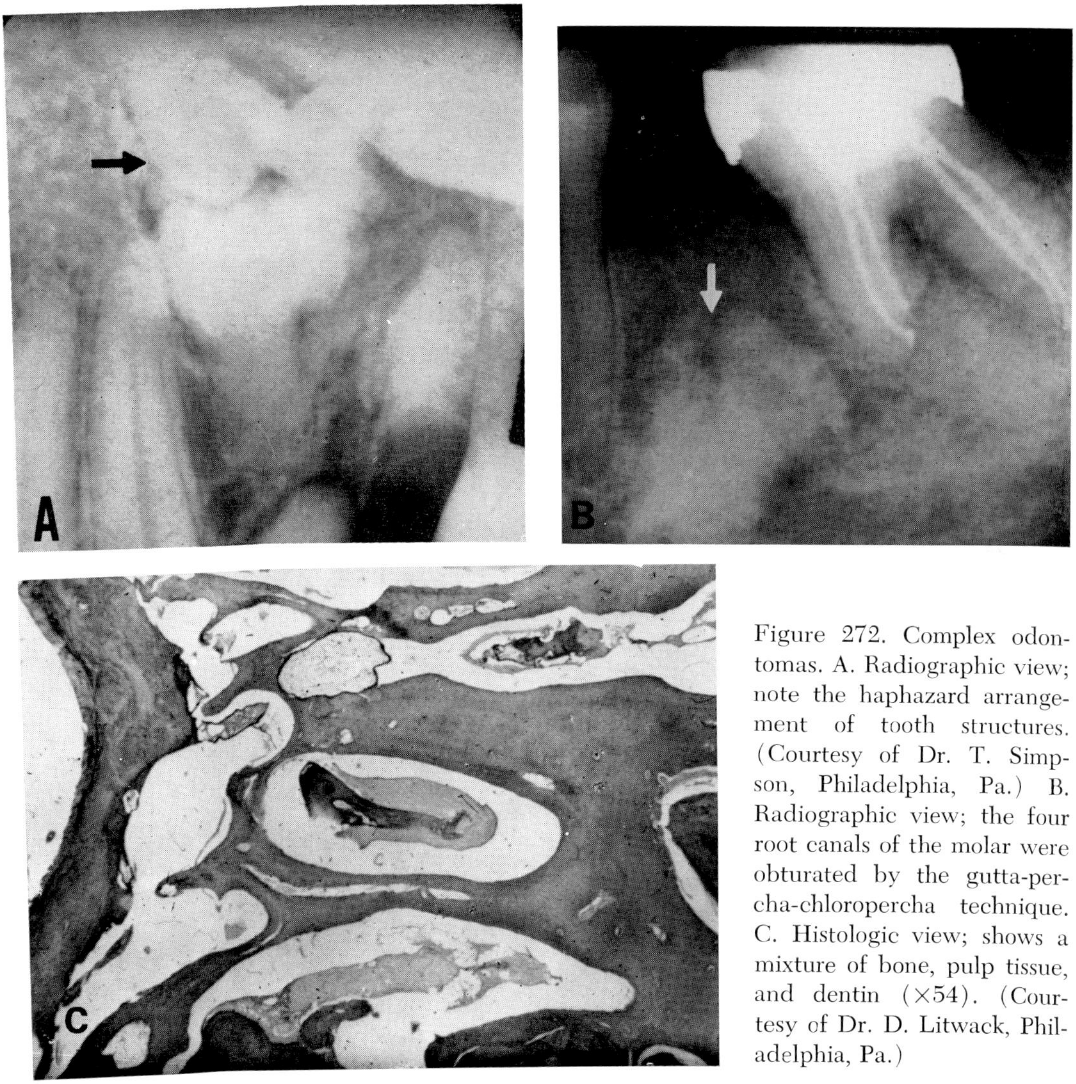

Figure 272. Complex odontomas. A. Radiographic view; note the haphazard arrangement of tooth structures. (Courtesy of Dr. T. Simpson, Philadelphia, Pa.) B. Radiographic view; the four root canals of the molar were obturated by the gutta-percha-chloropercha technique. C. Histologic view; shows a mixture of bone, pulp tissue, and dentin (×54). (Courtesy of Dr. D. Litwack, Philadelphia, Pa.)

CALCULUS. When there is a large amount of vertical bone loss, subgingival calculus can appear in the apical region. Pocket probing will detect the calculus.

OSTEOSCLEROSIS. Aside from systemic diseases already mentioned, osteosclerotic jaw changes can result from trauma, prolonged administration of estrogens, phosphorus exposure, and from an excessively strong biting pressure.

Odontogenic Tumors

These are slow growing, benign, usually symptomless, lesions. They include odontomas and dentinomas.

COMPLEX ODONTOMA. This is an odontogenic tumor composed of a haphazard arrangement of tooth structures. It is more common in the mandibular second and third molar areas. Usually, there are no symptoms. The radiographic appearance generally shows irregular radiopacities that are bounded by a thin radiolucent line (Fig. 272A, B). The histology reveals a mass of intertwined enamel, enamel matrix, dentin, cementum, pulp, and predentin (Fig. 272C).

COMPOUND ODONTOMA. This is another odontogenic tumor composed of tooth structures. However, in this case, there is a normal arrangement of tooth components. It is more common in the upper anterior region and is usually symptomless. The roentgenogram usual-

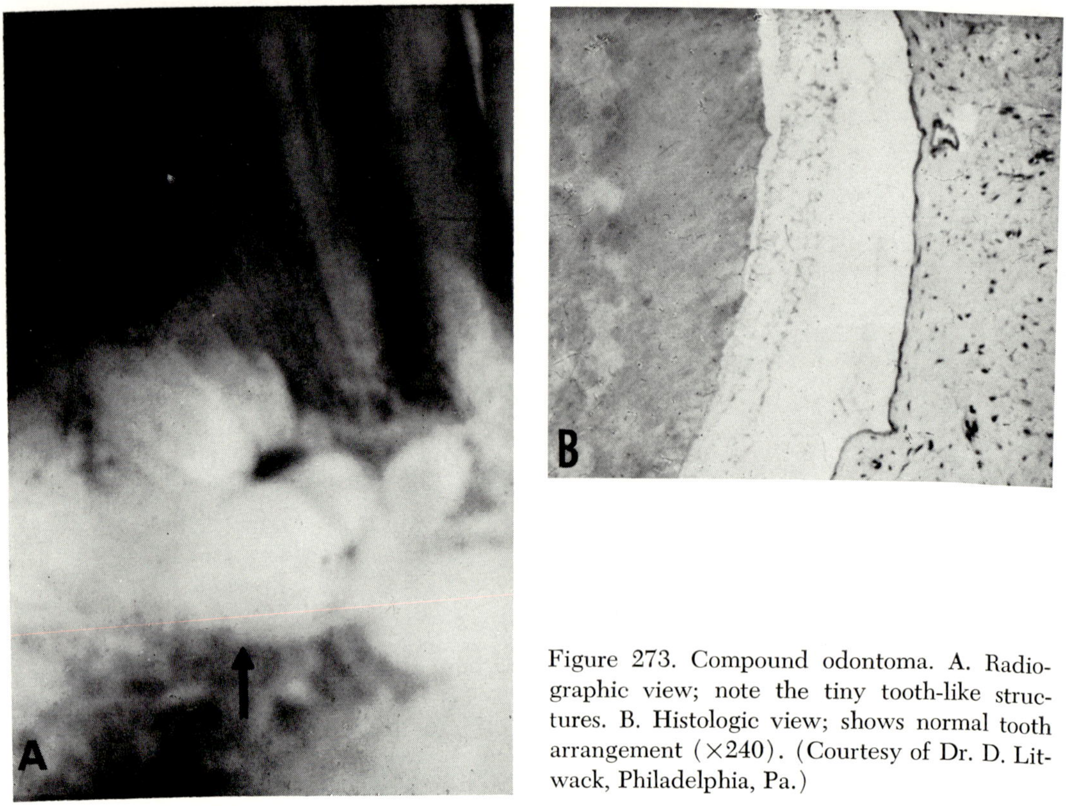

Figure 273. Compound odontoma. A. Radiographic view; note the tiny tooth-like structures. B. Histologic view; shows normal tooth arrangement (×240). (Courtesy of Dr. D. Litwack, Philadelphia, Pa.)

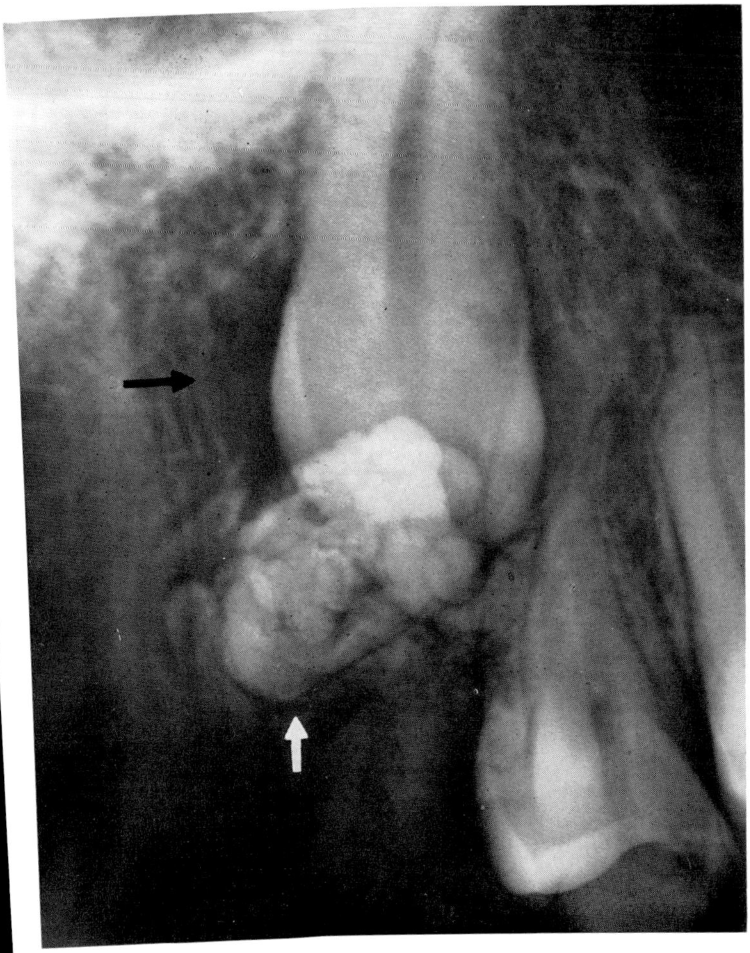

Figure 274. A cystic odontoma; black arrow indicates the cyst; white arrow points to the odontoma. (Courtesy of Dr. W. Updegrave, Philadelphia, Pa.)

ly reveals a mass of tiny tooth-like structures surrounded by a fine radiolucent line (Fig. 273A). Microscopically, the units have a normal tooth arrangement (Fig. 273B).

Cystic Odontoma. In rare cases, a cyst is associated with one of the previously described odontomas. The radiograph reveals a round, radiolucent area, in addition to the radiopacities (Fig. 274). Histologically, a lesion similar to a dentigerous cyst is found along with the tooth-like structures.

Dentinoma. This is a mesodermal odontogenic tumor composed primarily of dentin or osteodentin. It occurs predominantly in the lower molar area. The radiographic image shows a radiopaque structure. Histologically, the tumor is composed of osteodentin or dentin with few or irregular tubules enmeshed in a fibrous connective tissue stroma.

Non-odontogenic Tumors

These are benign, slow growing, and usually symptomless lesions. They include osteoma and Gardner's syndrome.

Osteoma. This is a tumor consisting of mature bone. It may be periosteal or endosteal. The bone may be either compact or cancellous. Osteomas may occur in the jaws (usually mandible) and can cause swelling and pain of the involved area. The roentgenogram reveals a dense, radiopaque area (Fig. 78). Histologically, the lesion is composed of normal bone.

Gardner's Syndrome. This is a genetically-induced syndrome in which there are epidermoid inclusion cysts of the skin, multiple polyps of the large intestine, and multiple osteomas of the cranial and facial skeleton, including the jaws. Compound odontomas can occur, along with hypercementosis of roots.

Cysts

Oral cysts are radiolucent but a mucous cyst of the antrum can be superimposed over the apexes of upper posterior teeth. The radiographic appearance shows a somewhat radiopaque hemispherical shaped or dome-shaped structure, with the sinus wall at the base.

BIBLIOGRAPHY

General

Bhaskar, S. N.: *Synopsis of Oral Pathology,* 2nd ed. St. Louis, Mosby, 1965.

Burket, L. W.: *Oral Medicine: Diagnosis and Treatment,* 6th ed. Philadelphia, Lippincott, 1971.

Gorlin, R. J., and Goldman, H. M.: *Thoma's Oral Pathology,* 6th ed. St. Louis, Mosby, 1970.

Seltzer, S.: *Endodontology: Biologic Considerations in Endodontic Procedures.* New York, McGraw, 1971.

Shafer, W. G., Hine, M. K., and Levy, B. M.: *A Textbook of Oral Pathology,* 2nd ed. Philadelphia, Saunders, 1963.

Dentinal, Pulpal, and Periapical Conditions

Bender, I. B.: A commentary on General Bhaskar's hypothesis. *Oral Surg, 34:*469, 1972.

Bhaskar, S. N.: Nonsurgical resolution of radicular cysts. *Oral Surg, 34:*458, 1972.

Cameron, C. E.: Cracked-tooth syndrome. *JADA, 68:*405, 1964.

Grossman, L. I.: *Endodontic Practice,* 7th ed. Philadelphia, Lea & Febiger, 1970.

Holcomb, J. B., and Gregory, W. B.: Calcific metamorphosis of the pulp: its incidence and treatment. *Oral Surg, 24:*825, 1967.

Ingle, J. I.: *Endodontics.* Philadelphia, Lea & Febiger, 1965.

Johnson, R. H., Dachi, S. F., and Haley, J. V.: Pulpal hyperemia—A correlation of clinical and histologic data from 706 teeth. *JADA, 81:*108, 1970.

Jorkjend, L., and Tronstad, L.: Treatment of hypersensitive root surfaces by calcium hydroxide. *Scand J Dent Res, 80:*264, 1972.

Jurist, B.: The cracked tooth. Presented at the Annual Meeting of the American Association of Endodontists, April, 1973, Dallas, Texas.

Mann, A. W.: Nutrition as it affects the teeth. *Med Clin North Am, 27:*545, 1943.

Morse, D. R., Patnik, J. W., and Schacterle, G. R.: Electrophoretic differentiation of radicular cysts and granulomas. *Oral Surg, 35:*249, 1973.

Oehlers, F. A. C.: Periapical lesions and residual dental cysts. *Br J Oral Surg, 8:*103, 1970.

Priebe, W. A., Lazansky, J. P., and Wuehrmann, A. H.: The value of the roentgenographic film in the differential diagnosis of periapical lesions. *Oral Surg, 7:*979, 1954.

Seltzer, S.: *Endodontology: Biologic Considerations in Endodontic Procedures.* New York, McGraw, 1971.

Seltzer, S.: Hypothetic mechanisms for dentine sensitivity. *Oral Surg, 31:*388, 1971.

Seltzer, S., and Bender, I. B.: *The Dental Pulp: Biologic Considerations in Dental Procedures.* Philadelphia, Lippincott, 1965.

Simon, P.: Periapical pulpo-osteosclerosis. *Dent Radiogr Photogr, 39:*75, 1966.

Endodontic-Periodontic Considerations

Bender, I. B., and Seltzer, S.: The effect of periodontal disease on the pulp. *Oral Surg, 33:*458, 1972.

Blair, H. A.: Relationships between endodontics and periodontics. *J Periodontol, 43:*209, 1972.

Hiatt, W. H.: Discussion of Periodontically and Endodontically Involved Teeth. In Grossman, L. I.: Trans. Third Inter. Conf. Endo., Philadelphia, Univ. Penn., 1963.

Mazur, B., and Massler, M.: Influence of periodontal disease on the dental pulp. *Oral Surg, 17:*592, 1964.

Ross, I. F.: The relation between periodontal and pulpal disorders. *JADA, 84:*134, 1972.

Simon, J. H. S., Glick, D. H., and Frank, A. L.: The relationship of endodontic-periodontic lesions. *J Periodontol, 43:*202, 1972.

Simring, M., and Goldberg, M.: The pulpal pocket approach: retrograde periodontitis. *J Periodontol, 35:*22, 1964.

Stallard, R. E.: Periodontic-endodontic relationships. *Oral Surg, 34:*314, 1972.

Oral Pathways of Infection

Banerjee, S. C.: Temporal osteitis and infratemporal space infection following dental extraction. *Oral Surg, 21:*15, 1966.

Birn, H.: Spread of dental infections. *Dent Pract, 22:*347, 1972.

Cogan, M. I. C.: Necrotizing mediastinitis secondary to descending cervical cellulitis. *Oral Surg, 36:*307, 1973.

El-Sheikh, M. M., and El-Hak, R. Y.: Infections of the infratemporal space. *Br J Oral Surg, 9:*189, 1972.

Hollin, S. A., and Gross, S. W.: Intracranial abscesses of odontogenic origin. *Oral Surg, 23:*277, 1967.

Kaye, D.: Bacteremia and disease. Presented at the Meeting of the Eastern Pennsylvania Chapter of the American Society for Microbiology, Oct. 1973, Philadelphia, Pennsylvania.

Laskin, D. M.: Anatomic considerations in diagnosis and treatment of odontogenic infections. *JADA, 69:*308, 1964.

Levitt, G. W.: Cervical fascia and deep neck infections. *Laryngoscope, 80:*409, 1970.

Marlette, R. H., Gerhard, R. C., and Conley, J.: Brain abscess of dental origin: report of case. *J Oral Surg, 28:*134, 1970.

Morse, D. R.: Oral pathways of infection: with special reference to endodontics. *J Br Endo Soc, 6:*13, 1972.

Shafer, W. G., Hine, M. K., and Levy, B. M.: *A Textbook of Oral Pathology,* 2nd ed. Philadelphia, Saunders, 1963.

Smith, R. W., Taylor, R. G., and O'Connor, J. F.: Dental infection: a source of pulmonary emboli. *Oral Surg, 24:*158, 1967.

Spilka, C. J.: Pathways of dental infections. *J Oral Surg, 24:*111, 1966.

Stones, H. H.: *Oral and Dental Diseases: Aetiology, Histopathology, Clinical Features and Treatment,* 4th ed. Baltimore, Williams and Wilkins, 1962.

Osteomyelitis

Degnan, E. J.: Current oral surgical opinion concerning the value of preirradiation exodontia. *Oral Surg, 18:*307, 1964.

Killey, H. C., Kay, L. W., and Wright, H. C.: Subperiosteal osteomyelitis of the mandible: a clinical survey and experimental study. *Oral Surg, 29:*576, 1970.

Kinman, J. E. G., and Lee, H. S.: Chronic osteomyelitis of the mandible: clinical study of thirteen cases. *Oral Surg, 25:*6, 1968.

Leake, D. L.: Bacteroides osteomyelitis of the mandible: a report of two cases. *Oral Surg, 34:*585, 1972.

Mopsik, E. R.: Infections and antibiotics. *Dent Clin North Am, 15:*327, 1971.

Narang, R., and Wells, H.: The avoidance of osteoradionecrosis of the mandible after extraction of a number of teeth in a patient given radio-therapy for oral carcinoma. *Oral Surg, 29:*656, 1970.

Panders, A. K., and Hadders, H. N.: Chronic sclerosing inflammations of the jaw. *Oral Surg, 30:*396, 1970.

Roane, J. B., and Marshall, F. J.: Osteomyelitis: a complication of pulpless teeth; report of a case. *Oral Surg, 34:*257, 1972.

Genetic Conditions

Baer, P., Brown, N. C., and Hamner, J. E.: Hypophosphatasia: report of two cases with dental findings. *Periodontics, 2:*209, 1964.

Bencze, J., and Walawska, J.: Dominant inheritance of hemifacial hyperplasia associated with strabismus. *Oral Surg, 35:*489, 1973.

Beumer, J., Trowbridge, H. O., Silverman, S., and Eisenberg, E.: Childhood hypophosphatasia and the premature loss of teeth: a clinical and laboratory study of seven cases. *Oral Surg, 35:*631, 1973.

Chabora, A. J., Berkman, M. D., Horowitz, S. L., and Nahoum, H. I.: Hereditary hypocalcified amelogenesis imperfecta. *Oral Surg, 33:*922, 1972.

Gardner, D. G.: The oral manifestations of Hurler's Syndrome. *Oral Surg, 32:*46, 1971.

Gardner, D. G., and Majka, M.: The early formation of irregular secondary dentine in progeria. *Oral Surg, 28:*877, 1969.

Gardner, D. G., and Sapp, J. P.: Regional odontodysplasia. *Oral Surg, 35:*351, 1973.

Gigliotti, R., Harrison, H., Reveley, R. A., and Drabkowski, A. J.: Familial vitamin-D-resistant rickets. *JADA, 82:*383, 1971.

Goldstein, E., and Gottlieb, M. A.: Taurodontism: familial tendencies demonstrated in eleven of fourteen case reports. *Oral Surg, 36:*131, 1973.

Halstead, C. L.: Oral manifestations of hemoglobinopathies: a case of homozygous hemoglobin C disease diagnosed as a result of dental radiographic changes. *Oral Surg, 30:*615, 1970.

Hayashi, S., Tomioka, T., Aoki, H., Nakakuki, K., and Mekaru, K.: Hemifacial hypertrophy: report of two cases. *Oral Surg, 35:*750, 1973.

Hintz, C. S., and Peters, R. A.: Odontodysplasia: report of an unusual case and a review of the literature. *Oral Surg, 34:*744, 1972.

Kennett, S., and Pollick, H.: Jaw lesions in familial hyperparathyroidism. *Oral Surg, 31:*502, 1971.

Michanowicz, A. E., Michanowicz, J. P., and Stein, G. M.: Gaucher's disease: report of a case. *Oral Surg, 23:*36, 1967.

Michelson, R. K., and Whitmore, R. B.: Sickle-cell anemia in the dental patient: report of two cases. *Oral Surg, 23:*19, 1967.

Neal, C. J.: Multiple osteomas of the mandible associated with polyposis of the colon (Gardner's Syndrome). *Oral Surg, 28:*628, 1969.

Petersson, A.: A case of dentinal dysplasia and/or calcification of the dentinal papilla. *Oral Surg, 33:*1014, 1972.

Poyton, H. G., and Davey, K. W.: Thalassemia: changes visible in radiographs used in dentistry. *Oral Surg, 25:*564, 1968.

Rao, S. R., Witkop, C. J., and Yamane, G. M.: Pulpal dysplasia. *Oral Surg, 30:*682, 1970.

Short, E. M., Binder, H. J., and Rosenberg, L. E.: Familial hypophosphatemic rickets: defective transport of inorganic phosphate by intestinal mucosa. *Science, 179:*700, 1973.

Simon, J. H. S., Glick, D. H., and Frank, A. L.: Predictable endodontic and periodontic failures as a result of radicular anomalies. *Oral Surg, 31:*823, 1971.

Ulmansky, M., and Hermel, J.: Double dens in dente in a single tooth: report of a case and radiologic study of the incidence of small dens in dente. *Oral Surg, 17:*92, 1964.

Via, W. F.: "Spontaneous" degeneration of the dental pulp associated with phosphate diabetes. *Oral Surg, 24:*623, 1967.

Witkop, C. J.: Manifestations of genetic diseases in the human pulp. *Oral Surg, 32:*278, 1971.

Various Lesions and Conditions

Adkins, K. F., Martinez, M. G., and Robinson, L. H.: Cellular morphology and relationships in giant-cell lesions of the jaws. *Oral Surg, 28:*216, 1969.

Albers, D. D.: Median mandibular cyst partially lined with pseudostratified columnar epithelium: report of a case. *Oral Surg, 36:* 11, 1973.

Andsberg, W., and Axéll, T.: Mediastinal emphysema as a complication of dental treatment. *Odontol Revy, 23:*21, 1972.

Barnes, P.: Submandibular sinus of dental origin treated as glandular tuberculosis. *J Dent Aux* (Malaysa), *9:*17, 1971.

Baughman, R. A.: Lingual thyroid and lingual thyroglossal tract remnants: a clinical and histopathologic study with review of the literature. *Oral Surg, 34:*781, 1972.

Beatty, R. E.: Case report: median mandibular cyst. *Dent Surv, 48:*27, 1972.

Bianco, R. P., Smith, P. J., Keen, R. R., and Jordan, J. E.: Iodine intoxication: report of a case. *Oral Surg, 32:*876, 1971.

Blevins, C., Dahlin, D. C., Lovestedt, S. A., and Kennedy, R. L. J.: Oral and dental manifestations of histiocytosis X. *Oral Surg, 12:*473, 1959.

Bottomley, W. K., Giorgini, G. L., and Julienne, C. H.: Oral extension of regional enteritis (Crohn's Disease): report of a case. *Oral Surg, 34:*417, 1972.

Christ, T. F., Cavalaris, C. J., and Crocker, D. J.: Papilliferous ameloblastic fibroma. *Oral Surg, 34:*806, 1972.

Curry, J. T., and Zallen, R. D.: Ossifying fibroma of the maxilla occurring with hyperthyroidism. *Oral Surg, 35:*28, 1973.

Dick, H. M., and Simpson, W. J.: Dental changes in osteopetrosis. *Oral Surg, 34:* 408, 1972.

Dutescu, N., Georgescu, L., and Hary, M.: Lipoma of submandibular space with osseous metaplasia: report of a case. *Oral Surg, 35:*611, 1973.

Eisenbud, L., Katzka, I., and Platt, N.: Oral manifestations in Crohn's disease; report of a case. *Oral Surg, 34:*770, 1972.

Eversole, L. R., Schwartz, W. D., and Sabes, W. R.: Central and peripheral fibrogenic and neurogenic sarcoma of the oral regions. *Oral Surg, 36:*49, 1973.

Gamble, J. W., and Stanley, H. R.: Hand-Schüller-Christian Disease with involvement of the dental pulp. *Oral Surg, 18:* 272, 1964.

Gardner, A. F., Drescher, J. T., and Goodreau, G. J.: Study of 24 cases of Paget's Disease involving the maxilla and mandible with reference to dentistry. *J Calif Dent Assoc, 39:*1, 1963.

Giunta, J., and Cataldo, E.: Lymphoepithelial cysts of the oral mucosa. *Oral Surg, 35:*77, 1973.

Glass, R. T.: Oral manifestations in primary hyperoxaluria and oxalosis: report of a case. *Oral Surg, 35:*502, 1973.

Gold, L.: The keratinizing and calcifying odontogenic cyst. *Oral Surg, 16:*1414, 1963.

Gormley, M. B., Jarett, W., and Seldin, R.: Ranulas: a series of eighteen cases of extravasation cysts. *J Acad Gen Dent, 21:*29, 1973.

Gross, M. A., and Green, D. B.: Fordyce's granule: a differential diagnosis of a sinus tract. *Oral Surg, 28:*885, 1969.

Hoggins, G. S., and Marsland, E. A.: Developmental abnormalities of the dentine and pulp associated with calcinosis. *Br Dent J, 92:*305, 1952.

Ingle, J. I. (Interview): Screening for the medical links to facial pain. *Clin Dent, 1:* 6, 1973.

Knewitz, K. W., Devine, K. D., and Waite, D. E.: Differential diagnosis of cervicofacial swellings. *Oral Surg, 25:*43, 1968.

Knight, W. O., and Caulfield, J. J.: Abbreviated case report: odontogenic fibroma. *Oral Surg, 34:*381, 1972.

Krook, L., and Lutwak, L.: Symposium on marginal mineral nutrition in man. Presented at meeting of Fed. Amer. Soc. Exper. Biol., April, 1972, Atlantic City, N.J.

Listgarten, M. A.: Periodontal Wound Healing. Presented to the Post-Graduate Departments of Periodontology and Endodontology; Temple University School of Dentistry, Jan., 1974, Philadelphia, Pa.

O'Donnell, J. P., and Shiere, F. R.: Oral manifestations of the histiocytosis X syndrome: report of two cases. *J Dent Child, 15:*33, 1973.

Oliver, L. P.: Aneurysmal bone cyst: report of a case. *Oral Surg, 35:*67, 1973.

Patterson, S. S., and Hillis, P. D.: Scar tissue

associated with the apices of pulpless teeth prior to endodontic therapy. *Oral Surg, 33:* 450, 1972.

Physicians Desk Reference, 27th ed. Oradell, N.J., Medical Economics Co., 1973.

Poyton, H. G.: Maxillary sinuses and the oral radiologist. *Dent Radiogr Photogr, 45:*43, 1972.

Poyton, H. G.: The simple bone cyst. *Oral Surg, 20:*188, 1965.

Poyton, H. G., and Arora, B. K.: Radiologic evidence of surgical emphysema: report of a case. *Oral Surg, 35:*129, 1973.

Sanger, R. G., and Kirby, J. W.: The oral and facial manifestations of dermatomyositis with calcinosis: report of a case. *Oral Surg, 35:*476, 1973.

Sedano, H. O.: Ameloblastic fibroma: report of two cases. *Oral Surg, 17:*475, 1964.

Selden, H. S., and August, D. S.: Maxillary sinus involvement—an endodontic complication. *Oral Surg, 30:*117, 1970.

Sigala, J. L., Silverman, S., Jr., Brody, H. A., and Kushner, J. H.: Dental involvement in histiocytosis. *Oral Surg, 33:*42, 1972.

Silverman, S., Ware, W. H., and Gillooly, C., Jr.,: Dental aspects of hyperparathyroidism. *Oral Surg, 26:*184, 1968.

Sirsat, M. V., Sampat, M. B., and Shrikhande, S. S.: Primary intra-alveolar squamous-cell carcinoma of the mandible: report of a case. *Oral Surg, 35:*366, 1973.

Sleeper, E. R.: Collective review: eosinophilic granuloma of bone; relationship to Hand-Schüller-Christian and Letterer-Siwe's diseases; with emphasis on oral symptoms and findings. *Oral Surg, 4:*896, 1951.

Smith, J. F.: The controversial ameloblastoma. *Oral Surg, 26:*45, 1968.

Smith, N. H. H.: Albers-Schönberg Disease: report of a case and review of the literature. *Oral Surg, 22:*699, 1966.

Stanley, H. R.: The effect of systemic diseases on the human pulp. *Oral Surg, 33:*606, 1972.

Weathers, D. R., and Waldron, C. A.: Unusual multilocular cysts of the jaws (Botryoid Odontogenic Cysts). *Oral Surg, 36:*235, 1973.

Weitzner, S.: Abbreviated case report: lymphoepithelial (Branchial) cyst of parotid gland. *Oral Surg, 35:*85, 1973.

Wright, J. A., and Kuehn, P. G.: Fibrosarcoma of the mandible: report of a case. *Oral Surg, 36:*16, 1973.

Young, L. L., Dolan, C. T., Sheridan, P. J., and Reeve, C. M.: Oral manifestations of histoplasmosis. *Oral Surg, 33:*191, 1972.

DIVISION TWO

TREATMENT PLANNING

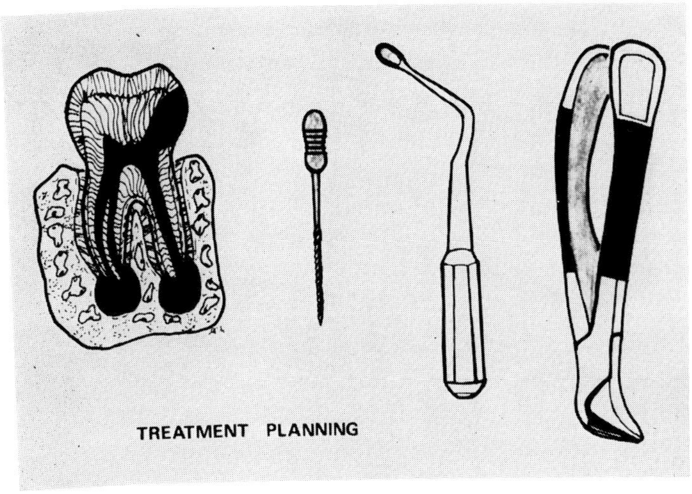

CHAPTER 3

TREATMENT PLANNING

GENERAL CONSIDERATIONS

In all cases, the practitioner must consider the following factors before beginning endodontic therapy.

The Strategic and Esthetic Value of the Tooth

It is usually preferable to extract an unopposed third molar, or a tooth that could not be as esthetically restored as a fixed bridge pontic. Also, if a partial denture is required because of missing teeth on one side and the other side has a full complement of teeth, it might be beneficial to extract an endodontically-involved tooth on the full complement side and then have a bilateral partial denture fabricated.

The Resistance of the Host

For most systemic diseases, endodontic therapy is preferable to extraction. A possible exception is prior to head and neck radiation. Most authorities recommend extractions to prevent the development of osteoradionecrosis. Also, some cardiologists request the removal of all teeth before transplant or valvular prosthesis procedures. Generally, patients have to be well enough to come to the dental office for treatment, although under certain conditions, treatment can be performed in the home or hospital. Treatment should not be performed when patients have a communicable disease or if they are febrile.

The Physical Condition of the Host

As discussed previously, patients with certain neuromuscular skeletal disorders may have to have short appointments and special handling. Occasionally, it may be necessary to treat chronically ill or disabled patients in their homes or in the hospital.

The Patient's Age

Pulpal and periapical repair is generally better in the young because of a good blood supply. In the aged, healing is often delayed, but endodontic therapy can be successful in any age group.

The Periodontal Health of the Supporting Tissues

Patients with untreatable periodontal conditions should not have endodontic therapy performed. With less than 3 mm of supporting bone remaining, even endodontic implants are contraindicated.

The Restorability of the Tooth

Nonrestorable teeth should not be treated endodontically.

The Mental Outlook of the Patient

Is the patient apprehensive? calm? or indifferent? Will the patient be cooperative? It may be necessary to use sedatives or tranquilizers before treatment or nitrous oxide analgesia, chemical analgesia, or hypnosis during treatment. Some patients salivate excessively because of fear, and in these patients, it may be necessary to use antisialogogues before treatment. Unmanageable patients shouldn't be treated, or may have to be treated in the operating room under general anesthesia. Patients who cannot or will not keep appointments should not be treated.

The Patient's Reasons for Seeking Treatment

Is the patient expecting alleviation of pain and/or swelling alone or does he (or she) desire complete therapy? The dentist should realize that regardless of what the patients state, a certain small proportion of patients do not return for treatment after the acute symptoms have been alleviated. The dentist should inquire about the patient's expectations from the treatment. Some patients believe the endodontic treatment will cure possible focal diseases like arthritis, etc. The patient should be informed that only very rarely, if ever, does this occur. Other patients expect the dentist to treat problems aside from their dental ones. For example, neurotic patients may expect alleviation of various nonanatomical facial pains or nonexistent facial swellings.

The Time Availability of the Patient

The dentist should ascertain whether the patient will be available in order to have complete therapy performed.

The Subsequent Therapy That Must Be Performed

If an endodontist is to treat the patient, the patient should be informed that permanent restorations are to be inserted by the general practitioner. Badly broken down teeth usually require crowns and posts. Upper premolars, because of the necessary access preparations, should have full crown restorations. Fractures often occur post-endodontically unless crowns are made. For other teeth, many factors have to be considered for the determination of the type of restoration. These include type of occlusal stress on the tooth, amount of tooth structure remaining, age of the patient, the patient's oral hygiene, the capabilities of the practitioner who must restore the tooth, the patient's desires, and the financial ability of the patient. If periodontal therapy must be performed, a consultation with the periodontist (or general practitioner) should first be obtained, to determine the order of treatment. Also, determination of order of surgical procedures, such as removal of an impacted third molar adjacent to a second molar requiring endodontic therapy, should be planned with the practitioner who will be performing the surgery. Teeth with completed endodontic therapy can be moved orthodontically as well as normal teeth. Also, from experience with a limited number of cases, it appears that teeth with endodontic implants can also be moved orthodontically, but care must be taken that tipping does not cause the implant to be displaced out of bone into the alveolar mucosa.

It also is apparent that endodontically treated teeth are somewhat more brittle than normal teeth. However, as long as there is sufficient tooth structure remaining, these teeth can be used as abutments for fixed or removable bridges.

The Financial Ability of the Patient

The dentist should try to help the patient have the service performed if the patient truly desires to have his (or her) tooth retained. If possible, payment plans should be used. The practitioner might want to adjust the fee for financially-deficient patients.

VARIOUS CLINICAL CONSIDERATIONS

In each of the various clinical conditions, one or more treatment plans are given. The proposed treatments and rationale are defined and the most probable prognosis is stated.

Pulposis

The patient has no pain, swelling or other symptoms and there is no radiographic evidence of periapical pathosis. The tooth may give a slight or no response to pulp testing. *No treatment* should be rendered, but the tooth should be checked periodically as it is difficult to differentiate this condition from pulpal necrosis without clinical manifestations.

An Immature Tooth (Wide Open Apex)

The patient has no pain, swelling or other symptoms and there is no radiographic evidence of periapical pathosis. The tooth may give a mild or no response to pulp testing. The tooth should *not be treated,* but should be checked periodically. If it is a normal tooth, as it matures, the pulp should respond to the electric pulp tester.

Traumatic Injury to Enamel Only

Edges should be polished and the tooth should be checked periodically (Fig. 275A).

Trauma Without Obvious Tooth Damage

No treatment should be rendered, but the tooth should be checked periodically, as pulpal necrosis can occur months or even years later. Also, immediately after a traumatic incident a tooth may give no response to the electric pulp tester. In this case, again, no treatment should be performed, because it is possible for the pulp to recover at a later date.

Previous Endodontic Therapy Which Radiographically Appears to Be of Poor Quality

If the patient has no pain, swelling or other symptoms and there is no radiographic evidence of periapical pathosis (Fig. 342) then *no treatment* should be rendered. The tooth should be checked periodically. However, if the tooth is to be used for an abutment, to prevent later complications, the endodontic therapy should be redone.

Acute Pulpitis

This is manifested as slight pulpalgia following insertion of a restoration or following a crown preparation. *No treatment* is necessary as the pain usually abates within a day or so.

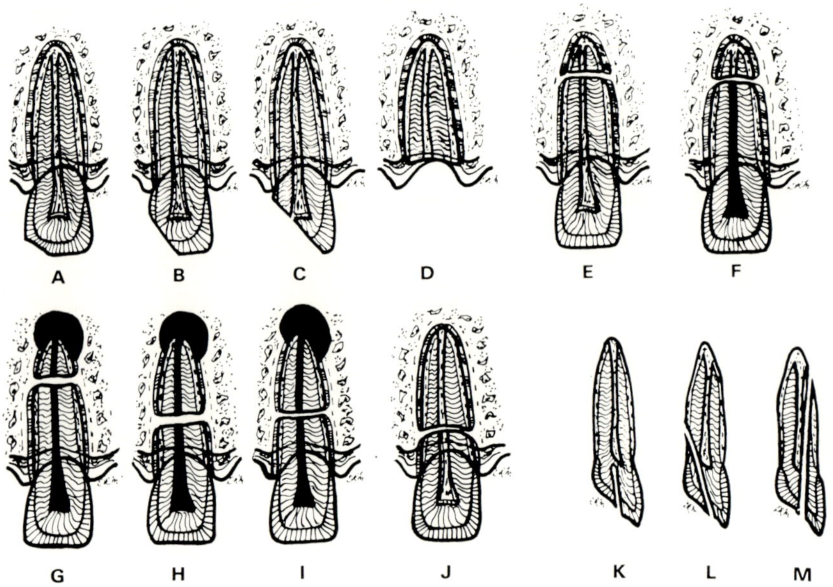

A— Polish rough edges
B— Acid-etch technique
C— Endodontics; post & crown
D— Gingivectomy, post & crown following endodontics
E— No treatment; if mobile, splint
F— Endodontics on incisal portion
G— Endodontics & apicoectomy
H— Endodontic implant & apicoectomy
I — Endodontic implant through both sections
J — Remove incisal portion, gingivectomy, ostectomy, post & crown
K — Crown
L — Remove lingual portion, endodontics, gingivectomy, ostectomy, post & crown
M— Remove labial portion & amalgam seal or extraction

Figure 275 A-M. Various considerations of fracture treatments.

Hypersensitive Dentin or Cementum

If it occurs on exposed roots, treatment is one of the possible methods previously described for treatment of hypersensitive dentin. These include use of *orangewood stick, fluoride treatments,* and *Sensodyne and Thermodent tooth pastes.*

Diffuse Pain in Jaw(s) That Cannot Be Localized to Any Particular Tooth

The pain is apparently of pulpal or periapical origin. *No treatment* should be rendered until the pain localizes. The tooth should be checked regularly.

Systemic, Neurologic, Psychiatric, or Non-endodontic Condition Causing Facial Pain, Swelling, or Lesion

If the dentist is certain that the signs and symptoms are not caused by an endodontic condition, then the patient should be *referred to the appropriate medical or dental specialist.*

Nonrestorable, Nontreatable, or Nonstrategic Tooth

The tooth should be *extracted* and consideration should be given for a replacement, if the latter is necessary (Fig. 122).

Periodontally Involved Tooth That Doesn't Require Endodontic Treatment

The periodontal condition should be treated (if it is treatable). Occasionally teeth with infra-bony pockets and no manifestations of endodontic disease, do not respond to periodontal therapy alone. In these cases, it is possible that there is a retrograde periodontitis present that originated from an undetected pulpal condition. Therefore, performing endodontic therapy may help in the resolution of the periodontal condition. However, as it is only conjecture that the pulp is involved, prognosis is not always good.

Acute Apical Periodontitis

If this condition is caused by a high cusp or filling, then simple *occlusal adjustment* should be performed and it is usually curative. Treatment for those cases occurring during endodontic therapy is discussed under treatment procedures.

Traumatic Injury to Enamel and Dentin with No Exposure

If there is pain, a sedative restoration should be placed and the tooth should be checked periodically. If an angle is destroyed, it can be restored by an acid-etch resin technique, or an acid-etch U-V sealant technique (Figs. 275B, 276). The results are generally good.

Vertical Fracture That Is Only Detectable After Special Tests

These are cases of the cracked tooth syndrome. If only *enamel and dentin are involved,* a *full crown restoration* can usually bring the parts together (Fig. 275K). If the *pulp* is also involved, then *nonsurgical endodontic therapy* is also necessary (Fig. 275L). If the *vertical fracture* extends the *whole extent of the root* then *extraction* is usually indicated (Fig. 275M). In rare cases, periapical surgery may be attempted (see section on pulpless fractured root apex).

Caries Without Pulp Exposure

The patient may have slight pain. This condition is most probably hypersensitive dentin; histologically the pulp may show a transitional pulp. The caries should be removed and a *sedative restoration* should be placed (Fig. 277). Periodic check-ups are necessary. The results are usually good.

Caries Without Pulpal Exposure, but Removal of Last Bit Would Result in an Exposure

The patient may have mild pain. Histologically the pulp would show a normal pulp, transitional pulp, or chronic pulpitis. *Indirect pulp capping* is the preferred treatment, and the results are good in most cases. Indirect pulp capping is the removal of the soft caries, leaving the hard, stained or leathery caries, in order to prevent an exposure. Most investigations have shown good results provided that there was a good coronal seal. The majority of studies revealed that the deepest layers of decay were sterile and that remineralization of demineralized collagen fibrils can occur. Calcium hydroxide appears to induce sclerosis of primary dentin and one study showed that even if microbes were present, they die under a calcium hydroxide base. Zinc oxide-eugenol is more apt to cause an increased deposition of reparative dentin. Although it is debatable which process is more advantageous, most investigators have found that reparative dentin is more porous than sclerotic dentin. A recent study has shown that the use of 10 per cent stannous fluoride causes a remineralization of the dentin, and this may prove to be the treatment of choice. However, as for now, it is preferable to place calcium hydroxide immediately over the deepest layer of caries. Zinc oxide-eugenol is inserted over the calcium hydroxide because of its sedative

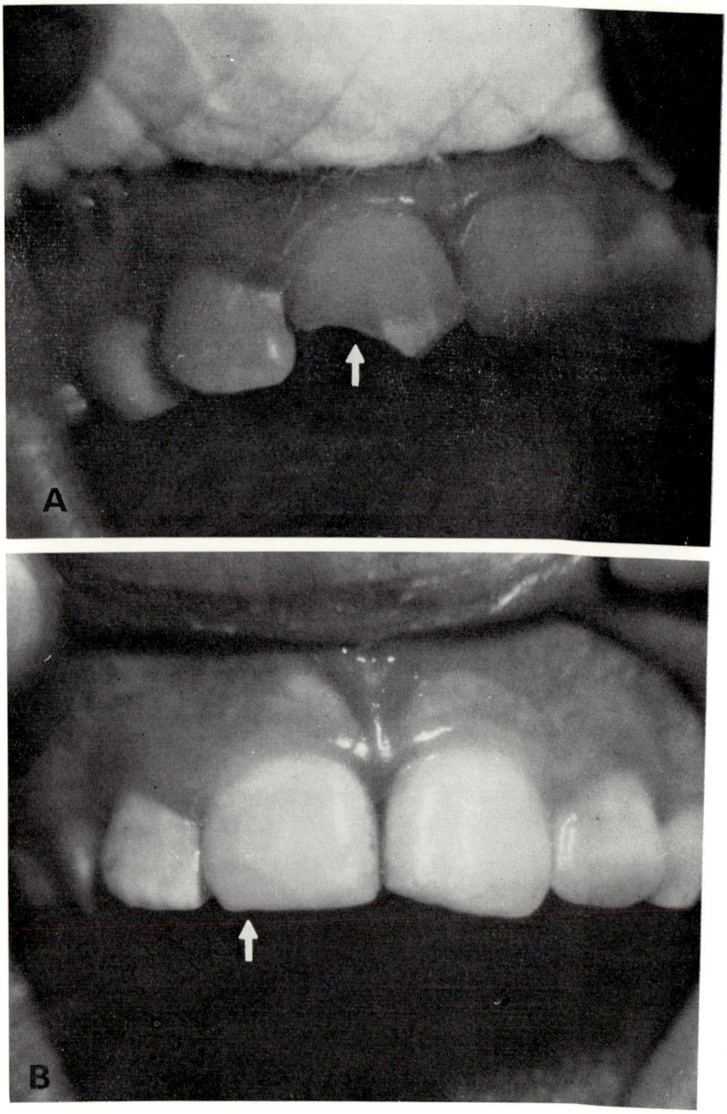

Figure 276. Acid-etch resin technique for restoration of a fractured angle. A. Before. B. After. (Courtesy of Dr. K. Bomze, Cherry Hill, N. J.)

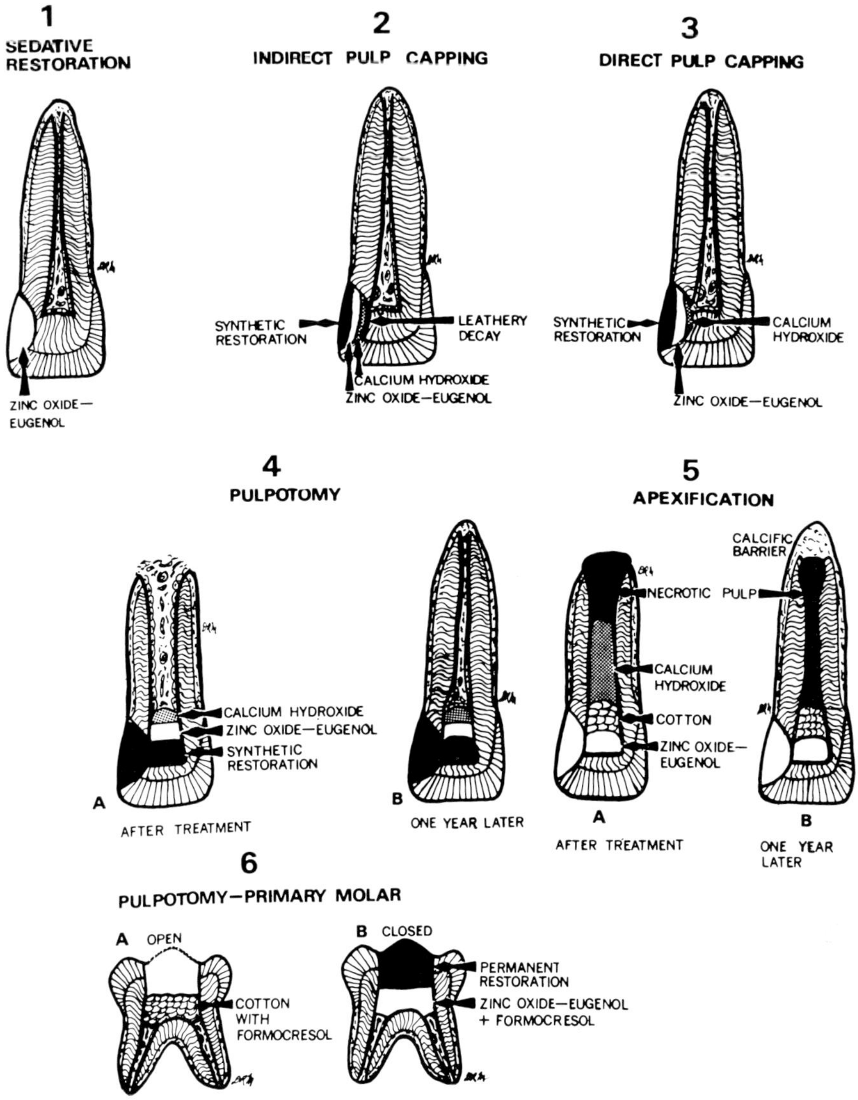

Figure 277. Sedative restoration, pulp cappings, pulpotomies, and apexification.

effect. An amalgam or synthetic restoration is then placed (Fig. 277). Although many clinicians advocate reentering the tooth weeks or months later to see if there is any evidence of caries or remineralization, this procedure is not recommended. The redrilling causes an added insult to the pulp. If there are microbes remaining, provided that the restoration maintains a good seal, they should die or remain dormant. Also, it is advantageous to the patient to have a serviceable restoration right from the start. Periodic radiographs, other clinical tests, and history taking will help verify if the treatment is successful.

Small Pulp Exposure Under Rubber Dam

The patient may have slight pain. Histologically, the pulp would show a normal pulp, an acute pulpitis, a transitional pulp, or a chronic pulpitis. If the hemorrhage is controllable, *direct pulp capping* should then be attempted. This procedure entails the placing of a cement, usually calcium hydroxide, directly over a pulpal exposure. Various authorities advocate different types of calcium hydroxide pastes. These pastes have additives such as methyl cellulose, opaquing agents, resins, antibacterial agents, and zinc oxide. Some commercially available brands are Dycal®, Pulpdent®, Hypocal®, Hydrex® and MPC®. Although there may be differences in the efficacy of these types, the clinical findings are controversial. Calcium hydroxide and water may be as effective as the other types. An important consideration in choosing a type is to use the one that is the easiest to administer. This may vary with the individual.

A sedative restoration of zinc oxide and eugenol (ZOE) is generally placed over the calcium hydroxide base, although some investigators advocate the use of zinc oxide and eugenol alone. As with the indirect pulp capping cases, it is suggested that the permanent restoration be placed at the same visit (Fig. 277). Use of a temporary restoration will not prevent a failure. The results of this treatment procedure are only fair. The presence of a dentin bridge is not indicative of success. It has been reported that internal resorption and pulp canal calcification occur in approximately two thirds of the cases. The dentin bridge that may form is usually quite porous (as has been shown in histological examinations). Under ZOE cements, pulpal abscesses can occur. There have been recent studies using gluteraldehyde, antibiotics, polycarboxylate cement, isobutyl cyanoacrylates, and dentin powder or chips as pulp capping agents. Preliminary findings with some of these methods have been good, but it is premature to advocate any of them. Results of direct pulp capping are superior in immature teeth because of the better blood supply. With large or contaminated pulp exposures, failure invariably occurs. With deep caries cases, it is preferable to do indirect pulp capping.

Large or Contaminated Pulp Exposure in an Immature Vital Permanent Tooth or a Vital Primary Molar

A chronic pulpitis would be present histologically. There is a method available entailing histological examination of the first drop of blood from the pulp. This is called a dental pulp hemogram. Differential examination of leucocytes and microbe evaluation is done with the consideration that this could aid in determination of the method of treatment. If only a few neutrophiles, lymphocytes, and no microbes were present, then a direct pulp capping could conceivably be successful. As this method involves immediate microscopic examination, it is not yet a clinically applicable method. Hence, with large or contaminated exposures a *pulpotomy* should be performed. This procedure is defined as the removal of the pulpal tissue from the pulp chamber. Calcium hydroxide is generally placed in the chamber up to the level of the orifice(s) after partial pulpal extirpation. A ZOE paste is placed over the calcium hydroxide. The remainder of the tooth is restored with a permanent-type filling (Fig. 277). As was discussed with the pulp capping procedures, there is no advantage in placing a temporary restoration. It is preferable to do the entire procedure in one sitting. Aside from calcium hydroxide, the use of ZOE has been advocated for pulpotomies. However, most histological studies have shown the development of chronic inflammatory responses under ZOE pulpotomies. The results of calcium hydroxide pulpotomies are only fair, as complete root formation doesn't always occur and calcification of the pulp canals and/or internal resorption may take place. As with direct pulp capping, the formation of a dentin bridge is not indicative of success. The prognosis is better in primary teeth, as the teeth have a shorter life cycle. Formocresol is also being used successfully for pulpotomies in primary molars (Fig. 277), and there have been reports of clinical success using this modality in permanent teeth. However, it is not recommended for permanent teeth because of the possible long range deleterious effects from the formocresol. From the evidence to date, it appears that the formocresol pulpotomy is clinically more successful than the calcium hydroxide pulpotomy in primary teeth. A permanent tooth that has had a pulpotomy should be checked at least every six months and when *root formation is complete, nonsurgical endodontic therapy* should be performed. Certain practitioners advocate the use of pulpotomy for all cases of vital pulpal exposure in permanent teeth. They state that the area where the pulpotomy was performed should be checked approximately 6 weeks post-treatment. If an intact barrier is felt with an explorer, then a permanent restoration can be subsequently placed with the assurance that the result will be successful. However, the findings are debatable. Therefore, pulpotomy should be used only for cases of vital exposures in immature permanent teeth as a temporary measure.

Pulpless Immature Permanent Tooth With or Without a Periapical Area of Rarefaction

An *apexification* procedure should be attempted. Apexification is a treatment procedure in which an attempt is made to affect continuous development of the root apex. The necrotic contents of the root canal are removed and instrumentation and irrigation are completed. An intracanal medicament such as camphorated monochlorophenol (CMCP) or formocresol is placed on a cotton pellet and inserted in the chamber. However, no medication may be necessary (as has been shown in some studies). At the following visit, a paste of calcium hydroxide and water, or calcium hydroxide and camphorated monochlorophenol, is placed in the root canal, usually about two thirds the way up the canal. The remainder of the chamber and occlusal opening are filled with a

Figure 278. Lentulo spiral paste filler.

zinc oxide and eugenol paste (Fig. 277). In a good proportion of cases, continuous development of the apex occurs, but often in an irregular manner. There are reports of good results, even with the use of no paste. Once the root has completed its development, the tooth is reopened, and the entire root canal is instrumented, irrigated and obturated. This treatment may also be attempted in older individuals in which the pulp became necrotic many years previously and the apex remained wide open. Some studies have shown success even in middle aged patients with this treatment.

Pulpless Primary Molar with or Without a Periapical Area of Rarefaction

There are five possible treatments for these pulpless cases:

(1) The regimen which is the most popular is the use of a *pulpotomy,* with formocresol as the medicament. This has been called a nonvital pulpotomy, but it re-

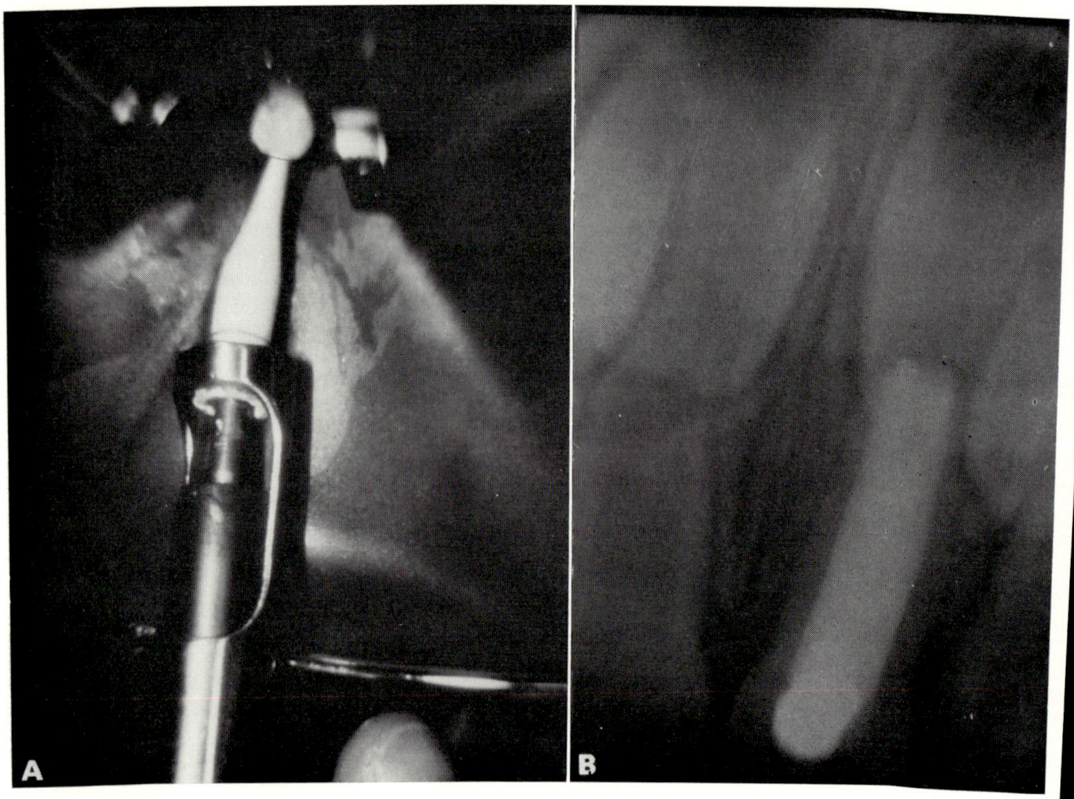

Figure 279. Nonsurgical endodontic therapy with a ZOE paste filling on a primary incisor. A. Paste being inserted. B. Radiograph of completed obturation. (Courtesy of Dr. K. Bomze, Cherry Hill, N. J.)

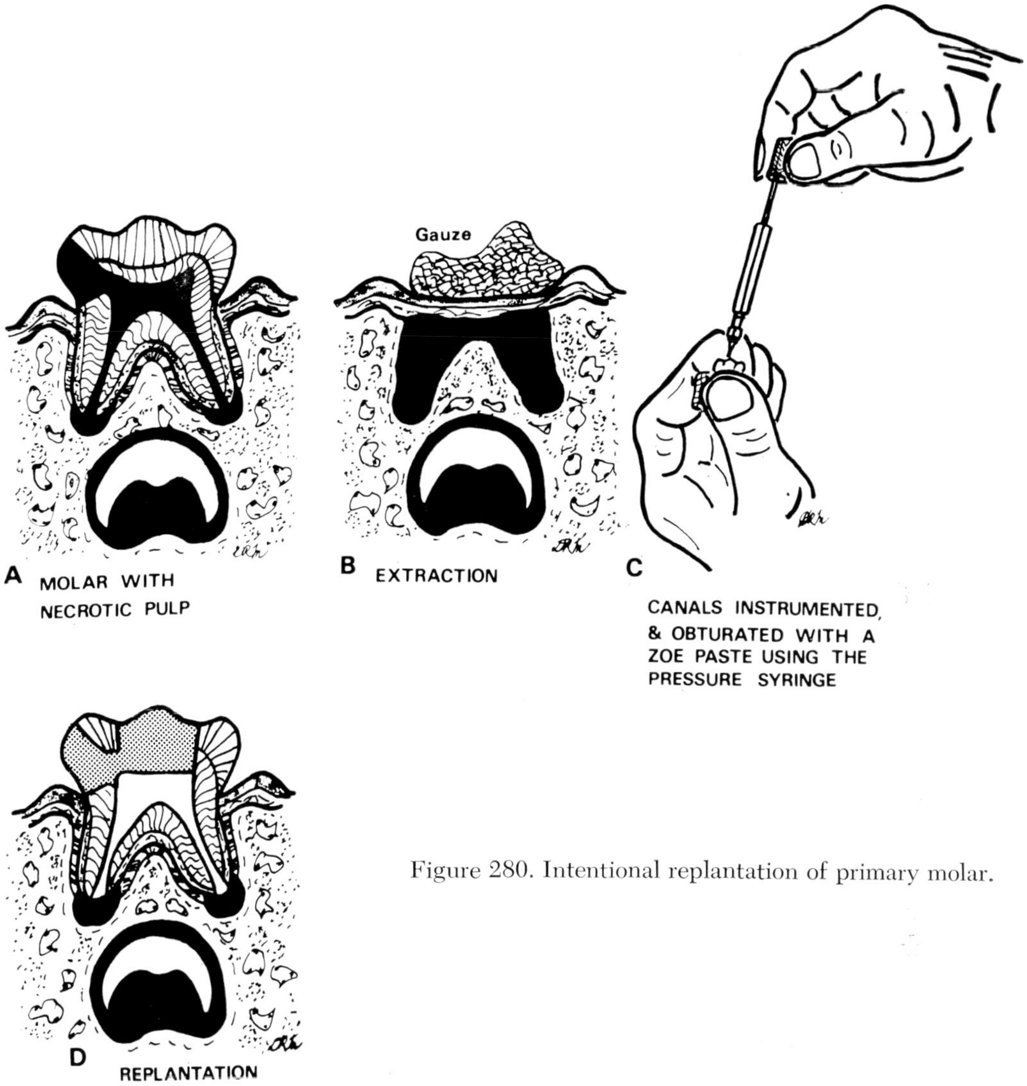

Figure 280. Intentional replantation of primary molar.

ally is not a pulpotomy at all; it is rather a mummification-type procedure. Some authorities advocate a two visit procedure, others state that one visit is sufficient. One visit treatment is apparently just as successful and it is therefore recommended. Clinical success can even be achieved with teeth with periapical *areas* and/or sinus tracts. The formocresol is placed in the chamber for a few minutes, after which a mix of ZOE with one drop of formocresol is inserted. A permanent-type restoration is placed at the same visit (Fig. 277).

(2) Other practitioners advocate *complete nonsurgical therapy*

with a paste filling. This method entails complete root canal instrumentation, followed by filling of the root canals and chamber with a ZOE paste. This can be done with either a lentulo spiral (Fig. 278) or a pressure syringe (Fig. 279B). This technique is usually indicated for those primary molars that have to be retained for longer than one year and for primary teeth that have no permanent successors. For psychological reasons, anterior teeth can also have this treatment (Fig. 279).

(3) Another method of management of these cases is *intentional replantation*. Intentional replantation is the act of deliberately extracting a tooth, performing endodontic therapy in the hands, and then reinserting the tooth into its socket (Fig. 280). Prognosis for all these modalities has been reported as good. The simplest to execute of the three procedures is the formocresol *pulpotomy*.

(4) There are practitioners who advocate *extracting pulpless teeth* with the subsequent insertion of *space maintainers*. However space maintainers are not always easy to insert, they often become loose or break, and there may not be teeth available (e.g. first molars might not be sufficiently erupted) for attachment of the bands (or crowns).

(5) Finally, some dentists state the best treatment is *no treatment* at all. The rationale is that the teeth do not have to last too long and at any rate cannot cause any damage. However, many investigators have shown that there can be deleterious effects from leaving infected primary teeth *in situ*. Among the effects are enamel hypoplasia of the underlying permanent tooth, cyst formation around the permanent tooth bud, changed eruption sequence or malposed eruption of the permanent tooth, retarded root development of the permanent tooth, exfoliation of the permanent tooth bud through a sinus tract (rare), formation of periapical granulomas, cysts, or abscesses, and development of osteomyelitis (rare).

Pulp Cannot Be Anesthetized or Hemorrhage Is Dangerous

These are the cases in which pulpal anesthesia cannot be obtained and general anesthesia, analgesia, and/or hypnosis cannot be used. Also included are cases in which hemorrhage can be very dangerous (e.g. hemophilia). The treatment of choice is *mummification*. This procedure entails sealing into the pulp cavity, either a paraformaldehyde paste, formocresol, or phenol, in order to cause pulpal necrosis (Fig. 281). The patients usually have severe pain for approximately one day. For a predictably successful result, complete nonsurgical endodontic therapy must be performed after the removal of the necrotic pulp.

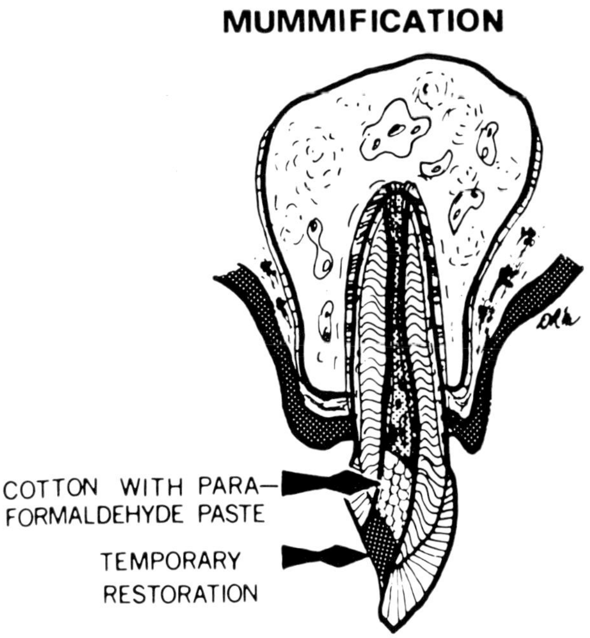

Figure 281

Permanent Tooth with Completely Formed Root Canals That Has a Contaminated Pulpal Exposure or a Painful Pulpitis with or Without an Exposure

A painful pulpitis usually means that the pulp has an area of liquefaction necrosis present. The histologic designation may be chronic pulpitis or acute exacerbation of chronic pulpitis. The cause of the exposure can be caries, trauma, dentistogenic, abrasion, attrition, or erosion. Treatment of these cases is *nonsurgical endodontic therapy for a vital case*. This procedure entails pulpectomy (complete removal of the pulp) followed by instrumentation and irrigation within the confines of the root canal. Root canal obturation (filling) with gutta-percha and chloropercha by lateral-apical condensation (the technique that I use, however other techniques can be used) is then placed ideally to the level of the root canal preparation, which should be approximately 1 mm from the radiographic apex. However, this is only a guide, with the most important consideration being a well prepared canal and a well condensed filling. In the treatment of a vital (or partially vital) case, it is important to maintain the integrity of the apical periodontal ligament and the pulp tissue in lateral and accessory canals. Therefore, determination of the exact measurement is important, as well as the use of a nonirritating irrigant, intracanal medicament, root canal filling, and root canal cement. As it is important not to introduce microbial contamination, which is probably the most deleterious periapical tissue irritant, vital cases should be completed in as few visits as possible. Depending upon the skill of the operator and the time availability of the patient, anterior and premolar teeth can be completed in one or two visits. Molars can be finished in two or three visits. Vital molars have even been completed in one sitting. Contrary to what has been reported by some investigators, extreme patient discomfort from completing cases in one visit has not occurred. This is provided that treatment is confined within the root canal limits. This finding has been verified by other clinical studies. In our one-visit cases, no problem was encountered in controlling hemorrhage following pulpal extirpation.

A culture test is not used as an aid in the determination of when to fill a root canal for the following reasons:

(1) There are numerous ways that a false positive culture can occur. These include incomplete sterilization of the field, incomplete sterilization of instruments, rubber dam leaks, use of unsterile absorbent points, forcing surface microbes apically, air contamination, hand contamination, breath contamination, root fractures, patent sinus tract, infected maxillary sinus, unsterile cotton tube plug, periodontal disease with exposure of lateral canals, and incomplete seal of temporary restoration.

(2) A false negative culture can result from incomplete penetration of absorbent point, use of too narrow an absorbent point, a canal with insufficient moisture, undetectable microbes (hidden in dentinal tubules, lateral or accessory canals, cementum lacunae), only phagocytes in sample, culturing at the conclusion of the visit, dormant microbes in sample that fail to grow, insufficient incubation time, presence of antimicrobial substances in the canal, reliance on visual determination of growth, failure to consider culture reversal (culture that was negative at the pre-filling visit becomes positive at the filling visit), and use of only one culture medium that does not allow for growth of obligate anaerobic microbes, and other difficult to culture species.

(3) A culture test tells nothing about the virulence of the microbes, the population of the microbes, and the resistance of the host. The host's response is of primary importance in the determination of when to fill a root canal.

(4) There is no positive correlation between any root canal microbe or product with any endodontic disease or clinical manifestation. Hence, there is no need to eradicate any particular microbe, as there is in a systemic disease such as syphilis.

(5) A deleterious host response (swelling, fluid exudation, pain) may result from a hypersensitivity reaction to the host's own cel-

lular products as well as from microbes or their products. Therefore if one considers the host's response as one of the major factors in "when to fill," the original etiology is not important as long as the host's response becomes normal. Several indices of readiness for obturation are little or no exudation, absence of pain, no sensitivity to hot, cold, or sweets (presence could indicate an undetected canal), no sensitivity to percussion or palpation, no malodor (malodor can be caused by proteolytic products of tissue cells or microbes, both of which can be periapical tissue irritants), removal of clean, white shavings, and a smooth, tapered canal preparation. In pulpless cases, additional manifestations of a return to normal are absence of swelling, decrease of mobility (if it was of endodontic origin), and disappearance of sinus tract (if one was originally present).

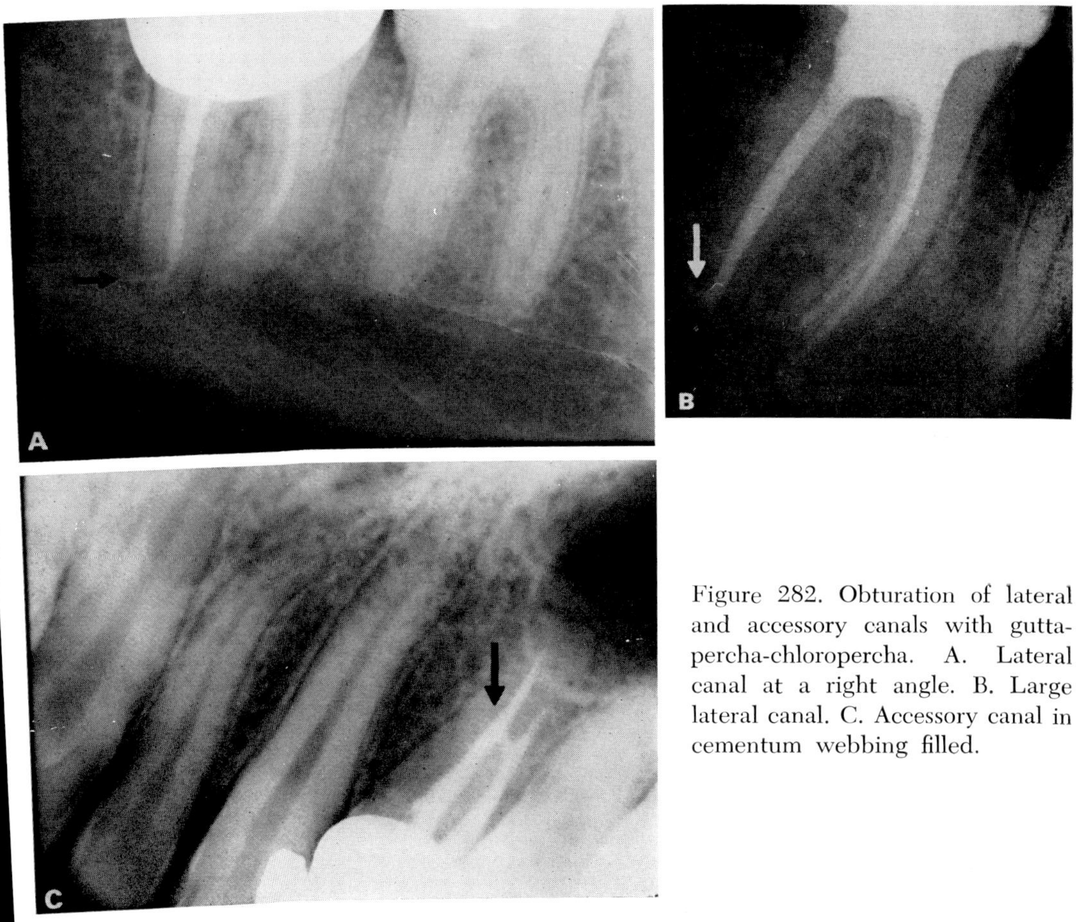

Figure 282. Obturation of lateral and accessory canals with gutta-percha-chloropercha. A. Lateral canal at a right angle. B. Large lateral canal. C. Accessory canal in cementum webbing filled.

(6) Most studies have shown that those microbes remaining in lateral and accessory canals, dentinal tubules, and cementum lacunae either remain dormant or tend to die (probably resulting from lack of nutrients).

(7) The results of clinical studies of success and failure relating to positive and negative culture findings are debatable. Most studies had numerous pitfalls, making interpretation very difficult. The study with the greatest number of cases showed no statistically significant difference between success and failure and the results of culture tests.

The technique of obturation advocated is gutta-percha-chloropercha (described in Chapter 9) in which chloropercha is placed only on the apical region of the master cone. No cement or chloropercha is used on any auxiliary cone or to line the walls of the canal. Chloropercha on auxiliary cones would tend to interfere with the seating of the cones. Only using chloropercha on the apex of the master cone obviates the biggest problem with chloropercha usage, that is shrinkage. The small amount of chloropercha on the initial cone softens that cone enough to allow for a good apical seal. Any shrinkage tends to be minimal because of the small amount of material used. Chloro-

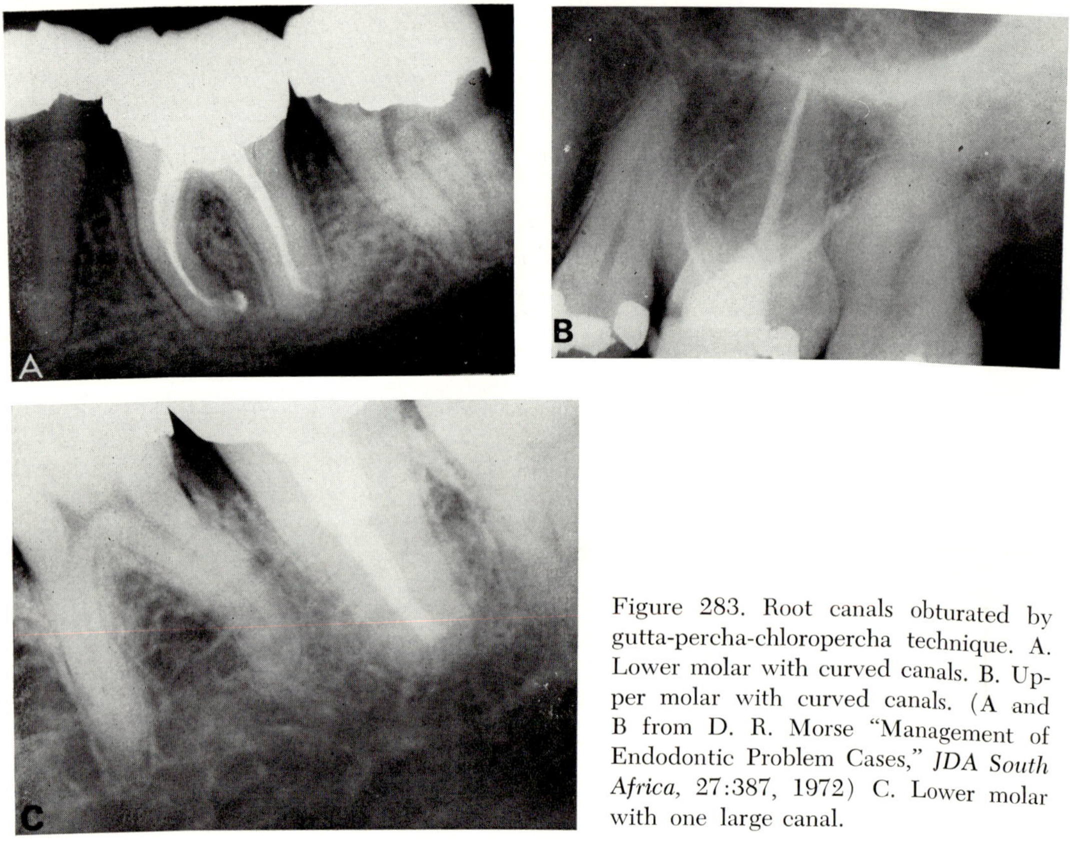

Figure 283. Root canals obturated by gutta-percha-chloropercha technique. A. Lower molar with curved canals. B. Upper molar with curved canals. (A and B from D. R. Morse "Management of Endodontic Problem Cases," *JDA South Africa*, 27:387, 1972) C. Lower molar with one large canal.

percha is used instead of cements because all the currently used cements are periapical tissue irritants. Also recent studies have shown that the various root canal cements shrink upon setting and leak *(in vitro)*. Although chloroform is irritating, once it evaporates from the mass (which should occur rapidly *in vivo*), it becomes inert. This technique has been used for over thirteen years in many thousands of cases by the author. All nonsurgical endodontic cases were treated with this method with a reported clinical success rate of over 90 percent. The advantage gained from using clean auxiliary cones (without cement) as far as ability to insert them into the full extent of the paths created by the spreader, offsets the possible advantage cement would give in filling voids and lateral canals. Numerous instances have been found of lateral and accessory canals being filled by this technique (Figs. 180, 282), and practically never is there any radiographic evidence of voids (Figs. 92, 96A, 283). Therefore, considering the detrimental effect of cements (tissue toxicity), the present technique is apparently as histologically

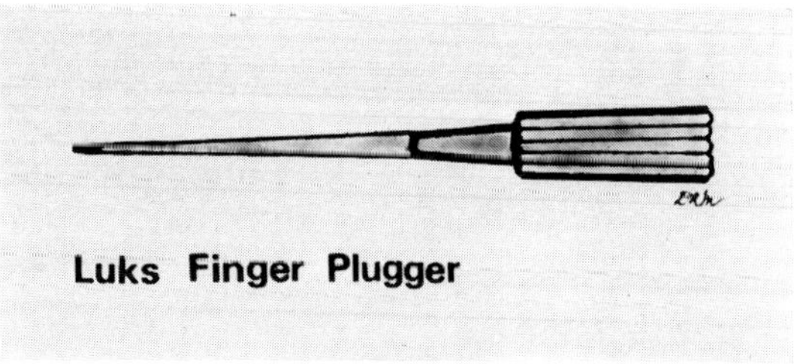

Figure 285

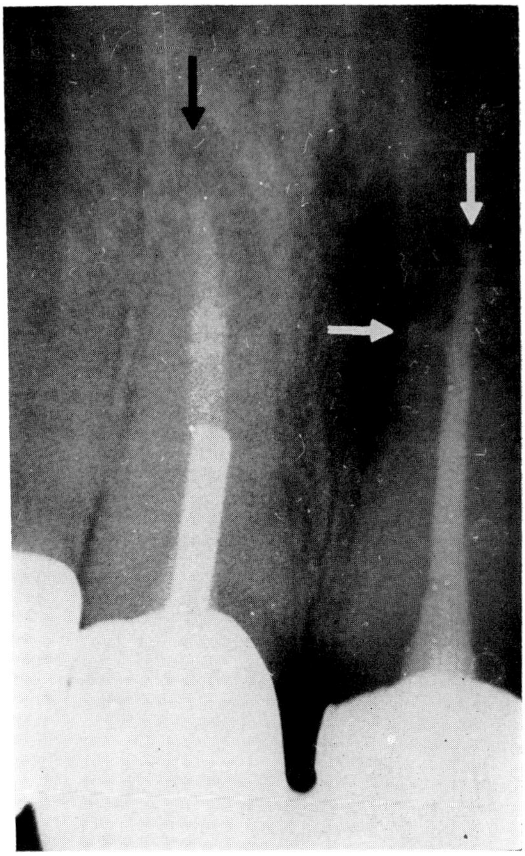

Figure 286. Two upper centrals: one filled by warm gutta-percha technique (black arrow); one filled by gutta-percha-chloropercha technique (white arrows).

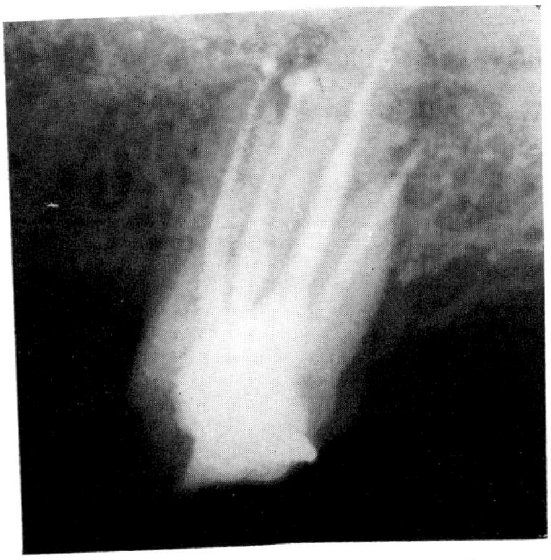

Figure 284. Lateral condensation with gutta-percha and root canal cement; four canals in an upper molar filled by this technique. (Courtesy of Dr. R. Loeb, Babylon, N. Y.)

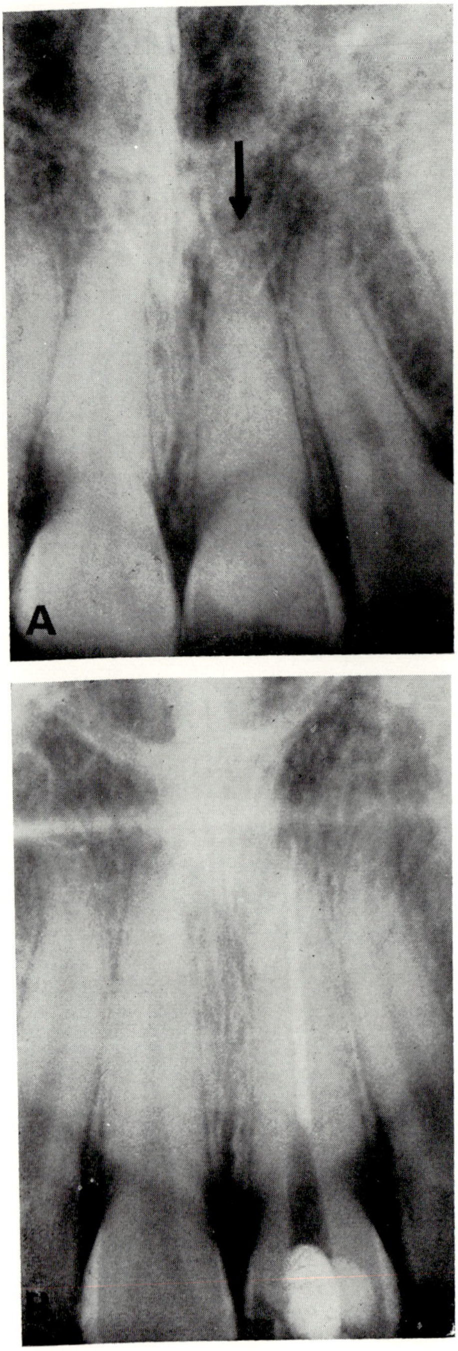

Figure 287. Root canal filled by sectional technique. (From D. R. Morse, "Management of Endodontic Problem Cases," *JDA South Africa,* 27:387, 1972) A. Canal was almost calcified. B. Canal filled by sectional technique; space left for post insertion.

acceptable and clinically effective as any in current usage.

There are other excellent techniques that can be used very successfully. Different techniques that have been used include lateral condensation with gutta-percha and root canal cement (Fig. 284) with or without the use of finger pluggers (Fig. 285), warm gutta-percha (Fig. 286), sectional gutta-percha (Fig. 287), gutta-percha-chloropercha diffusion (Fig. 288), cemented in root canal instruments (Fig. 289), "N_2 method," using a lentulo spiral (Fig. 278), silver cones (Fig. 290), ZOE pastes inserted with a pressure syringe (Fig. 279B), sectional silver cone technique (Fig. 291), absorbable paste filling (e.g. iodoform paste) (Fig. 292A), inverted gutta-percha cone (Fig. 293A), custom made gutta-percha cone (Fig. 293B, C), and polycarboxylate cement inserted with a pressure syringe (Fig. 292B, C).

The use of silver cones is not advocated because of the following reasons:

(1) A clinical study has shown that silver cones become corroded and these corroded cones show tissue toxicity. This was true for flush-filled, short-filled, and overfilled cones. The contact of the tissue fluid with the cone set up corrosion currents. As overfilled cones had more surface contact with tissue fluids, these cases showed the greatest corrosion.

(2) It is difficult to obtain a good

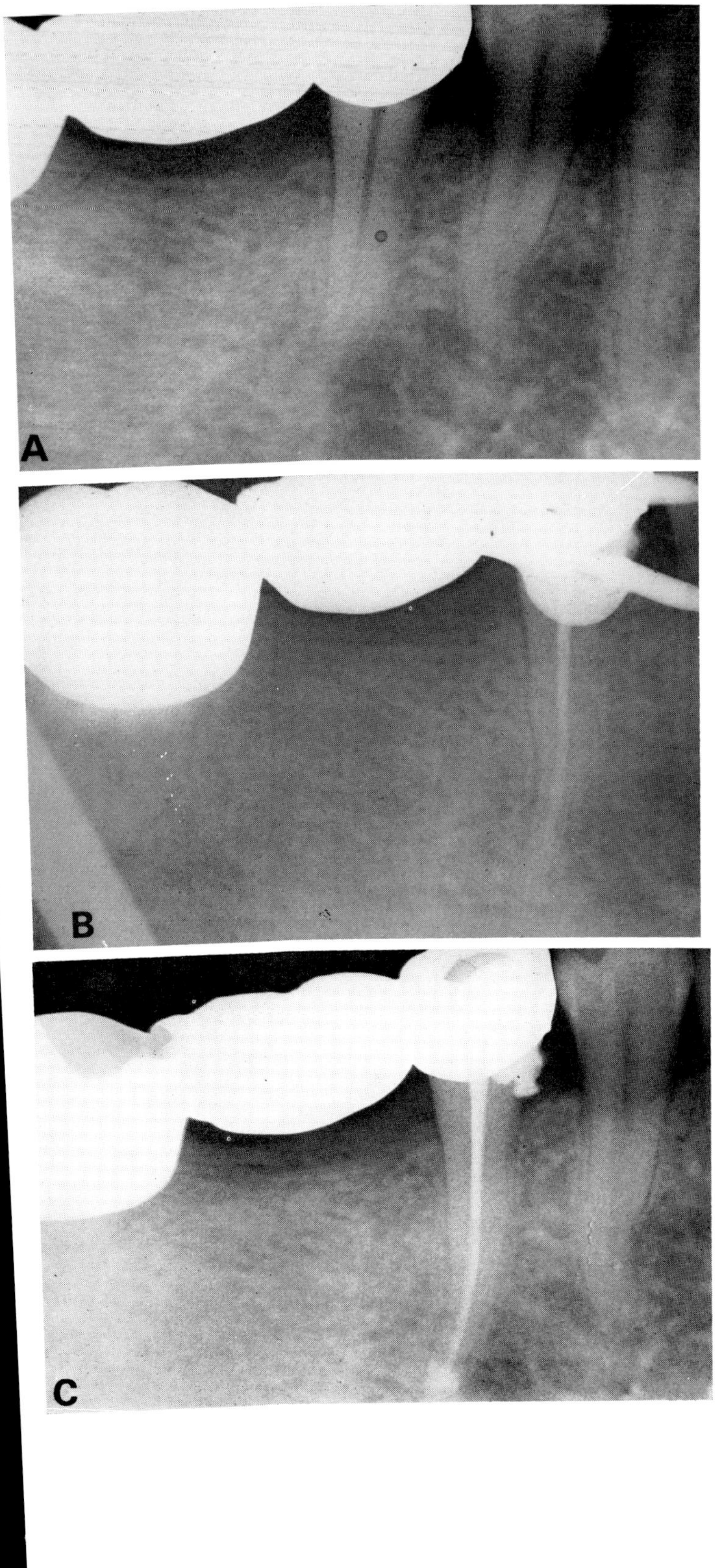

Figure 288. Obturation with the gutta-percha-chloropercha diffusion technique. A. Before treatment. B. After master cone is fitted; penetration of apical region is not possible. C. After obturation by diffusion method; apical region is sealed. (From D. R. Morse, "Management of Endodontic Problem Cases," *JDA South Africa*, 27:387, 1972)

apical seal with a round cone and therefore great reliance is placed on the cement for the seal. Cements are irritating and can wash out with a subsequent loss of seal.

(3) Overextended silver cones can cause periapical irritation that is enhanced when the patient bites on the tooth.

(4) Silver cones cut off at the level of the orifice are very difficult to remove, and it is practically impossible to remove sectional silver cones.

(5) In contradistinction, during crown or cavity preparation, silver cones can loosen.

(6) It is difficult to make a post preparation in a case with a silver cone in position.

With the use of broken instruments, we are again depending upon the cement for the seal. Also, instruments can corrode and give off irritating products.

Techniques which only use a paste filling rely on the paste for the seal. Although recent studies with the scanning electron microscope show that paste fillings can seal well (Fig. 294), the use of a paste alone is difficult to control, especially with the use of a lentulo spiral, and pastes can be absorbed. The more cement that is expressed into the periapical region, the greater is the potential for irritation. Also to be considered are the ingredients of the paste, as some materials are more irritating than others

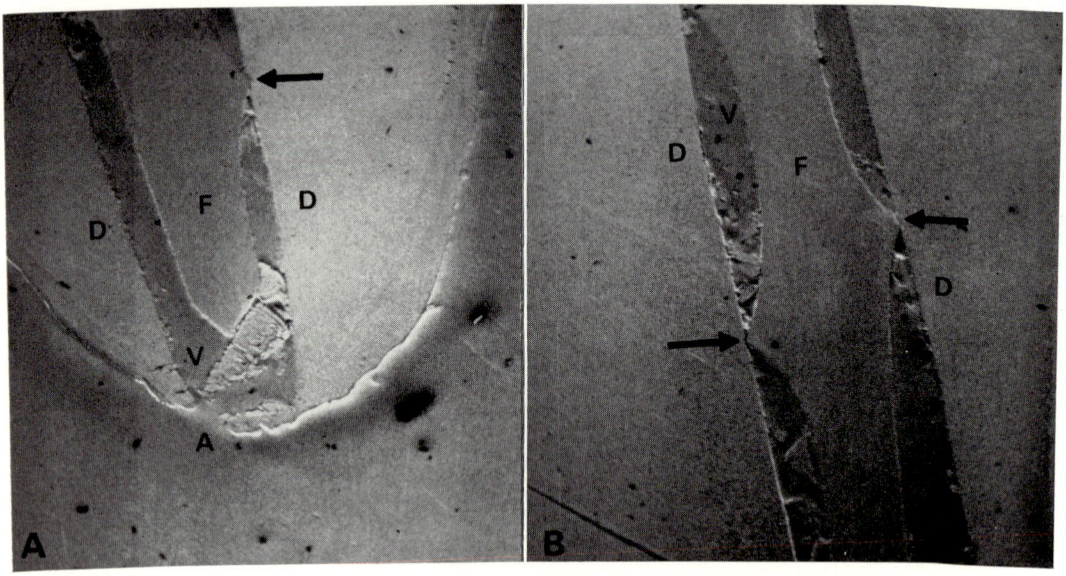

Figure 289. Scanning electron microscope pictures of root canal obturated with a file (×37). A. Apex; D = dentin, F = file, V = void, A = apex, arrow indicates the only region where the flutes of the file are in contact with the dentin. B. Mid-root region; D = dentin, F = file, V = void, arrows indicate places of contact of flutes of file with dentin wall. (Courtesy of Dr. S. Seltzer, Philadelphia, Pa.)

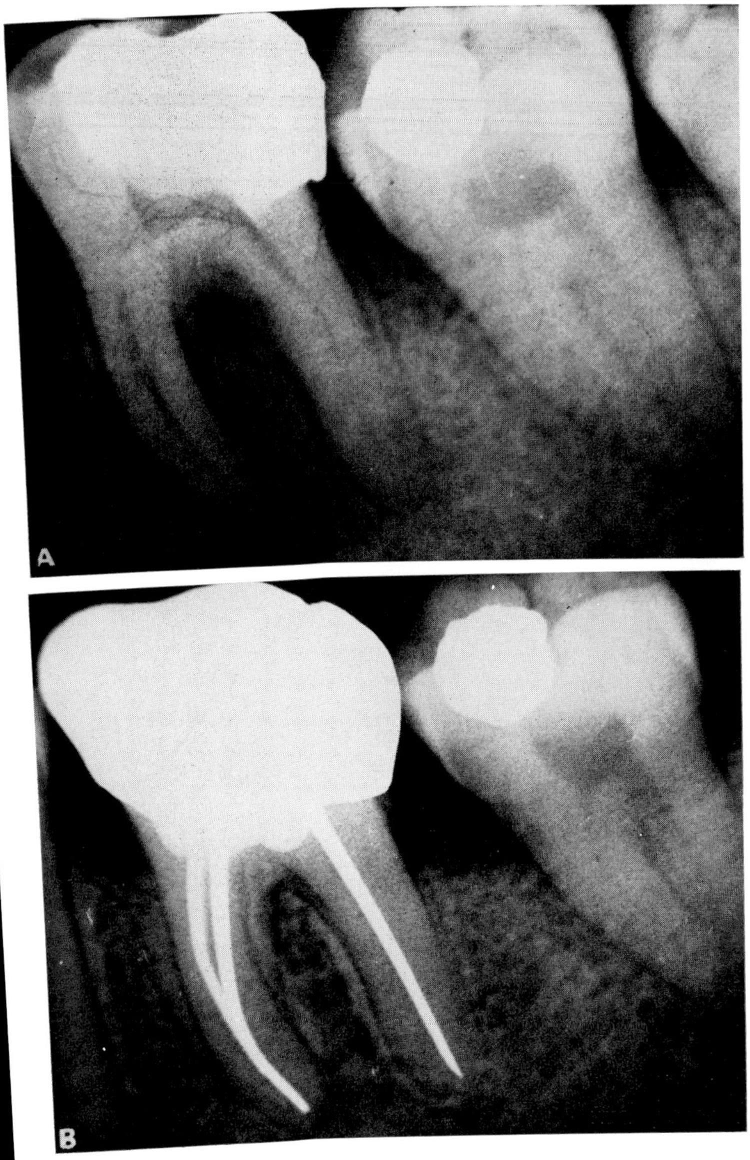

Figure 290. Obturation with silver cones. A. Before treatment; periapical *area* present on mesial root. B. Over one year after canals had been sealed with silver cones and root canal cement; periapical repair is evident. (Courtesy of Dr. A. Cetron, Cherry Hill, N. J.)

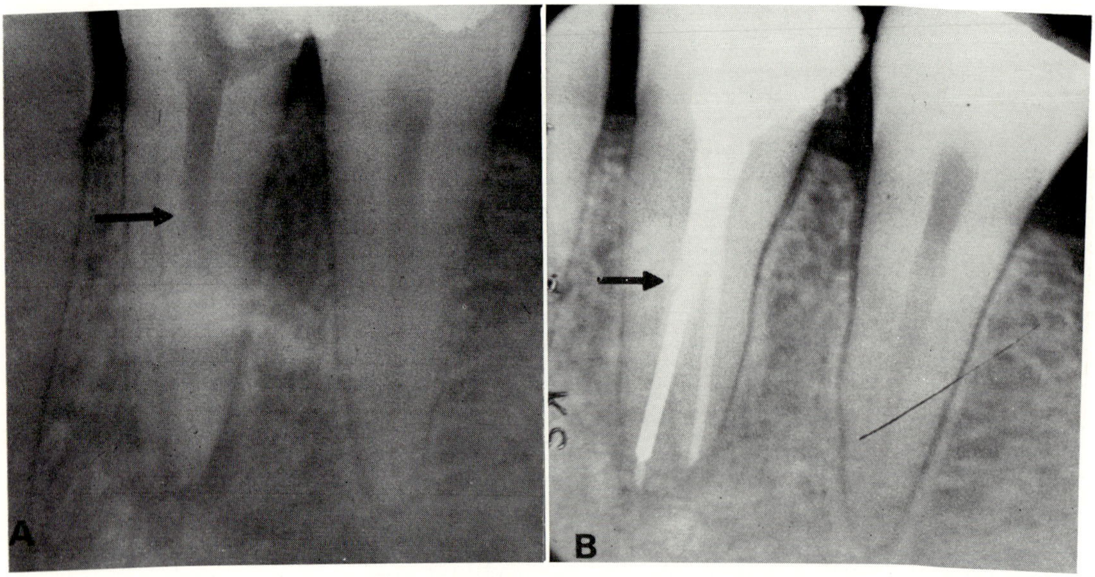

Figure 291. Sectional silver cone technique on a lower first premolar with a bifurcating canal. A. Before treatment; canal bifurcates approximately one-half way down the root. B. Over one year later; mesial canal obturated by a sectional silver cone; distal canal sealed with gutta-percha and root canal cement. (Courtesy of Dr. J. Levy, Philadelphia, Pa.)

(both locally and systemically). However, if the ingredients were not irritating or toxic, it is conceivable that adequate endodontic therapy can be performed with a paste technique. With the use of absorbable pastes, it is possible for the absorption to continue into the canal, with the concomitant loss of the apical seal.

The custom fitted gutta-percha cone and the inverted cone techniques are excellent for wide open apex cases, but generally these teeth are better handled by the use of a pulpotomy (vital) or an apexification procedure (pulpless), subsequently followed by conventional nonsurgical obturation. However, recent findings have shown the use of a polycarboxylate cement inserted with a pressure syringe can seal the canal extremely well in these wide open cases (Fig. 295).

The warm gutta-percha technique, the sectional gutta-percha technique, and lateral condensation with gutta-percha and root canal cement are all excellent methods but the gutta-percha-chloropercha method is just as effective and easier to do. The gutta-percha-chloropercha diffusion technique has its indications (e.g. by-passing obstructions as discussed in section on endodontic aids). However, it has the disadvantage of possible excessive shrinkage due to the large amount of chloroform that is used.

Although the technique discussed in this textbook is recommended, it is re-

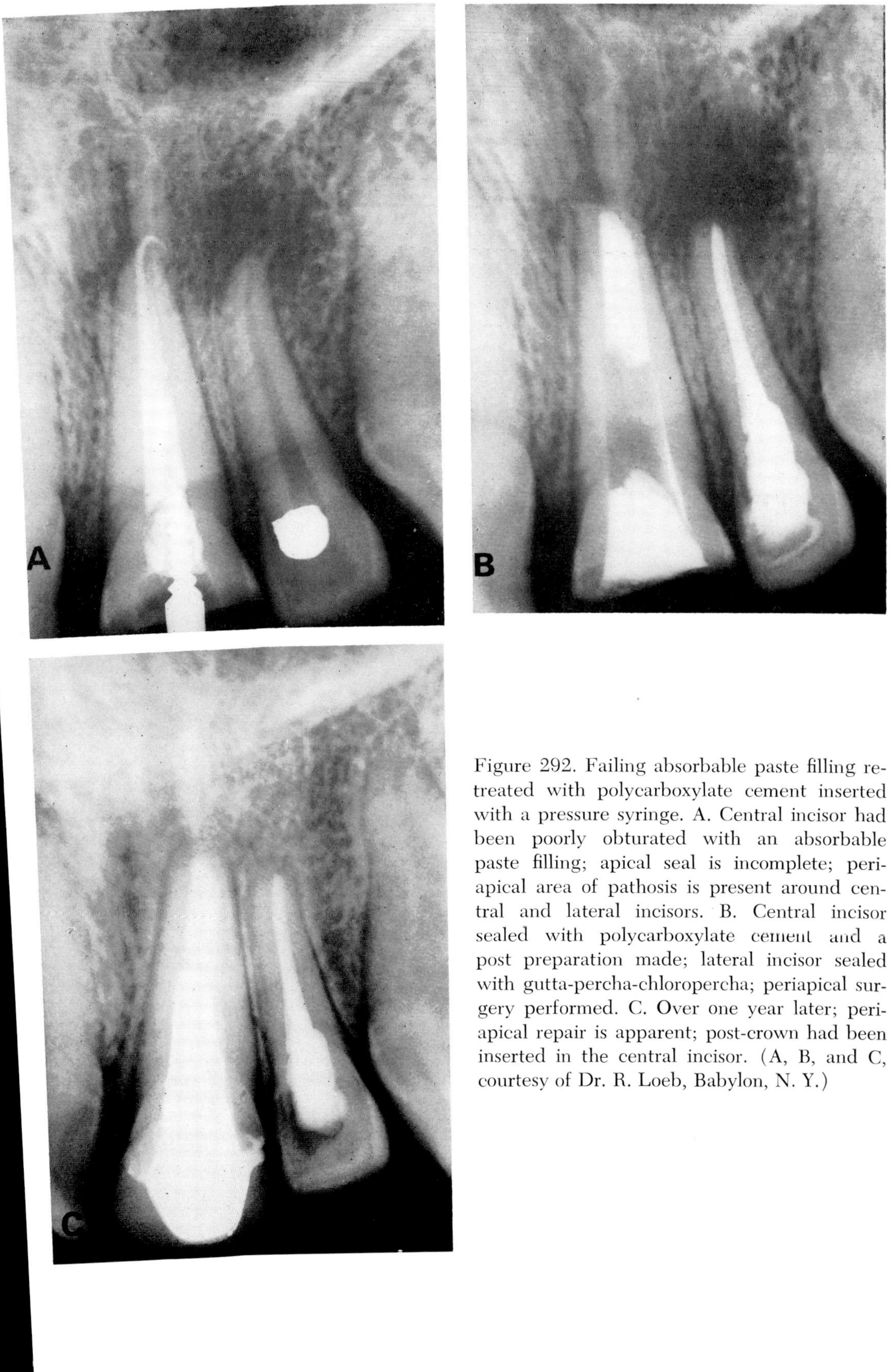

Figure 292. Failing absorbable paste filling retreated with polycarboxylate cement inserted with a pressure syringe. A. Central incisor had been poorly obturated with an absorbable paste filling; apical seal is incomplete; periapical area of pathosis is present around central and lateral incisors. B. Central incisor sealed with polycarboxylate cement and a post preparation made; lateral incisor sealed with gutta-percha-chloropercha; periapical surgery performed. C. Over one year later; periapical repair is apparent; post-crown had been inserted in the central incisor. (A, B, and C, courtesy of Dr. R. Loeb, Babylon, N. Y.)

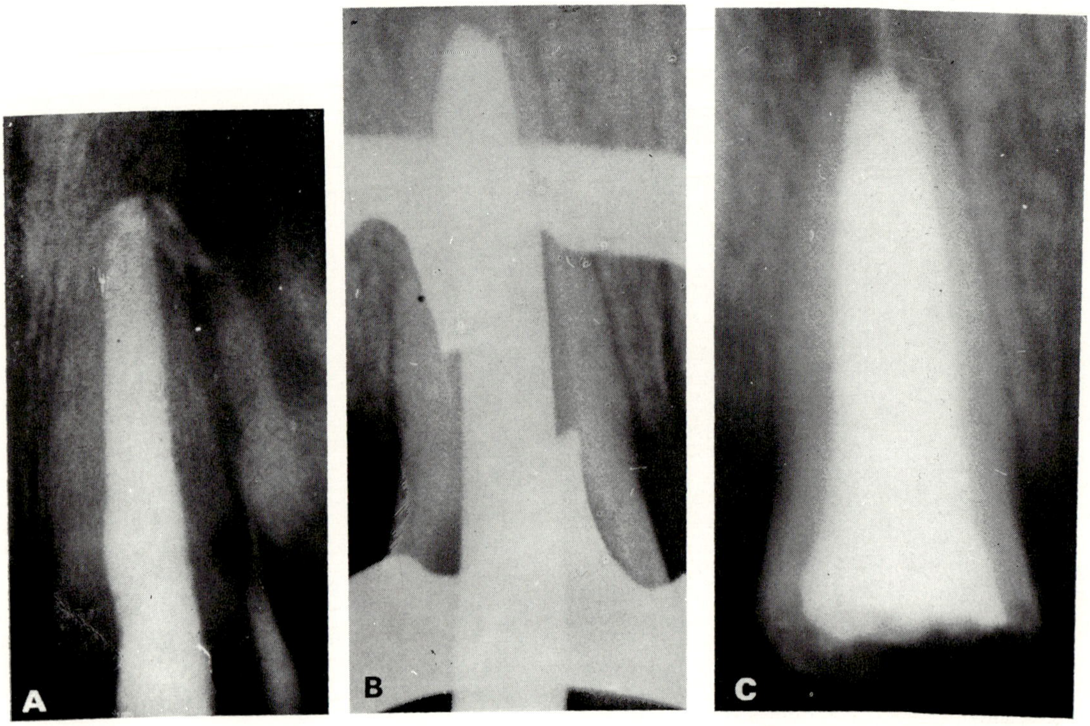

Figure 293. Inverted and custom made gutta-percha cone fillings. A. Wide open canal in central incisor sealed with inverted gutta-percha cone and chloropercha. B. Custom made gutta-percha fitted in wide open canal in central incisor. C. Custom made gutta-percha obturating the canal. (B and C, courtesy of Dr. L. Muldorf, Philadelphia, Pa.)

alized that it is not ideal. As a result, currently under investigation are several other approaches to root canal obturation. These techniques are the use of titanium cones (practically no corrosion) inserted with adhesive cements, the use of cyanoacrylates, the use of polycarboxylate cement alone (Fig. 296), the use of a polymer that expands as it sets, and could conceivably fill all of the interstices of the root canal system and the use of dentin chips to seal the apex, followed by one of the aforementioned materials. Hopefully, one of these methods will prove to be superior to the currently accepted techniques.

There have been studies that reported clinical success using combinations of antibiotics and corticosteroids as pulp capping or pulpotomy agents in cases of contaminated pulpal exposures or painful pulpitis. However, most histological studies and long-term clinical studies have shown poor results. Also, there have been reports of the deleterious effects of corticosteroids, even when placed on dentin. Therefore, this procedure is not recommended. Nonsurgical endodontic therapy is a much more predictably successful procedure.

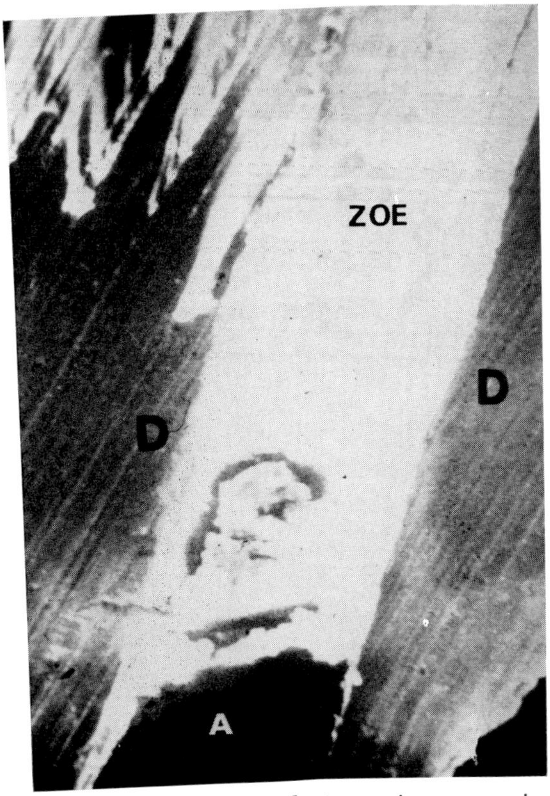

Figure 294. Scanning electron microscope picture of a ZOE paste filling in an incisor root canal; the canal is well obturated. A = apex, D = dentin, ZOE = zinc oxide-eugenol paste (×100). (Courtesy of Dr. S. Seltzer, Philadelphia, Pa.)

A possible indication for a calcium hydroxide pulpotomy would be a patient that for psychologic or financial reasons does not want complete endodontic therapy at the time of the visit. If the possibilities of failure are explained to the patient, a pulpotomy could be completed. It is certainly preferable to perform a pulpotomy rather than extract the tooth. The tooth should be checked at six month intervals for any signs of calcification, internal resorption or other pulpal or periapical disease manifestations. When it is apparent that complete endodontic therapy must be performed, then the patient should be informed. At that time, the situation may be more favorable for the patient to have complete endodontic therapy. If that is not the case, then either an intentional replant (discussed in a later section) or an extraction must be done.

Permanent Tooth with Completely Formed Root Canals and Condensing Osteitis

One or both of the roots may be involved. The histologic appearance usually is that of chronic pulpitis, but the pulp may be necrotic. Clinically, caries or a restoration is present. The tooth may test vital or not, depending upon the underlying histological condition. Treatment is *nonsurgical endodontic therapy for a vital case.* The results are usually good, with the return of the bone to a normal appearance (see Chapter 2, condensing osteitis).

Permanent Tooth with Negotiable Root Canals and a Necrotic Pulp with or without Radiographic Evidence of Periapical *Areas* of Pathosis

In these cases, the pulp is either completely necrotic, or it can contain some vital tissue with or without a periapical *area* present. It is rare but possible to have a periapical *area* present with some vital tissue remaining in the pulp. If the apical region of the pulp is vital and there is no area of rarefaction present, then treatment should be the same as is described for the vital cases. For the other cases discussed, treatment is

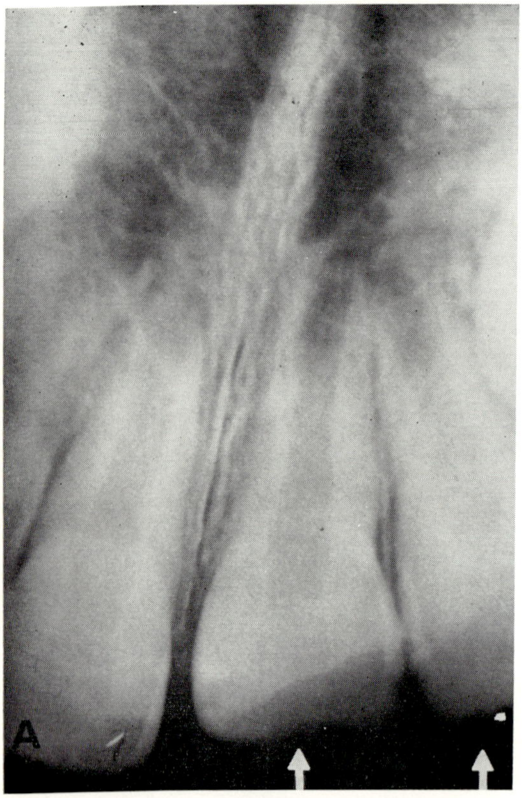

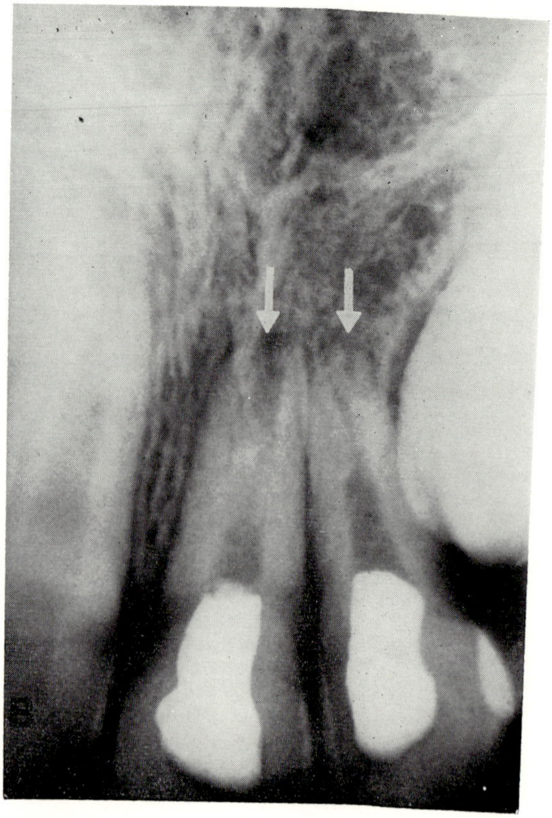

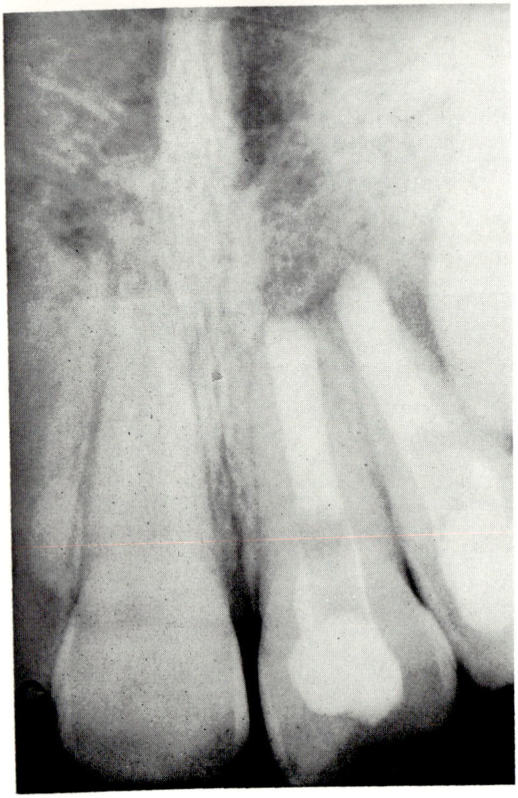

Figure 295. Failure of apexification; canals sealed with polycarboxylate cement inserted with a pressure syringe. A. Wide open apexes with necrotic pulps. B. One year after apexification procedure with calcium hydroxide paste, apexes developed irregularly, but sinus tracts developed. C. Cases retreated and canals sealed with polycarboxylate cement (inserted with a pressure syringe). (Courtesy of Dr. R. Loeb, Babylon, N. Y.)

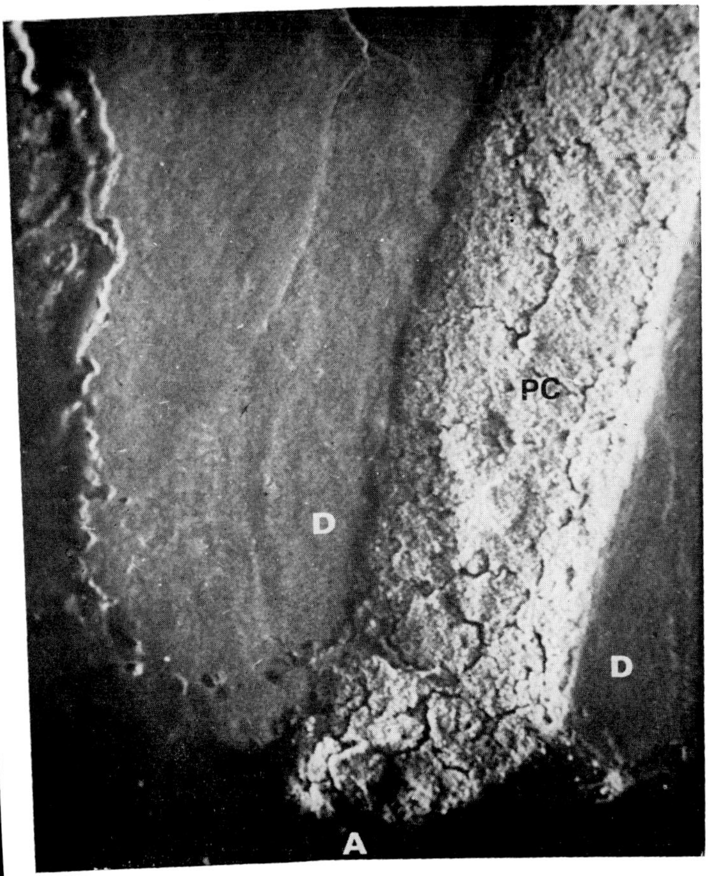

Figure 296. Scanning electron microscope picture of a polycarboxylate cement filling in an incisor canal; the canal appears to be well obturated; A = apex, D = dentin, PC = polycarboxylate cement (×100). (Courtesy of Dr. S. Seltzer, Philadelphia, Pa.)

nonsurgical endodontic therapy for a pulpless case. Generally, these cases should not be treated in one visit, as irritating products in the root canal can cause a flare-up. Anterior teeth and premolars usually can be treated in two to three visits and molars two to four visits. In selected cases, it is possible to do a tooth in one visit. In these instances, a trephination is performed at the same visit (see section on unbearable pain later in this chapter). Also in the cases where a sinus tract is present (a naturally trephinated area), one visit treatment is permissible. The sinus allows for the escape of fluids, gases, or microbial products. In nonsurgical endodontic therapy for a pulpless case, instrumentation goes beyond the apex into the periapical area of pathosis. In the pulpless cases without an *area,* instrumentation is to the radiographic apex. In the latter case, there may be a radicular cyst or granuloma present, but it may not yet have destroyed cortical bone and therefore would not be visible on a radiograph. In pulpless cases with definite periapical radiolucencies, overinstrumentation should be at least into the center of the lesion, but not beyond the lesion. The penetration should be verified by a periapical radiograph. The reason to overinstrument into the depth of the lesion is that cyst formation sometimes occurs at a site several millimeters beyond the root apex. The instrumentation beyond the apex is for three possible reasons: (1) to help in the evacuation of fluid, as fluid exudates impair healing, (2) to set up an inflammatory reaction which might help in the destruction or entrapment of epithelium, and (3) to perform an *inner apicoectomy* which helps in the removal of necrotic resorbed dentin and cementum.

It is debatable whether an intracanal medicament is necessary. In pulpless cases, the prime use of a medicament is to help destroy microbes. Other uses are fluid removal and anodyne effect. In a three year study at Temple University, no intracanal medication was used in the graduate clinic. Results were similar to those obtained in the years before and after the study. Although it has been claimed that periapical healing is faster after the use of a polyantibiotic root canal paste, a controlled study showed no difference in healing between cases treated with polyantibiotics and nonspecific intracanal medicaments. In a recent study on developing monkey incisor teeth, it was found that root formation was delayed and periapical healing was interfered with in cases in which an intracanal medicament was used. The controls were cases left open to the oral environment. However, if the practitioner decides to use an intracanal medicament, medicaments that can be used are camphorated parachlorophenol (CMCP) and formocresol, PBSC (a polyantibiotic) has been withdrawn from *the market* by the action of the FDA. It is not recommended because of the allergy-inducing possibilities of penicillin. Care must be exercised in using formocresol as it is highly irritating and therefore should be placed diluted (1:50) and relatively dry (Fig. 297). However, formocresol appears to be effective as an anti-microbial agent in the gaseous phase. A recent *in vitro* study has shown that 2% Iodine-Potassium Iodide is the most tissue tolerant medication that is still antimicrobial. Clinical testing may show that this is the medicament of choice. Disadvantages of all intracanal medicaments are that they can cause tissue damage, be antigenic (especially true for penicillin and formocresol), and get into the systemic circulation. Hence they must be used sparingly, if at all.

In these pulpless cases because of the overinstrumentation and the presence of a periapical *area*, it is extremely difficult to have a well condensed filling that does not extend into the periapical *area*. However, it is not essential that the root canal obturation remain within the confines of the root canal, as there is no vital tissue to impinge upon. Although it is preferable not to have excess (even with gutta-percha) because any foreign body can act as a potential irritant. Nevertheless, excess gutta-percha is often absorbed (Fig. 298). Prognosis is good, although some studies have reported a somewhat lowered success rate for teeth with periapical areas of rarefaction as compared to teeth without periapical *areas*. In a clinical

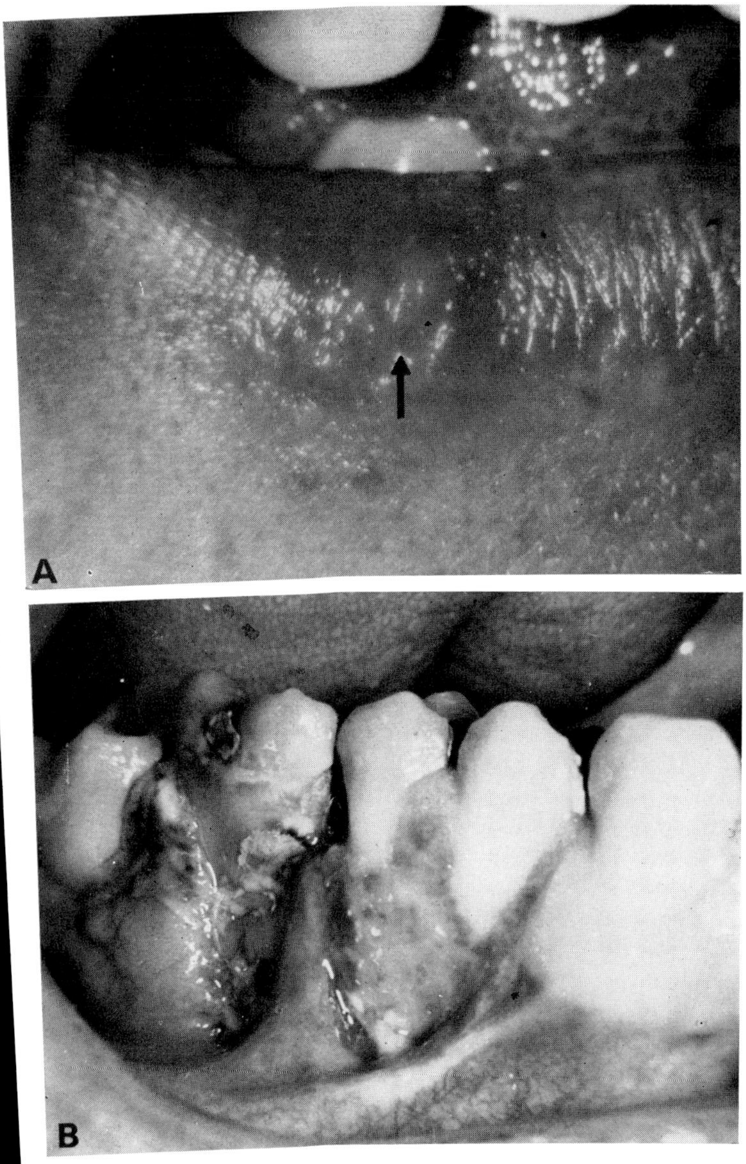

Figure 297. Destructive action of formocresol. A. Lip burn caused by formocresol seeping under the rubber dam. B. Destruction and sloughing of gingiva, alveolar mucosa, and bone, caused by formocresol seeping through a perforation in a lower molar. (Courtesy of Dr. R. Wollard, Philadelphia, Pa.)

study by the author, this was not the case.

Some practitioners advocate a formocresol pulpotomy (really a mummification-type procedure) as a temporary procedure for those patients who cannot afford complete endodontic therapy. This may be utilized in rare instances, but calcium hydroxide is preferable because of its less deleterious effects (both locally and systemically). However, it must be emphasized to the patient that the treatment is temporary. The tooth should be checked every six months and

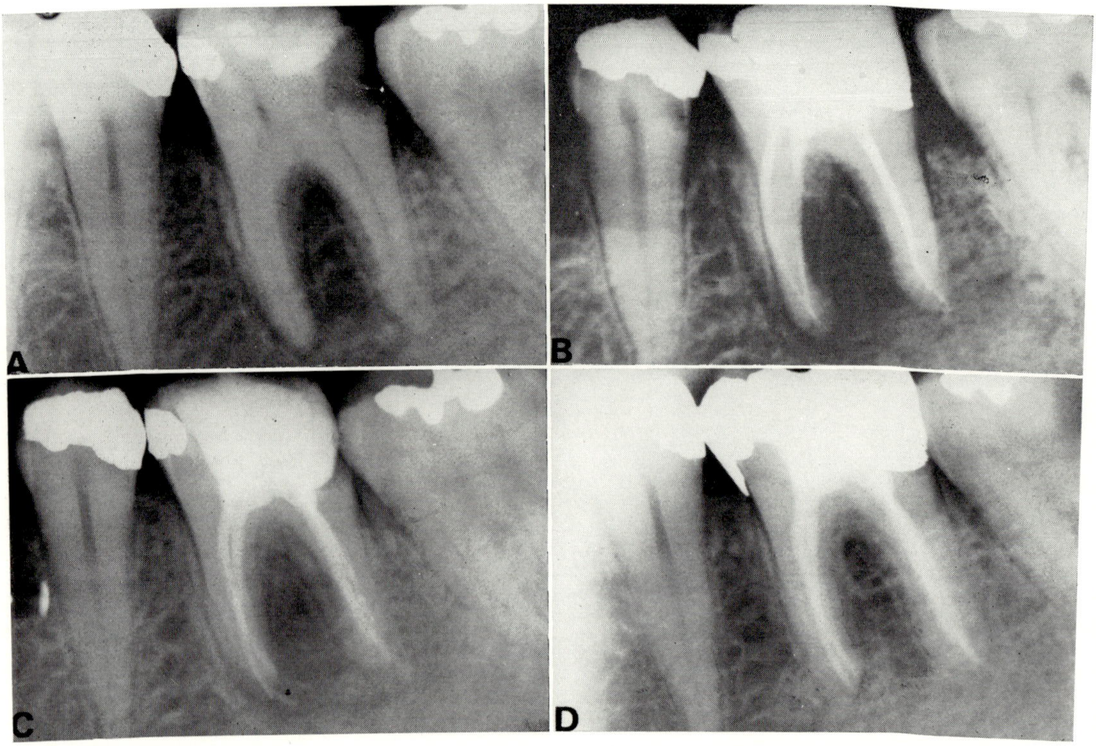

Figure 298. Retreatment of a lower molar with gutta-percha-chloropercha; excess gutta-percha was absorbed. A. Before treatment; lower right molar with caries into the pulp. B. One and one-half years after endodontic treatment with gutta-percha-chloropercha; bone breakdown is evident. C. Canals were reinstrumented and refilled with gutta-percha-chloropercha; excess extruded beyond the apex. D. Three years later; excess has been absorbed and periapical repair is evident. (From D. R. Morse, "The Management of Endodontic Problem Cases," *JDA South Africa*, 27:387, 1972)

if there is any sign of continuation of the disease process, then the patient should be informed. If finances are still a consideration and allowances cannot be made, then intentional replantation is preferable to extraction.

Permanent Tooth That for Strategic, Esthetic, or Psychologic Reasons Must Be Intentionally Devitalized

The treatment is *nonsurgical endodontic therapy for a vital case.* If a tooth has erupted beyond the occlusal table, it may be necessary to perform endodontic therapy in order to be able to use that tooth as an abutment. Often malposed teeth that cannot be treated orthodontically have intentional devitalization performed. If a tooth is in labial protrusion, it may be necessary to devitalize it in order to make a more esthetic crown. Teeth with large coronal fractures without pulpal exposures may have to have intentional devitalization. This is because in preparing for a coronal restoration, the pulp would be exposed. The results on these cases is usually very good. In certain cases of presumed psychosomatic pain (atypical facial pain), performing endodontic therapy on a vital uninflamed pulp affords the patient relief from the pain (usually temporary). This result depends primarily on the authoritarian role that the practitioner assumes toward the patient, and the response of the patient to that role. Usually, this type treatment is undertaken only as a last resort, as results are unpredictable.

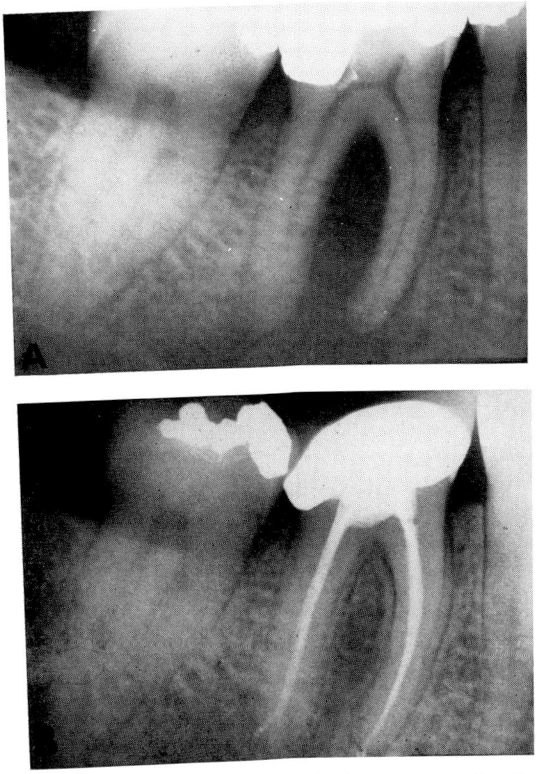

Figure 299. Case of endodontic-periodontic syndrome; endodontic origin. A. Before; bone breakdown in furca and periapical areas. B. Two years after obturation with gutta-percha-chloropercha; no periodontal treatment was performed; complete bony repair has occurred. (From D. R. Morse, "The Management of Endodontic Problem Cases," *JDA South Africa*, 27:387, 1972)

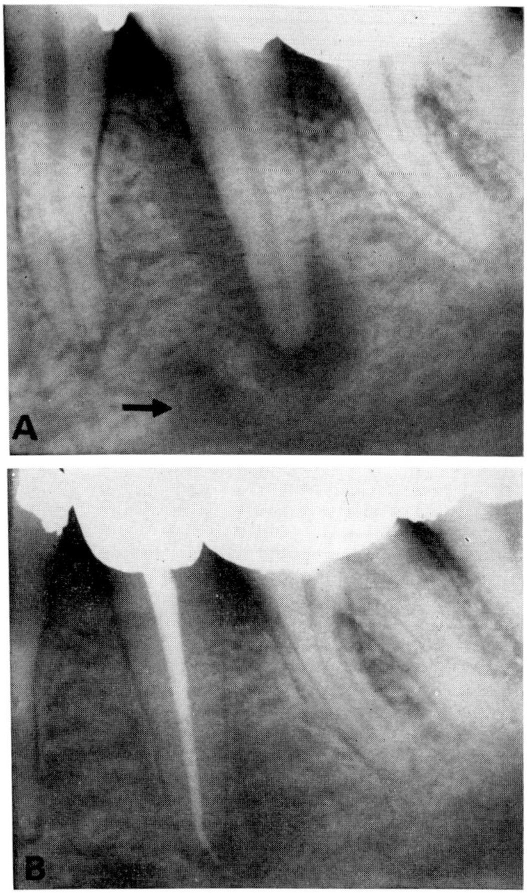

Figure 300. Case of endodontic-periodontic syndrome; endodontic origin. A. Before; bone breakdown periapically and along the mesial aspect of the root up to the alveolar crest; the pocket could be probed to the apex; arrow points to the mental foramen. B. Over one year after obturation with gutta-percha-chloropercha, no periodontal treatment was performed; almost complete bony repair has occurred.

Endodontic-Periodontic Syndrome Cases and Other Cases Requiring Endodontic-Periodontic Treatment

If the syndrome case is of endodontic origin, then the treatment is *nonsurgical*

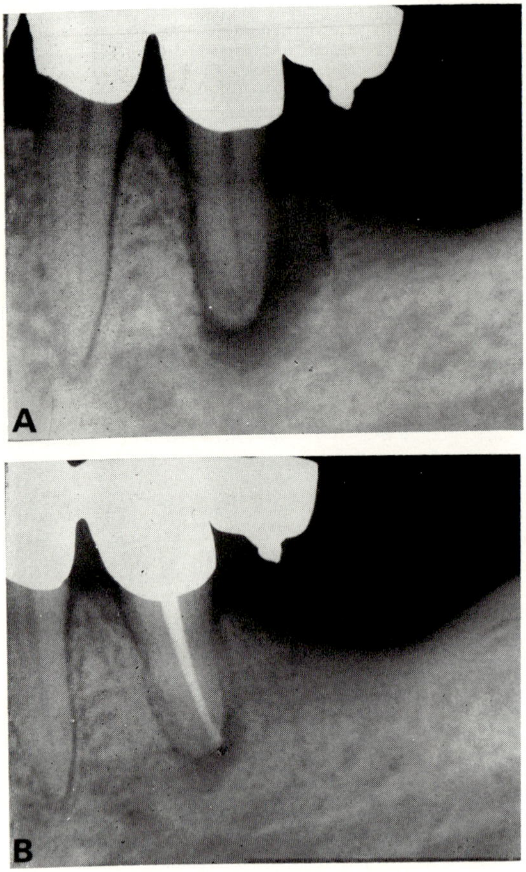

Figure 301. Case of endodontic-periodontic syndrome; endodontic origin; periodontal treatment was required. A. Before; bone breakdown periapically and along the distal aspect of the root up to the alveolar crest; the pocket could be probed to the apex. B. Over one year after obturation with gutta-percha-chloropercha and periodontal surgery; bone repair is progressing well.

endodontic therapy for a pulpless case. If repair of the periodontal bone defect takes place, then no subsequent periodontal treatment is necessary (Figs. 299, 300). If repair does not take place, then periodontal therapy should be attempted (Fig. 301). Generally, the results of cases of endodontic origin are

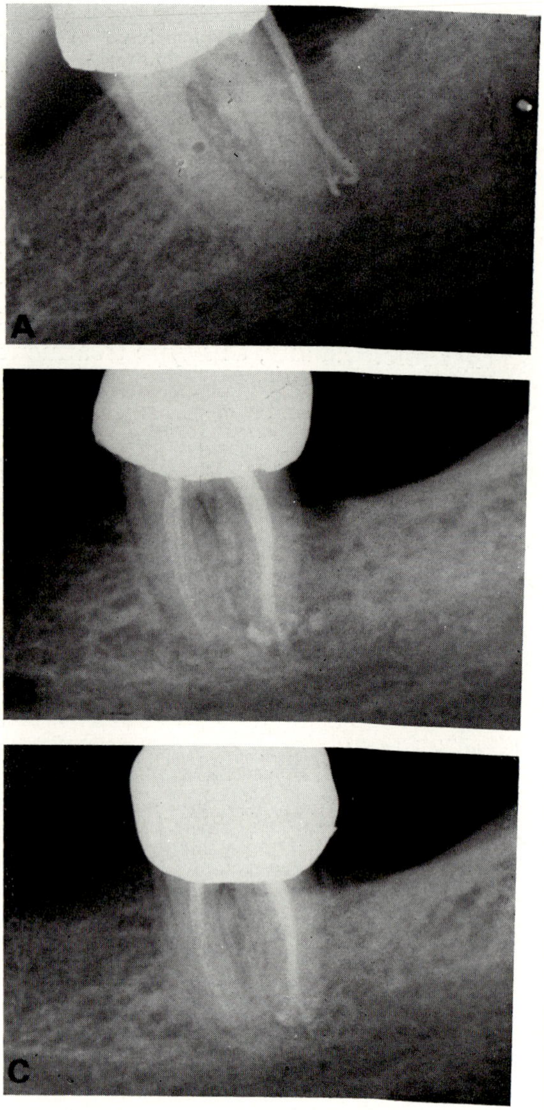

Figure 302. Case of endodontic-periodontic syndrome; combined origin. A. Before; bone breakdown periapically and along the distal aspect of the root; gutta-percha cone inserted through the pocket to the apex. B. After obturation with gutta-percha-chloropercha (note the accessory canals sealed at the distal apex) and periodontal surgery. C. One year later; complete bone *fill in* is evident; excess gutta-percha has been absorbed. (From D. R. Morse, "The Management of Endodontic Problem Cases," *JDA South Africa*, 27:387, 1972)

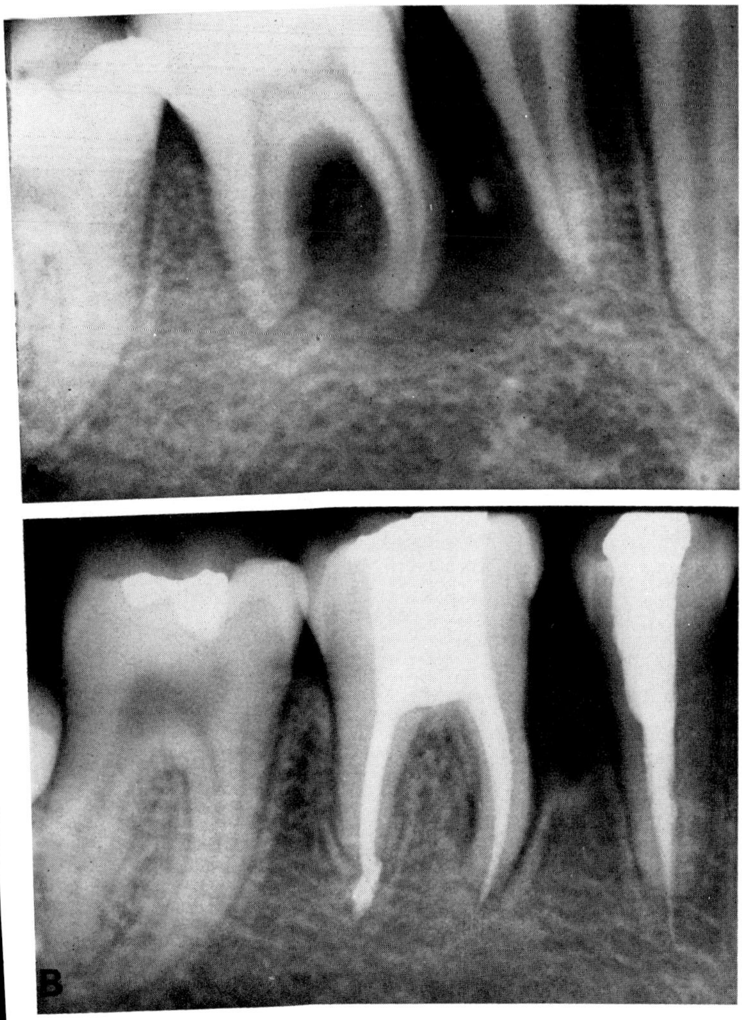

Figure 303. Case of endodontic-periodontic syndrome; etiology unphysiologic orthodontic movement; treatment —obturation with gutta-percha-chloropercha and combined periodontal and periapical surgery. A. Before treatment; extensive bone destruction evident. B. More than one year later, bone repair is evident, although at a lower level interproximally.

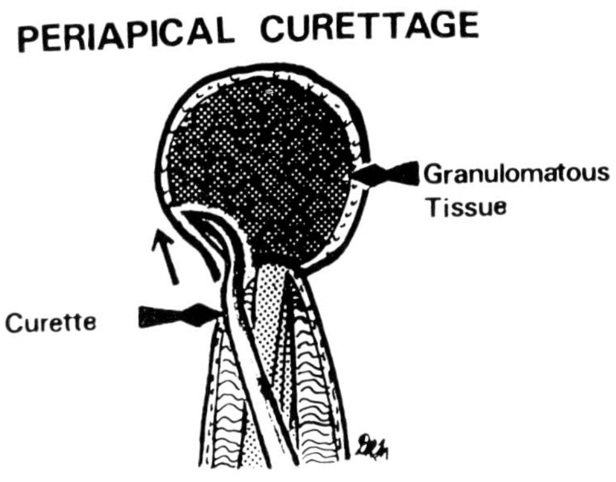

Figure 304

good. If the case is of *periodontic* or *combined* origin, then the same *endodontic treatment* is performed after the completion of *periodontal therapy* (Fig. 302). However, if pain or swelling of endodontic origin is present, then endodontic therapy should be initiated prior to the periodontal therapy. The periodontal treatment usually entails curettage, gingivectomy, ostectomy, or gingival repositioning procedures. If there will be *surgical periodontal therapy*

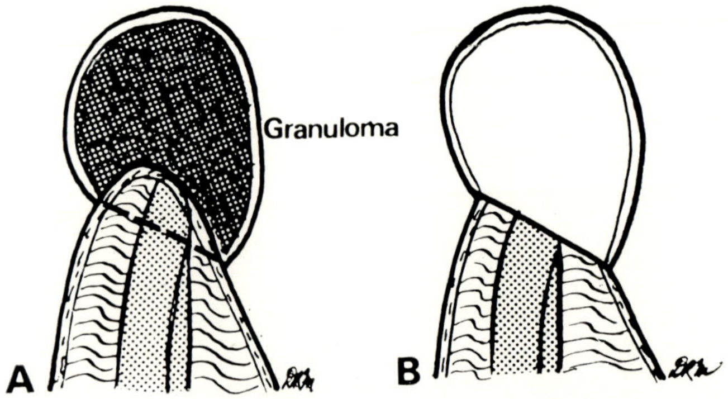

Figure 305 A and B. Apicoectomy; before and after.

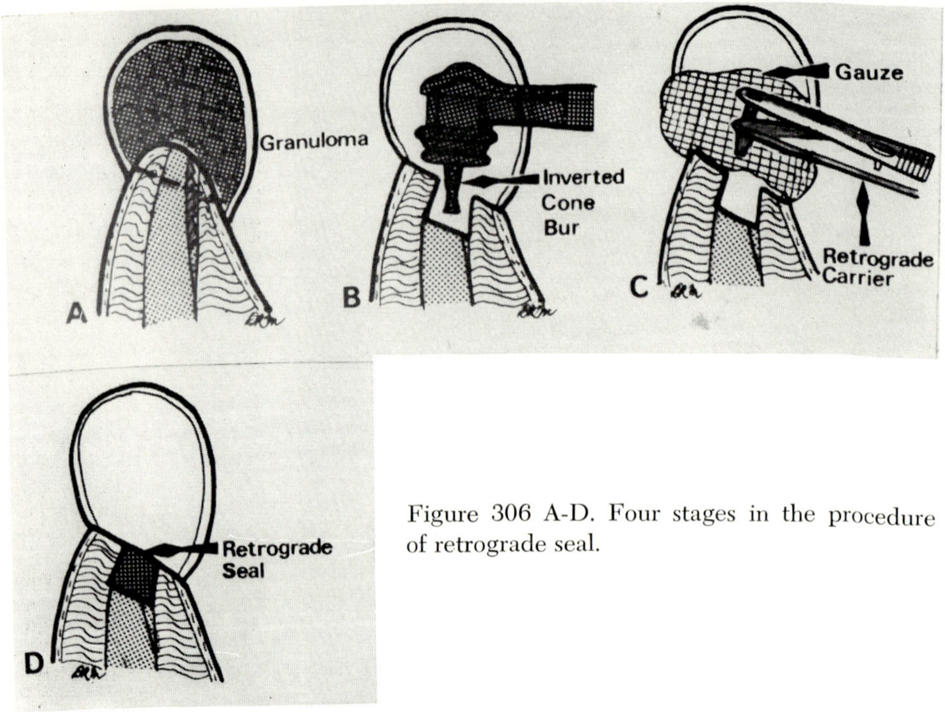

Figure 306 A-D. Four stages in the procedure of retrograde seal.

performed, and there is an associated periapical lesion present that is accessible with the periodontal flap, then a *periapical curettage* is usually done at the same time (Fig. 303). A periapical curettage is a surgical endodontic procedure in which granulomatous tissue is removed with curettes from around the apex of an endodontically-involved tooth. It is usually done after the root canal(s) has been instrumented and obturated (Fig. 304). If it is necessary to remove a portion of the apex in order to more readily remove this tissue, or because the apex is fractured or necrotic, then the procedure is called an *apicoectomy* (Fig. 305). Most often this is not necessary, as complete enucleation of the inflamed tissue is not essential for repair to take place. There is good evidence from the success of nonsurgical endodontic therapy that the inflammatory response itself will set up a reaction allowing for the removal and then replacement of granulomatous tissue by fibrous tissue and bone. If during the root canal obturation it is not possible to adequately seal the apical portion of the canal, then a small preparation is made in the apex with a bur. This is then sealed with either amalgam, gold foil, or polycarboxylate cement. The procedure is called a *retrograde seal* (Fig. 306). It is used for any surgical case in which there is doubt about the completeness of the apical seal. The usual retrograde material used is amalgam (Fig. 307), but there are some

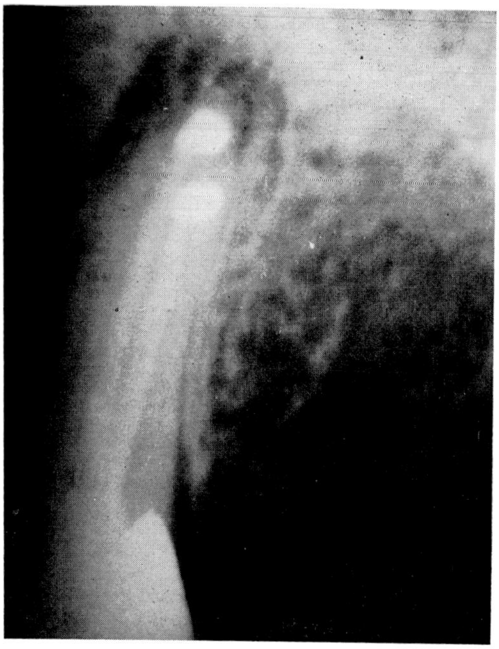

Figure 307. Retroseal with amalgam at upper premolar apexes.

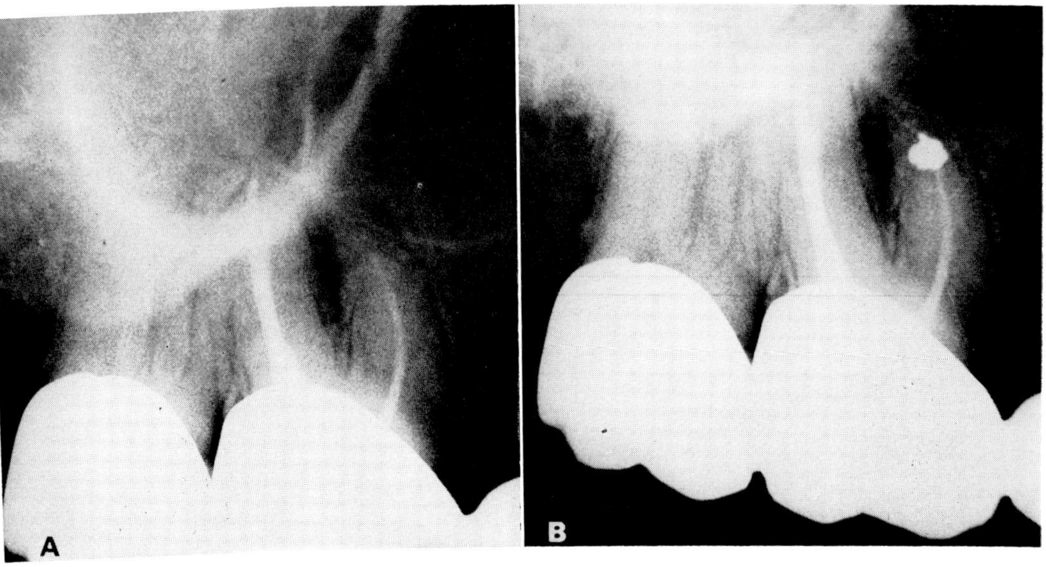

Figure 308. Retroseal with gold foil at apex of mesio-buccal root of upper first molar. A. Obturation with gutta-percha of three canals; apical region of M-B canal was calcified. B. After retroseal with gold foil at the M-B apex. (From W. K. Kopp and H. Kresberg, "Apicoectomy with Retrograde Gold Foil: A New Technique," *New York State Dental Journal*, 39:8, 1973)

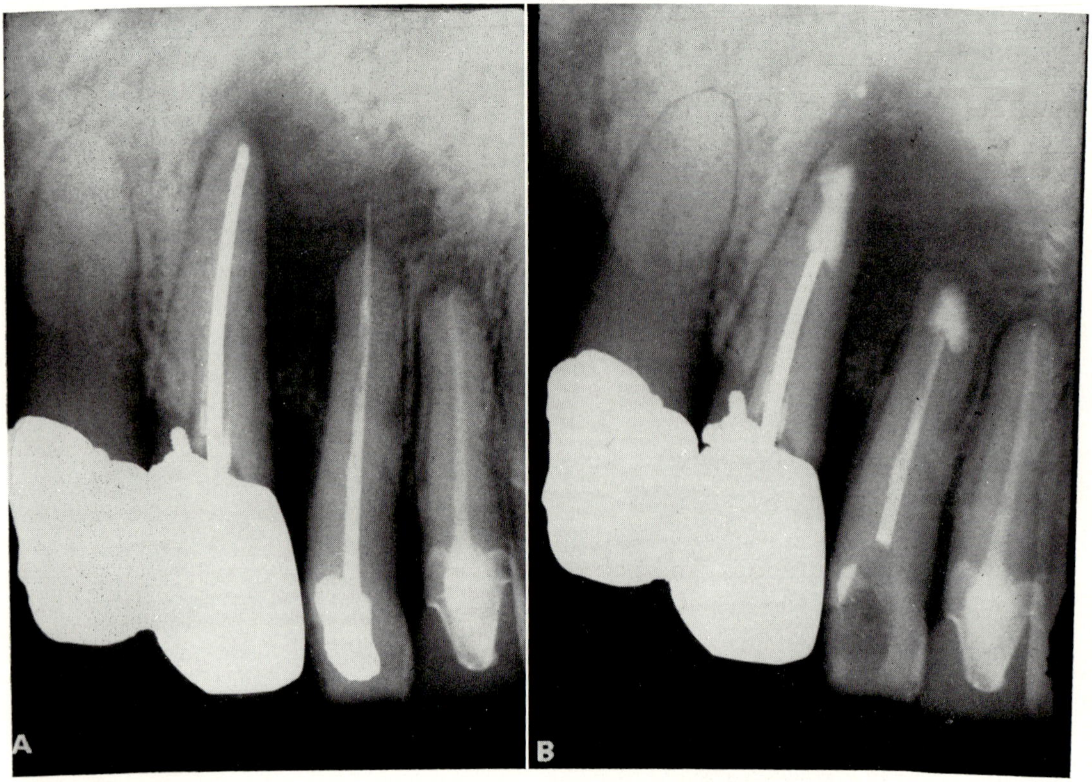

Figure 309. Retroseal with polycarboxylate cement. A. Before. B. After; three months later, periapical healing is beginning. (Courtesy of Dr. R. Loeb, Babylon, N. Y.)

problems inherent in the use of amalgam. These are release of irritating corrosion products into the surrounding tissues, difficulty of control of hemorrhage, scatter of particles (cause of amalgam tattoo), and the possibility of subsequent loosening of the apical seal.

Gold foil is practically noncorrosive, nonirritating, and if it is inserted correctly, it should not loosen (Fig. 308). The disadvantages are that it is difficult to insert, a dry field is essential, and it is relatively expensive. Polycarboxylate cement is relatively nonirritating, is very adhesive, and is not difficult to insert if mixed properly (Fig. 309).

Some investigators have suggested that in teeth with roots that bulge toward the labial (especially upper canines), and are prone to dehiscences and fenestrations (due to lack of bony covering), it is a good idea to reduce the bulge of the root. This can be done by a chisel or by the use of a bur. Approximately one and one-half mm of the overlying root is removed. This should then give a more favorable environment for new bone to grow into. Also in furcas and infrabony pockets, the use of autogenous and allogeneic bone grafts and even plaster of paris may help in restoring bone.

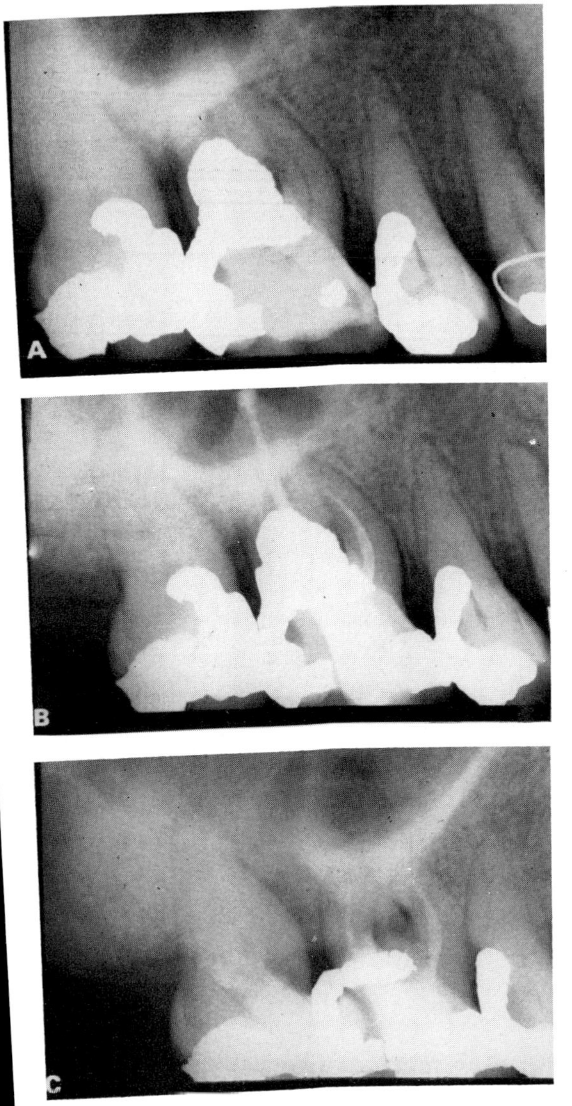

Figure 310. Case of endodontic-periodontic syndrome; combined etiology; palatal root (*halo* at apex) has bone destruction completely to the apex; treatment is endodontic therapy and radisectomy of palatal root. A. Before treatment; upper left first molar is pulpally-involved and palatal root is involved periodontally. B. Three canals obturated with gutta-percha-chloropercha. C. Palatal root amputated. (From D. R. Morse, "The Management of Endodontic Problem Cases," *JDA South Africa*, 27:387, 1972)

The results of treatment of the combined endodontic-periodontic syndrome cases and the cases of periodontal origin are fair and are not as predictable as the cases of endodontic origin. The following conditions are not related to the endodontic-periodontic syndrome, but still require combined endodontic-periodontic treatment. In molars (usually uppers), if one root has an *untreatable periodontal condition,* or a root that doesn't respond to treatment, and the remaining roots have satisfactory bony attachment or a treatable periodontal condition then a *radisectomy* (root amputation) can be performed. A radisectomy is a surgical procedure in which one root is removed from a multirooted tooth. The crown is not severed. The *area* where the root is removed from the remainder of the tooth is usually sealed with amalgam. Endodontic therapy is generally performed first on these radisectomy cases (Fig. 310). However, there have been recent reports of successful cases in which vital root amputations were performed. Endodontic therapy was not performed on the remaining roots. As there have not been any controlled studies to substantiate these claims of success, it is still recommended that endodontic therapy be performed on the remaining roots. The results of root amputation generally are good provided that no periodontal disease exists on the remaining roots or the periodontal condition is treatable. Also, the tooth must have a coronal restoration that is serviceable and there must not be undue trauma on the tooth.

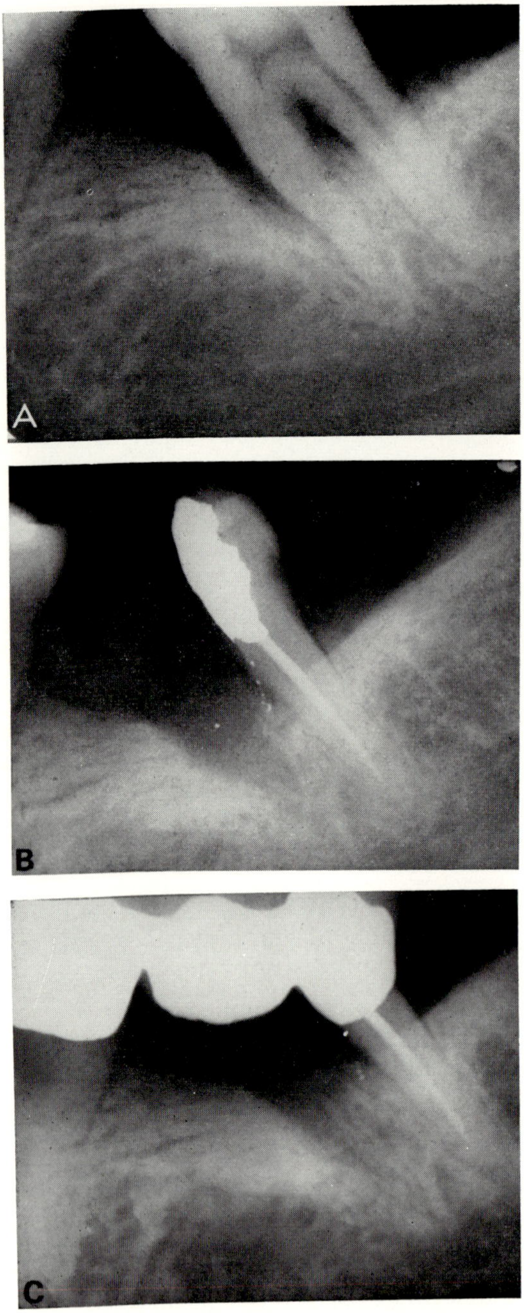

Figure 311. Hemisection following endodontic therapy on a lower molar. A. Before treatment; mesial root has inadequate bony support and there is a bifurcation involvement. B. Following root canal obturation with gutta-percha-chloropercha, hemisection, removal of the mesial crown-root complex, and contouring of the distal crown-root complex. C. Nine months later, fixed bridge is in position. (From D. R. Morse, "The Significance of Endodontics in Plantation Procedures," *JDA South Africa*, 26:263, 1971)

In periodontally-involved molars (usually lowers) with *untreatable furcation involvements* or furca that are unresponsive to treatment, the teeth may be saved by a procedure called *hemisection*. A hemisection is a surgical procedure in which a tooth is sectioned into two equal parts after endodontic therapy has been completed. The tooth is sectioned through the furcation area. One crown-root section may be extracted or both may be retained, depending upon the restorative procedures that might be entailed, the amount of supporting bone remaining, and the remaining space between the sections, after hemisection has been done. If a full complement of teeth is present, and other conditions are favorable, then both sections are kept and full crowns are made. In other cases, one section is retained and is used as a bridge abutment (Fig. 311). If there is a potential abutment with good bony support adjacent to the tooth that is to be sectioned and there is any doubt about the adequacy of the crown-root section that is to be retained, then it is more practical to extract the doubtful molar. However, if a crown-root section is to be retained, then temporary *external splinting* is necessary until the permanent splint is ready. Splinting is the act of horizontal stabilization of teeth that are either mobile, or have poor bony support. The methods in use include silk,

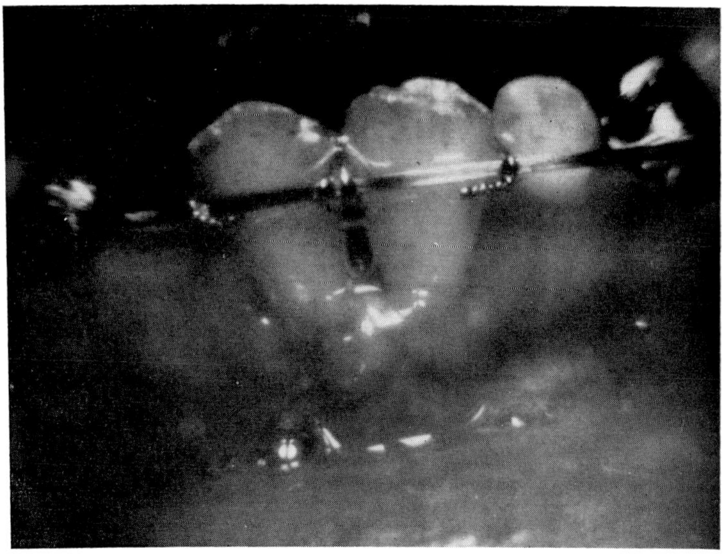

Figure 312. Orthodontic wire splint with brackets. (Courtesy of Dr. K. Bomze, Cherry Hill, N. J.)

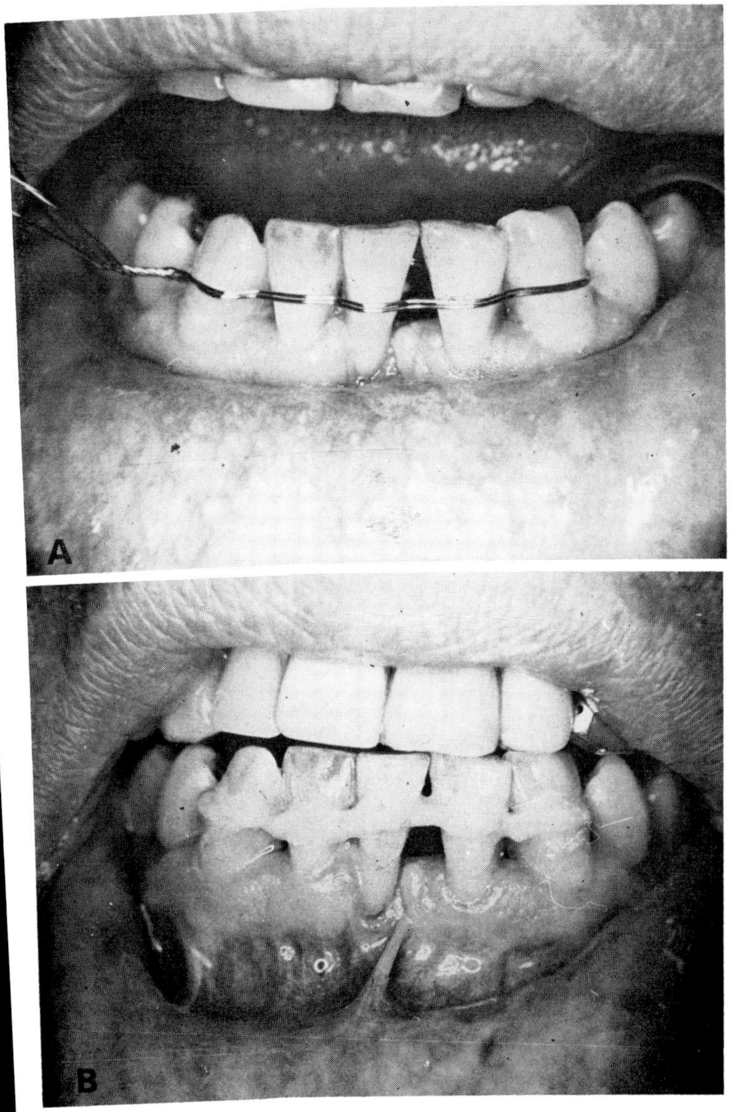

Figure 313. Wire-acrylic splint. A. Wire being inserted. B. Acrylic covers wire; no sharp edges are exposed. (Courtesy of Dr. M. Gross, Philadelphia, Pa.)

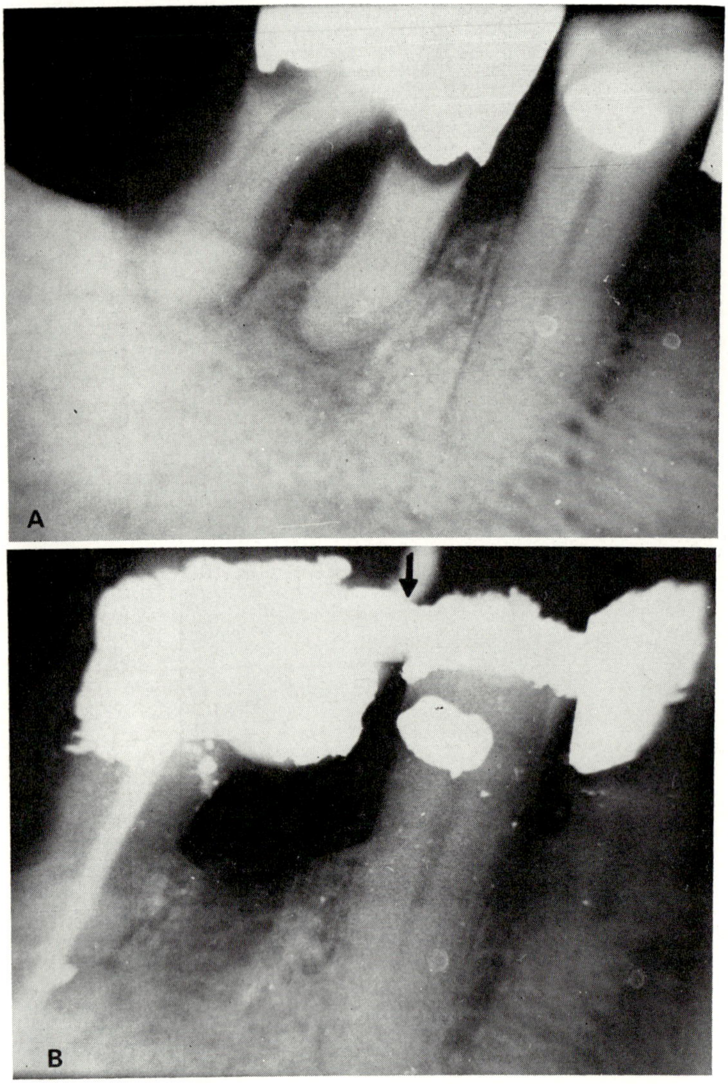

grassline, wire (orthodontic type) with or without brackets (Fig. 312), acrylic, wire-acrylic (Fig. 313), pin reinforced amalgam or acrylic (A-splint, Figs. 314, 315), cemented steel crown-bar type, U-V-activated plastic splint (Fig. 316), and orthodontic bands or wires that are cemented along the labial (buccal) surface (Fig. 317). For posterior teeth, the simplest splints to use are wire, and for anterior teeth, wire-acrylic or acrylic. The strongest are the cemented steel crown type and the pin-reinforced amalgam.

Results are good for hemisection cases, provided that periodontal disease is either not present or controllable for the remaining root. Also, the tooth must not be overloaded.

Another type of case requiring both

←

Figure 314. Amalgam A. Splints. A. Lower molar requiring caries removal, hemisection, an endodontic implant, and a temporary splint (provisional splint). B. After caries removal, hemisection, endodontic implant insertion and pin-reinforced amalgam splint placement (arrow). C. Clinical picture of an amalgam A splint. (Courtesy of Dr. M. Gross, Philadelphia, Pa.)

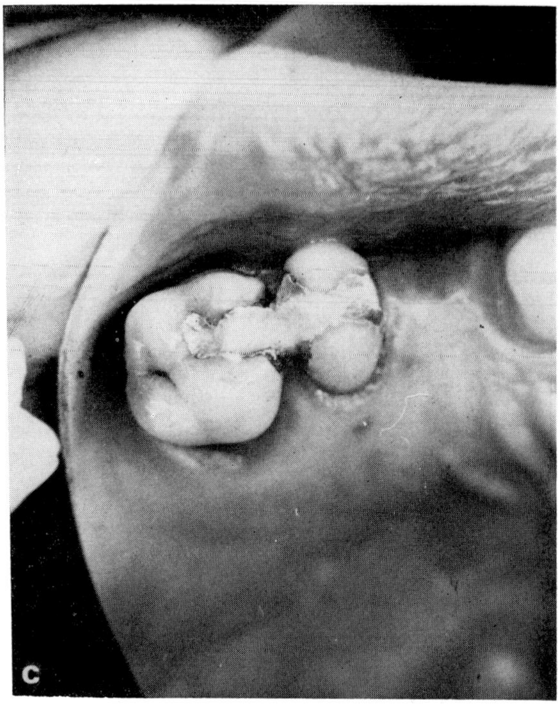

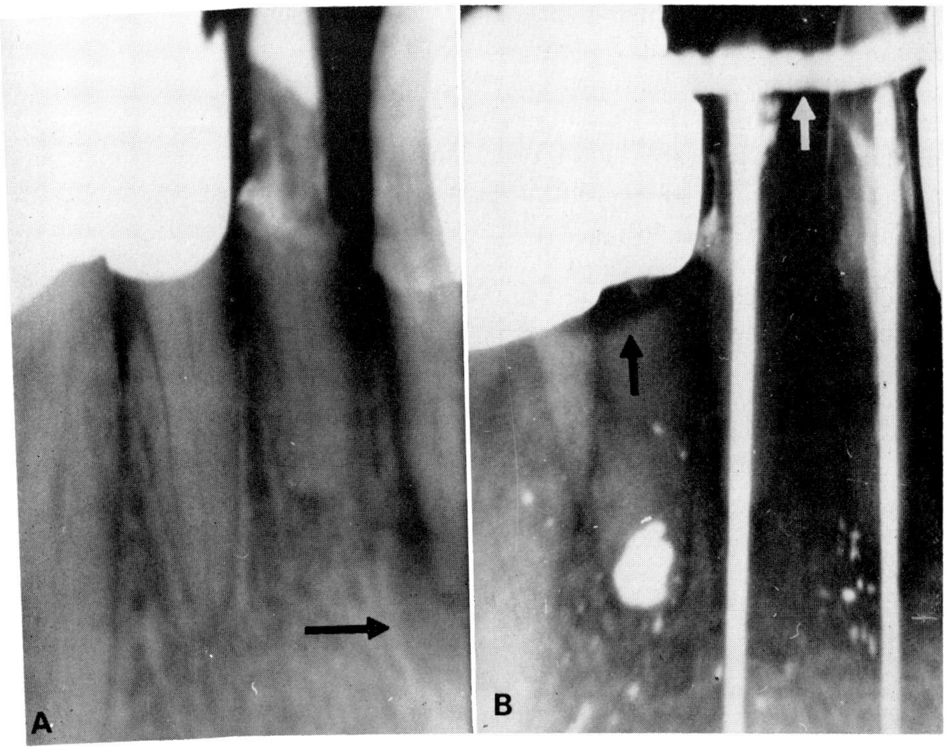

Figure 315. Lower anterior region requiring endodontic implants, a retrograde amalgam seal, and temporary splinting. A. Before treatment; periapical *area* present (arrow). B. Four years after endodontic implants and a retroseal were placed; periapical healing is evident; an acrylic A splint is in position (white arrow); recurrent caries is evident (black arrow). (From D. R. Morse, "Endodontic Implants: A Review and New Approach," *New York State Dental Journal*, 35:5, 1969)

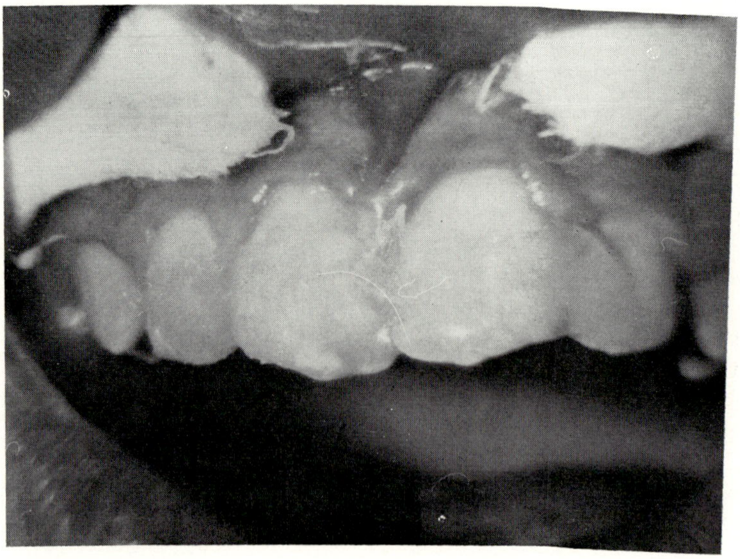

Figure 316. A U-V activated plastic splint. (Courtesy of Dr. K. Bomze, Cherry Hill, N. J.)

endodontic and periodontal treatment is the *periodontal case showing either excessive mobility or minimal bone support* (about 3 mm of remaining bone attachment) (Fig. 175L). Periodontal treatment alone is not satisfactory in decreasing the mobility or in restoring the bone level. Provided that it is important to save the tooth, an *endodontic implant* can be inserted through the root to increase the crown-root ratio and stabilize the tooth (Fig. 318). An endodontic implant is a smooth or threaded (screw-type) tapered metal rod of either chrome-cobalt alloy (Vitallium) or titanium alloy (Plantanium). Both these alloys are relatively inert but in research at Temple University School of Dentistry with dogs and tissue culture, titanium has been found to be less corrosive. There have been more clinical results with the smooth-type as compared to the threaded-type of implants, and the author's clinical experience has been primarily with the smooth-type. However, recent papers have stated that threaded implants are more effective. Under current investigation at Temple University are both the screw and smooth-type implants and when these experiments are completed a more thorough evaluation of the threaded type can be made.

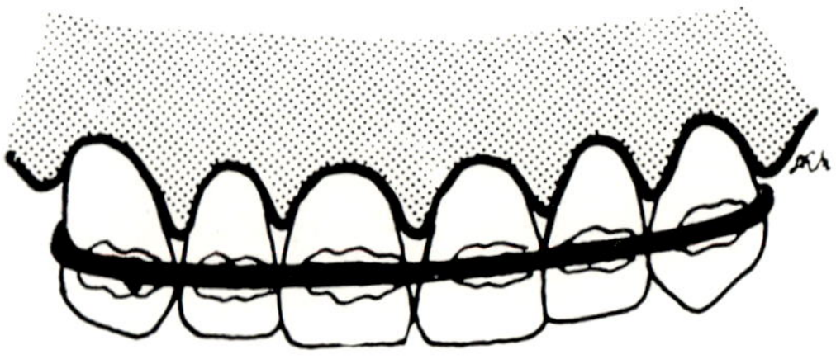

Figure 317. Splinting using rectangular orthodontic wire and zinc polycarboxylate cement.

An endodontic implant is usually inserted several millimeters beyond the apex of a prepared root canal into periapical bone (apical endodontic implant) (Fig. 319A). In cases where ana-

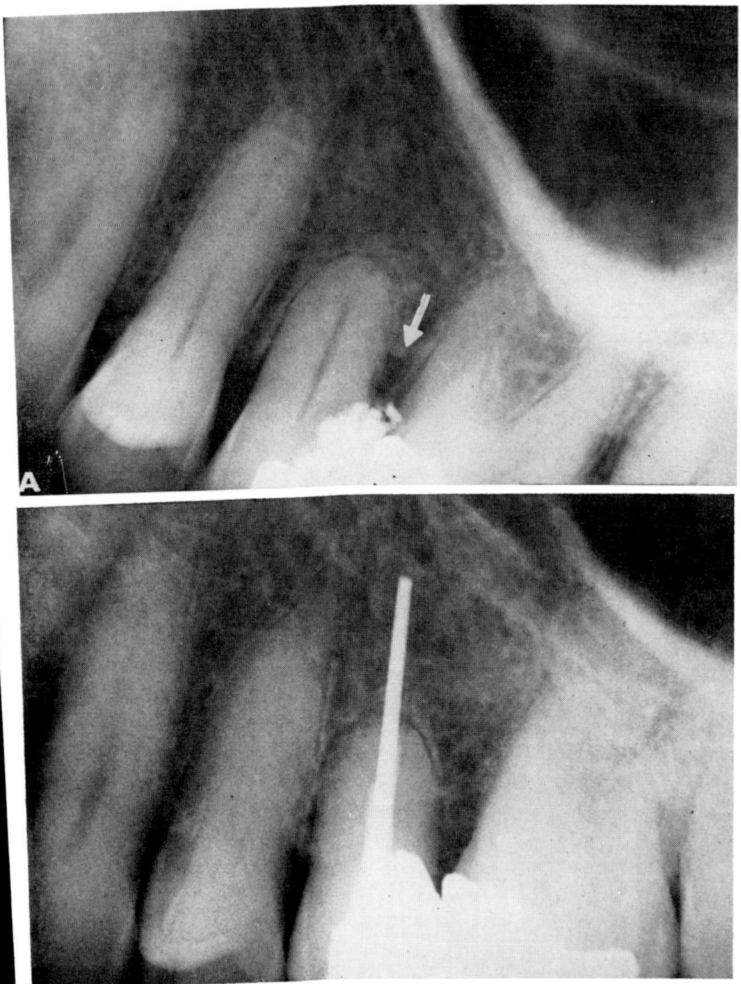

Figure 318. Periodontally involved upper second premolar with minimum bone support; tooth stabilized and crown-root ratio restored by means of an endodontic implant. A. Before treatment; arrow indicates bone destruction. B. Almost four years later, bone level is good; no mobility is evident and the tooth is symptom-free. (From D. R. Morse, "The Significance of Endodontics in Plantation Procedures," *JDA South Africa,* 26:263, 1971)

tomic landmarks might interfere (mental foramen, inferior alveolar canal, maxillary sinus, nasal fossa) or adjoining roots are in the path, then implants are inserted through the sides of the root (lateral root endosteal implant) after the root canal(s) is conventionally filled. Lateral-type implants are also used for cases where the inclination of the tooth is such that periapical extension would cause alveolar mucosa penetration and for cases with calcified or otherwise obstructed canals (Fig. 319B). In connection with the former indication, implants should never be bent in order to avoid alveolar mucosal penetration. A bent implant can act as an orthodontic appliance and cause labial displacement of an anterior tooth. In order to do a lateral-type implant, bone must be available, either proximally or palatally.

Endodontic implants are cemented into position with a root canal cement.

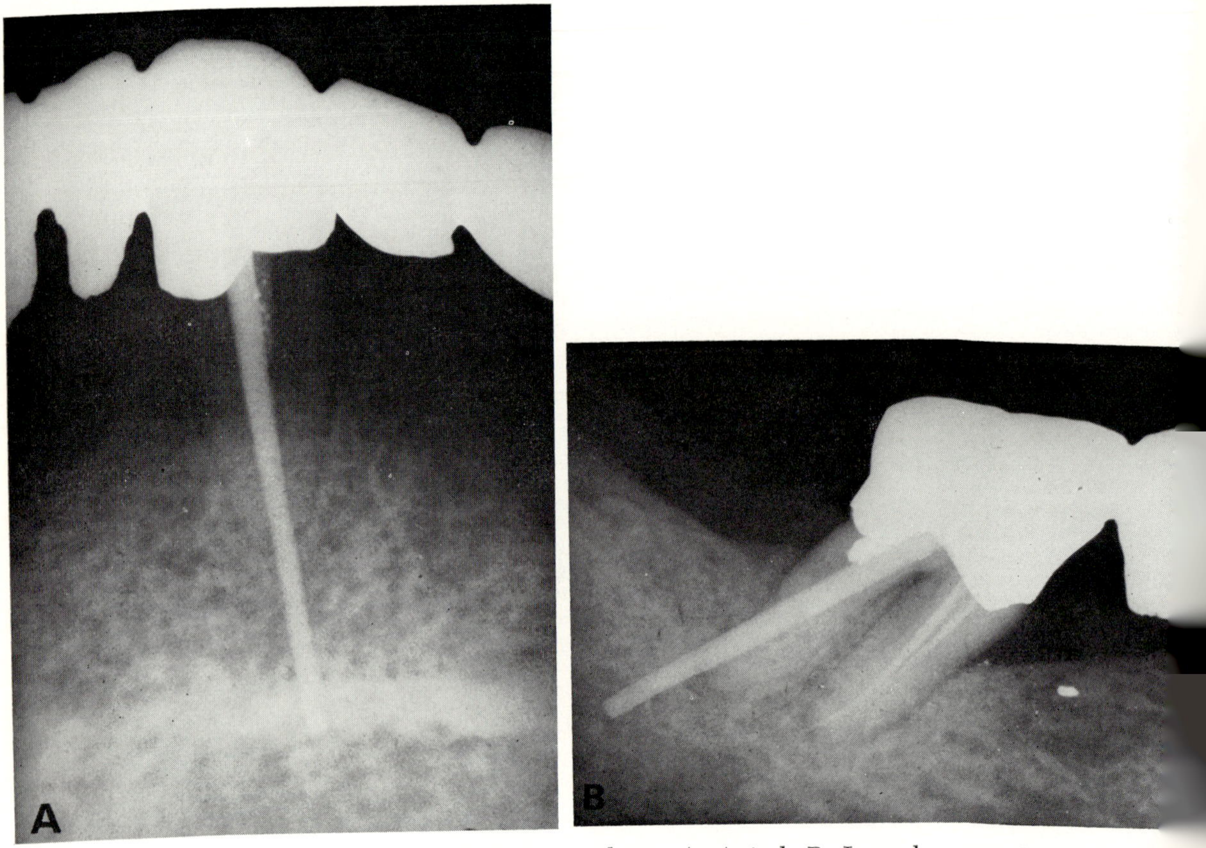

Figure 319. Two types of endodontic implants: A. Apical. B. Lateral root endosteal. (From D. R. Morse, F. Nislow, and N. Busch, "The Full Arch Splint Using Endodontic Implants: Report of Case," *Journal of the American Dental Association*, 85:351, 1972, copyright by the American Dental Association, reprinted by permission.)

The cases are usually treated nonsurgically. Indications for periapical surgery are cases in which a periapical or combined periapical and periodontal pathosis exists or when a fractured root apex has to be removed. The results for endodontic implant treatment of periodontally involved cases depend greatly upon the outcome of the periodontal therapy. If the latter can be successfully performed, and the patient can maintain good oral hygiene, then often the prognosis is fairly good. If periodontal treatment cannot be successfully undertaken, then the prognosis is poor. Usually *external splinting* should be performed along with the implant insertion. The splint should be kept in position while the periodontal healing is taking place (up to 6 weeks).

Localized Fluctuant Abscesses

These abscesses may be located on the buccal mucosa, the floor of the mouth, the palatal region, or the skin. Treatment is *incision and drainage* (I&D).

This surgical procedure entails a scalpel incision through the most dependent part of the swelling. The incision is made through to the bone (if possible). The fluid is then aspirated and a drain of either iodoform gauze or rubber dam is inserted (Fig. 320). If the swelling is indurated and not localized, drainage is poor and the patient usually does not get symptomatic relief. In the usual case, relief is dramatic. Along with the drainage through the alveolar mucosa, the lingual or occlusal aspect of the tooth should be opened. If there is a *purulent or sanguinous exudate* that does not stop after a few moments, then the *tooth should be left open for drainage*. Occasionally, swelling of the gingiva or alveolar mucosa can be drained through the gingival sulcus. This is true for *periapical abscesses* that communicate with the gingival sulcus. Treatment is *currettage* until drainage is established (Fig. 321).

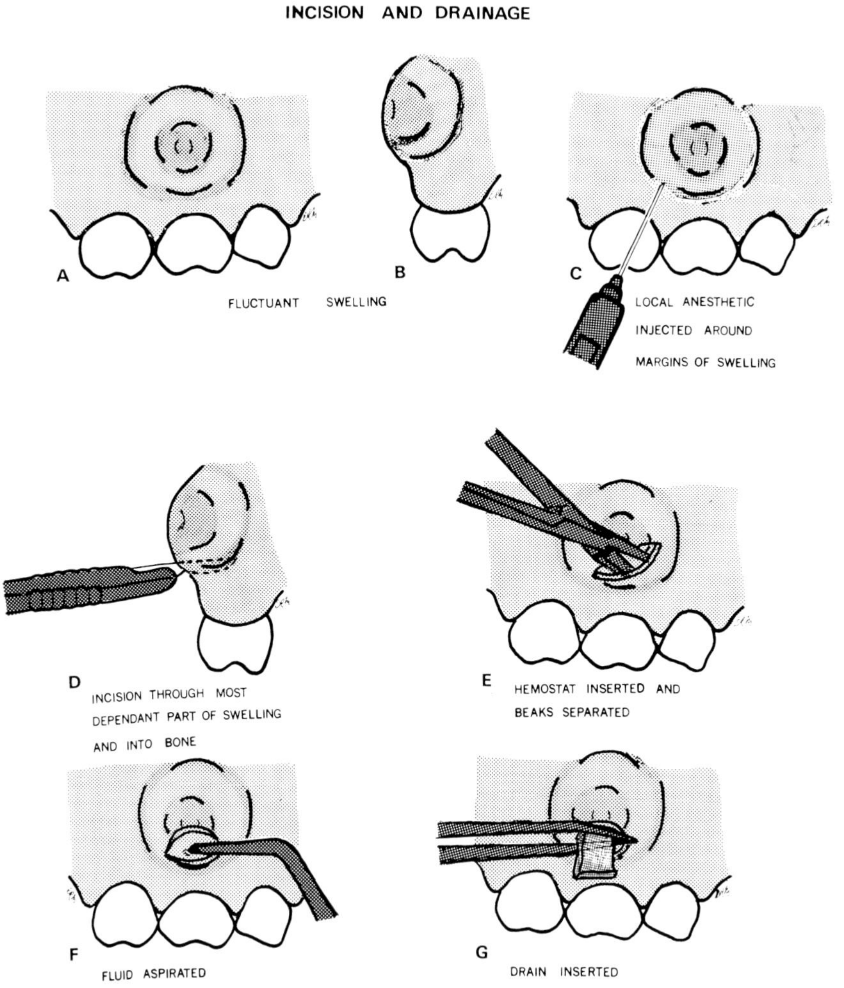

Figure 320 A-G. Incision and drainage; various stages in the procedure.

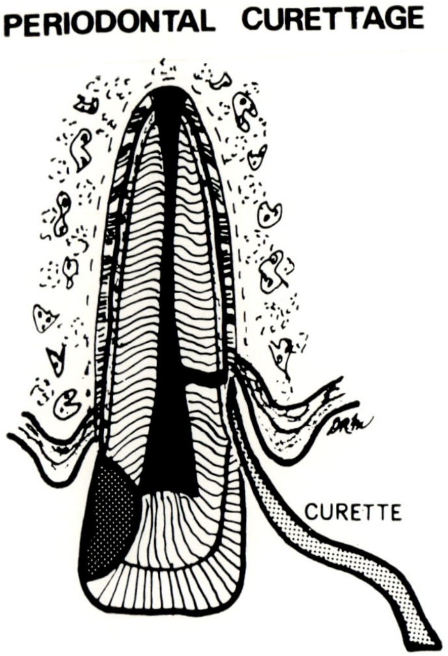

Figure 321

Unbearable Pain, Before, During, or After Completion of Endodontic Therapy That Cannot Be Controlled by Instrumentation, Medication, Analgesic Drugs, and Antibiotics

Provided that the root canal obturation is apparently well done (if pain occurs after completion of therapy), and there is no apparent swelling (this could be treated by incision and drainage and/or antibiotics), then *trephination* (artificial fistularization) should be performed and the tooth should be taken out of occlusal contact. Trephination is a surgical procedure in which an artificial opening is made through the cortical bone in the vicinity of the root apex. Usually a small incision is made with a scalpel, which is followed by bur penetration to the desired area (Fig. 322). There is an instrument available called a Sargenti Fistulator® (Medidenta) that is used for trephination. It is an effective alternative method to the use of the scalpel and bur (Fig. 323). The purpose of trephination is to allow for possible drainage and relief of pain. The results are usually good. If success is not achieved, then periapical surgery is necessary. If periapical surgery is not possible, then an intentional replant can be tried. Other indications for trephination are the presence of a post that cannot be removed, silver cones or root canal instruments lodged within canals, and an apparently calcified canal. Endodontic therapy must be performed later (nonsurgical or surgical).

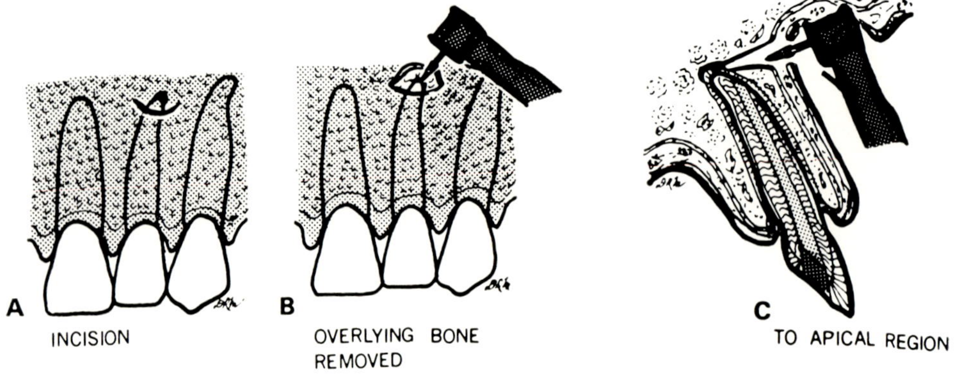

Figure 322 A-C. Three stages in the procedure of trephination.

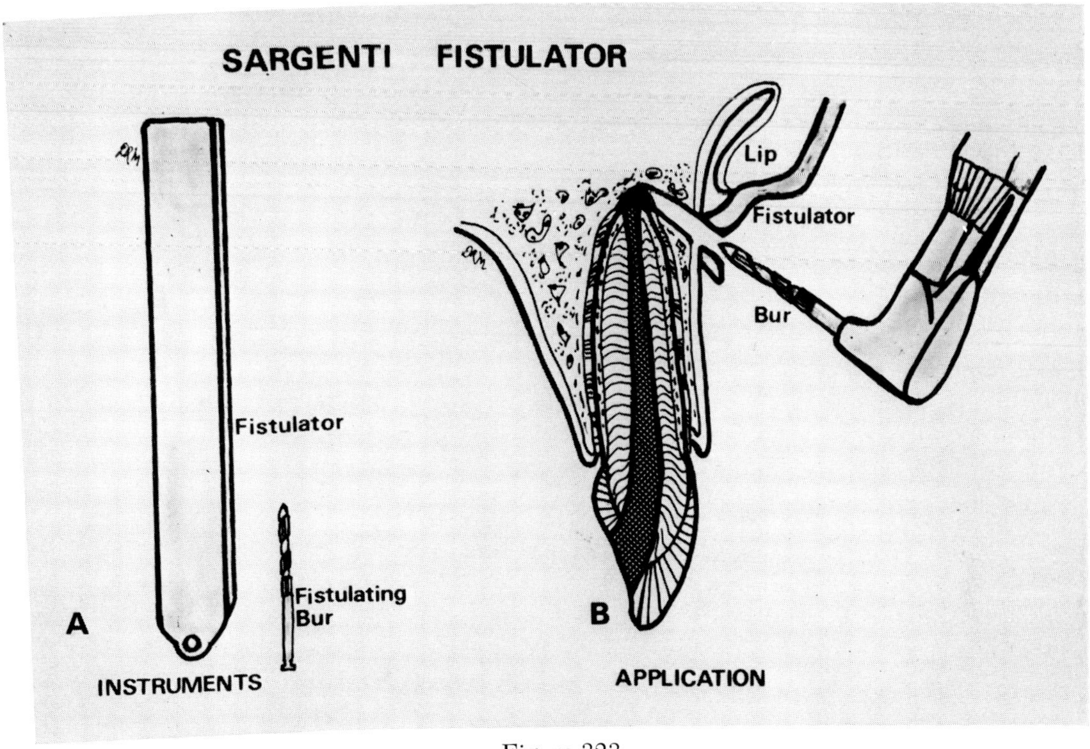

Figure 323

Drainage Cannot Be Controlled and There Is a Large Periapical *Area* Present

If drainage cannot be diminished by instrumentation and medication and periapical surgery is not the primary treatment choice, then the procedure of *marsupialization* can be attempted. A true marsupialization procedure entails an incision into a lesion (usually a cyst), exposure of the anterior wall and overlying skin or mucous membrane, and suturing of the cut edges of the remaining anterior section to the adjacent skin or mucous membrane. The purpose is to evacuate the fluid and allow for shrinkage and possible complete regression of the lesion. In endodontics, a polyvinyl or polyethylene tube is periodically inserted and cut back until the lesion shrinks sufficiently and exudation ceases. Then, nonsurgical endodontic therapy for a pulpless tooth is performed (Fig. 324).

Cases in Which Nonsurgical Endodontic Therapy Is Either Not the Treatment of Choice, or Is Not Successful

The indicated treatment is *periapical surgery*, including periapical curettage, apicoectomy, and retrograde seal (Fig. 325). The definitions for each have been given under the section on the endodontic-periodontic syndrome. When root canal instrumentation and obturation is done at the same visit as the periapical surgery, the procedure is called *immediate surgical endodontics*. Whenever possible, both procedures should be performed at the same visit to pre-

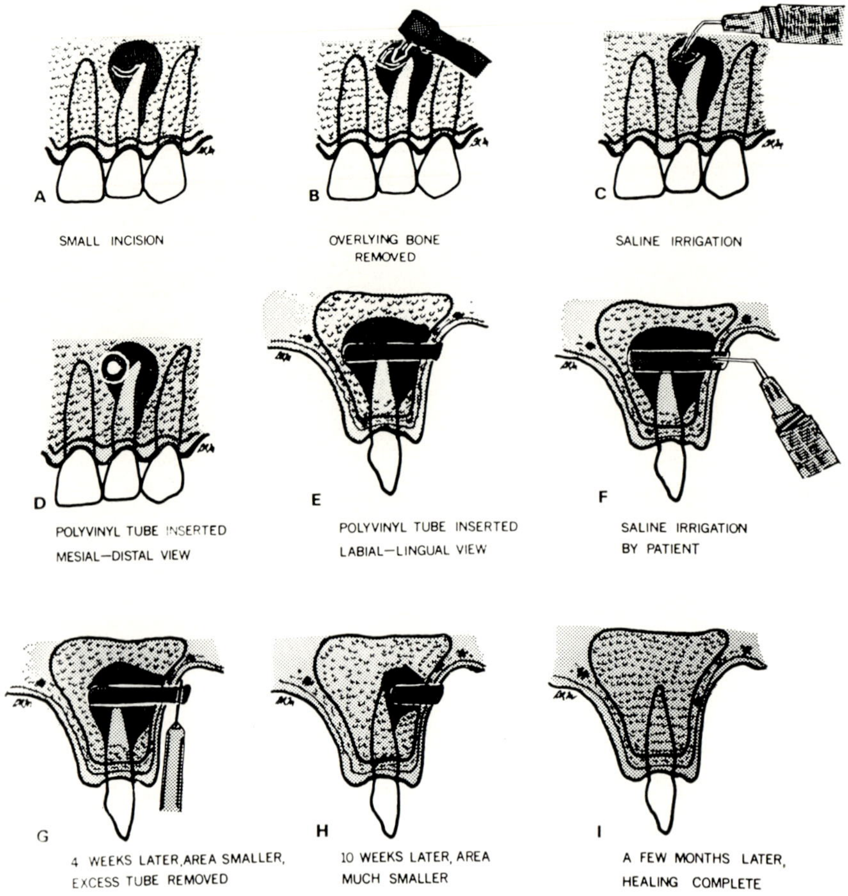

Figure 324 A-I. Various stages in marsupialization.

vent development of pain and/or swelling. All tissues removed should be placed in 10 percent formalin and sent to a pathology laboratory for histological diagnosis. The various indications for periapical surgery include the following:

(1) Failure to control exudation during treatment (an alternative to marsupialization).

(2) Failure to control pain during treatment (an alternative to trephination).

(3) Instrument broken in canal, it cannot be bypassed, and there is a periapical *area* present (Fig. 326).

(4) Ledge created in canal, it cannot be bypassed, and there is a periapical *area* present.

(5) Pulp stone or dentin debris in canal, it cannot be bypassed, and there is a periapical *area* present (Fig. 327).

(6) Previous root canal filling or post that cannot be removed, and there is a periapical *area* present (Fig. 328).

(7) Calcified canals or lateral canals that are impenetrable, and

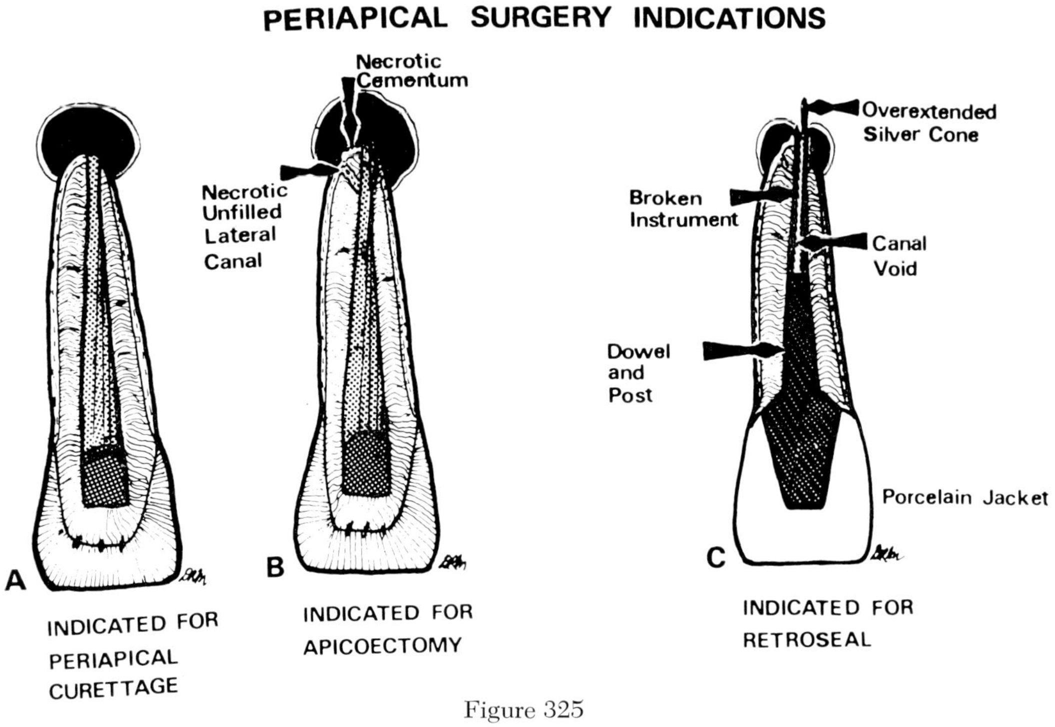

Figure 325

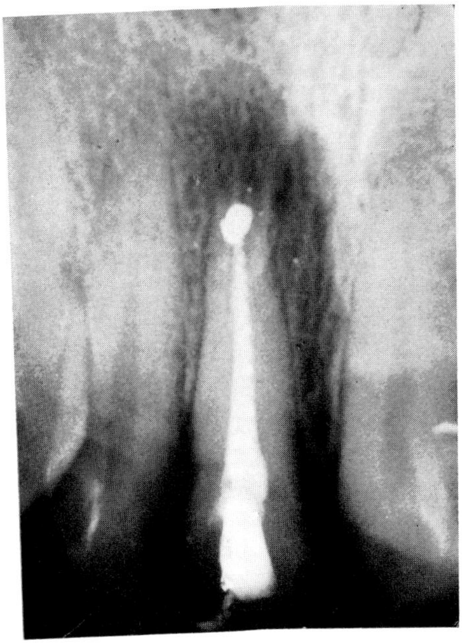

Figure 326. Upper left central incisor; reamer was broken in canal; gutta-percha-chloropercha condensed along the instrument and an amalgam retroseal is placed. (From D. R. Morse "The Management of Endodontic Problem Cases," *JDA South Africa,* 27:387, 1972)

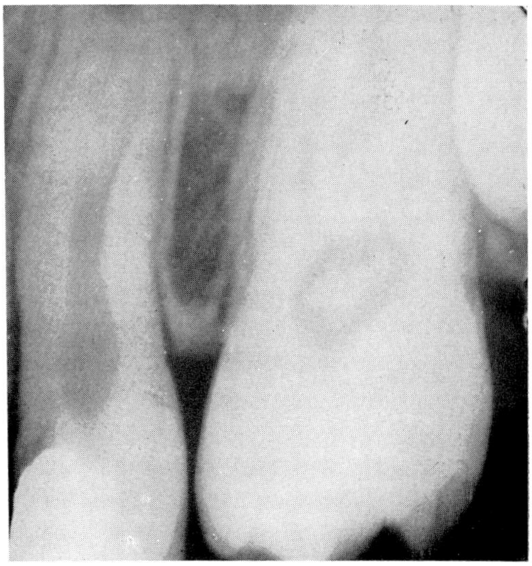

Figure 327. Large pulp stone in chamber; if it cannot be removed or bypassed, retrograde obturation may be necessary.

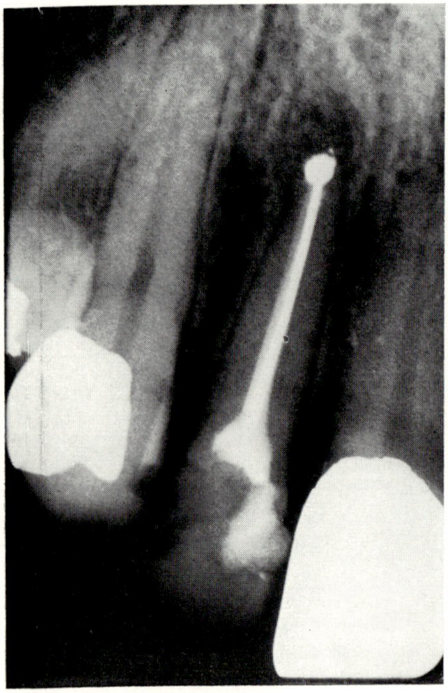

Figure 328. Previous silver cone was present that could not be dislodged; an amalgam retroseal is placed. (From D. R. Morse, "The Management of Endodontic Problem Cases," *JDA South Africa*, 27:387, 1972)

there is a periapical or lateral *area* present (Fig. 329). If a lateral canal is on the lingual (palatal) aspect, it is usually not possible to treat it surgically and failure can occur.

(8) Extreme root curvature (dilaceration) in which the canal(s) are not negotiable to the apex, and there is a periapical *area* present (Fig. 330). In these last six indications, first an attempt should be made to negotiate the canal using a calcium chelating agent complex (R-C Prep®, Premier®).

(9) Impenetrable bifurcating canals; occasionally on lower premolars, lower canines, and lower incisors, the main canal bifurcates into two or more branches far down in the root (Figs. 291A, 331A). It is rarely possible to instrument and obturate both of the branches (Figs. 291B, 331B, 400). Only those cases with definite *areas* should be treated surgically, the others should be observed periodically. If periapical areas of

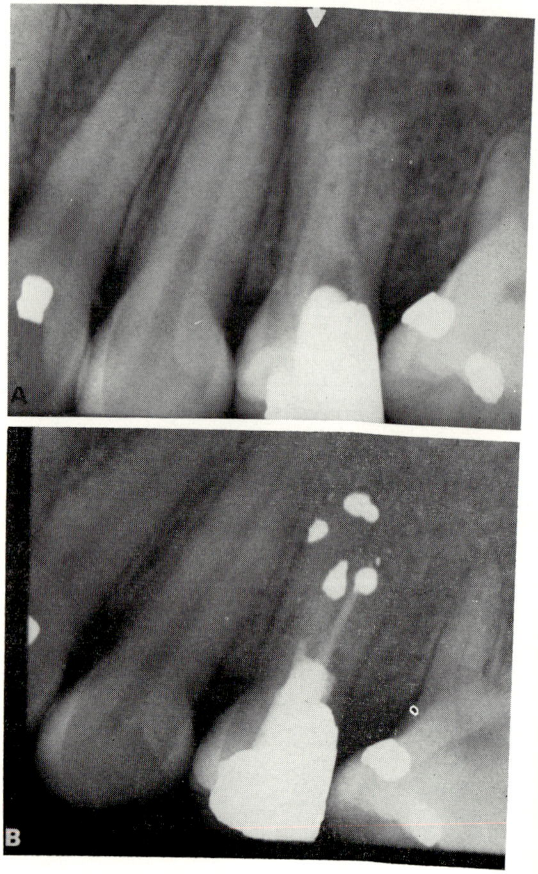

Figure 329. Upper first premolar with three roots and impenetrable canals; periapical area of pathosis is present. A. Before; arrow indicates area of pathosis. B. Over two years later; four apexes had been sealed with amalgam; bone repair is evident.

rarefaction develop, then surgery should be done. Periapical surgery is extremely difficult in the lower premolar area, and if the mental foramen is close to the root apex, periapical surgery should not be attempted, and the involved tooth should be extracted or an intentional replant should be attempted.

(10) External resorption that doesn't cease after nonsurgical endodontic therapy has been performed or following transplantation or replantation procedures. The prognosis with periapical surgery on these cases is only fair (Fig. 171).

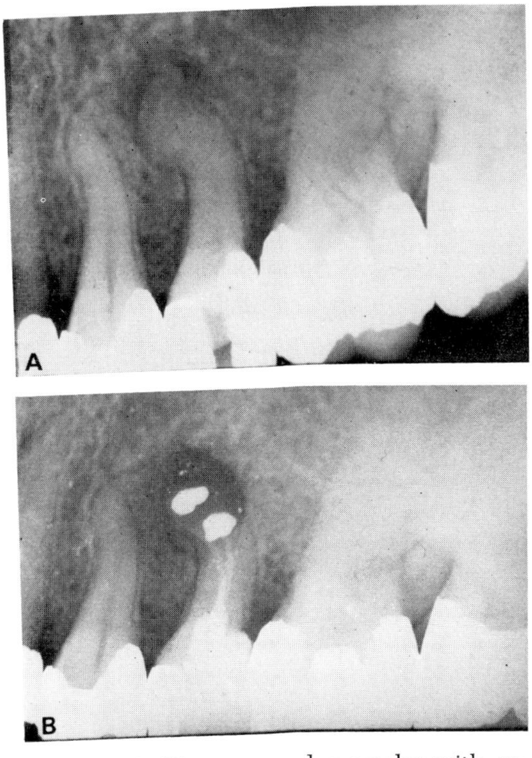

Figure 330. Upper second premolar with extreme root curvature; canals not negotiable to the apexes, and periapical *area* is present. A. Before treatment. B. One year following therapy with gutta-percha-chloropercha and amalgam retroseals; periapical repair is occurring. (From D. R. Morse, "The Management of Endodontic Problem Cases," *JDA South Africa*, 27:387, 1972)

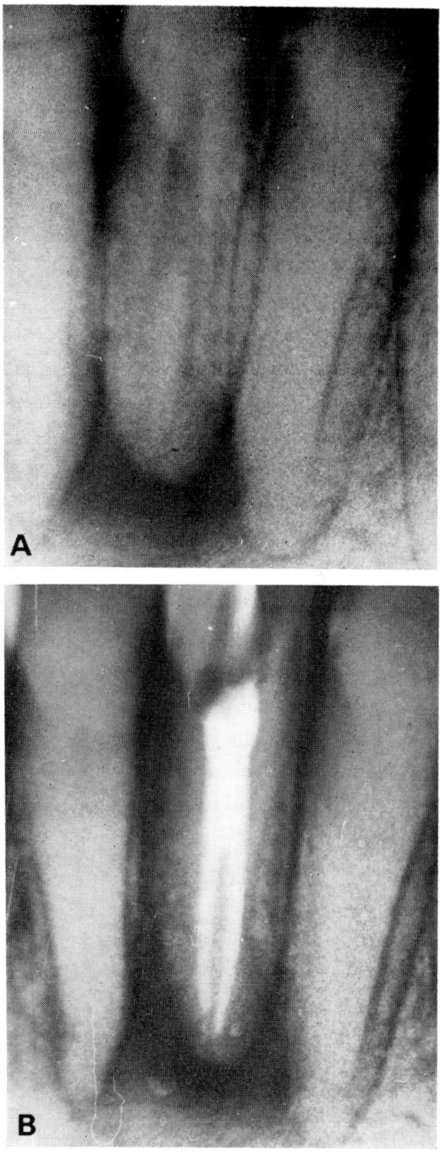

Figure 331. Bifurcating lower central incisor treated by nonsurgical endodontic therapy. A. Before treatment. B. After obturation with gutta-percha and root canal cement. (Courtesy of Dr. L. Muldorf, Philadelphia, Pa.)

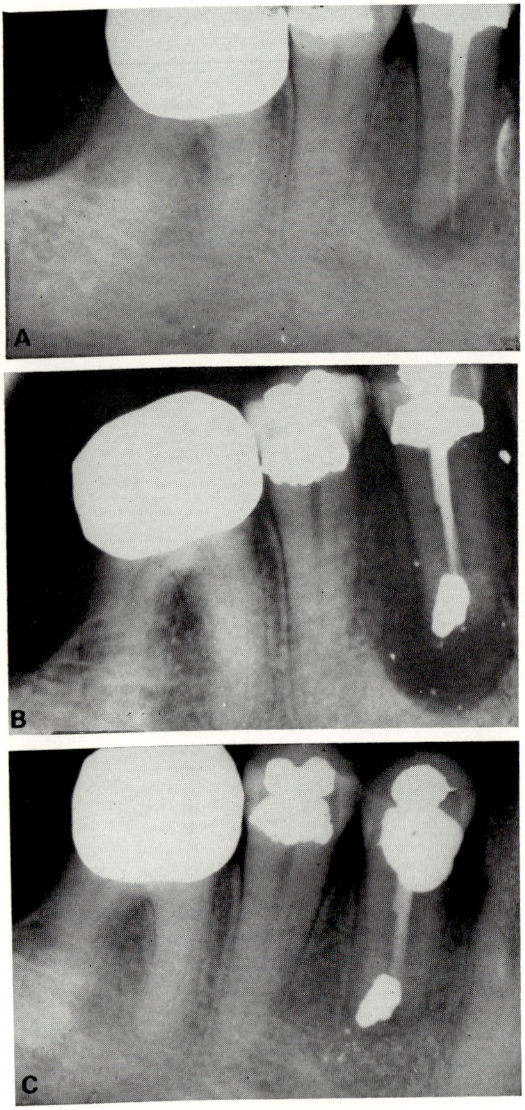

Figure 332. Perforation of lower first premolar; perforation could not be sealed by nonsurgical endodontic therapy; periapical surgery and a retroseal was done. A. After obturation with gutta-percha-chloropercha; a perforation is evident (*area* had enlarged after the obturation). B. After apicoectomy (performed at a 45° angle from above to avoid the mental foramen) and a retrograde amalgam seal. C. Over two years later; repair is evident; patient did not develop paresthesia. (From D. R. Morse, "The Management of Endodontic Problem Cases," *JDA South Africa*, 21:387, 1972)

(11) Perforation or internal resorption that cannot be sealed by nonsurgical endodontic therapy (the latter should be tried first). In the previous two cases, the prognosis is good provided that the root canal is well sealed to the apex and that the perforation or internal resorption is above the level of the attached bone (for maxillary teeth). If the defect is below the level of the attached bone (for maxillary teeth), then a periodontal pocket will occur to the level of the perforation or internal resorption (the reverse is true for mandibular teeth) (Figs. 332, 333). If the *internal resorption* causes a *complete severance of the root,* then the severed apical root section should be removed and an *endodontic implant* should be inserted (Fig. 334). If external or internal resorption is so extensive that there would not be enough tooth structure remaining for either an *endodontic implant* or a coronal restoration, then the tooth should be extracted. Also, if the resorption occurs close to the coronal aspect of the tooth, then there could not be enough supporting bone remaining in the incisal portion and the tooth must be removed. If the remaining root can be exposed by gingivectomy and ostectomy procedures, then a post, core, and crown can be made and the tooth can be saved. The prob-

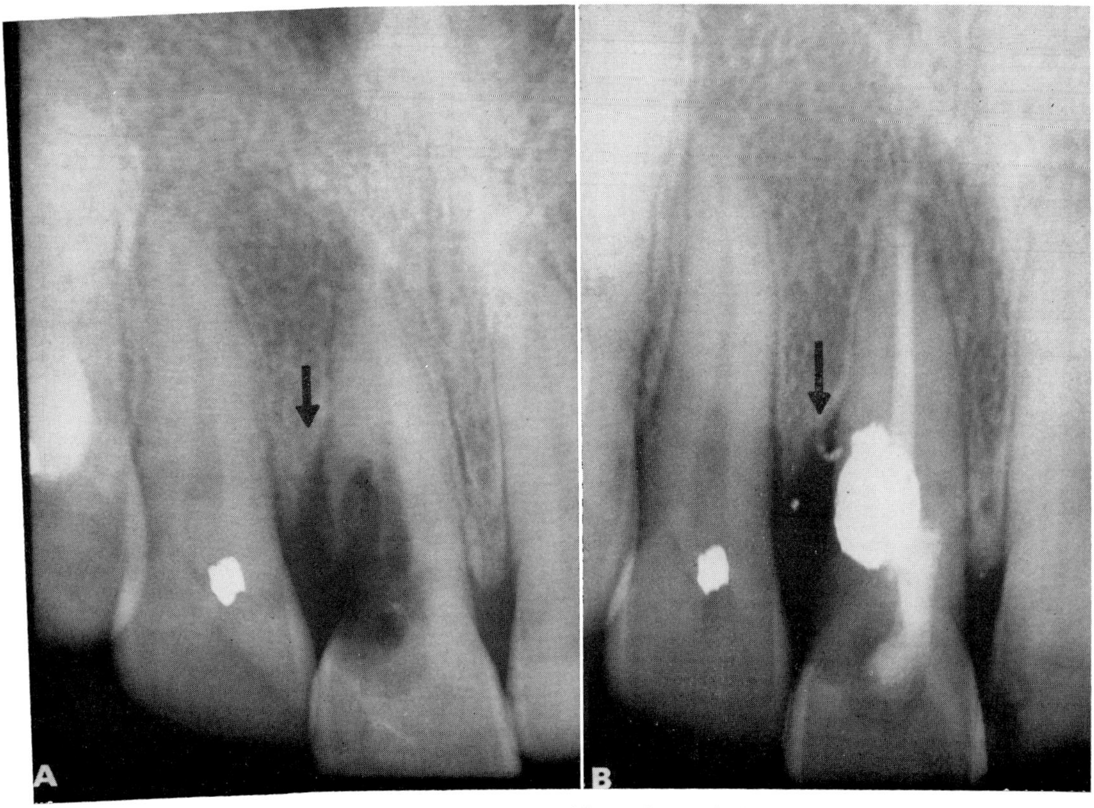

Figure 333. Internal resorption case that could not be sealed by nonsurgical endodontic therapy; defect was sealed with amalgam. A. Before treatment; upper left central incisor has periodontal pocket (arrow). B. Two years after obturation of the root canal with gutta-percha-chloropercha and surgical repair of the defect with amalgam; pocket is still present to the level of the defect. (From D. R. Morse, "The Management of Endodontic Problem Cases," *JDA South Africa,* 27:387, 1972.)

lem then would be whether the esthetic result is satisfactory.

(12) Porcelain jacket or crown that has esthetic value, and there is a possibility of a fracture occurring during the access preparation. If the remainder of the root canal is not treated and filled the prognosis is only fair. It is therefore preferable to do nonsurgical endodontic therapy and risk fracture of the restoration.

(13) Fixed bridge or partial denture attachment, such as a precision attachment, that is on the involved tooth and is in the pathway of the access preparation. In this case, it also must be realized that chances for success are not as good because the root canals are not filled in their entirety when only a retrograde seal is placed.

(14) Foreign bodies such as paper points, cotton, cement, and sil-

ver cones pushed beyond the apex.

(15) Pulpless fractured root apex. If there is a discernible radiographic image of a *root fracture,* and the *tooth tests vital* and no symptoms are present, then *no treatment should* be done. The tooth should be checked periodically. If the tooth is *mobile,* a splint should be inserted for approximately six weeks and then the case should be re-evaluated. If the tooth tests *nonvital,* then *nonsurgical endodontic therapy* should be performed on the incisal portion of the tooth, and radiographs should be taken every six months. It is possible in these described cases, for fibrous or cementum repair of the fractured portions to occur. If the fractured portions separate and a *periapical area of rarefaction* and/or a *sinus tract* occurs, then *nonsurgical endodontic therapy* should be done followed by *removal* of the *apical section.* If the same conditions are present and the remaining incisal-root section would leave a very short root, then there are two possibilities. One is the *removal* of the *apical section,* followed by insertion of an *endodontic implant* (Figs. 335,

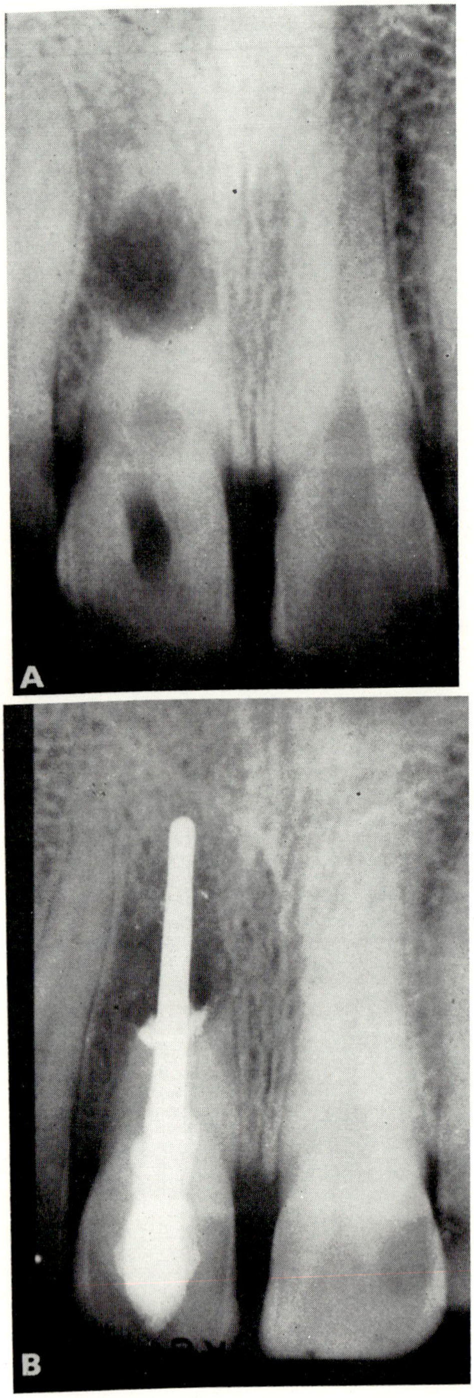

Figure 334. Internal resorption resulted in complete severance of the root; apical section was removed and an endodontic implant was inserted. A. Before treatment. B. Over two years after removal of apical section of root and insertion of endodontic implant (cemented in with polycarboxylate cement). (From D. R. Morse, "The Management of Endodontic Problem Cases," *JDA South Africa,* 27:387, 1972)

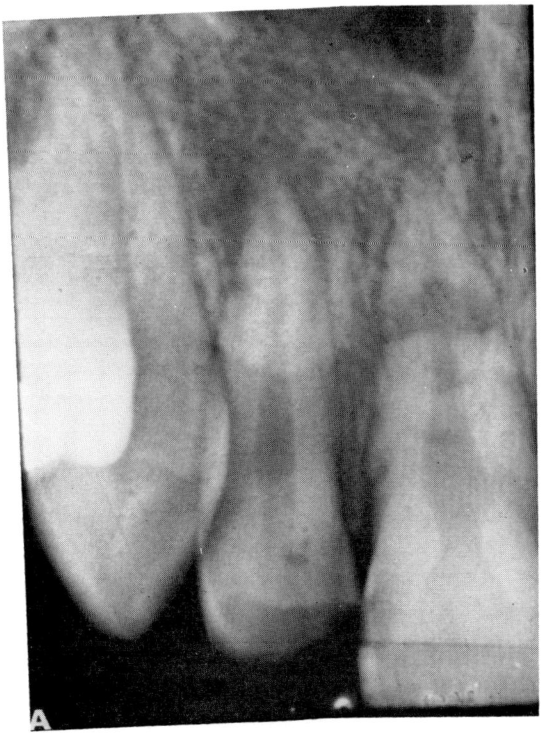

Figure 335. Upper central incisor with fractured root apex, excessive mobility and a draining sinus tract; lateral incisor had a necrotic pulp and a periapical area of pathosis. A. Before treatment; note displaced root fracture of the central incisor. B. For lateral incisor, obturation was by gutta-percha-chloropercha; for the central incisor, the apical portion was removed, a periapical curettage was performed, and an endodontic implant was inserted. C. Over four years later; bone repair is evident and the central incisor has remained firm and symptomless; unfortunately caries has occurred on the lateral incisor. (From D. R. Morse, "The Management of Endodontic Problem Cases," *JDA South Africa*, 27:387, 1972)

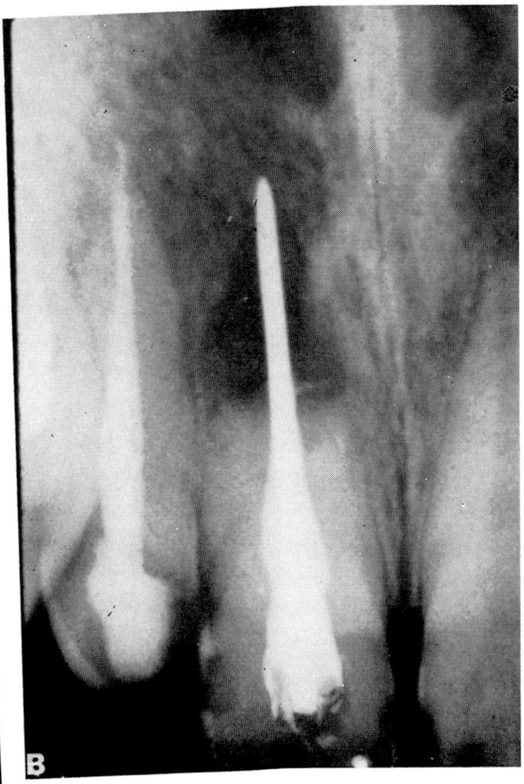

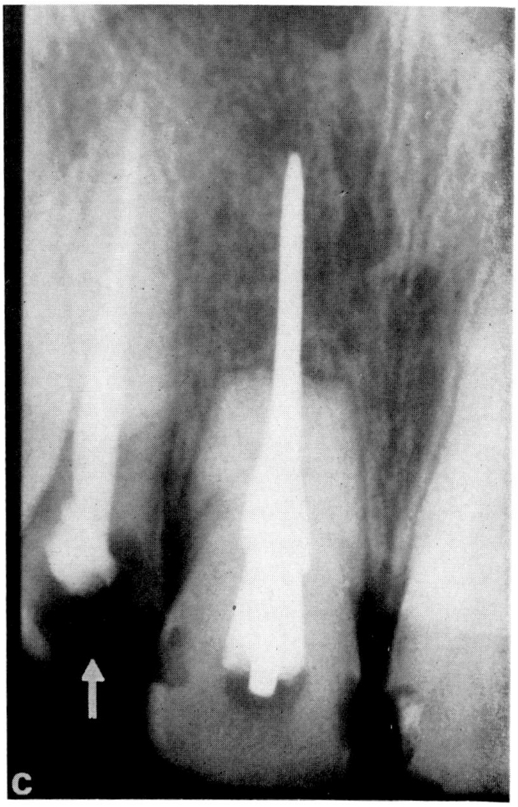

345A). The results are good if the apex is well sealed. A second possibility is instrumentation and *implant insertion* through both *root sections.* This is usually performed when the *separated portions are close to each other,* and there is no sinus tract present (Fig. 336). As very few cases of this type have been performed, it is too early to evaluate success. If the root fracture is close to the incisal part of the tooth and there is wide separation of the parts, then the incisal portion is removed because there would be insufficient supporting bone remaining for this portion. It then would be possible to perform a gingivectomy, ostectomy, post and crown insertion and still save the tooth. The problem in this case is primarily an esthetic one, as an extremely long clinical crown would result. Recently, an interesting new technique has been devised for these type cases. It involves the use of orthodontic therapy to bring the fractured root closer to the gingival margin to allow for a better esthetic result. If a vertical root fracture extends the entire cervical-apical distance, usually extraction is indicated. It is possible

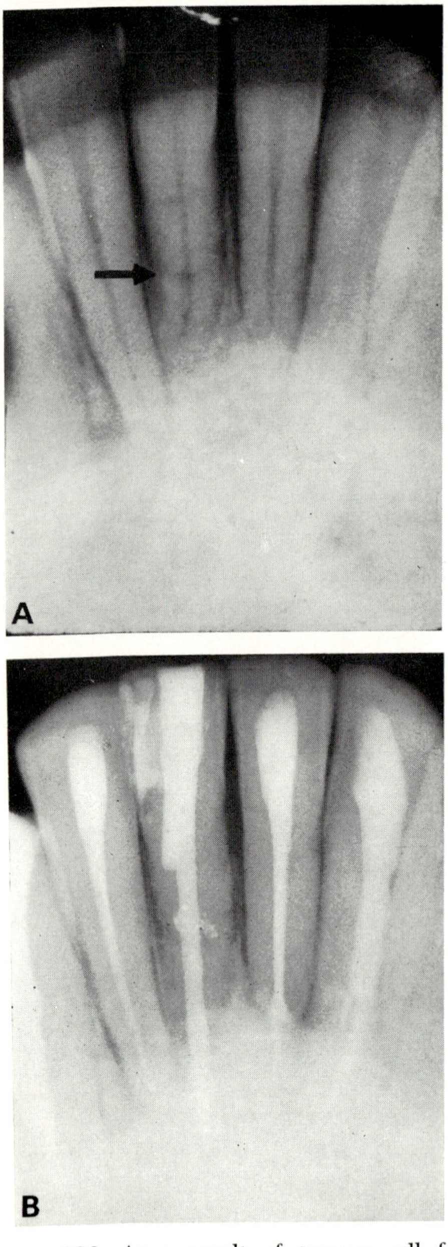

Figure 336. As a result of trauma, all four lower anteriors developed necrotic pulps; the lower left central incisor had a fractured root. A. Before treatment; arrow indicates root fracture. B. The right central incisor and the lateral incisors were obturated with gutta-percha-chloropercha; an endodontic implant was inserted through both sections of the left central incisor. (From D. R. Morse, "The Management of Endodontic Problem Cases," *JDA South Africa,* 27:387, 1972)

to attempt to save the tooth by removing the fractured part, and preparing the remaining part of the canal for an amalgam seal. The results are successful 50 percent of the time or less, as no attachment occurs to the amalgam and a periodontal pocket results. It is also possible that the weak root may fracture further (Fig. 337). A root with a partial vertical fracture can be treated by removal of the fractured part followed by a retroseal (Fig. 338).

(16) Impossibility to keep canal(s) uncontaminated because of fracture beneath the gingiva. If it is not possible to prevent the ingress of fluids into the canal so that a well filled root canal can be obtained, then microbes can lodge in canal spaces and failure may result, even with a good retrograde seal.

(17) Apparently well filled root canal, but patient has persisting pain and/or swelling. This may not be successful because the cause of the symptoms may be a vertical fracture or a canal branch that cannot be reached.

(18) Failure of pulpotomy or apexification procedure to close wide open apex.

(19) Sinus tract that persists after retreatment and/or cauterization. The cause might be overfilling into the alveolar mucosa. However if the cause is a ver-

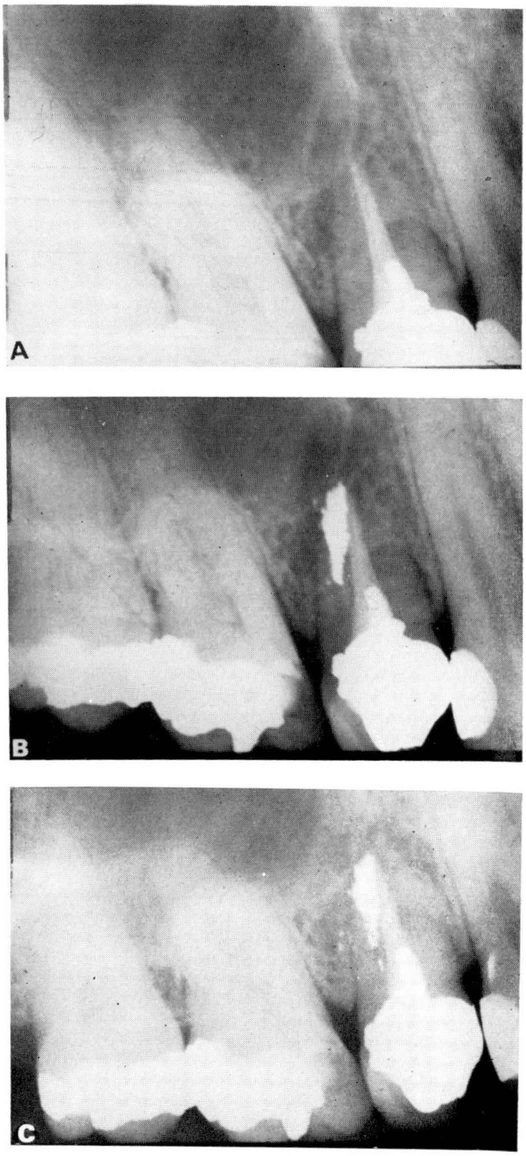

Figure 337. Upper second premolar with a vertical root fracture probably resulting from delay in placement of a permanent restoration. A. Before treatment. B. Fractured section removed; amalgam seal placed in a prepared trough. C. Over one year later; repair is evident. (From D. R. Morse, "The Management of Endodontic Problem Cases," *JDA South Africa*, 27:387, 1972)

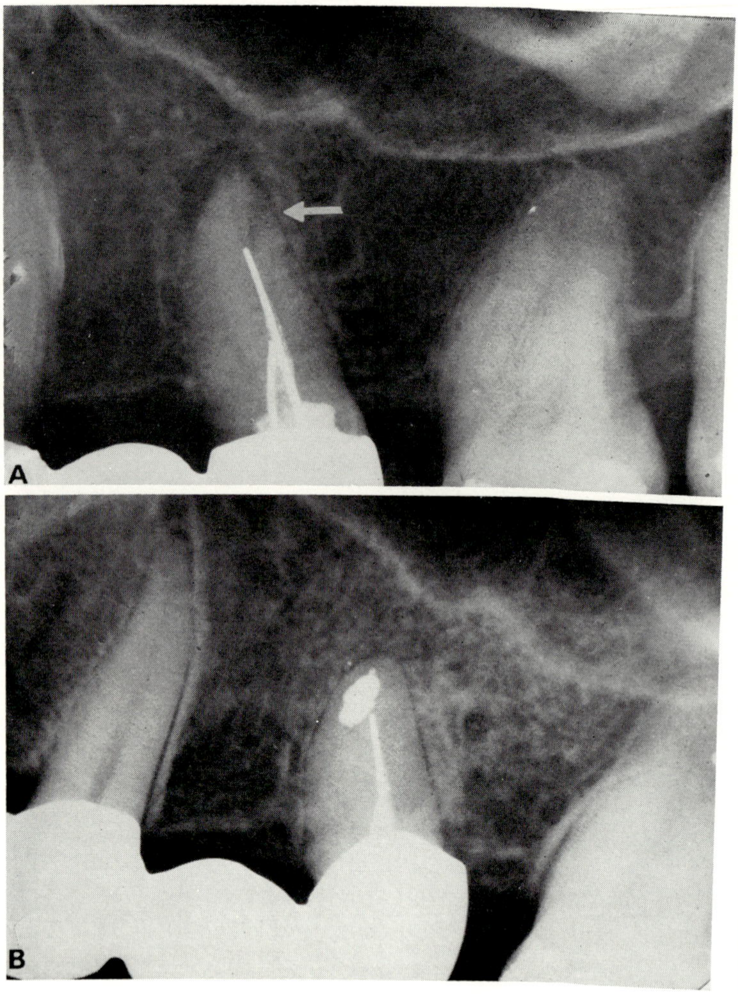

Figure 338. Upper second premolar with a small vertical root fracture; root canals had been sealed with silver cones, which could not be retrieved. A. Before treatment, arrow indicates fracture. B. Three years following removal of fractured portion and placement of amalgam in a prepared trough.

tical fracture, then failure would most probably result.

(20) As previously discussed, when there is planned simultaneous endodontic and periodontic surgery (see endodontic-periodontic syndrome).

(21) For those patients who have a cancerphobia, removal of the periapical lesion and tissue analysis should tend to allay their fears of cancer.

(22) For those cases in which the periapical lesion is associated with a pulpless tooth, but the radiographic appearance is not like the typical appearance of a radicular cyst or periapical granuloma. There are suspicions of a nondental cause of the lesion and therefore a histological analysis of the lesion is necessary.

(23) One visit procedure would be

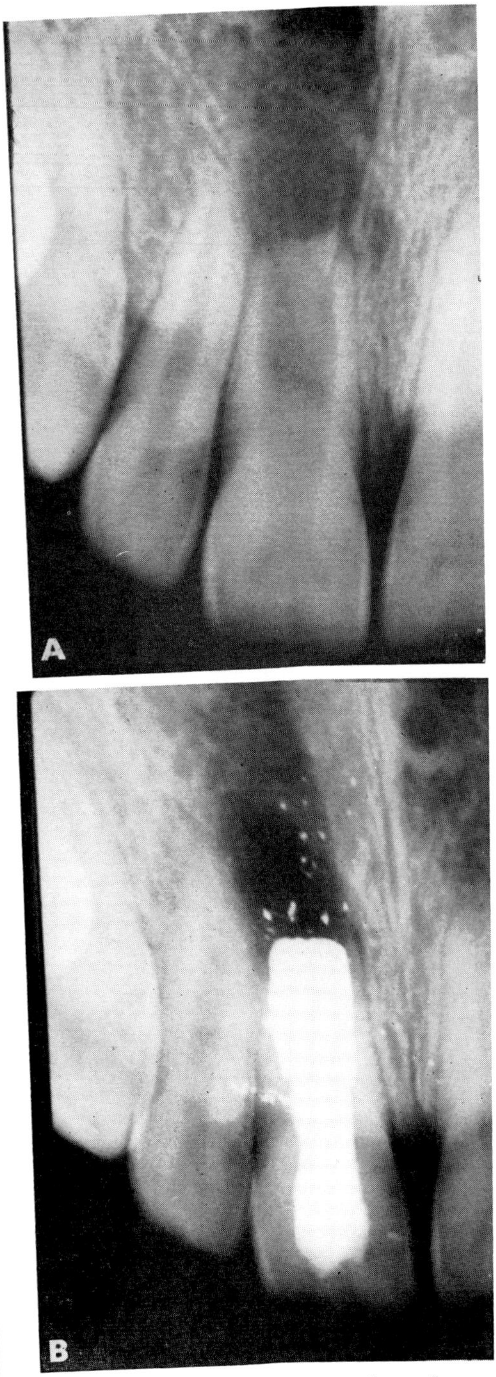

Figure 339. Central incisor with wide open apex; case was treated in one visit by immediate surgical endodontics because of time availability (patient was relocating out of the district). A. Before treatment. B. Canal sealed with gutta-percha-chloropercha and retrograde amalgam. (From D. R. Morse, "The Management of Endodontic Problem Cases," *JDA South Africa*, 27:387, 1972)

more feasible because of time and/or previous symptoms (pain and swelling) (Fig. 339).

(24) One tooth has to be treated surgically for one of the reasons listed above and there is an adjacent tooth with a periapical area of rarefaction that could be treated nonsurgically. However, as long as a surgical procedure is being performed in the vicinity, both teeth can be treated surgically at the same visit (Fig. 340).

Other indications for periapical surgery that have been given include gross overfilling, very large periapical *areas*, and extensive root resorption. I have not found these to be indications for periapical surgery. The possible harmful effects from overfilled silver cones has been discussed, and periapical surgery and a retroseal should be performed in those cases. Overfilled gutta-percha fillings are not recommended but if the canals are well sealed, the overfilling is usually no clinical problem and often it is absorbed (Figs. 80, 298, 341). Cases with large periapical *areas* (Fig. 342) and teeth with extensive root resorption (Figs. 80, 342) often heal after nonsurgical endodontic therapy. Only if these cases do not respond should periapical surgery be done. It is interesting to speculate on whether heal-

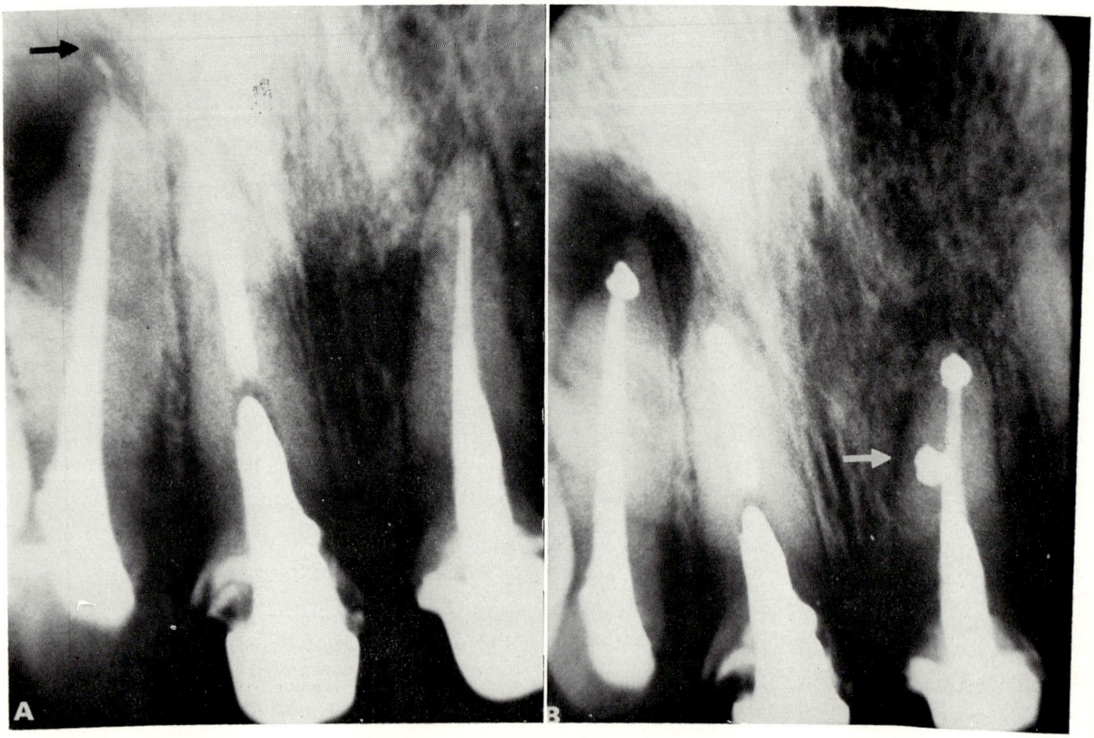

Figure 340. Central incisors require retroseals, lateral incisor could be retreated nonsurgically but is also being retreated surgically during the same surgical procedure. A. Before retreatment; arrow indicates the lateral incisor that could have been retreated nonsurgically; the central incisors have posts and crowns in position. B. Retroseal gold foils have been placed at the apexes and at a lateral canal (arrow) for all the involved teeth. (From W. K. Kopp and H. Kresberg, "Apicoectomy with Retrograde Gold Foil; A New Technique," *New York State Dental Journal,* 39:8, 1973)

ing is faster with or without periapical surgery. It has been taught that periapical granulomatous tissue is a precursor to healing tissue and therefore shouldn't be removed. However, recent radioisotope evidence shows that before repair takes place, the granulomatous tissue is removed by the host. Therefore, if this is the case, it may actually expedite healing if the granulomatous tissue is removed surgically. Nevertheless, as nonsurgical endodontic therapy is generally less traumatic (but not always), and as periapical repair usually occurs with this method, it should be considered first in treating teeth with periapical areas of pathosis.

Multirooted Teeth in Which One Root Has Either Untreatable Caries, Erosion, Perforations, External or Internal Resorption, a Fracture, or Is a Nontreatable Endodontic Failure

The other root(s) has adequate bone support, can be treated by endodontic therapy, and the tooth is restorable. The treatment is radisectomy or hemisection, if the bifurcation area of lower molars is involved. The root planned for sectioning should not be fused to another root, as this would make root amputation difficult, if not impossible. The periodontal indication for these procedures have been discussed under endodontic-periodontic syndrome. . . . The results of these procedures are good, provided that no undue trauma occurs, and the periodontal conditions are treatable.

Cases Where Neither Nonsurgical nor Surgical Endodontic Therapy Can Readily Be Performed and the Tooth Has an Adequate Clinical Crown

Typical cases are lower molars with nonnegotiable root canals and proximity of the root apexes to the in-

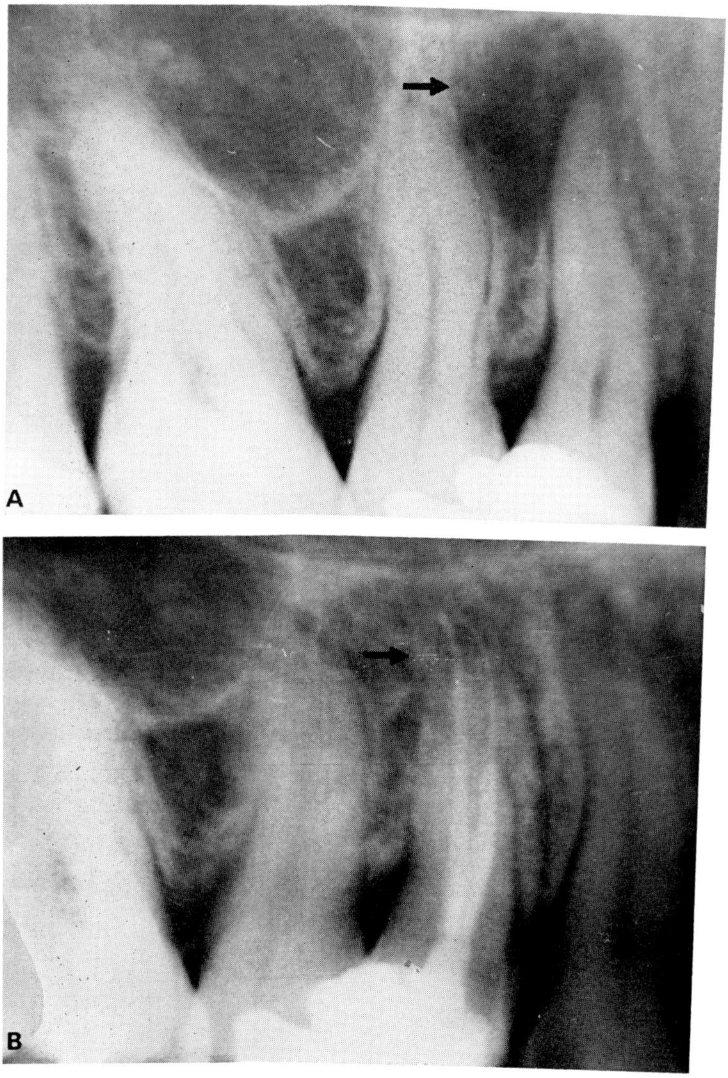

Figure 341. Upper first premolar with large periapical *area* present; treated by nonsurgical endodontic therapy. A. Before treatment. B. Two years after obturation with gutta-percha-chloropercha; even though there was some overfilling, canals were apparently well obturated and periapical repair is evident.

ferior alveolar canal. Possible causes are that the canals may be clinically calcified, the canals may be obstructed because of a ledge, debris, a broken instrument, or a pulp stone, there may be a previous root canal filling or post that cannot be dislodged, there may be an extreme root curvature that cannot be negotiated, and resorptions or perforations may have occurred. Other possible indications are unbearable pain that cannot be alleviated by other methods, and for patients who cannot keep their mouths open wide enough or for a long enough time to have nonsurgical or periapical surgical endodontic therapy performed. The treatment is *intentional replantation and splinting.* (For definition, see section on pulpless primary molar.) Some investigators state that they ob-

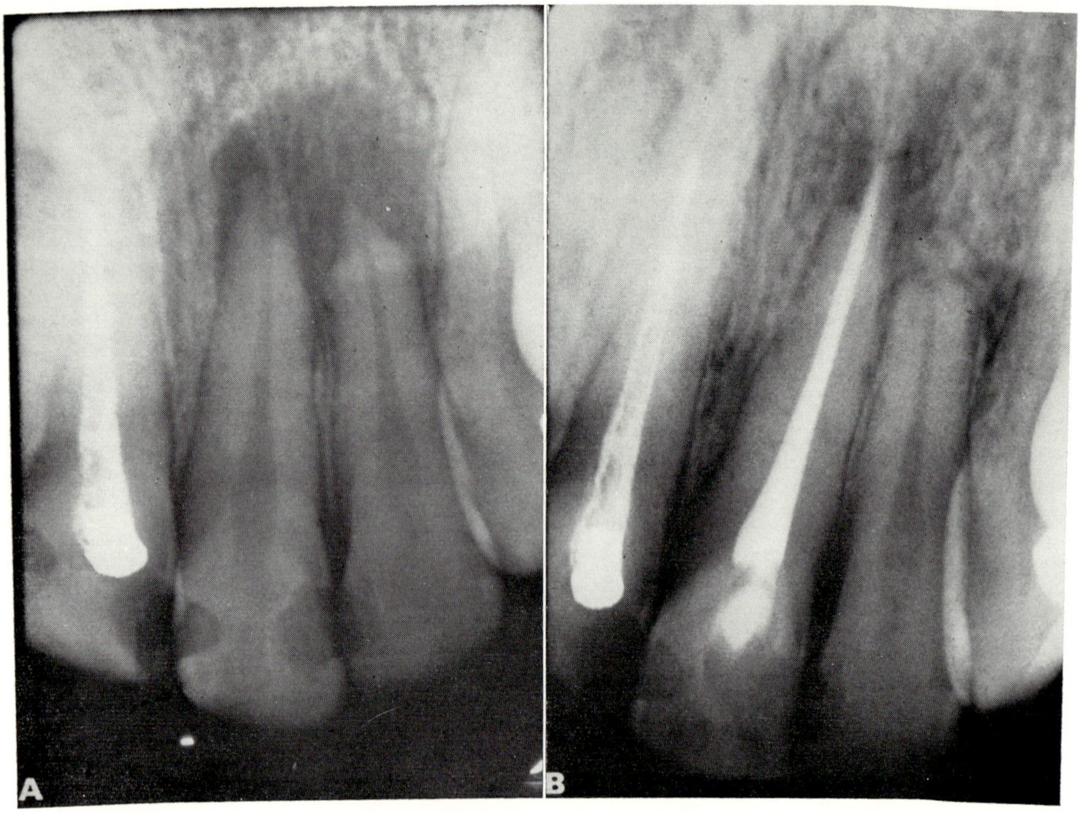

Figure 342. Large periapical *area* around apex of central and lateral incisor; apex of lateral incisor shows root resorption; case treated by nonsurgical endodontic therapy of the central incisor, as the lateral incisor responded normally to pulp testing. A. Before treatment. B. Two years following obturation with gutta-percha-chloropercha; periapical repair is evident and resorption apparently has stopped around the lateral incisor (tooth remained vital); although the left central incisor had a poorly obturated root canal, as there was neither clinical manifestations nor radiographic evidence of breakdown, no retreatment was performed.

tain good retention without the use of any splint; others advise a splint. Each case should be judged individually. If retention is adequate, no external splinting is necessary. If the roots are too curved, fracture may result and the procedure cannot be attempted. These cases are sometimes performed for patients who cannot afford nonsurgical *endodontic therapy* and would have the teeth extracted anyway. It is possible for tray set-ups to be arranged so that intentional replantation could be performed in only a few minutes more than a conventional extraction. This should lower the cost of the procedure, as compared to nonsurgical endodontics. Although the results are not as good as those with nonsurgical endodontics or periapical surgical procedures, it is certainly a worthwhile procedure, especially for those patients who would normally have the teeth extracted. Five year success rates have been reported as between 74 and 82 percent.

Acute Apical Abscess, Acute Exacerbation of Granuloma or Cyst, or Cellulitis

Treatment is *drainage through the tooth* as discussed under treatment of localized fluctuant abscess and the tooth should be taken out of occlusal contact. If no drainage occurs and no drainage is possible through the alveolar mucosa (I&D), then the patient should be given a *strong analgesic drug* and a systemic *antibiotic* (preferably penicillin V, or phenethicillin, if the patient is not allergic). See Chapter 4 for details. The patient should also be advised to rinse his (or her) mouth with warm saline as often as possible. As a result of the antibiotics and saline rinses, the swelling may localize and then an *I* and *D* can be performed. When the painful symptoms abate, nonsurgical endodontic therapy can be completed. If the pain still persists then *trephination* should be attempted. If this is to no avail, then *immediate surgical endodontics,* should be performed. If the involved tooth is a lower molar where surgery is not feasible, then *intentional replantation* can be attempted. Finally, if all else fails then *extraction* must be done. For cases where swelling does not diminish after two days, a fluid sample should be obtained if possible, for antibiotic sensitivity testing. While waiting for the results, the patient should be put on a second antibiotic such as erythromycin or a penicillinase-resistant penicillin. If the condition doesn't improve, and the results of the antibiotic sensitivity testing indicate that a different antibiotic is preferable, then the new antibiotic should be used (provided that it is safe and no allergy exists). In nonresponding cases, it may be necessary to extract the tooth to allow for drainage, and even hospitalize the patients, and institute intravenous antibiotic therapy.

Teeth That Have Been Intruded, Extruded, Labially Displaced, or Lingually Displaced

The teeth should be *repositioned and splinted.* Repositioning is the manual replacement of a tooth into its approximate previous position (prior to the trauma) (Fig. 343). Splinting can be by

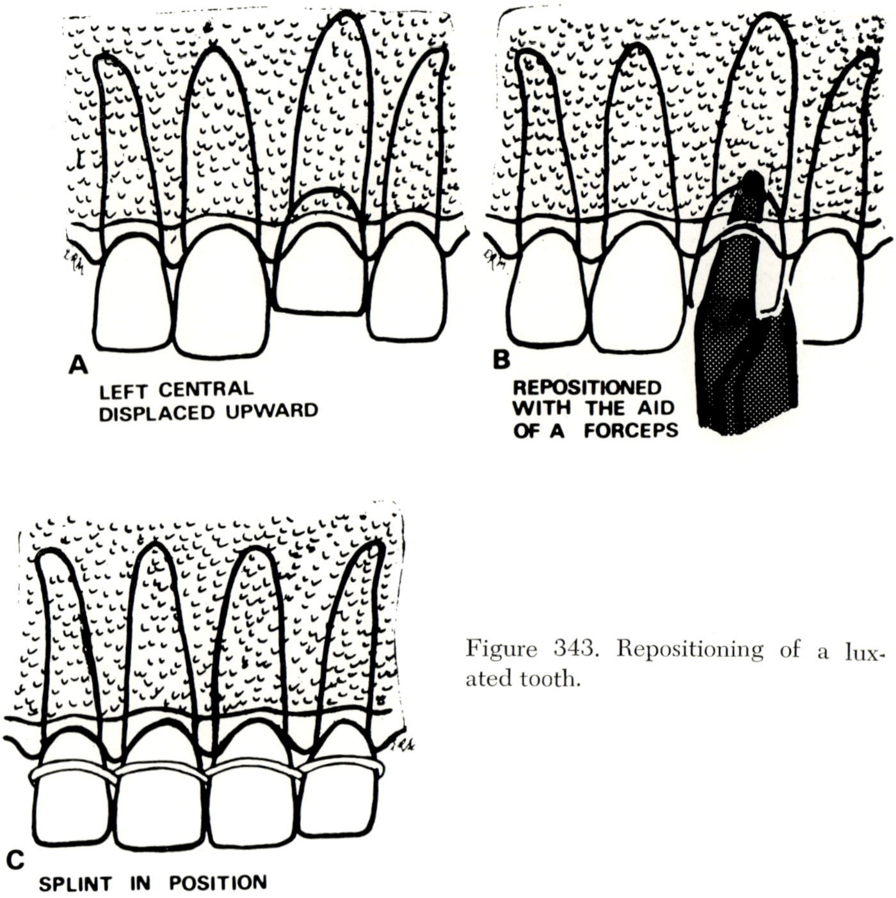

Figure 343. Repositioning of a luxated tooth.

any of the methods previously discussed. The repositioned teeth should be checked periodically, as the pulps can become necrotic, and then endodontic therapy would be necessary.

Teeth That Have Been Avulsed

Treatment is *replantation and splinting*. Replantation is the replacement of an avulsed tooth back into its socket in as close to the previous position as possible. The replanted tooth may or may not have endodontic therapy performed (Fig. 344). The most important consideration is the time of the replantation. Most authorities consider the chances of success to be good if replantation occurs within thirty minutes. If the parent or patient calls the office, they should be informed that if they cannot get to the office within thirty minutes from the time of the avulsion, they should replant the tooth themselves. If the tooth has been out of the mouth for a longer period, then they should be told to bring the tooth, wrapped in wet gauze, along with the patient to the office. If the dentist has the avulsed tooth and the time period is less than thirty minutes, then the

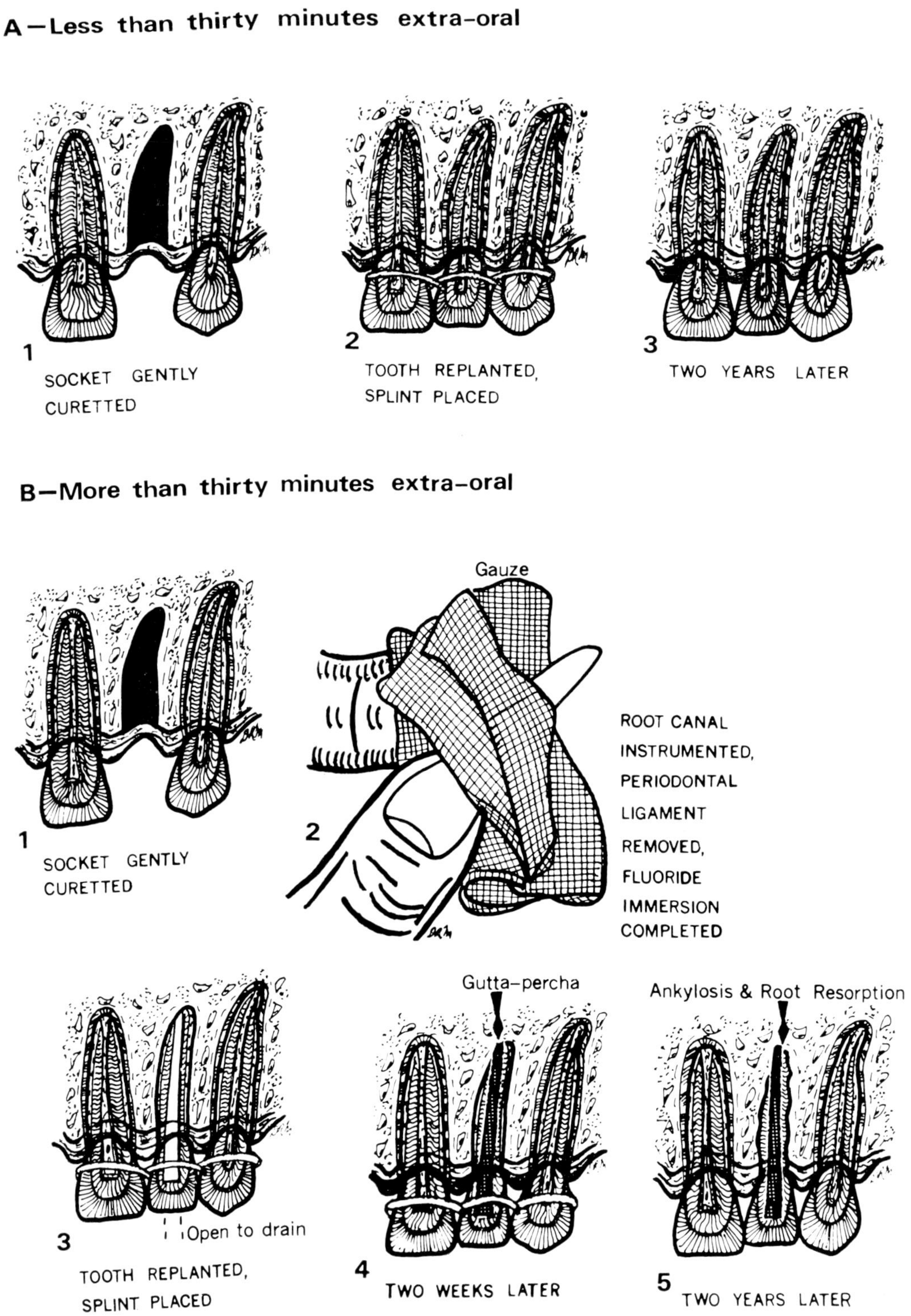

Figure 344. Replantation of avulsed tooth.

treatment is simple replantation and splinting as described previously. The splint should be kept in place for approximately six weeks, and the tooth should be checked radiographically by pulp testing, and other clinical tests at least every three months. There has been some recent evidence that firm splinting may not be necessary or may even be detrimental, with the added risk of resorption and ankylosis. This may be related to the inhibition of tooth movement during function. If the tooth *snaps* back into place, splinting is not necessary. However, if it is mobile, then a splint should be placed, but firm pressure should be avoided. If after the replantation, pain becomes severe, analgesics should be prescribed. If pain doesn't abate after a few days, then the pulp must be removed and if necessary the tooth should be left open. It also may be necessary to do a trephination procedure, if other pain relieving methods fail.

If any radiographic sign of a *periapical area of rarefaction or external resorption develops,* then *nonsurgical endodontic therapy for a pulpless tooth should be performed.* If the root is short, or if mobility hasn't ceased after splint removal then an *apical endodontic implant* should be inserted (Fig. 345G). Also if the patient develops pain, swelling, a sinus tract, or a nonvital response to pulp testing, then en-

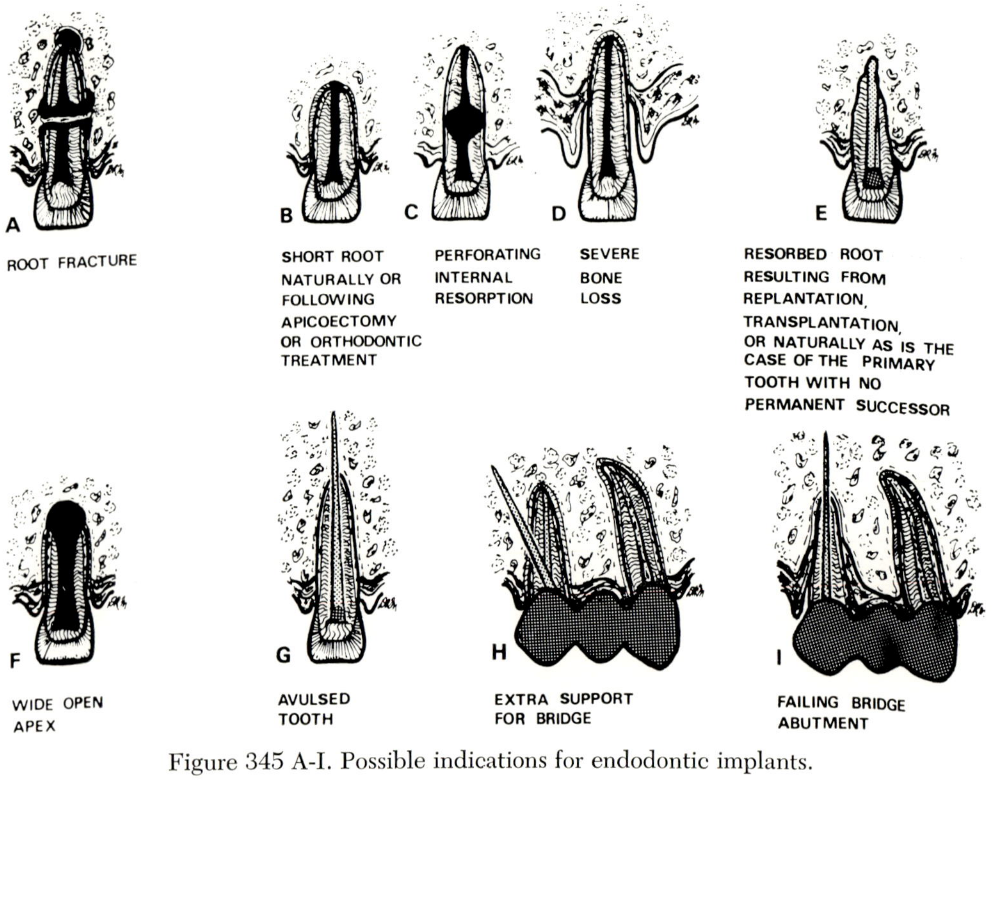

Figure 345 A-I. Possible indications for endodontic implants.

dodontic therapy should be performed as described above.

If the tooth has been out of the mouth longer than thirty minutes, then the pulp is removed and instrumentation is completed, with the access remaining open. Leaving the tooth open affords an orifice for venting of gases and drainage of fluids. An alternative to leaving the tooth open is to close the access opening and perform a trephination.

The periodontal ligament should be removed by scraping and immersion in a proteolytic solution, like trypsin. This should be followed by immersion in 2.4% phosphate-sodium fluoride solution for twenty minutes (pH 5.5). This is to help prevent root resorption. Without this treatment, root resorption and ankylosis occurs, apparently because the periodontal ligament becomes necrotic or altered enough to act as a foreign antigen. After the treatments, the tooth is replanted and splinted. After a week or two, when the soft tissue lacerations have healed (if they were present), nonsurgical endodontic therapy for a pulpless tooth or an endodontic implant should be completed (as indicated above).

As the treatment regimen using the fluoride solution is a relatively new procedure, it is not yet possible to predict the long term prognosis. Past experience with replanted teeth that have been out of the mouth for a prolonged period, have shown that in most cases rapidly produced external root resorption occurs, and the teeth generally do not last longer than five years. Other new techniques that are being investigated as methods to inhibit resorption are the use of calcium hydroxide root canal fillings and the use of cell cultures of the patient's own cells covering the root surfaces.

Teeth with Extremely Short Roots That Require Endodontic Therapy

Treatment is *endodontic implantation* (Figs. 318, 345B). Prognosis is good provided that there is no associated periodontal disease. With periodontal disease, the prognosis depends upon how well the periodontal condition can be controlled. If several adjacent periodontally involved teeth are being treated, it is necessary for additional stabilization, to have temporary horizontal splinting along with the endodontic implants until the periodontal treatments are completed. Endodontic implant treatment can be used for primary teeth that have no permanent successors. Prognosis depends upon the rate of root resorption, which is unpredictable.

Replanted Teeth with Resorbing Roots

In teeth that have had previous replantation and presently show resorption and mobility, the use of *endodontic implants* can prolong the life of these teeth (Fig. 345E). The resorption process may slow down after the procedure, but the prognosis still has to be considered questionable.

Teeth That Are to Be Used as Bridge Abutments but Need Extra Support

For teeth with short roots, straight roots, or single roots that may not be sufficient to carry the load as bridge abutments, the use of *endodontic implants* can provide extra support (Fig. 345H). Temporary splints should be in position before implant insertion. This prevents excessive movement of the tooth-implant complex. The prognosis is fairly good and depends greatly upon how much stress the teeth will have to bear.

Failing Bridge Abutments

For cases where the bridge abutments are failing because of mobility and loss of bone support, *endodontic implants* inserted through the crowns can prolong the life of these abutments (Fig. 345I). Prognosis is fair, as it is often difficult to control the underlying periodontal condition.

Endodontically Nontreatable Tooth and in the Same Mouth There Is an Available Partially Developed Tooth That Is Nonfunctional

A typical case is an untreatable lower first molar with a partially formed third molar available. The treatment is *autogenous tooth transplantation,* and *splinting.* Autogenous tooth transplantation is a procedure in which a partially developed tooth (usually with approximately 4-5 mm of roots developed beyond the furcation area) is surgically removed, and then inserted into the site of a previously extracted tooth (Fig. 346.1). It is essential that the mesiodistal width of the tooth to be transplanted must be less than the tooth that is to be extracted. However, it should not be too narrow or else there will be no proximal contact of the transplanted tooth to adjoining teeth. As the transplanted tooth is from the same mouth, signs of apparent rejection, like ankylosis, and root resorption do not occur, unless the tooth has been kept out of the mouth longer than one-half hour. Prognosis is doubtful however, as the roots rarely complete their development, and mobility usually follows. The pulps can become necrotic which would then necessitate endodontic therapy (Fig. 347). If the roots are short and the teeth are mobile, then consideration should be given to the adjunctive use of endodontic implants. This could increase the usefulness of these teeth.

Nontreatable Endodontic Case Where There Is no Available Transplantable Tooth in the Same Mouth

The patient does not want a fixed or removable bridge and a similar size mature tooth (to replace the nontreatable one) is available either from a suitable donor or a tooth bank. The treatment is *allogeneic tooth transplantation and splinting.* Allogeneic tooth transplantation is a procedure in which a tooth from one individual is transferred to an extraction site in a second individual (Fig. 346.2). Current studies indicate that the same treatment should be performed on these teeth as was mentioned for prolonged replantation cases (periodontal ligament removal and fluoride treatment). Without that treatment, prognosis is poor, as no long term favorable results have been published. The usual occurrence is root resorption and ankylosis (clinical signs of a probable

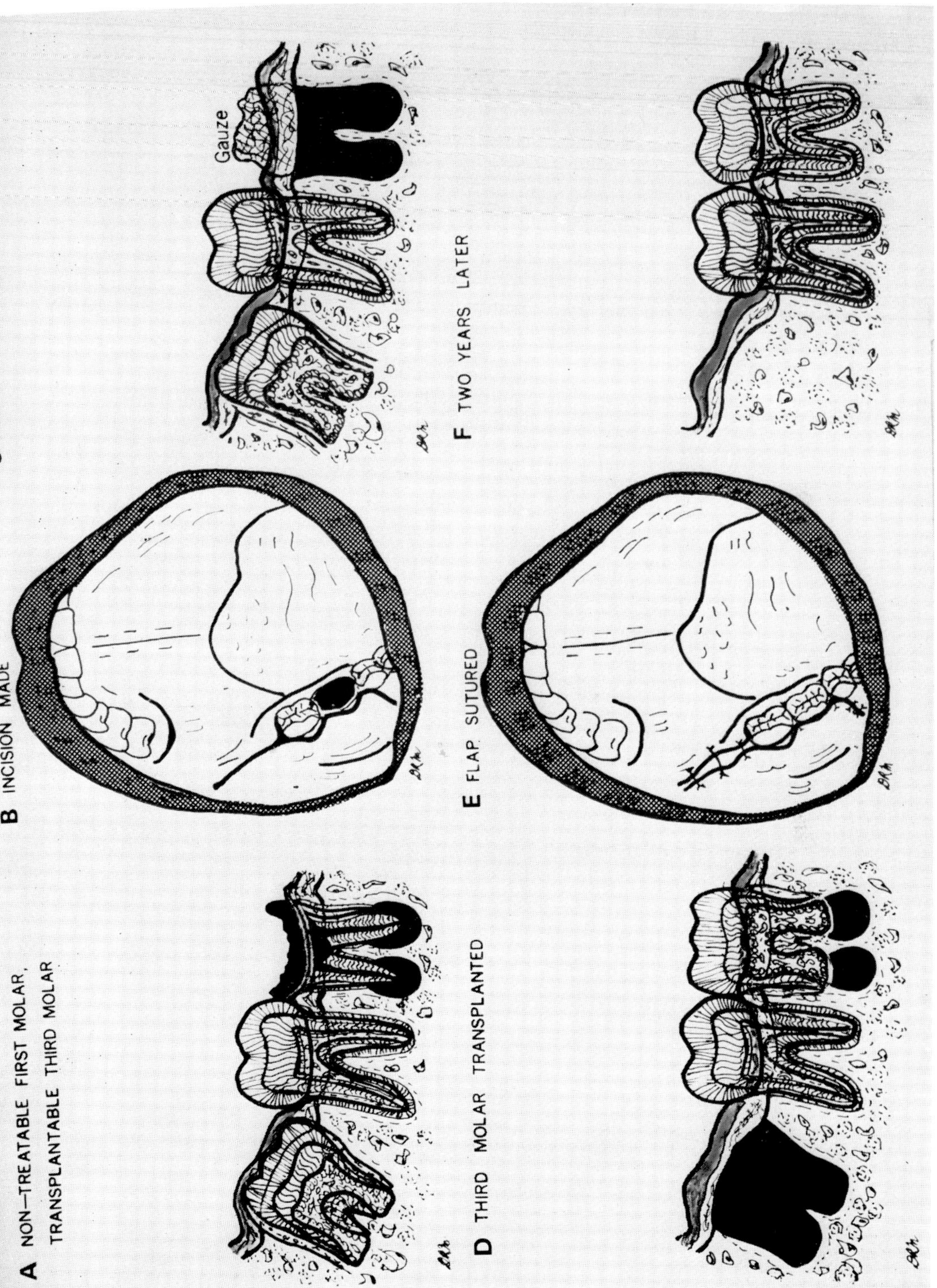

Figure 346. A-F. Autogenous tooth transplantation. A-D. Allogeneic tooth transplantation.

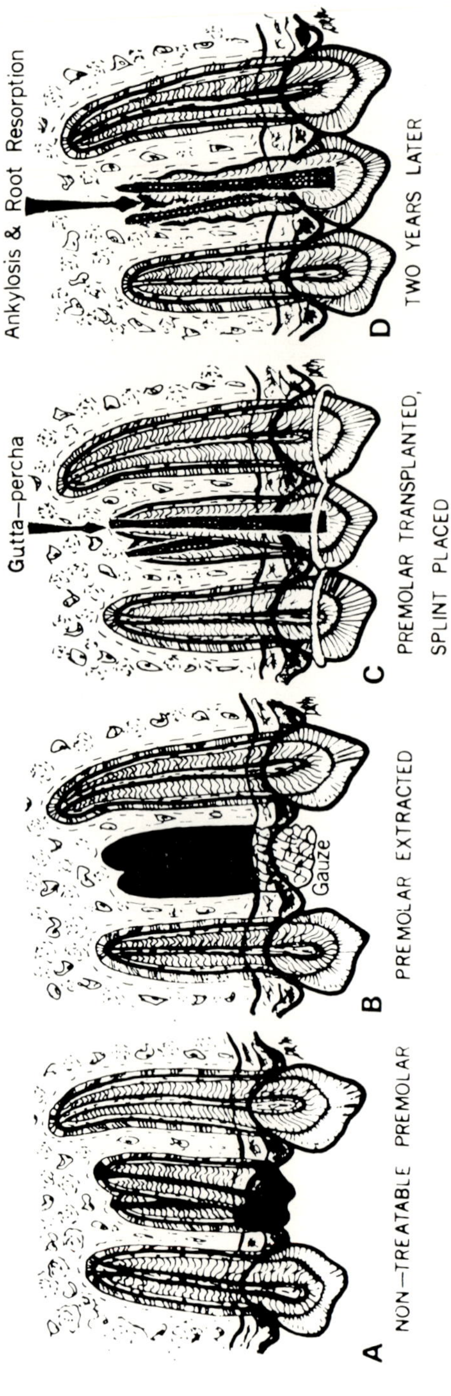

Figure 346. A-D

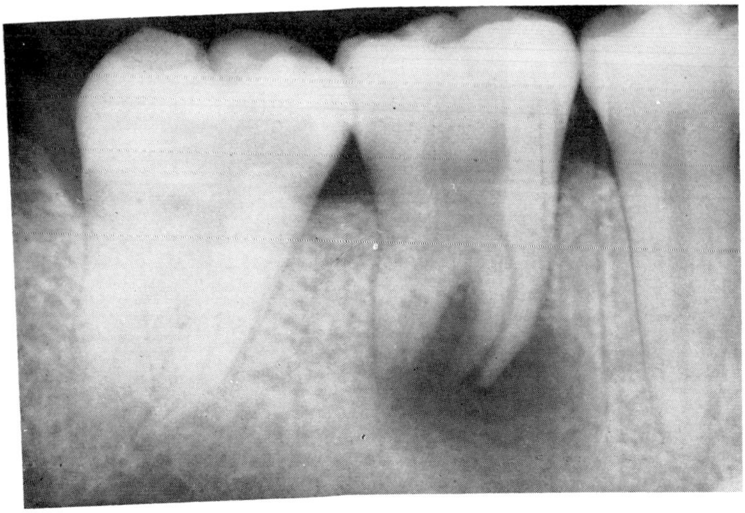

Figure 347. Autogenous tooth transplant in which the pulp became necrotic. (Courtesy of Dr. D. Levinson, Philadelphia, Pa.)

rejection mechanism). It is possible with the newer treatment methods (see previous discussion under section "teeth that have been avulsed") that transplanted teeth may last for at least five years. However, the prognosis is still considered questionable.

Roots That Are Buried Beneath the Gingiva

If the roots have adequate length and are close enough to the alveolar ridge, then they can be exposed and treated endodontically. The first stage is either *periodontal surgery* or *electrosurgery* to remove the overlying mucosa and expose the roots. It may be necessary to remove some bone by the use of a bur in an ultra-high speed handpiece. For an isolated root, nonsurgical endodontic therapy is done, followed by a post preparation and insertion, and crown cementation (Fig. 348). Multiple roots can be exposed, treated endodontically, and then used for attachments to dentures to give extra retention for the dentures (overlay dentures). The maintenance of the roots also prevents the loss of alveolar bone and hence gives more supporting bone. A reasonable

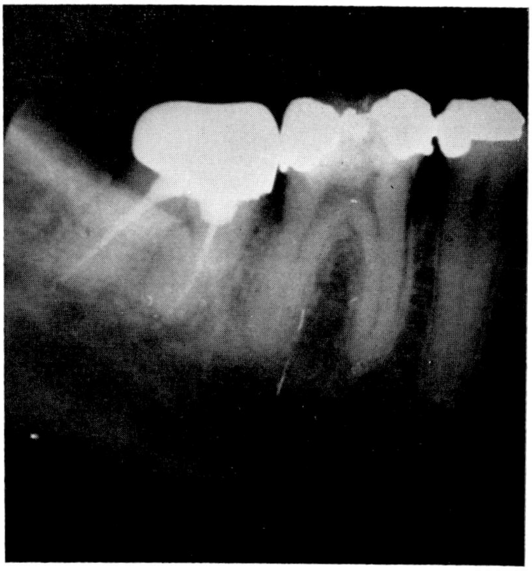

Figure 348. Lower second molar was fractured subgingivally. Periodontal surgery was performed to expose the crown and the canals were obturated with gutta-percha-chloropercha and posts and a crown were inserted. (From D. R. Morse, "The Significance of Endodontics in Plantation Procedures," *JDA South Africa*, 26:263, 1971)

question is that if the roots could be uncovered, and posts, cores, and crowns made, should not a partial denture be inserted? The answer is that there might not be sufficient teeth remaining for a partial denture (e.g. only four lower incisors present) and the use of a partial denture (repeated insertion and removal) would cause more trauma to the abutments by the clasp action, than would a full denture.

Discolored Endodontically-Treated Teeth with Relativcly Intact Clinical Crowns and no Large Restorations Present

Treatment is *bleaching*. Bleaching is a process of restoring the approximate natural color to discolored teeth by the use of a oxygenating solution (some form of peroxide). The solution is usually placed on both the external and internal coronal surfaces of these teeth

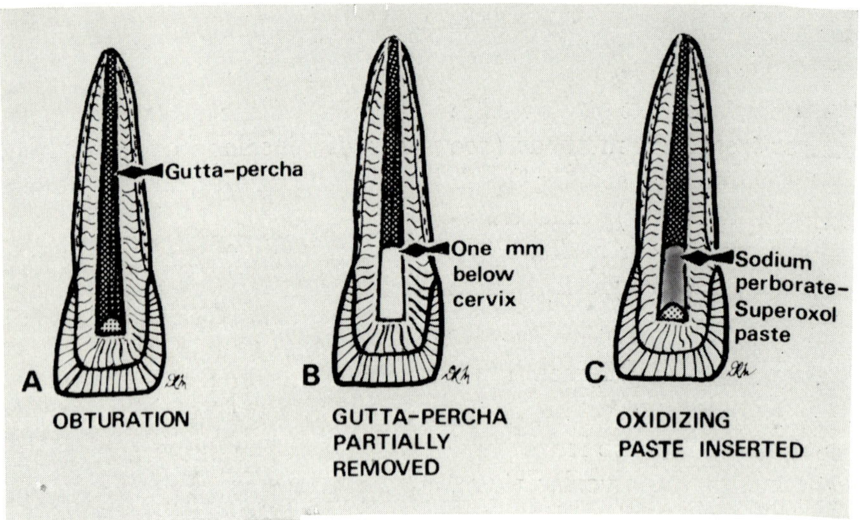

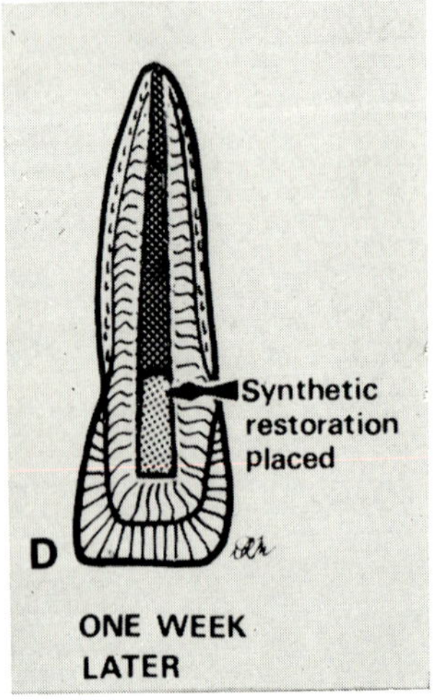

Figure 349. Bleaching technique following endodontics.

(Fig. 349). Treatable teeth include those with discolorations resulting from products of erythrocytic and tissue decomposition, products of chromogenic microbes, and products of decomposing food residues. More difficult cases to treat are those in which discolorations result from metallic stains, and long standing cases. Recently, there have been reports of successful bleaching of tetracycline-stained teeth. There are various techniques for bleaching including use of Superoxol® (a 30% by weight solution of hydrogen peroxide, Merck) with a bleaching lamp (a No. 1 photoflood lamp is satisfactory), Superoxol plus activation by a red hot plugger or burnisher, sodium perborate (Amosan® or Vince® will do) plus water, and sodium perborate plus Superoxol. There are also a few methods used to restore translucency including use of chloral hydrate solution, acrylic monomer, and silicone fluid. The technique that I find to give satisfactory results with the least complications is the use of sodium perborate with either water or Superoxol plus a silicate or plastic seal of the access opening. Care must be taken in the use of Superoxol, as it is highly irritating. It should not be allowed to touch the patient's tissues or clothes (or the doctor's either). Superoxol should not be kept near heat, as explosions can occur. It can last up to four months, if refrigerated. Results with the use of Superoxol may be better than with plain water but this has not been documented. With either technique results are usually good, but it may be necessary to have two or three sessions. Also, retreatments may be necessary at a future date. If the results are not good, then consideration should be given to the use of a porcelain jacket restoration.

BIBLIOGRAPHY

General

Grossman, L. I.: *Endodontic Practice,* 7th ed. Philadelphia, Lea & Febiger, 1970.

Ingle, J. I.: *Endodontics,* Philadelphia, Lea & Febiger, 1965.

Seltzer, S.: *Endodontology: Biologic Considerations in Endodontic Procedures.* New York, McGraw, 1971.

Sommer, R. F., Ostrander, F. D., and Crowley, M. C.: *Clinical Endodontics: A Manual of Scientific Endodontics,* 3rd ed. Philadelphia, Saunders, 1966.

Weine, F. S.: *Endodontic Therapy,* St. Louis, Mosby, 1972.

Apexification, Pulp Capping, and Pulpotomy

Anneroth, G., and Bang, G.: The effect of allogeneic demineralized dentin as a pulp capping agent in Java monkeys. *Odontol Revy, 23:*315, 1972.

Berger, J. E.: A review of the erroneously labeled "mummification" techniques of pulp therapy. *Oral Surg, 34:*131, 1972.

Bhaskar, S. N., Beasely, J. D., Ward, J. P., and Cutright, D. E.: Human pulp capping with isobutyl cyanoacrylate. *J Dent Res, 51:*58, 1972.

Canby, C. P., and Burnett, G. W.: Clinical management of deep carious lesions. *Oral Surg, 16:*999, 1963.

Dylewski, J. J.: Apical closure of nonvital teeth. *Oral Surg, 32:*82, 1971.

Fisher, F. J.: The effect of a calcium hydroxide/water paste on micro-organisms in carious dentine. *Br Dent J, 133:*19, 1972.

Frank, A. L.: Therapy for the divergent pulpless tooth by continued apical formation. *JADA, 72:*87, 1966.

Guthrie, T. J., McDonald, R. E., and Mitchell,

D. F.: Dental pulp hemogram. *J Dent Res, 44:*678, 1965.

Ham, J. W., Patterson, S. S., and Mitchell, D. F.: Induced apical closure of immature pulpless teeth in monkeys. *Oral Surg, 33:*438, 1972.

Hannah, D. R.: Glutaraldehyde and calcium hydroxide: a pulp dressing material. *Br Dent J, 132:*227, 1972.

Jordan, R. E., and Suzuki, M.: Conservative treatment of deep carious lesions. *J Can Dent Assoc, 37:*337, 1971.

Kelley, M. A., Bugg, J. L., and Skjonsky, H. S.: Histologic evaluation of formocresol and oxpara pulpotomies in Rhesus monkeys. *JADA, 86:*123, 1973.

King, J. B., Jr., Crawford, J. J., and Lindahl, R. L.: Indirect pulp capping: a bacteriologic study of deep carious dentine in human teeth. *Oral Surg, 20:*663, 1965.

McWalter, G. M., El-Kafrawy, A. H., and Mitchell, D. F. Pulp capping in monkeys with a calcium-hydroxide compound, an antibiotic and a polycarboxylate cement *Oral Surg 36:*90 1973.

Sayegh, F. S.: The dentinal bridge in pulp-involved teeth: part 1. *Oral Surg, 28:*579, 1969.

Sekine, N., Asai, Y., Nakamura, Y., Tagami, T., and Nagakubo, T.: Clinico-pathological study of the effect of pulp capping with various calcium hydroxide pastes. *Bull Tokyo Dent Coll, 12:*149, 1971.

Shovelton, D. S., Friend, L. A., Kirk, E. E. J., and Rowe, A. H. R.: The efficacy of pulp capping materials: a comparative trial. *Br Dent J, 130:*385, 1971.

Shröder, U.: Evaluation of healing following experimental pulpotomy of intact human teeth and capping with calcium hydroxide. *Odontol Revy, 23:*329, 1972.

Stanley, H. R., and Lundy, T.: Dycal therapy for pulp exposures. *Oral Surg, 34:*818, 1972.

Steiner, J. C., and VanHassel, H. J.: Experimental root apexification in primates. *Oral Surg, 31:*409, 1971.

Torneck, C. D., Smith, J. S., and Grindall, P.: Biologic effects of endodontic procedures on developing incisor teeth. II. Effect of pulp injury and oral contamination. *Oral Surg, 35:*378, 1973.

Torneck, C. D., Smith, J. S., and Grindall, P.: Biologic effects of endodontic procedures on developing incisor teeth. IV. Effect of débridement procedures and calcium hydroxide-camphorated parachlorophenol paste in the treatment of experimentally induced pulp and periapical disease. *Oral Surg, 35:*541, 1973.

Trask, P. A.: Formocresol pulpotomy on (young) permanent teeth. *JADA, 85:*1316, 1972.

Wei, S. H. Y., Kaqueler, J. C., and Massler, M.: Remineralization of carious dentin. *J Dent Res, 47:*381, 1968.

Wei, S. H. Y., and Massler, M.: Pulp capping with stannous fluoride. Submitted for publication.

Trauma

Andreasen, J. O., and Hjørting-Hansen, E.: Intraalveolar root fractures: radiographic and histologic study of 50 cases. *J Oral Surg, 25:*414, 1967.

Cvek, M.: Pedodontic-Endodontics. Presented at the Fifth International Conference on Endodontics, Sept. 1973, Philadelphia, Pennsylvania.

Feldman, G., Solomon, C., Notaro, P., and Moskowitz, E.: Endodontic management of the subgingival fracture. *Dent Radiogr Photogr, 45:*3, 1972.

Hargreaves, J. A.: The traumatized tooth. *Oral Surg, 34:*502, 1972.

Michanowicz, A. E., Michanowicz, J. P., and Abou-Rass, M.: Cementogenic repair of root fractures. *JADA, 82:*569, 1971.

Natkin, E.: The traumatized tooth: a synthesis. *Oral Surg, 34:*516, 1972.

Rabinowitch, B. Z.: Internal resorption. *Oral Surg, 33:*263, 1972.

Stanley, H. R.: The Cracked Tooth Syndrome. *JAAGFO, 11:*36, 1968.

Irrigation, Intracanal Medication, and Culturing

Brown, J. I.: An evaluation of the antimicrobial effectiveness of intracanal medicaments. *JSCDA, 40:*845, 1972.

Frank, A. L., Glick, D. H., Weichman, J. A., and Harvey, H.: The intracanal use of sulfathiazole in endodontics to reduce pain. *JADA, 77:*102, 1968.

Morse, D. R.: The endodontic culture technique: an impractical and unnecessary procedure. *Dent Clin North Am, 15:*793, 1971.

Morse, D. R.: Resolved that culturing is contributory to endodontic success. Con. *In* Grossman, L. I.: Trans. Fifth Inter. Conf. Endo., Philadelphia, Univ. Penn., 1974. In Print.

Page, D. O., Trump, G. N., and Schaeffer, L. D.: Pulpal Studies. 1. Passage of ^{3}H-Tetracycline into circulatory system through rat molar pulps. *Oral Surg, 35:* 555, 1973.

Penick, E. C., and Osetek, E. M.: Intracanal drugs and chemicals in endodontic therapy. *Dent Clin North Am., 14:*743, 1970.

Seltzer, S., Bender, I. B., and Turkenkopf, S.: Factors affecting successful repair after root canal therapy. *JADA, 67:*671, 1963.

Senia, E. S., Marshall, F. J., and Rosen, S.: The solvent action of sodium hypochlorite on pulp tissue of extracted teeth. *Oral Surg, 31:*96, 1971.

Spangeberg, L.: Cellular Reaction to Intracanal Medicaments. Presented at the Fifth International Conference on Endodontics, Sept. 1973, Philadelphia, Pennsylvania.

Stewart, G. G., Kapsimalas, P., and Rappaport, H.: EDTA and urea peroxide for root canal preparation. *JADA, 78:*335, 1969.

Strindberg, L. Z.: Lokal Användning av Antibiotika vid Konserverande Rotbehandling. En Jämförande Klinisk, Bakteriologisk och Röentgenologisk Undersökning. *Svensk Tandläk J, 56:*639, 1963.

Tinkelman, C. I.: *Personality of a Dentist as It Relates to His Interpretation of Pain.* Thesis, Post-Graduate Program in Endodontics, Temple University School of Dentistry, Philadelphia, 1972.

Torneck, C. D., Smith, J. S., and Grindall, P.: Biologic effects of endodontic procedures on developing incisor teeth. III. Effect of débridement and disinfection procedures in the treatment of experimentally induced pulp and periapical disease. *Oral Surg, 35:* 532, 1973.

Treanor, H. F., and Goldman, M.: Bactericidal efficiency of intracanal medications. *Oral Surg, 33:*791, 1972.

VanderWall, G. L., Dowson, J., and Shipman, C., Jr.,: Antimicrobial efficacy and cytotoxicity of three endodontic drugs. *Oral Surg, 33:*230, 1972.

Nonsurgical Endodontic Therapy, General Considerations

Bhaskar, S. N.: Periapical lesions—types, incidence, and clinical features. *Oral Surg, 21:* 657, 1966.

Clem, W. H.: Posttreatment endodontic pain. *JADA, 81:*1166, 1970.

Compton, D. E., and Mitchell, D. F.: Pharmacologic treatment of painful pulpitis: a five year report. *J Dent Res, 49:*183, 1970.

Crump, M. C., and Natkin, E.: Relationship of broken root canal instruments to endodontic case prognosis: a clinical investigation. *JADA, 80:*1341, 1970.

de Deus, Q. D., and Han, S. S.: The fate of H^3-Cortisone applied on the exposed dental pulp. *Oral Surg, 24:*404, 1967.

Fox, J., Atkinson, J. S., Dinin, A. P., Greenfield, E., Hechtman, E., Reeman, C. A., Salkind, M., and Todaro, C. J.: Incidence of pain following one-visit endodontic treatment. *Oral Surg, 30:*123, 1970.

Lawson, B. F., and Mitchell, D. F.: Pharmacologic treatment of painful pulpitis: a preliminary, controlled double-blind study. *Oral Surg, 17:*47, 1964.

Melcher, A. H.: Mechanisms of Wound Healing and Repair. Presented at the Louis I. Grossman Endodontic Study Club Meeting, Oct. 1971, Philadelphia, Pennsylvania.

Morse, D. R., Patnik, J. W., and Schacterle, G. R.: Electrophoretic differentiation of radicular cysts and granulomas. *Oral Surg, 35:*249, 1973.

Nonsurgical Endodontic Therapy, Obturation

Castagnola, L., and Orlay, H. G.: *A System of Endodontia,* London, Pitman Medical Publishing Co. Ltd., 1956.

Barker, B. C. W., and Lockett, B. C.: Reaction of dog pulp and periapical tissue to two glucocorticosteroid preparations. *Oral Surg, 33:*249, 1972.

Erausquin, J.: Periapical tissue response to the apical plug in root canal treatment. *J Dent Res, 51:*483, 1972.

Fink, H. D.: Simplified obturation of molar root canals with gutta-percha: description of technique. *NY J Den, 37:*12, 1967.

Fox, J., Moodnik, R. M., Greenfield, E., and Atkinson, J. S.: Filling root canals with files: radiographic evaluation of 304 cases. *NY State Dent J, 38:*154, 1972.

Geiser, M. W., and Jensen, J. R.: Comparative sealability of four root canal cements. *Am IADR Abs. No. 713,* 1972.

Krakow, A. A., and Berk, H.: Efficient endodontic procedures with the use of the pressure syringe. *Dent Clin North Am, 9:*387, 1965.

Leuck, M. H., and La Vette, W. E.: Preservation of the mandibular ridge through root retention. *J Acad Gen Dent, 21:*29, 1973.

Luks, S.: Guttapercha versus silver points in the practice of endodontics. *NY State Dent J., 31:*341, 1965.

Morse, D. R.: The endodontic culture technique: an impractical and unnecessary procedure. *Dent Clin North Am, 15:*793, 1971.

Sargenti, A. G.: Endodontics, Switzerland, Angelo G. Sargenti; Endodontic Education Service, 1973.

Schilder, H.: Filling root canals in three dimensions. *Dent Clin North Am, 11:*723, 1967.

Seltzer, S., Bender, I. B., and Turkenkopf, S.: Factors affecting successful repair after root canal therapy. *JADA, 67:*671, 1963.

Seltzer, S., Green, D. B., Weiner, N., and De Renzis, F.: A scanning electron microscope examination of silver cones removed from endodontically treated teeth. *Oral Surg. 33:*589, 1972.

Soltanoff, W., and Parris, L.: Controlled silver point filling technique for endodontically involved teeth. *JADA, 65:*301, 1962.

Spangberg, L., and Langeland, K.: Biologic effects of dental materials. 1. Toxicity of root canal filling materials on hela cells *in vitro. Oral Surg, 35:*402, 1973.

Weine, F. S., Healey, H. J., and Lippert, J. L.: Use of silver points with improved digital control. *JADA, 83:*125, 1971.

Wiener, B. H., and Schilder, H.: A comparative study of important physical properties of various root canal sealers. II. Evaluation of dimensional changes. *Oral Surg, 32:* 928, 1971.

Surgery

Amen, C. R.: Hemisection and Root Amputation. *Periodontics, 4:*197, 1966.

Bergenholtz, A.: Radectomy of multirooted teeth. *JADA, 85:*870, 1972.

Bier, S. J. (Interview): Plaster of paris is reported adequate substitute to bone for filling periodontal defects. Clin Dent, 2:1 1974.

Kopp, W. K., and Kresberg, H.: Apicoectomy with retrograde gold foil: a new technique. *NY State Dent J, 39:*8, 1973.

Freedland, J. B.: Conservative reduction of large periapical lesions. *Oral Surg, 29:*455, 1970.

Haskell, E. W.: Vital root resection. *Oral Surg, 27:*266, 1969.

Heithersay, G. S.: Combined endodontic-orthodontic treatment of transverse root fractures in the region of the alveolar crest. *Oral Surg, 36:*404, 1973.

Hiatt, W. H.: Periodontal pocket elimination by combined endodontic-periodontic therapy. *Periodontics, 1:*152, 1963.

Hiatt, W. H.: Regeneration via flap operation and the pulpal periodontal lesion. *Periodontics, 4:*205, 1966.

Rakower, W.: Indications and technique for the root end amalgam seal. *NY State Dent J, 34:*609, 1968.

Schlagel, E., Seltzer, R. J., and Newman, J. J.: Apicoectomy as an adjunct to diagnosis. *NY State Dent J, 39:*156, 1973.

Soltanoff, W.: Apical sealing procedures. *JNJ Dent Assoc, 44:*36, 1973.

Plantation Procedures

Andreasen, J. O., Hjørting-Hansen, E., and Jølst, O.: A clinical and radiographic study of 76 autotransplanted third molars. *Scand J Dent Res, 78:*512, 1970.

Deeb, E., Prietto, P. P., and McKenna, R. C.: Reimplantation of luxated teeth in humans. *JSCDA, 33:*194, 1965.

Emmertsen, E., and Andreasen, J. O.: Replantation of extracted molars: a radiographic and histological study. *Acta Odontol Scand, 24:*327, 1966.

Frank, A. L.: Improvement of the crown-root ratio by endodontic endosseous implants. *JADA, 74:*451, 1967.

Grossman, L. I.: Intentional replantation of teeth. *JADA, 72:*1111, 1966.

Judy, K. W. M., Eilberg, R., Lew, I., and Greene, D.: Cement leakage and retention of threaded and non-threaded endodontic implants. *Oral Implant, 3:*28, 1973.

Kingsbury, B. C., and Wiesenbaugh, J. M.: Intentional replantation of mandibular premolars and molars. *JADA, 83:*1053, 1971.

Mezrow, R. R.: Homologous viable tooth transplantation. *Oral Surg, 17:*375, 1964.

Morse, D. R.: Endodontic implants: a review and new approach. *NY State Dent J, 35:*5, 1969.

Morse, D. R.: The significance of endodontics in plantation procedures. *JDA South Africa, 26:*263, 1971.

Orlay, H. G.: Endodontic splinting treatment in periodontal disease. *Br Dent J, 108:*118, 1960.

Price, P. J., and Cserepfalvi, M.: Pulp viability and the homotransplantation of frozen teeth. *J Dent Res, 51:*39, 1972.

Soder, P. O.: Transplantation of teeth. Presented at the Fifth International Conference on Endodontics, Sept. 1973, Philadelphia, Pennsylvania.

Shulman, L. B.: Allogeneic tooth transplantation. *J Oral Surg, 30:*398, 1972.

Shulman, L. B., and Kalis, P. J.: A comparison of autologous and allogeneic tooth transplants in Rhesus monkeys. *J Oral Surg, 28:* 168, 1970.

Restorations and Bleaching

Arens, D. E., Rich, J. J., and Healey, H. J.: A practical method of bleaching tetracycline-stained teeth. *Oral Surg, 34:*812, 1972.

Brown, G.: Factors influencing successful bleaching of the discolored root-filled tooth. *Oral Surg, 20:*238, 1965.

Buonocore, M. G., and Davilla, J.: Restoration of fractured anterior teeth with ultraviolet-light-polymerized bonding materials: a new technique. *JADA, 86:*1349, 1973.

Cohen, S., and Parkins, F. M.: Bleaching tetracycline-stained vital teeth. *Oral Surg, 29:* 465, 1970.

Zamikoff, J. I.: Overdentures—theory and technique. *JADA, 86:*853, 1973.

DIVISION THREE

TREATMENT

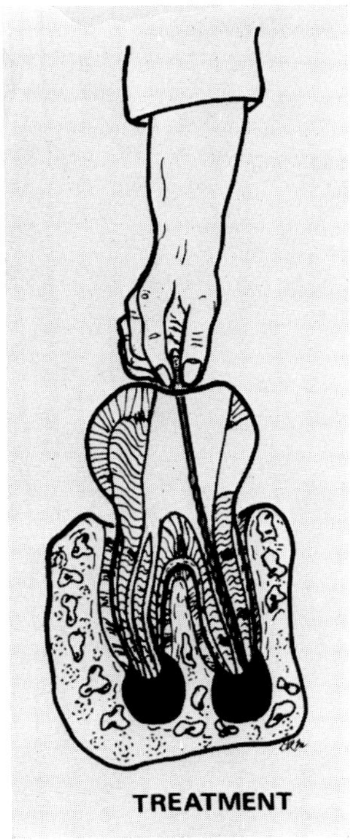

CHAPTER 4

DRUG THERAPY

TYPICAL SYSTEMIC DRUGS AND SUPPLEMENTS USED IN ENDODONTICS

THE CATEGORIES CONSIDERED in this chapter are analgesics, antibiotics, sedatives and anti-anxiety agents, anti-inflammatory agents, antisialogogues, nutritional supplements, and nasal decongestants.

For each category is given indications, contraindications, side effects, and dosages. When writing prescriptions, the dentist should indicate to the pharmacist on the prescription "LABEL AS SUCH." Then the bottle will have the name of the drug labeled. This is important in cases of drug toxicity, drug interactions, and allergic reactions.

Analgesics

Analgesics are used for pain relief before, during, or after treatment. A summary chart of typical analgesics is shown in Table IV. Drugs are discussed under the sections of "for mild to moderate pain" and "for severe pain."

For Mild to Moderate Pain—Nonnarcotics

Drugs included are aspirin, phenacetin, propoxyphene formulations, ethoheptazine compound, acetaminophen, mefenamic acid, and dihydrocodeine formulation.

ASPIRIN (ACETYLSALICYLIC ACID, ASA). Aspirin is still the most widely used analgesic. It should not be used for patients on anticoagulants or corticosteroids, ulcer patients, gout patients, asthmatics, or patients allergic to it. The various effects from aspirin interaction have been discussed in Chapter 1. Typical dosage is 300 to 600 mg (one to two tablets) every three to four hours. Some common aspirin compounds are Anacin® (aspirin 324 mg and caffeine 32 mg), Empirin compound (aspirin 230 mg, phenacetin 150 mg, and caffeine 30 mg), Bufferin® (aspirin 324 mg, aluminum glycinate 49 mg, and magnesium carbonate 97 mg), Coricidin® (aspirin 390 mg, chlorpheniramine maleate 2 mg, and caffeine 30 mg), Excedrin® (aspirin 192 mg, salicylamide 128 mg, and caffeine 64 mg), Phenaphen® (aspirin 162 mg, phenacetin 194 mg, phenobarbital 162 mg, and hyoscyamine sulfate 0.031 mg), Sal-Fayne capsules (aspirin 228 mg, phenacetin 162 mg, and caffeine 32.5 mg). It has not been proven that these combinations are any more effective than aspirin alone. The purported advantages are that Bufferin causes less stomach upset than aspirin, Coricidin provides an antihistamine also, if that drug is needed, Phenaphen has a sedative action, and the other formulations

TABLE IV
TYPICAL ANALGESICS*

Analgesics	*Use*	*Usual Dose*
Aspirin	Mild pain	300-600 mg every 3-4 hrs
Phenacetin	Mild pain	300 mg every 3-4 hrs
Darvon Compound 65	Mild pain	One capsule every 4-6 hrs
Darvon-N with A.S.A.	Mild pain	One capsule every 4-6 hrs
Darvocet-N	Mild pain	Two tablets every 4 hrs
Darvon 32 mg	Mild pain	One capsule every 4 hrs
Tylenol	Mild pain	325-650 mg (1-2 tablets) every 3-4 hrs
Zactirin Compound-100	Mild pain	One tablet every 4-6 hrs
Zactane	Mild pain	One tablet (75 mg) every 4-6 hrs
Ponstel	Mild pain	Two tablets at start (500 mg), then one tablet every 6 hrs
Talwin	Moderate pain	One tablet (50 mg) every 3-4 hrs
Codeine and in combination with other analgesics	Moderate pain	30 mg every 4 hrs
Synalgos-DC	Moderate pain	Two capsules every 4 hrs
Percodan	Moderate pain	One tablet every 6 hrs
Percodan-Demi	Less severe pain	One tablet every 3 hrs
Demerol	More severe pain	One tablet (50 mg) every 4 hrs
Methadone	Extreme pain	One to two tablets (25 to 50 mg) every 4 hrs

* Should rarely be necessary for more than three days use.

give a combination of more than one analgesic.

PHENACETIN (ETHOXYACETANILIDE). This analgesic drug is a component of many proprietary drug compounds including Empirin compound, Phenaphen, Sal-Fayne (see ingredients under aspirin), and Synalgos®. It may be used alone in a 300 mg dose every three to four hours for individuals who are allergic to aspirin. It should not be used for a prolonged period as it can cause the formation of methemoglobin and cyanosis. Other reported effects are acute hemolytic anemia and kidney failure. Hence, it should not be used for any patient with kidney, liver, or blood diseases, and it should not be used regularly for anyone for longer than ten days.

PROPOXYPHENE FORMULATIONS (DARVON COMPOUND-65®, DARVON COMPOUND-32®, DARVON N WITH A.S.A.®, DARVON, AND DARVOCET-N®). These are different formulations of propoxyphene hydrochloride, propoxyphene napsylate, aspirin, and acetaminophen. Darvon alone can be given to patients who are allergic to aspirin. The most popular formulation was Darvon Compound-65 which is a capsule containing propoxyphene hydrochloride 65 mg, aspirin 227 mg, phenacetin 162 mg, and caffeine 32.4 mg. However, late studies have shown that it may be no more effective than aspirin, although the evidence is not incontrovertible. It previously was thought not to have addictive properties, but recent reports have shown that individuals can become habituated to it. Darvon-N with A.S.A. contains 100 mg propoxyphene napsylate and 325 mg aspirin. It had been formulated to prevent addicts from injecting the drug into their veins (mainlining). A new formulation of these drugs (without aspirin) is Darvocet-N. This contains 50 mg of propoxyphene napsylate and 325 mg of acetaminophen. This formulation has been incorporated to give the advantages of Darvon and acetaminophen. Hence, it is especially useful for patients who cannot and/or should not take aspirin. Side effects are euphoria, gastrointestinal disturbances, skin rash (occasional), dizziness, and sedation. Usual dosage is one capsule every four to six hours for Darvon Compound 65 and Darvon-N with A.S.A., and two tablets of Darvocet-N every four hours. As propoxyphene can cause dizziness and euphoria, patients should be cautioned against operating a motor vehicle.

ETHOHEPTAZINE COMPOUND (ZACTIRIN® COMPOUND-100). This combination contains ethoheptazine citrate 100 mg, aspirin 227 mg, phenacetin 162 mg, and caffeine 32.4 mg. This preparation is purported to be as effective as 30 mg of codeine with 650 mg of aspirin. However, the evidence for this is not convincing, and this combination may be only slightly more effective than aspirin alone. Side effects are minimal and include nausea, vomiting, epigastric distress, and rarely a rash, euphoria, dizziness, and mental stimulation. Contraindication is for those individuals who might be allergic to any of the constituents. Average dose is one tablet every four to six hours. Zactane®, which is ethoheptazine citrate alone (75 mg) can be given to patients who are allergic to aspirin.

ACETAMINOPHEN. This analgesic is chemically N-acetyl-para-aminophenol which is the active break-down product of phenacetin. It is much less likely than phenacetin to induce the formation of methemoglobin and cause cyanosis. Acetaminophen can also be given to patients who are allergic to aspirin or who are taking uricosuric drugs for the treatment of gout. Unlike aspirin, acetaminophen does not promote gastrointestinal bleeding nor affect the action of anticoagulants. It is contraindicated for prolonged use in patients with kidney or liver diseases, because of the slight tendency to cause methemoglobulinemia and agranulocytosis. Preparations containing acetaminophen are Tylenol tablets (acetaminophen 325 mg), Percogesic® tablets (acetaminophen 325 mg, and phenytoxamine citrate 30 mg), Nebs (acetaminophen 325 mg), Trigesic tablets (acetaminophen 125 mg, aspirin 230 mg, and caffeine 30 mg), and the previously mentioned Darvocet-N. The typical dose is 325 to 650 mg (one to two tablets) every three to four hours. As Trigesic contains aspirin, it should not be given to any individual who should not take aspirin.

MEFENAMIC ACID (PONSTEL). The usual preparation is Ponstel Kapseals (mefenamic acid 250 mg). This drug has recently been introduced into dentistry, but it doesn't appear to be much more effective than aspirin. It can be used for patients who are allergic to aspirin. Ponstel is contraindicated in individuals with intestinal ulcers, in women in the child-bearing age (or who are pregnant), in children under 14 years of age, in asthmatics, and in patients with gastrointestinal inflammations or with abnormal kidney function. Side effects are headache, drowsiness, nausea, dizziness, and nervousness. Ponstel has also been reported to occasionally cause liver, kidney, and bone marrow damage. The preferred dosage is 500 mg (two tablets) at the start, followed by 250 mg (one tablet) every six hours. It should not be used for longer than one week. Because of possible side effects, patients should be advised against operating a motor vehicle.

Dihydrocodeine Formulation (Synalgos-DC). This combination is supplied as a capsule and contains dihydrocodeine bitartrate (Drocode®) 16 mg, promethazine hydrochloride 6.25 mg, aspirin 194.4 mg, phenacetin 162 mg, and caffeine 30 mg. The purported uses of the various components are dihydrocodeine for analgesia and sedation, aspirin and phenacetin for analgesia and anti-pyresis, promethazine for sedation, and caffeine for mild stimulation. Although dihydrocodeine can be prescribed without a narcotic blank, both physical and psychic dependence, as well as tolerance can occur. Synalgos-DC should not be given to individuals allergic to any of the components. Safe usage for children or during pregnancy has not been established. Side effects are dizziness, drowsiness, sedation, lightheadedness, nausea, vomiting, pruritis, constipation, skin reactions, and rarely hypotension. The usual dosage is two capsules every four hours as is needed. The patient should not drive a motor vehicle while under the influence of the compound. Although this combination has been in use for a relatively short period, it appears to be effective for mild to moderate pain with apprehension.

For Severe Pain

Drugs included are the nonnarcotic and narcotic analgesics.

Nonnarcotic Analgesics. The only drug to be considered in this category is Talwin. Talwin (pentazocine hydrochloride) is apparently as effective in a 50 mg dose as 60 mg of codeine and can be given to patients who are allergic to codeine. It appears to have a more rapid onset and somewhat shorter duration of action than codeine. It is contraindicated for patients with head injuries, brain diseases or lesions; asthmatics and other lung disease patients; patients with cyanosis; and children under twelve (not enough clinical trials with children). Adverse reactions include dizziness, nausea, vomiting, headache, constipation, emotional disturbances, hallucinations, anorexia, tachycardia, dermatitis, and respiratory depression. Talwin also has been claimed to cause sedation in about 30 percent of patients. This can be advantageous. It had been believed that Talwin was not addicting, but recently there have been reports of dependence on this drug. The oral dosage form is not as reliable as the parenteral form. The recommended dose is 50 mg every three to four hours. For severe pain, 100 mg may have to be administered. Patients should be advised not to drive because of possible side effects. Because of its possible adverse effects, Talwin should be used with caution.

NARCOTICS. These drugs are used for moderate to extreme pain, as well as for sedation. The range is from codeine and oxycodone hydrochloride (Percodan®) for moderate pain, through meperidine hydrochloride (Demerol® hydrochloride), dihydromorphinone hydrochloride (Dilaudid®), and anileridine (Leritine®) for more severe pain, to methadone hydrochloride (Dolophine® hydrochloride) and morphine sulphate, for extreme pain. The narcotics should be administered with caution to patients with respiratory diseases and hypotension. Patients should be advised not to operate a motor vehicle while under the influence of these drugs, because of the possible depressant effects. Also as described in Chapter 1, narcotics should not be given to patients who have taken a monoamine oxidase inhibitor within the previous two weeks, because of the possibility of severe depression. They also should not be given to patients with cerebral lesions, diseases and injuries because of the cerebral effect of the narcotics.

Codeine. Codeine by itself, with aspirin, or as a component of proprietary products is the most commonly used analgesic in dentistry for pain relief of moderate to severe nature. Of the narcotics, codeine is the least addictive, nauseating, constipating, sedative, respiratory depressing, and analgesic. People can be allergic to codeine, but generally it is the safest of the strong analgesics. Some of the commonly used forms and dosages are codeine phosphate 30 mg (one tablet) with aspirin 600 mg (two tablets) every four hours, Empirin compound no. 3 (contains 30 mg of codeine), one tablet every four hours, Phenaphen with codeine phosphate ½ grain (contains 32.4 mg of codeine), one capsule every four hours, and Tylenol with codeine, ½ grain (contains 30 mg of codeine). Tylenol is useful in patients allergic to aspirin and Phenaphen is used because the phenobarbital induces a degree of sedation.

Oxycodone Formulation (Percodan). This compound contains the narcotic oxycodone. Its analgesic effect is similar to codeine's, but it appears to have a longer duration. The side effects of Percodan include nausea, vomiting, constipation, and rarely, hypotension. Its addiction potential is greater than that of codeine. The formula is oxycodone hydrochloride, 4.5 mg; oxycodone terephthalate, 0.38 mg; aspirin 224 mg; phenacetin 160 mg; and caffeine 32 mg. The compound should not be administered to any patient who is hypersensitive to any of the ingredients. The usual dose is one tablet every six hours. For less severe pain, or children over twelve, Percodan-Demi can be used. It contains approximately one-half the normal adult dose.

Meperidine Hydrochloride (Demerol Hydrochloride). This narcotic is a more potent analgesic than codeine or Percodan. It also has good sedative properties. Side effects include dizziness, drowsiness, nausea, vomiting, constipation, and rarely respiratory depression. Demerol also has stronger addiction potential than codeine. The usual dosage is 50 mg (one tablet) every four hours. For severe pain, 100 mg can be given. For children under 16, 25 mg is the dose. Oral administration is not as effective as the parenteral route. For IM injection, Demerol hydrochloride sterile aqueous solution 5% can be used. Each ml contains 50 mg of meperedine hydrochloride.

Hydromorphone Hydrochloride (Dilaudid). This analgesic is apparently as effective as 100 mg of Demerol. Side effects are similar to the other narcotics. These include diarrhea, vomiting, nausea, somnolence, euphoria, and respiratory depression. The dosage is 2 mg every five hours (one tablet). As there is greater addiction potential and respiratory depression than with codeine or Demerol, it is rarely necessary to use this drug in endodontics.

Anileridine (Leritine). This drug resembles Demerol in its action and side effects, but it is more potent. The average dose is 25 mg (one tablet) every four to six hours. For severe pain, an initial oral dose of 50 mg may be necessary. The same precautions are necessary as discussed under Dilaudid.

Dolophine Hydrochloride (Methadone Hydrochloride). This is a strong analgesic that is comparable to morphine, but has less of a sedative effect. It also has less addiction potential and causes less respiratory depression than morphine. Other side effects include nausea, vomiting, constipation, and meiosis. The average dose is 2.5 mg every four hours. For more severe pain, 5 mg can be given. It is rarely necessary to use this analgesic in endodontics.

Morphine Sulphate. This is one of the most potent analgesics. However, it also produces sedation or hypnosis (depending upon the dose), the most respiratory depression, and has the most addiction potential of any of the narcotics. Interaction between morphine and alcohol can be lethal. Morphine is also much less effective orally than by injection. The average oral dose is 5 mg every four hours. Considering all these factors, it is rarely indicated for nonhospitalized patients.

Antibiotics

These drugs should not be used routinely because of the possibilities of allergic reaction, toxicity, iatrogenic diseases, and development of resistant microbes. There is no hard and fast rule when to use antibiotics. Generally, if the swelling can be relieved by drainage through the tooth or soft tissues, then antibiotics should not be used. As discussed in Chapter 1, cases of deep cellulitis, nonresponding superficial cellulitis, and osteomyelitis should be treated with antibiotics. Patients with diabetes, Cushing's disease (or under treatment with corticosteroids), cardiovascular diseases (especially rheumatic heart disease, congenital heart disease, bacterial endocarditis, or history of these conditions), uremia, valvular prosthesis or grafts, leukemia, granulocytopenia, multiple myeloma, hypothyroidism, and Paget's disease, should be covered with antibiotics during treatment. Provided that there is no known allergy, penicillin G, V or phenethicillin (if taken orally) are the drugs of choice. If penicillin cannot be used, erythromycin is then indicated. Other antibiotics that may be effective are clindamycin (Cleocin®), lincomycin (Lincocin®) and the cephalosporins (Keflex®). As explained in Chapter 1, antibiotic sensitivity testing is not infallible, but it does have its uses. If after 36 to 48 hours, the original antibiotic is not effective, then antibiotic sensitivity testing should be performed using aspirated fluid (if it is available). If possible, it would be advantageous to withdraw fluid for sensitivity testing when the patient first presents with the cellulitis symptoms (before any antibiotic is prescribed). The reason is that antibiotics in circulation can interfere with the results of subsequent antibiotic sensitivity testing because the presence of the first antibiotic can seriously affect the microbes' response to any other antibiotic. If the results of the test show penicillinase-producing organisms as the most probable etiological agents, then the newer semi-synthetic penicillinase resistant penicillins should be used. They should not be used if they are not needed, as they are not as effective as penicillin G, V or phenethicillin (Syncillin, Darcil) against most oral microbes. Other antibiotics that may be active against penicillinase-producing microbes are erythromycin, lincomycin, clindamycin, and the cephalosporins. If a patient has a very severe cellulitis (toxic, high fever, droopy eyes and dry, parched skin), it is a good idea to give both penicillinase-sensitive and penicillinase-resistant penicillins simultaneously, until a sample of the exudate can be tested. Broad spectrum antibiotics, like ampicillin (a broad-spectrum semi-synthetic penicillin) and the tetracyclines are less frequently indicated. The reason is that most acute apical abscesses and cellulitises are caused by Gram positive microbes, which are usually most susceptible to penicillin. The tetracyclines are bacteriostatic and hence microbes can recover, while penicillin and erythromycin (in high concentration) are bactericidal (the microbes are destroyed). However, the clinical effectiveness of an antibiotic is also related to dose, and site of action (concentration gradient between plasma and the involved tissue). Ampicillin has a broader spectrum than penicillin G or V, but it is less effective than the latter drugs against Gram positive microbes. Antibiotics should generally be prescribed for seven to ten days in order to effectively eradicate the microbes. Prolonged therapy (two weeks or longer) can lead to drug toxicity, allergic reactions, and superinfection. A summary of typical antibiotics for use in endodontics is given in Table V.

Potassium Penicillin G (Pentids/400), Phenoxymethyl Penicillin (V-cillin K, Pen-Vee K, Compocillin-VK) and Potassium Phenethicillin (Darcil, Marpen, Syncillin)

Penicillin G is not as effective orally as parenterally. The average oral dose is 400,000 units (one tablet) every four hours for seven days. It should be given at least one hour before eating or two hours after eating to prevent inactivation by the gastric juices. If the patient will reliably adhere to this schedule, the dentist can save the patient money and still give him (or her) effective therapy by prescribing penicillin G. If the cost is not too crucial, penicillin V or phenethicillin are much more reliable forms of oral penicillin, as they have greater resistance to acid deactiva-

TABLE V
TYPICAL ANTIBIOTICS*

Antibiotic	*Use*	*Usual Dose*
Penicillin V	Antibiotic of choice if patient is not allergic to it	One tablet (250 mg) every 6 hrs
Erythromycin	Antibiotic of choice if patient is allergic to penicillin	250 mg (one tablet or capsule) every 6 hrs
Penicillinase-resistant penicillins (Staphcillin; Resistopen, Unipen, etc.)	Antibiotic sensitivity testing shows pencillinase producing microbes are involved and are sensitive to these antibiotics	One tablet (250 mg) every 6 hrs
Ampicillin	Antibiotic sensitivity tests shows Gram negative organisms are present and are sensitive to this antibiotic	One capsule (250 mg) every 6 hrs
Tetracyclines	Antibiotic sensitivity tests show Gram negative organisms are present and are sensitive to these antibiotics	250 mg (one tablet or capsule) every 6 hrs
Clindamycin (Cleocin)	A good substitute if patient is allergic to penicillin; first choice after erythromycin	One tablet (150 mg) every 8 hrs
Lincomycin (Lincocin)	Can also be used for patient who is allergic to penicillin; second choice after erythromycin	Two capsules (500 mg) every 8 hrs
Cephalexin (Keflex)	New antibiotic; wider spectrum than penicillin, less affected by penicillinase, more side effects than penicillin, can't be used in patient allergic to penicillin	Two tablets (500 mg) every 6 hrs

*Usually taken for seven days.

tion than penicillin G. An average dose of penicillin V (or phenethicillin), is 250 mg (one tablet of 400,000 units), every six hours. For the average infection, the patient should be covered for seven days. For more severe cases, 500 mg every six hours should be given for the first one to two days. Once noticeable improvement occurs, the dosage can be decreased to 250 mg every six hours for approximately five more days. It is rarely necessary to use injectable penicillin in endodontic practice. However, if the patient is toxic, febrile, and has a severe cellulitis, an injectable form of penicillin should be used. A good choice for a high initial blood level plus a prolonged effect is Bicillin® All Purpose Injection (2 ml) which contains benzathine penicillin G, 600,000 units (prolonged effect), procaine penicillin G, 300,000 units (maintains good blood level for 24 hours), and potassium penicillin G, 300,000 units (rapid effect).

Penicillin is the least toxic of all the commonly used antibiotics. Its greatest disadvantages are the hypersensitivity reactions that can occur, and the emergence of microbial strains resistant to penicillin. Hypersensitivity reactions include erythema multiforme-like lesions, urticaria, serum sickness, angioneurotic edema, and anaphylactoid reactions (asthma, shock, and even death). Oral administration is much less likely to produce severe reactions. Treatment of these reactions is discussed in Chapter 16.

Penicillinase-Resistant Penicillins

These include methicillin (Staphcillin®), oxacillin (Prostaphlin®, Resistopen®), cloxacillin (Tegopen®), nafcillin (Unipen®), and dicloxacillin (Dynapen®). These drugs appear to be bound to a greater extent to serum proteins than is penicillin G. Hence, they are not as active as penicillin G against microbes which are not resistant. These penicillins cross react with penicillin G and therefore shouldn't be given to patients allergic to penicillin G. Bone marrow depression has been reported in isolated cases from ingestion of methicillin. Also superinfections from nonaffected microbes have been reported with methicillin. Average dose is similar to penicillin V, 250 mg every six hours and 500 mg for severe infections. The dose should be given one hour before meals or two hours after meals.

Ampicillin (Penbritin, Omnipen, Polycillin)

This penicillin has a broader spectrum than penicillin G but as stated before, is less effective against Gram positive microbes, and it is not resistant to the action of penicillinase-producing microbes. Ampicillin should not be used in patients with liver damage, and it has been reported to occasionally cause severe rashes and nephrotoxicity. Ampicillin also cross reacts with penicillin G and can cause hypersensitivity reactions in patients allergic to penicillin G. Typical dosage is 250 mg (in capsule form) every six hours for seven days.

Erythromycin

Erythromycin and its salts have an antibacterial spectrum similar to penicillin. Dosage forms are erythromycin (Ilotycin®, E-mycin) enteric coated tablets (100 and 250 mg), erythromycin stearate (Erythrocin S), 100 and 250 mg tablets, erythromycin estolate (Ilosone), capsules of 125 and 250 mg and 500 mg tablets, and chewable tablets of 125 mg, and erythromycin ethyl succinate (Erythrocin E, Pediamycin®), chewable tablets of 200 mg. Patients who are allergic to penicillin can take erythromycin because there is no cross reactivity between the two drugs. However, patients can become allergic to erythromycin and some bacteria can become resistant to its actions. Reactions that may occur include mild gastrointestinal effects, and in case of the estolate salt (Ilosone), liver impairment (which is usually reversible). The latter complication is characterized by jaundice, nausea, vomiting, and stomach pain, and it rarely occurs unless the patient is on the drug for more than 10 to 14 days. The advantage of the estolate salt is more reliable absorption. Usual dosage is 250 mg every six hours for 5 to 8 days. Ilosone also comes in a 500 mg tablet that only has to be taken every 12 hours. For the first one or two days in severe infections, 500 mg every six hours should be used. If the form of erythromycin used doesn't contain a buffer or an acid-resistant coating, then it should be given one hour before meals, or two hours after meals.

Lincomycin (Lincocin Capsules)

Lincomycin hydrochloride is effective against most oral Gram positive microbes. As most endodontic infections are caused by these microorganisms, lincomycin is usually an effective antibiotic. It can be given to patients who are allergic to penicillin. Hypersensitivity reactions are not frequent with lincomycin. The chief side effect is diarrhea, which may become so severe that the drug has to be discontinued. Lincomycin has the property of good bone penetration, but it is a bacteriostatic agent. Hence, if the patient is not allergic and the microbes are sensitive, penicillin is still preferable. Average dosage is 500 mg every 8 hours for seven days.

Clindamycin (Cleocin)

This antibiotic is related to lincomycin, but it has two advantages over it. It does not cause as severe a diarrhea, and it is effective in smaller doses. The antibacterial spectra are similar. Usual dose is 150 mg every 8 hours for seven days.

Tetracyclines

These broad spectrum antibiotics (effective against Gram positive and Gram negative microbes) have recently declined in favor because of the occurrence of undesirable side effects and adverse drug interactions. The various classes of tetracyclines include chlortetracycline (Aureomycin®), oxytetracycline (Terramycin®, Oxy-Kesso-Tetra®), tetracycline (Achromycin®, Tetracyn®), demethylchlortetracycline (Declomycin®), methacycline (Rondomycin®) and doxycycline (Vibramycin®). Microbial resistance can develop to these agents and allergic reactions can also occur. Tetracyclines should not be given to patients with the disease porphyria, because of severe reactions that can occur. Undesirable side effects include nausea, vomiting, diarrhea, overgrowth by fungi and yeasts (moniliasis), photosensitivity skin reactions (especially with Declomycin), kidney and liver damage (rare), anemia (rare) and enamel hypoplasia. The degree of enamel hypoplasia and the number of teeth affected depends upon when the tetracyclines were administered (Fig. 51). Because of all the possible side reactions, drug interactions, and their bacteriostatic nature, tetracyclines should only be used when the previously described antibiotics are not indicated. Milk and other high calcium foods interfere with the absorption of tetracyclines. Hence, these foods should not be given within one hour of the administration of the tetracyclines. In order to avoid gastric irritation, a small amount of food should be taken with the antibiotic. A full meal should be avoided as this would interfere with absorption. Usual dosage is 250 mg four times daily for seven days, for Declomycin and methacycline either 150 mg four times daily or 300 mg twice a day, and for doxycline 50 mg four times daily or 100 mg twice a day.

Cephalosporins

These antibiotics are similar to penicillin. They have a somewhat broader spectrum and are less affected by penicillinase. There is cross-antigenicity between the cephalosporins and penicillin; hence the cephalosporins should not be used for patients who are allergic to penicillin. The commercially available injectable forms are cephalothin (Keflin®) and cephaloridine (Loridine®). There is a new oral form now available, cephalexin monohydrate (Keflex). Usual dose is 250 to 500 mg every four to six hours for seven days. Clinical results are promising. In high doses, cephaloridine can cause kidney damage. Other effects are similar to penicillin.

Sulfonamides

Before the advent of antibiotics, sulfonamides had been widely used. However, because of their side effects, and possible drug interactions, the systemic use of these agents is not recommended unless the patient is allergic to or cannot take any indicated antibiotic. Some of the toxic effects of sulfonamides are hepatitis, leukopenia, granulocytopenia, thrombocytopenia, agranulocytosis, hemolytic anemia, kidney disturbances, skin photosensitivity, blisters of the skin and mucous membranes, fever, rash, anorexia, nausea, vomiting, eye disorders, and serious allergic reactions. For the rare endodontic indication, a dose schedule would be four 500 mg tablets of sulfadiazine to start, then two tablets every four to six hours until the infection is under control. The patient should be carefully checked for any sign of toxicity.

Sedatives, and Anti-Anxiety Agents

These drugs are used for premedication of the apprehensive patient. They do not have analgesic action. The classes are barbiturates, non-barbiturate sedatives, and the anti-anxiety agents (phenothiazines, meprobamate, hydroxyzine, and the diazepines). The sedatives affect the cerebral cortex, while the anti-anxiety agents selectively depress sub-cortical structures. Hence, the latter drugs are less likely to cause a loss of mental alertness and they can also block aggressive actions. Patients who have had sedatives must not drive. Generally, patients taking the anti-anxiety agents can become drowsy or lethargic and therefore should also have an accomplice to drive them home. Sedatives can become hypnotics (sleep-inducing) by an increase in the dose. The dentist may want to give a hypnotic the night before an endodontic procedure in an extremely apprehensive patient. These drugs are also useful as premedicants before general anesthesia, by themselves, or in conjunction with narcotics. They may be also used in intravenous therapy for sedation and as a co-medication with nitrous-oxide analgesia. Patients who are on depressant drugs require a much lower dosage of sedatives or anti-anxiety drugs, and alcohol must be avoided as a combined effect can lead to serious depression. (See section on drugs in Chapter 1.) A summary of typical agents is given in Table VI.

TABLE VI

TYPICAL SEDATIVES AND ANTI-ANXIETY AGENTS

Agent	*Category*	*Usual Dose*
Pentobarbital (Nembutal)	Sedative	30 mg the night before the visit; 60 mg one-half hour before the visit
Secobarbital (Seconal)	Sedative	50 mg the night before the visit; 50 mg one-half hour before the visit
Ethinamate (Valmid)	Sedative	One to two tablets (500 mg to 1 gr) the night before the visit; one tablet one-half hour before the visit
Chloral hydrate (Noctec)	Sedative	500 mg (in syrup) one-half hour before the visit
Chlordiazepoxide (Librium)	Anti-anxiety agent	One capsule (5 mg) morning and evening starting two days before the visit; two capsules one hour before the visit
Diazepam (Valium)	Anti-anxiety agent	One capsule (5 mg) morning and evening starting two days before the visit; two capsules one hour before the visit
Hydroxyzine (Atarax, Vistaril)	Anti-anxiety agent	50 mg the night before the visit; 50 mg one-half hour before the visit
Meprobamate (Equanil, Miltown)	Anti-anxiety agent	One tablet (200 or 400 mg) four times daily beginning three days before the visit

Barbiturates

The short acting barbiturates, pentobarbital (Nembutal) and secobarbital (Seconal) have the greatest application in endodontics. However, there are possible disadvantages. These include contraindication in patients with porphyria, asthma, and liver disease because of damaging effect; side effects such as occasionally causing excitement rather than depression, dizziness, headache, nausea, diarrhea, and skin eruptions; potential for habituation (psychic dependence); possibility of deleterious drug interactions; and overdoses can cause respiratory depression and death. Typical dosage schedule is 30 mg (7.5 ml of elixir Nembutal), the night before the appointment and 60 mg (15 ml) one-half hour before the visit. If there is a great amount of pain, 60 mg of pentobarbital (15 ml) can be given with 50 mg of meperidine (Demerol), one hour before the dental appointment (given on empty stomach). This should give good sedation and analgesia. The dose for secobarbital is 50 mg, the night before and one-half hour pretreatment.

Non-Barbiturate Sedatives

For patients who have a tendency to become habituated to barbiturates or who cannot take a barbiturate for some other reason, the non-barbiturate sedative drugs may be used. They generally are less effective and produce more side effects than the barbiturates. In extreme doses, they can produce respiratory depression and death. Drugs in this class include ethinamate (Valmid®), ethchorvynol (Placidyl), glutethimide

(Doriden), methprylon (Noludar®), methaqualone (Quaalude, Soper®) chloral hydrate (Noctec®) and paraldehyde. Valmid can have the side effects of drowsiness, occasionally a residual hangover (less than with barbiturates), lethargy, gastrointestinal upsets, skin eruptions, and addiction. Typical dosage schedule is 500 mg to 1 gram (one to two tablets) the night before the visit and one tablet one-half hour before the appointment. Habituation can develop to Placidyl. A sedative dose is 100 to 200 mg. Reactions to Doriden include nausea, drowsiness, headache, lethargy, stomach upset, skin rashes, occasional residual hangover, and addiction. Average sedative dose is 125 to 250 mg; for hypnosis 500 mg is used. Noludar has side effects similar to Doriden. Typical sedative dose is 50 to 100 mg and the onset takes 30 minutes. Methaqualone (Quaalude) has a very high addiction-liability and it therefore doesn't appear to have a use in dentistry. Chloral hydrate is a relatively safe and effective sedative. It is contraindicated in patients with liver or kidney impairment. Side effects include nausea, vomiting, gastrointestinal upsets, and rashes. Prolonged use can lead to habituation. An average dose is 500 mg given in syrups, as the powder itself causes gastric irritation. Onset of action takes about thirty minutes. Paraldehyde is another relatively safe and effective sedative. It is not used too often because of a disagreeable odor and taste. This can be masked somewhat with syrups. However, the patient's exhaled air may have an odor due to the excretion of this drug by the lungs. It is contraindicated in patients with lung and liver disease. Habituation rarely occurs and prolonged use may lead to liver damage. Usual dose is 3 to 8 ml in a syrup such as orange or cinnamon.

Anti-Anxiety Agents

These include the agents formerly grouped as tranquilizers, and ataractics. Drugs considered are promethazine, meprobamate, hydroxyzine, and the diazepines.

PROMETHAZINE HYDROCHLORIDE (PHENERGAN HYDROCHLORIDE). This is a phenothiazine drug that possesses antihistaminic action as well as sedation. It can be used along with meperidine (Demerol) for sedation with analgesia. Adverse reactions are dizziness, drowsiness, nausea, headache, and xerostomia. Other phenothiazines can cause blood dyscrasias, jaundice, postural hypotension and epinephrine reversal, but these reactions have not been reported for Phenergan. However, they should be considered and it is good practice to use a local anesthetic without epinephrine when the patient is taking Phenergan. Typical dosage schedule is 25 to 50 mg 12 to 24 hours before the visit, and the same dose one hour before the procedure.

MEPROBAMATE (EQUANIL, MILTOWN). This is a good drug to suppress anxiety and tension, and it produces sedation and much less drowsiness than barbiturates. Adverse effects include dizziness, headache, drowsiness, xerostomia, gastrointestinal upsets, nausea, vomiting, and an occasional rash. Prolonged use can lead to habituation. Some studies have shown that meprobamate is no more effective than a placebo. For most effectiveness, meprobamate therapy should begin approximately three days before the procedure. The dose is one tablet (200 or 400 mg), four times a day.

HYDROXYZINE (ATARAX®, VISTARIL®). This is a sedative-type antihistamine. It is an effective, relatively safe drug that is useful in the management of anxiety and tension. Side effects include drowsiness, xerostomia, dizziness, nausea, vomiting, and gastrointestinal upsets. A common dosage schedule is 50 mg the night before the appointment, and 50 mg one-half hour before the visit.

DIAZEPINES. These anti-anxiety agents include three closely related compounds, chlordiazepoxide (Librium), diazepam (Valium) and oxazepam (Serax®).

Chlordiazepoxide (Librium). This is an agent widely used for the relief of anxiety, apprehension, and tension. Adverse effects are drowsiness, euphoria, excitement instead of calming (rare reaction), lethargy, nausea, headache, rash, agranulocytosis, and jaundice. Dependence can develop after prolonged use. A typical dose schedule is 5 mg (one Librium capsule) morning and evening, starting two days before the procedure, plus two capsules (10 mg) one hour before the appointment.

Diazepam (Valium). This is another widely used psychosedative. It is also used effectively for intravenous sedation. Diazepam is contraindicated in patients with glaucoma because of dangerous reactions. Side effects are similar to those described for Librium. Valium comes in 5 mg tablets and the schedule is similar to that described for Librium.

Oxazepam (Serax). The uses, effects, and contraindications are similar to those of chlordiazepoxide. Dose is 10 to 30 mg, three or four times daily.

Anti-Inflammatory Agents

These drugs have been and are being used for the control of post-surgical swelling in endodontics. However, there is a great deal of controversy about their effectiveness or necessity. It very well may be that it is not biologically sound to interfere with the inflammatory reaction, as the latter is the natural method to overcome injurious agents, and initiate the repair process. However in certain cases, for aesthetic and functional reasons, it may be necessary to decrease post-surgical swelling. If infection is present or suspected, an antibiotic must also be used. A summary of some anti-inflammatory agents is given in Table VII.

Antihistamines

These drugs have been considered as effective in the reversal of a low grade pulpititis provided that the causative factors were removed. The theory is that histamine is released as a result of damage to injured cells, and the antihistamines counteract this effect. However, there has never been any clinical documentation to verify this concept. Antihistamines have also been used to treat post-surgical swelling with equivocal results. Other uses of antihistamines are for treatment of allergic reactions (see Chapter 16, Medical Emergencies) and as local anesthetic agents (see Chap-

TABLE VII

TYPICAL ANTI-INFLAMMATORY AGENTS*

Agent	*Category*	*Usual Dose*
Brompheniramine maleate (Dimetane)	Antihistamine	4 mg four times daily for 5 to 7 days
Chlorpheniramine maleate (Chlortrimeton)	Antihistamine	4 mg four times daily for 5 to 7 days
Diphenhydramine HCl (Benadryl)	Antihistamine	25 mg four times daily for 5 to 7 days
Tripelennamine HCl (Pyribenzamine)	Antihistamine	25 mg four times daily for 5 to 7 days
Thonzylamine (Anahist)	Antihistamine	25 mg four times daily for 5 to 7 days
Aspirin	Analgesic	300-600 mg every 3-4 hrs
Streptokinase Streptodornase (Varidase)	Enzyme	One tablet four times daily
Papain (Papase)	Enzyme	One or two tablets one hour before visit; one tablet every two hours the first day; one tablet every 6 hrs the next 3 days
Alpha amylase (Buclamase)	Enzyme	Two tablets four times daily for 3 to 5 days
Trypsin (Chymoral)	Enzyme	Two tablets four times daily for the first day; one tablet four times daily for the the next few days
Prednisone	Corticosteroid	Not recommended

* This table is presented for informational use only, as anti-inflammatory agents are not usually necessary in endodontics.

ter 5, section on local anesthesia). Undesirable effects include sedation, convulsions (rare), and allergic reactions. Antihistamines have an additive effect with sedatives. Typical drugs and dosages are brompheniramine maleate (Dimetane®), 4 mg four times a day for 5 to 7 days; chlorpheniramine maleate (Chlor-Trimeton Maleate), 4 mg four times a day for 5 to 7 days; dexcholorpheniramine maleate (Polaramine® Maleate) 2 mg four times a day for 5 to 7 days; diphenhydramine hydrochloride (Benadryl) 25 mg four times a day for 5 to 7 days; tripelennamine hydrochloride (Pyribenzamine), 25 mg four times a day for 5 to 7 days; and thonzylamine (Anahist) 25 mg four times a day for 5 to 7 days.

Proteolytic Enzymes

These enzymes break down proteins. However, clinical studies have shown ambiguous results. Some of the agents used are chymotrypsin (Chymar®), trypsin (Chymoral®), alpha amylase (Buclamase®), and papain (Papase®). Allergic reactions are possible to these drugs. Side effects from alpha amylase and papain include development of a rash and gastrointestinal upset. The dose schedule for Papase is one or two tablets one hour before surgery, one tablet every two hours for the first day after surgery, and then one tablet every six hours for three more days. Buclamase dose schedule is two tablets four times daily for three to five days. For Chymoral, two tablets are taken four times a day for the first day; then for the next few days one tablet is taken four times a day. Chymar is given only by intramuscular injection. The dose is one-half to one ml three times a day starting the day of surgery and continuing till the swelling decreases noticeably.

Corticosteroids

The corticosteroids have the best anti-inflammatory response of any of the drugs previously described. However, they also have the most severe side effects. Not only do they interfere with inflammation, they also interfere with repair and if infection is present, a severe cellulitis can develop. The contraindications and other effects have been described in Chapter I. Patients have to be gradually taken off the steroid to prevent adrenal insufficiency. Because of all these reasons, the systemic administration of corticosteroids is not recommended. Local use was discussed in the sections on pulp capping and nonsurgical endodontic therapy in Chapter 3.

Electromagnetic Energy

A new modality that has been used on occasion is not a drug but it is reported to be effective in the reduction of post-surgical edema and ecchymosis. It is the use of nonthermal pulsed high-peak power electromagnetic energy (Diapulse®). The therapy is purported to be effective as a result of increased permeability of edematous tissues allowing for free flow of blood and other body fluids in the inflamed areas. This then should facilitate drainage and tissue repair. One clinical study has shown it to be effective, but further testing appears to be necessary as it has not been approved by the F.D.A.

Antisialagogues

There are patients who salivate excessively and this can be a problem during endodontic therapy. The use of antisialagogues can help in controlling salivation. Drugs considered are atropine, belladonna, methantheline, and propantheline.

Atropine Sulfate

Atropine effectively dries up secretions of the mouth, nose, and throat. It should be used with caution in patients with cardiovascular and pulmonary diseases, as there can be an increase in pulse and respiratory rate with these patients. Atropine should also be used cautiously in patients with glaucoma, although the small doses used in dentistry probably wouldn't precipitate an attack. Side effects are dryness of the throat, blurring or dimness of vision, dry skin sensation, reddening of the face, nausea, headache, and an increased pulse and respiratory rate. An average dose is between one-quarter to one mg (1/240 to 1/60 grain atropine sulfate tablets), taken two hours before the appointment.

Belladonna Tincture

This has atropine sulfate as its active component. Contraindications and effects are the same as for atropine. Usual dose is 0.6 ml about two to three hours before treatment.

Methantheline Bromide (Banthine® Tablets)

The effects of this drug are similar to atropine, but there is a greater tendency toward glaucoma and it is more dangerous to use for patients with cardiovascular disease. Usual dose is 50 mg, thirty minutes pre-operatively.

Propantheline Bromide (Pro-Banthine®)

Reactions and contraindications are similar to those for Banthine. A common dose is 15 mg taken thirty to forty-five minutes before treatment.

Nutritional Supplements

For patients that the dentist knows or suspects may have a nutritionally defective diet, it is good clinical judgment to prescribe nutritional supplements after surgery. This is also true following traumatic surgical procedures in which the patient may experience difficulty in masticating solid foods. To aid in repair the patient should receive sufficient proteins, minerals, vitamins A, C, and B complex, and fluid (about 2.5 liters of water daily). Recent research indicates that in stress, there is a severe depletion of the vitamin C level of the blood and most patients are under stress prior to surgery. Therefore, it is a good idea to give these patients vitamin C prior to the procedure and for a few days post-surgically (500 mg twice a day, preferably a sustained or slow release capsule). There is also some evidence to show that optimum levels of zinc are needed for repair, although the exact dosage needed is not definitely known. Zinc is rich in seeds (sesame, sunflower) and wheat germ. Recent research shows that vitamin A is needed for protein formation from amino acids. Good protein-vitamin-mineral food supplements are Carnation Instant Breakfast®, Nutrament®, Instant Nutrament®, and Meritene®. All except Nutrament should be mixed with 8 ounces of milk. Acceptable B complex and C preparations are Surbex-T®, Albee® with C, Albee-T®, Thera-Combex H-P Kapseals®, Novo Basic® (high potency B complex with C), Cebefortis® tablets, Cevi-Bid® capsules, B-C-Bid® capsules, and Stren-Tabs®. Adequate vitamin A can be obtained in milk, cheese, butter, and other dairy products.

Nasal Decongestants

As part of the treatment for a maxillary sinus perforation, the patient should receive a prescription for Neo-Synephrine® nose drops or nasal spray. The rationale is that the vasoconstrictor shrinks the nasal membranes which then keeps the ostium open and allows for adequate drainage through the nose from the sinus. The vasoconstrictor can control any hemorrhage that may be present. This should not be prescribed for any patient who cannot or should not take a vasopressor agent.

BIBLIOGRAPHY

General

American Dental Association: *Accepted Dental Therapeutics 1973/1974.* 35th ed. Chicago, American Dental Association, 1973.

Ellison, R.: Drug Considerations in Endodontics. Presented at the Louis I. Grossman Endodontic Study Club Meeting, Oct. 1972, Philadelphia, Pennsylvania.

Gurney, B. F.: Anesthesiology and pharmacology in endodontics. *Dent Clin North Am, 11:*615, 1967.

Weine, F. S.: *Endodontic Therapy,* St. Louis, Mosby, 1972.

Analgesics

Guernsey, L. H.: Analgesics in dental practice. *Dent Clin North Am, 14:*757, 1970.

Gurney, B. F.: Chemotherapy in dental practice: aspirin compounds; part one. *Dent Dig, 76:*439, 1970.

Gurney, B. F.: Chemotherapy in dental practice: aspirin compounds; part two. *Dent Dig, 76:*476, 1970.

Gurney, B. F.: Chemotherapy in dental practice: acetaminophen preparations. *Dent Dig, 76:*527, 1970.

Gurney, B. F.: Chemotherapy: nonnarcotic analgesics; part one, pentazocine. *Dent Dig, 77:*598, 1971.

Gurney, B. F.: Chemotherapy: nonnarcotic analgesics; part two, mefenamic acid. *Dent Dig, 77:*666, 1971.

Popkes, D. L., and Folsom, T. C., Jr.: Comparative study of three analgesic agents used in oral surgical procedures. *J Oral Surg, 27:*950, 1969.

Reynolds, D. C.: Pain control in the dental office. *Dent Clin North Am, 15:*319, 1971.

Walton, J. G., and Thompson, J. W.: Pharmacology for the dental practitioner. 10—The relief of pain: nonnarcotic analgesics and desensitising agents. *Br Dent J, 127:*472, 1969.

Walton, J. G., and Thompson, J. W.: Pharmacology for the dental practitioner. 11—The relief of pain: narcotic analgesics and premedication (including the use of psychotropic drugs). *Br Dent J, 127:*511, 1969.

Antibiotics

Booth, D. F.: Acute anaphylaxis from orally administered penicillin G: report of case. *JADA, 85:*1367, 1972.

Davis, W. M., Jr., and Balcom, J. H.: Lincomycin studies of drug absorption and efficacy. *Oral Surg, 27:*688, 1969.

Gurney, B. F.: Chemotherapy: cephalosporins; part one. *Dent Dig, 78:*98, 1972.

Gurney, B. F.: Chemotherapy: cephalosporins; part two. *Dent Dig, 78:*144, 1972.

Holroyd, S. V.: Clinical pharmacology of antibiotics of dental importance. *Dent Clin North Am, 14:*711, 1970.

Hooley, J. R.: Cloxacillin in the treatment of dental infection. *Oral Surg, 28:*485, 1969.

Mopsik, E. R.: Infections and antibiotics. *Dent Clin North Am, 15:*327, 1971.

Okun, R.: Use and abuse of antibiotics. *J Hosp Dent Pract, 2:*3, 1968.

Paterson, J. A., Cardo, V. A., Jr., and Stratigos, G. T.: An examination of antibiotic prophylaxis in oral and maxillofacial surgery. *J Oral Surg, 28:*753, 1970.

Tarsitano, J. J.: The use of antibiotics in dental practice. *Dent Clin North Am, 14:*697, 1970.

Walton, J. G., and Thompson, J. W.: Pharmacology for the dental practitioner. 13-chemotherapeutic agents (1). *Br Dent J, 128:*32, 1970.

Walton, J. G., and Thompson, J. W.: Pharmacology for the dental practitioner. 14-chemotherapeutic agents (2). *Br Dent J, 128:*85, 1970.

Walton, J. G., and Thompson, J. W.: Pharmacology for the dental practitioner. 15—chemotherapeutic agents (3); including their prophylactic use. *Br Dent J, 128:*134, 1970.

Sedatives and Anti-Anxiety Agents

Gurney, B. F.: Chemotherapy in dental practice: anti-anxiety agents; part one, meprobamate. *Dent Dig, 75:*327, 1969.

Gurney, B. F.: Chemotherapy in dental practice: anti-anxiety agents; part two, diazepines. *Dent Dig, 75:*368, 1969.

Gurney, B. F.: Chemotherapy in dental practice: barbiturate substitutes; part one, glutethimide, and methprylon. *Dent Dig, 75:*421, 1969.

Gurney, B. F.: Chemotherapy in dental practice: barbiturate substitutes; part two, hydroxizine, methapyrilene, and pyrilamine. *Dent Dig, 75:*467, 1969.

Small, E. W.: Preoperative sedation in dentistry. *Dent Clin North Am, 14:*769, 1970.

Anti-Inflammatory Agents

Aronsky, D. H.: Reduction of dental postsurgical symptoms using nonthermal pulsed high-peak-power electromagnetic energy. *Oral Surg, 32:*688, 1971.

Cranin, A. N., and Cranin, S. L.: A study of the effects of an antihistamine on oral surgical postoperative sequelae. *Oral Surg, 18:*432, 1964.

Galloway, C. R., Hinds, E. C., and Reid, R.:

Clinical and laboratory evaluation of streptokinase-streptodornase in oral surgery. *J Oral Surg, 25:*147, 1967.

Gurney, B. F.: Chemotherapy in dental practice. *Dent Dig, 71:*93, 1965.

Marlotte, R. H., and Amen, C. R.: An evaluation of two proteolytic enzymes and critique of the clinical study. *Oral Surg, 29:* 249, 1970.

Michanowicz, A. E., Michanowicz, J. P., and Watkins, E. B.: Clinical report on the use of alpha amylase (buclamase) following periapical surgery. *Oral Surg, 18:*377, 1964.

Nathanson, N. R., and Seifert, D. M.: Betamethasone in dentistry: a clinical report. *Oral Surg, 18:*715, 1964.

Young, H. R.: Resolution of postoperative swelling following oral surgery: chymoral. *Oral Surg, 23:*12, 1967.

Antisialagogues and Nutrition

Gurney, B. F.: Chemotherapy in dental practice: antisialagogues. *Dent Dig, 73:*270, 1967.

Jones, N. B.: Dietary needs of the oral surgery patient with comparison of dietary supplements. *J Oral Surg, 28:*892, 1970.

Nizel, A. E.: *The Science of Nutrition and Its Application in Clinical Dentistry,* 2nd ed. Philadelphia, Saunders, 1966.

Smith, J. F.: Nutritional maintenance of the dental patient. *Dent Clin North Am, 14:* 833, 1970.

CHAPTER 5

ANALGESIA AND ANESTHESIA

These are the techniques that allow the dentist to perform endodontic therapy in a relatively painless environment. Among the modalities discussed are nitrous oxide-oxygen relative analgesia, chemanalgesia, audio-analgesia, hypnosis, general anesthesia, acupuncture anesthesia, local anesthesia, mummification, electro-anesthesia, jet injection anesthesia, and topical anesthesia.

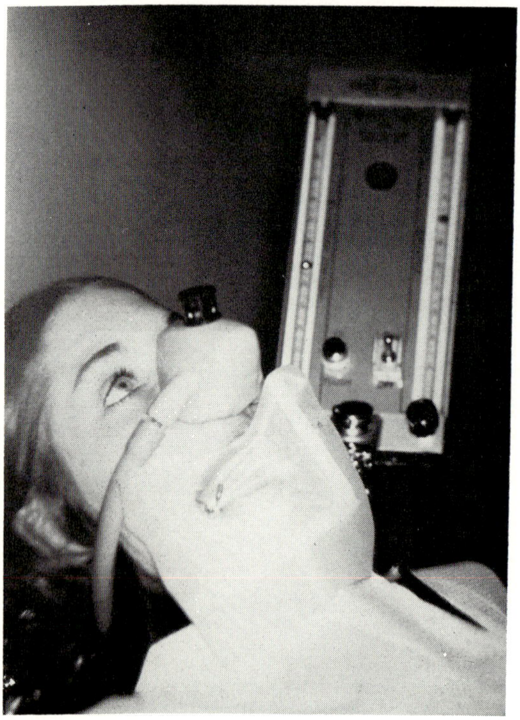

Figure 350. Nitrous oxide-oxygen relative analgesia in use with rubber dam in position.

NITROUS OXIDE-OXYGEN RELATIVE ANALGESIA (NITROUS OXIDE-OXYGEN PSYCHOSEDATION)

This is the most popular and safest form of psychosedation. It is a method of sedation, tranquilization and analgesia, using an inhalation technique with a small rubber nosepiece and the gaseous mixture of nitrous oxide and oxygen (Fig. 350). Nitrous oxide-oxygen analgesia is more effective and reliable than oral sedatives and anti-anxiety agents, but less effective than intravenous chemanalgesia. However, if combined with good local anesthesia, it is the treatment of choice for good sedation, anxiety reduction and analgesia. Most machines now in use are of the constant-flow, fail-safe type. The machines cannot deliver less than 2.5 liters/minute of oxygen, and if the oxygen supply runs out, the nitrous oxide automatically cuts off. Also, newer machines have settings, valves, and hoses that cannot be transposed from the nitrous oxide to oxygen tanks. Hence, the patient cannot inadvertently be given pure nitrous oxide. A typical setting is 2.5 liters/minute oxygen, 3.5 liters/minute nitrous oxide, and the nasal inhaler air vent left open. With this setting, the patients receive at least 50 per cent oxygen. Side effects are quite infrequent and include nausea, vomiting, persisting euphoria, and fright. Most patients feel an exhilarating, pleasant, relaxed feeling, somewhat akin to one or two *martinis.* However, an occasional patient will feel trapped. If the patient persists in this type of feeling, the nitrous oxide should be shut off, pure oxygen should be administered for about one to two minutes, and a different modality should be used. After a typical session, pure oxygen should be given for one to two minutes and most patients then feel perfectly normal. However, they should be assisted from the chair in case they are slightly dizzy. After a few minutes, the patient should be able to drive home unaccompanied. During endodontic therapy, radiographs can be taken and surgery can be performed with the small analgesic nose piece in position. For a routine vital case, nitrous oxide-oxygen relative analgesia is given, after the modality has been explained to the patient. When the patient has begun to have a *tingly,* warm feeling, after one to three minutes, a painless local anesthetic injection can be given. The analgesia is continued during the whole extent of the procedure. The patients usually feel no pain, and may actually enjoy the procedure. For a pulpless case, at the second visit of a vital case, or at the obturation visit, nitrous oxide-oxygen relative analgesia is used alone. Some other uses of nitrous oxide-oxygen relative analgesia in endodontics are incision and drainage (when local anesthesia is difficult to obtain), opening into a tooth when the patient has an acute exacerbation of a chronic pulpitis or periapical lesion, an acute abscess or cellulitis (also difficult to obtain local anesthesia), placement of rubber dam clamp, drain removal, suture removal (the last three are minor procedures that can be painful), removing a crown or a bridge, pulp testing a sensitive tooth (dentists can still get a response but the sensation is dulled), all surgical procedures, in conjunction with local anesthesia (takes a patient's mind off what is happening), caries removal, periodontal curettage for drainage, and in conjunction with other modalities, such as hypnosis, audio analgesia, chemanalgesia, and intrapulpal anesthesia. Dentists should use nitrous oxide-oxygen psychosedation only after they have taken a dental school or dental society-approved course.

CHEMANALGESIA

This is the use of chemical agents injected intravenously for the purpose of psychosedation and varying degrees of analgesia (Fig. 351). Nitrous oxide-oxygen relative analgesia may be used in conjunction with chemanalgesia. Local anesthetics are generally added to give good regional analgesia. The drugs and drug combinations that are currently used for chemanalgesia are diazepam (Valium); neuroleptanalgesia (Innovar®, which contains the tranquilizer droperidol, 2.5 mg per ml, and the narcotic analgesic fentanyl, 0.05 mg per ml); propiomazine (a phenothiazine, tranquilizer); hydroxyzine (Atarax); meperidine (Demerol); diazepam and meperidine; hydroxyzine and meperidine; hydroxyzine and fentanyl; pentobarbital and meperidine; pentobarbital, meperidine, and scopolamine; intermittent methohexital sodium (Brevital®

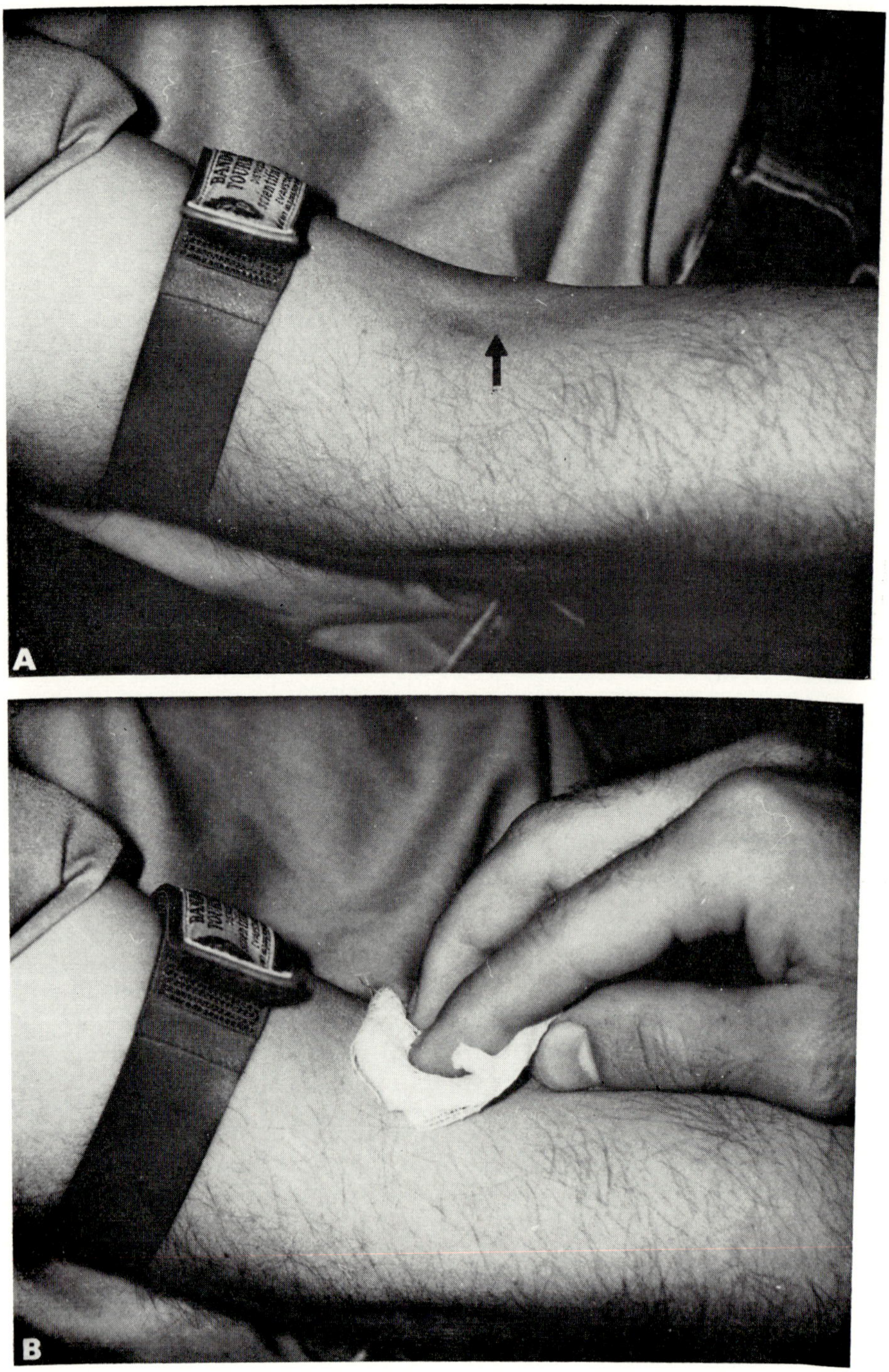
A
B

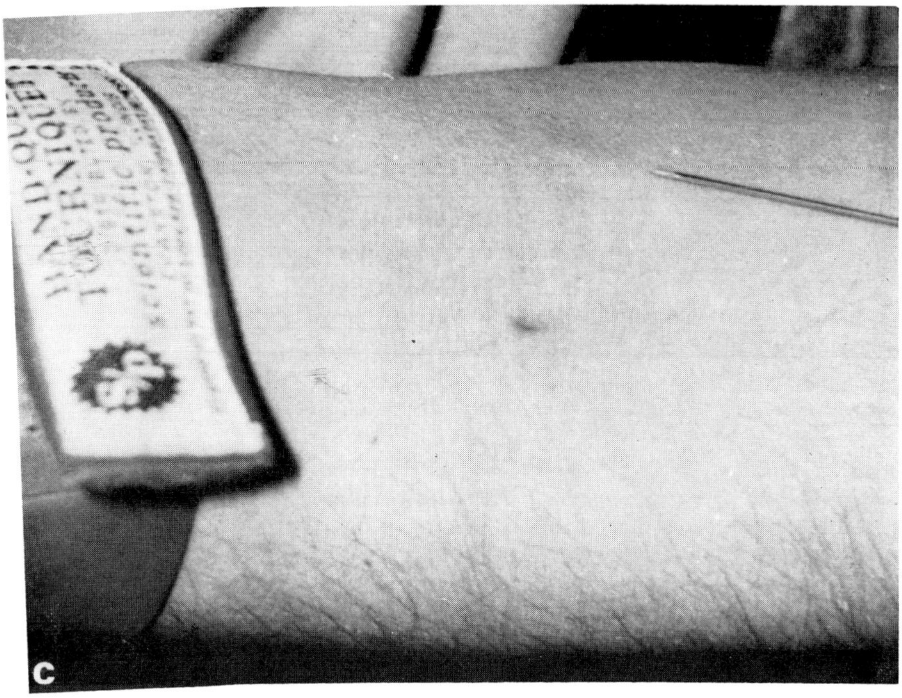

Figure 351. Chemanalgesia (IV sedation). A. Arrow points to site of injection. B. Site being decontaminated. C. Needle inserted into vein.

Sodium); intermittent propanidad; secobarbital, meperidine and methohexital; hydroxyzine, alphaprodine (Nisentil®), and methohexital; diazepam and methohexital. These drugs and drug combinations are all designed to give various degrees of sedation, analgesia, and amnesia. One of the safest and most widely used drugs is diazepam alone. Although chemanalgesia gives the greatest degree of sedation, as compared to oral and inhalation techniques, it also requires much greater care, expecially when combinations of drugs are used. Under *no* circumstances should chemanalgesia be used, unless the dentist has had adequate training in its use. There are now available one week dental society and dental school-sponsored courses. This is the minimum training that a dentist should have. The practitioner should not use those drugs that are also general anesthesics such as methohexital, unless he (or she) has had general anesthesia training. It is imperative that the dentist is knowledgeable of resuscitative methods when chemanalgesia is used, even though the dentist may rarely have to use these methods. It is important that a sphygmomanometer is available to record blood pressure changes, and it is advisable to have an audible pulse rate monitor. There must be adequate recovery room facilities available and someone must be present to drive the patient home. The dentist should be knowledgeable of the contraindications and side effects of the various drugs that may be used (see under the section for each of the drugs).

AUDIO ANALGESIA

This modality was popular a few years ago. The patients listened with headphones to a *white* sound and/or stereo music and supposedly the sound was able to diminish the intensity of painful impulses. This technique was never proven effective by double blind studies. However, some dentists do find that the use of stereophonic, semi-classical music with headphones, provides a calming effect to many patients. It has also been found that the use of nitrous oxide-oxygen relative analgesia and stereophonic music with headphones is an advantageous combination with certain patients. Audio analgesia has also been used successfully along with hypnosis to control fear and pain.

HYPNOSIS

This method of inducing analgesia, sedation, and amnesia by the use of suggestion is being practiced by certain dentists. There is no doubt that it can be successful in amenable patients. The disadvantages are that it may be time consuming, it may cause adverse psychological reactions on the part of the patient, and patients may object to the loss of control. Dentists should have adequate training in this method before employing it in their practice.

GENERAL ANESTHESIA

In this form of anesthesia, the patient is rendered unconscious, with analgesia, muscle relaxation, and amnesia occurring. There are various methods in use including nitrous oxide-oxygen with either trichlorethylene, halothane (Fluothane®), methoxyflurane (Penthrane®), or vinyl ether (Vinethene®); sodium thiopental (Pentothal® Sodium) or sodium methohexital (Brevital Sodium) with atropine sulfate; and ketamine hydrochloride. General anesthesia is rarely used in endodontic therapy. Some possible uses are for debilitated hospitalized patients, patients with uncontrollable fear, and patients in which acute pain cannot be relieved by any other method. General anesthesia should only be used under the supervision of a practitioner thoroughly trained in its use. If a dentist gives the anesthesia, he (or she) should first have had an anesthesia residency in an approved hospital or dental school program. There must be facilities for continuous monitoring of the patient and all emergency equipment and drugs must be readily at hand. Side effects and contraindications for these procedures must definitely be known. Because of all these considerations, endodontics under general anesthesia should only be performed in a hospital or in an office thoroughly set up for general anesthesia. It should *not* be performed in a general practitioner or endodontist's office without all these facilities.

ACUPUNCTURE ANESTHESIA

This is an oriental method of obtaining analgesia by the insertion of long, sterile needles into certain predetermined anatomical sites of the body. The needles are continuously rotated. It has been recently introduced into the

U.S. from China where it has been in use for several years. Acupuncture is being tested in several dental institutions in this country. It is too early to state whether acupuncture anesthesia will become an accepted method of analgesia that can be of use in endodontics. A recent study in New York involved thirty patients. The patients were being treated for operative dentistry, extractions, and endodontic therapy. Successful anesthesia was achieved in 80 per cent of the patients with another ten per cent showing partial analgesia. We are currently conducting a study at Temple University Hospital and Dental School.

LOCAL ANESTHESIA

This is the injection of a solution, usually a water soluble salt of a weak organic base, into the skin or mucous membrane for the purpose of obtaining regional analgesia of the involved tissues. The usual anesthetic agents used in dentistry are of two types, ester and amide. Examples of the ester type are procaine hydrochloride (Novocain®), butethamine hydrochloride (Monocaine® Hydrochloride), meprylcaine hydrochloride (Oracaine® Hydrochloride), isobucaine hydrochloride (Kincaine® Hydrochloride), tetracaine (Pontocaine®) hydrochloride (in Novocain® 2%, Pontocaine Hydrochloride 0.15%, Neo-cobefrin® 1:20,000), and propoxycaine (Ravocaine®), hydrochloride (in Ravocaine Hydrochloride 0.4%, Novocain 2%, and Neo-cobefrin 1:20,000 or Levophed® 1:30,000). Examples of the amide type are lidocaine hydrochloride (Xylocaine Hydrochloride, Octacaine® Hydrochloride, Lidocaton®, Lidothesin®), mepivacaine hydrochloride (Carbocaine® Hydrochloride), prilocaine hydrochloride (Citanest Hydrochloride), and pyrrocaine hydrochloride (Dynacaine® Hydrochloride). If a patient is allergic to an ester-type anesthetic, the dentist can then use an amide-type anesthetic. There is a much higher incidence of hypersensitivity to ester-type anesthetics as compared to amide-type anesthetics. There is cross allergenicity between members within each group of anesthetics. Therefore if a patient is allergic to one member of the ester series, he (or she) can also be allergic to any other members. The same is true for amide local anesthetics.

Most local anesthetics contain vasoconstrictors. These are used to prolong and intensify the reaction and delay the anesthetic from entering the systemic circulation. Vasoconstrictors also decrease hemorrhage in the local area. Some commonly used vasoconstrictors are epinephrine (Adrenalin®), phenylephrine (Neo-Synephrine), levonordefrin (Neo-cobefrin), and levarterenol (Levophed). Preservatives are also included in local anesthetic solutions. Reactions to local anesthetics or their additives are not common but they should be recognized and treated promptly, when they occur. Some dentists can develop contact dermatitis (an allergic reaction) by mere contact with local anesthetic solutions. Patient reactions can be psychogenic, systemic reactions to the local anesthetic, hypersensitivity reactions to the local anesthetic, vasoconstrictor, or preservative and systemic reactions to local anesthetics.

Psychogenic

This is the usual fainting reaction (syncope). Use of nitrous oxide-oxygen relative analgesia (high oxygen content) before giving the injection should prevent a fainting reaction. Other measures that would diminish the incidence of syncope and a painful injection are premedication, calm and reassuring manner by the practitioner, IV sedation, hypnosis, jet or topical anesthesia before injection, relaxing music, use of fine gauge sharp needles (preferably 25 bore disposable type), use of a slow injection technique, prewarming the anesthetic carpules, application of pressure by pulling the lip or cheek tight at the same time the injection is given, and applying pressure on the palate or lingual surfaces by pressing with a mirror as the injection is given.

Systemic Reactions

First reaction is central nervous system stimulation, which is followed by central nervous system depression. Diagnosis and treatment of these reactions is described in Chapter 16. Use of aspiration during injection can help prevent these systemic reactions. If blood is withdrawn, a new site should be selected and the injection repeated. It has been shown that with the use of a 27 gauge needle, as compared to the use of a 25 gauge needle, there is a higher incidence of intravascular injections for an inferior alveolar block injection. Premedication with a barbiturate offsets the central nervous system stimulation, but enhances the depression reaction, and is therefore not advantageous with amide-type local anesthetics.

Other Systemic Reactions

In patients with plasma cholinesterase deficiency, sudden collapse, followed by unconsciousness and cyanosis, may occur following local anesthetic injection. This occurs only after ester-type local anesthetic injections. One of the infrequent side effects of prilocaine (Citanest®) is the development of methemoglobinemia. As prilocaine can pass the placenta and cause methemoglobinemia in the fetus, it should not be used for pregnant women.

Hypersensitivity Reactions

True allergic reactions such as rash, angioneurotic edema, asthma, and anaphylactoid reactions can occur to the local anesthetic, vasoconstrictor, or preservative. Allergic reactions occur more readily with ester type local anesthetics.

Systemic Reaction to the Vasoconstrictor

Systemic reactions to the vasoconstrictor may occur, and include an increase in blood pressure and heart rate. Use of vasoconstrictors are contraindicated in patients with hyperthyroidism, and medical consultation should be obtained before using vasoconstrictors for cardiac patients. After a local anesthetic is given, the patient should always be kept under observation (either by the assistant or doctor). Treatment for these reactions is discussed in Chapter 16.

Other Local Anesthetic Considerations

For patients who cannot take any local anesthetics, consideration should be given to using antihistamine drugs for local anesthesia. Antihistamines that have been shown to have local anesthetic properties are diphenhydramine hydrochloride (Benadryl) and tripelennamine hydrochloride (Pyribenzamine). They can be obtained as 1% solutions (IM) containing 10 mg per ml. A dose that should give good local anesthesia is 5 ml (50 mg). The antihistamines are somewhat irritating at the site of injection, and some fibrosis may result. The latter may take ten to fourteen days to resolve.

In endodontic therapy, as with most dental procedures, the amide-type local anesthetics are used most frequently. They give good analgesia with adequate duration. Commonly used are lidocaine 2% (Xylocaine) with epinephrine 1:100,000, mepivacaine (Carbocaine) 2% with Neo-cobefrin 1:20,000, prilocaine (Citanest) 4%, prilocaine (Citanest) 4% with epinephrine 1:200,000 (Citanest Forte), mepivacaine (Carbocaine) 3%, and pyrrocaine (Dynacaine) 2% with epinephrine 1:150,000. For patients who cannot take epinephrine, good anesthesia without a vasoconstrictor can be obtained with Citanest 4%, and Carbocaine 3%. Duration is longer with Citanest than with Carbocaine.

Before giving a local anesthetic injection, one of the following should first be done: (1) use of nitrous oxide-oxygen psychosedation, (2) use of IV sedation, (3) use of hypnosis (may be effective alone), (4) use of topical anesthesia, (5) use of jet injection anesthesia, (4) and (5) to be discussed shortly, and (6) use of audio analgesia. The most effective is IV sedation, the easiest to use is topical anesthesia, but the one that is effective, and has few drawbacks is nitrous oxide-oxygen psychosedation.

Local anesthetics are used in endodontics for the following type injections: infiltration, block, intraseptal, intraosseous, sub-periosteal, intra-pulpal, and periodontal ligament. For each injection, a description and indications are given (Fig. 352).

Infiltration

This is a supraperiosteal injection (Fig. 352A). It is used on the labial (buccal) and palatal (lingual) surfaces of all upper teeth and lower anterior teeth. Most of the carpule is deposited on the labial (buccal) surface, with just a few drops deposited on the palatal (lingual) surface. Gently massaging the tissues facilitates the onset of anesthesia. This injection is usually sufficient for anesthesia of the above mentioned teeth. For refractory cases, other techniques are used which are discussed below.

Block Injections

In these supraperiosteal injections, the proximal part of the nerve axon is anesthetized by depositing the local anesthetic in the vicinity of the nerve trunk. Block injections considered are inferior alveolar, posterior superior alveolar, infraorbital, nasopalatine, anterior palatine, and mental.

INFERIOR ALVEOLAR. The principal block injection is the inferior alveolar (mandibular). For pulp extirpation to be painless, it is important that the solution is deposited on target, with a few drops deposited as the syringe is withdrawn for lingual nerve analgesia (Fig.

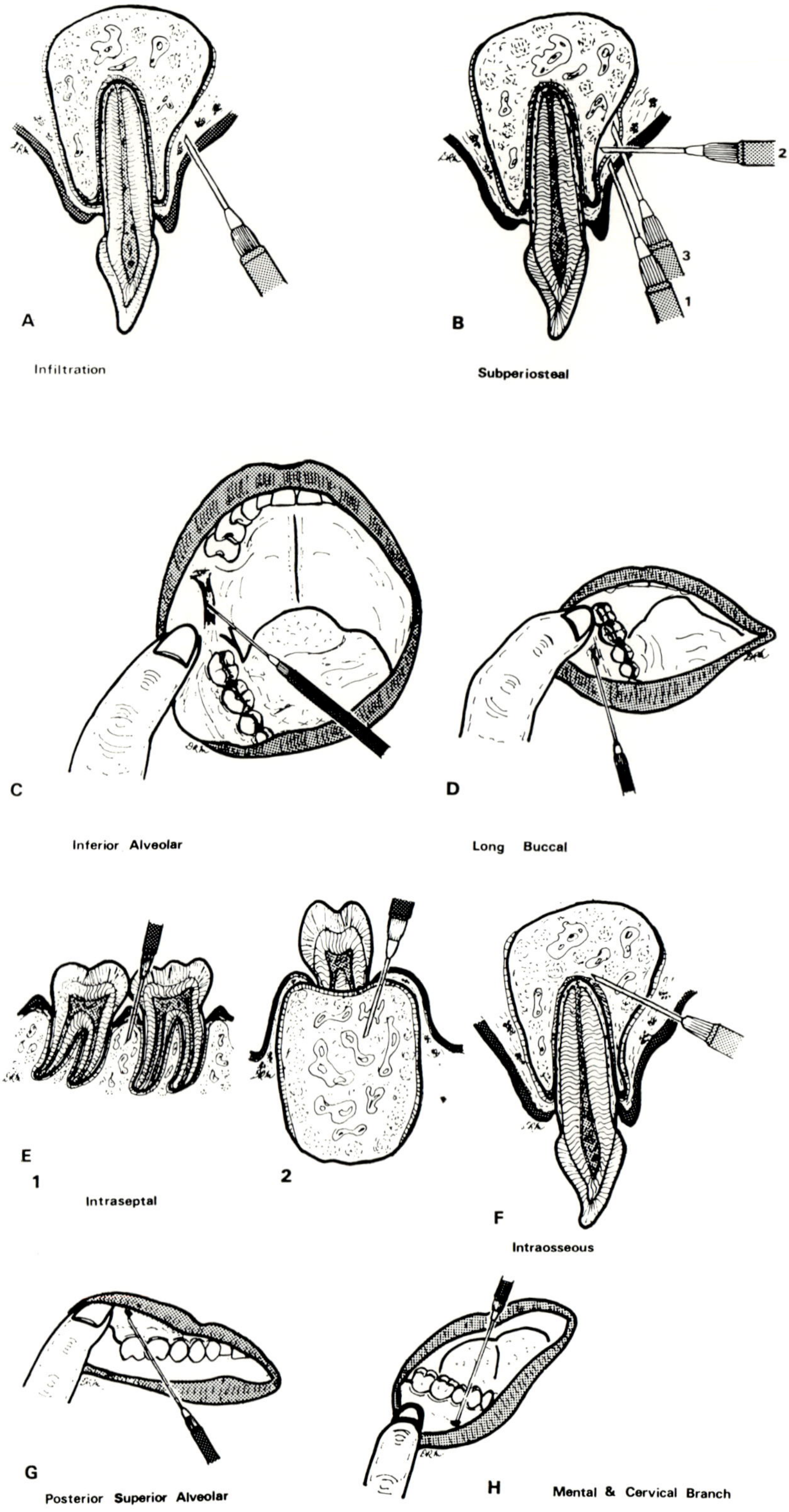

Figure 352. Local anesthetic techniques.

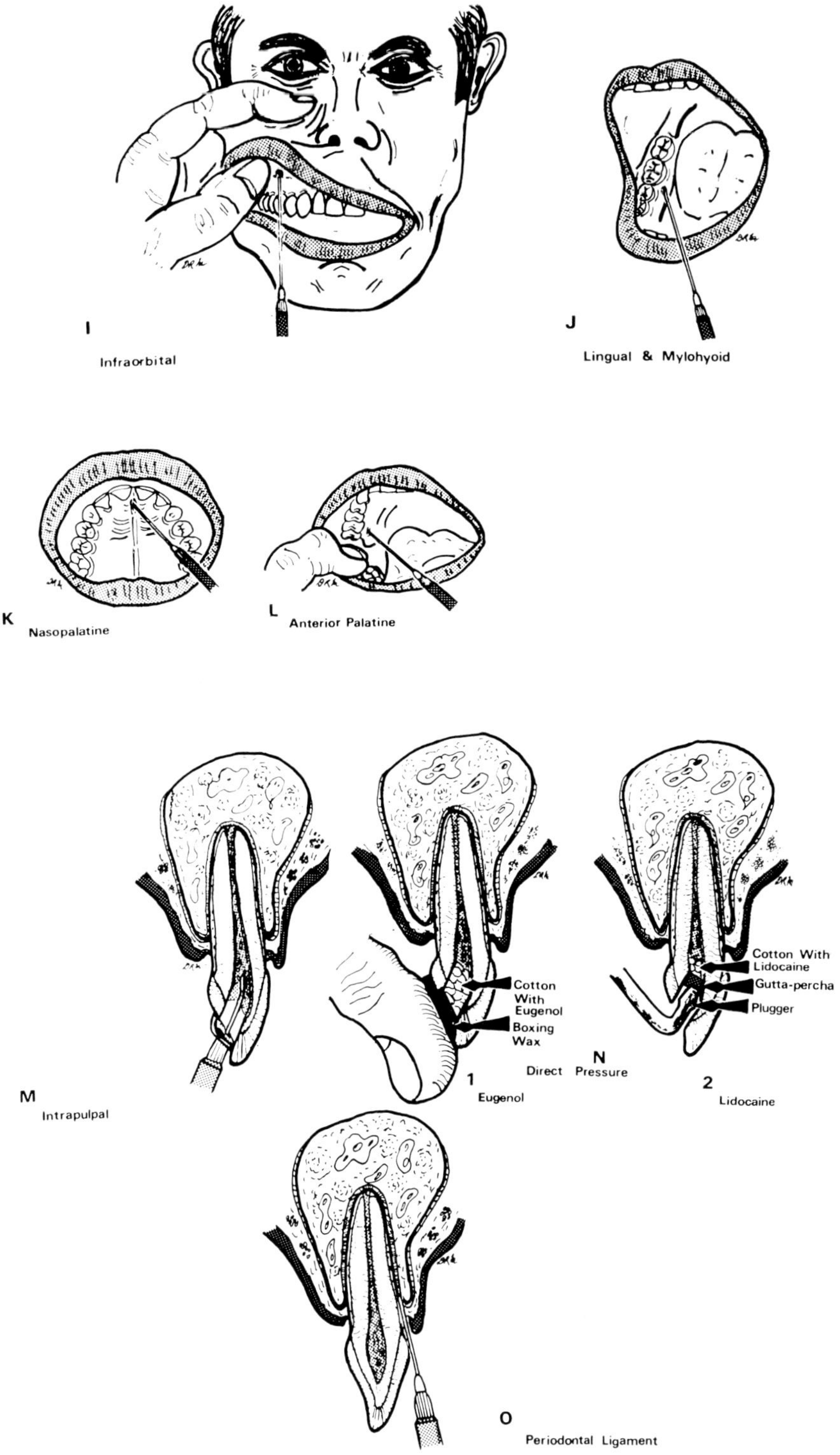
I
Infraorbital
J
Lingual & Mylohyoid
K
Nasopalatine
L
Anterior Palatine
M
Intrapulpal
Cotton With Eugenol
Boxing Wax
1
Eugenol
N
Direct Pressure
Cotton With Lidocaine
Gutta-percha
Plugger
2
Lidocaine
O
Periodontal Ligament

Figure 352.

352C). This injection is used for anesthesia of all lower teeth on one side. After symptoms of regional analgesia are apparent (numbness of lip and tongue), then a supplementary long buccal injection is given (Fig. 352D). Two methods to check for anesthesia are to blow air around all surfaces of the tooth (the patient should not feel any discomfort), and to use the electric pulp tester applied to the maximum number (again the patient should not feel discomfort). If anesthesia is still not complete, there may be some accessory innervation present from the mylohyoid nerve and/or the ascending branch of the transverse cutaneous cervical nerve (Fig. 40). To anesthetize the mylohyoid nerve, a few drops of anesthetic solution are placed on the lingual attached gingiva a few millimeters distal to the second premolar (Fig. 352J). For the cervical branch, a small amount of solution is deposited around the mental foramen area (Fig. 352H).

Posterior Superior Alveolar. This injection is used to obtain analgesia of the upper second and third molars and the distal-buccal and palatal root of the first molar (Fig. 352G). It usually is necessary to give supplemental infiltration around the mesio-buccal root to obtain analgesia of that root.

Infraorbital. This injection is useful for analgesia of the upper anterior teeth on the involved side, especially when infection makes it difficult to obtain anesthesia from infiltration injections (Fig. 352I).

Nasopalatine. This injection is used to obtain regional analgesia of the palatal surfaces of the upper anterior teeth (Fig. 352K). It is useful when the palatal surface of the anterior maxilla is involved by an infectious process. In patients with cleft palate, it is possible that innervation of the anterior teeth is by the nasopalatine nerve, rather than the anterior superior alveolar.

Anterior Palatine. This injection is used to obtain regional analgesia of the palatal surfaces of the upper posterior teeth (Fig. 352L). This is helpful in obtaining analgesia for infected palatal roots and associated periapical areas of pathosis.

Mental. This injection is used to obtain regional analgesia of the lower anteriors and premolars of the involved side (Fig. 352H). It is supplemented by a lingual injection (Fig. 352J).

Subperiosteal

If after one of the previous injections are given, there is still not good analgesia, then this injection is usually helpful. The solution (about 0.5 ml) is deposited beneath the periosteum until contact is made with the bony plate (Fig. 352B).

Intraseptal

This is an intraosseous injection made with a short needle through the interdental alveolar crest of bone. Injection is made through the mesial and distal interdental papilla on both labial (buccal) and lingual aspects (palatal). See Figure 352E. This injection is used when one of the previous injections is ineffective. The injection usually requires sustained pressure and the needle may have to be rotated in order to penetrate into the cancellous bone.

Periodontal Ligament

When the previous injections are not successful, or in place of the subperiosteal or intraseptal, injection can be made directly into the periodontal ligament (Fig. 352O). About .05 ml of solution is deposited slowly on both the labial (buccal) and lingual (palatal) aspects of the involved tooth. With this small amount of fluid, there is no discernible damage to the periodontal ligament. However, as the possibility of periodontal ligament damage exists, this injection should only be used as a last resort, unless the involved root is to be removed. The patient may feel some pain during the injection.

Intraosseous

This injection has two different indications:

(1) When it is not possible to obtain good analgesia by any of the previous injections, it may be necessary to drill with a 701 bur through the anesthetized mucous membrane directly into the bone in the region of the apex. A radiograph and visual examination is used to help in the location of the apex. As the bur is removed, the injection needle is made to penetrate to the vicinity of the apex and a small amount of fluid is deposited (Fig. 352F).

(2) During periapical surgery, it may be difficult to obtain good local analgesia and an injection directly into the cancellous bone is helpful.

Intrapulpal

When a tooth is highly inflamed, even with symptoms of good local analgesia, the first entrance into the pulp can be quite painful. The treatment to be used then is direct pulpal injection. The patient should be told that he (or she) will feel a sharp pain for just a moment, after which they will have complete loss of pain. After the rubber dam is placed on the involved tooth and partial access is gained (described in Chapter 9), the needle is placed into the chamber and a few drops of solution are deposited. If after the pulp is removed from the chamber, there is still pain upon entering the canals, then intrapulpal injections are made into each canal. Use of a sterile rubber plunger from an anesthetic carpule helps in giving a tight seal, so that the fluid will enter the canals under pressure and good analgesia will be obtained (Fig. 352M).

Direct Pressure Anesthesia

This is used when it is not possible to obtain pulpal anesthesia by any other technique. A topical anesthetic solution is pressed directly into the pulpal tissue. There are a few techniques. In one, eugenol-drenched cotton pellets are placed into the cavity or pulp chamber. Then a thick layer of boxing wax is placed over the tooth and firm pressure in exerted (Fig. 352N-1). In another technique, lidocaine-drenched cotton pellets are placed into the cavity or pulp chamber (an aqueous solution of cocaine is even more effective). Gutta-percha is warmed and placed on the end of an amalgam plugger so that the mass will just fit inside the coronal opening. The plugger is then forced firmly into the opening (Fig. 352N-2). In all of these techniques, the patients should be forewarned that they will have a momentary painful experience, that should soon disappear.

MUMMIFICATION

If the pulp cannot be anesthetized by any other means, a mummification procedure can be attempted. The rubber dam is placed on the tooth. Cotton pellets are saturated with either formocresol, paraformaldehyde paste, or phenol, and are placed into the cavity. The excess is blotted with cotton. A temporary restoration of zinc oxide-eugenol or Cavit is then used to seal the cavity (Fig. 281). The patient is told to expect pain (possibly severe) for about one day. He (or she) should be given a prescription for a narcotic (Percodan, codeine combinations, Demerol). A usual dose is 6 to 8 tablets, to be taken as one tablet every 4 to 6 hours. The patient is asked to return in about three days, at which time, either nitrous oxide-analgesia or chemanalgesia can be used as adjuncts. The rubber dam is placed on the involved tooth; the access preparation is completed, and the necrotic pulp is removed. Complete therapy is then performed at another sitting (described in Chapter 9).

ELECTROANESTHESIA

Recently a new instrument has been introduced into operative dentistry for the purpose of causing tooth desensitization during the operative procedure. It is called the Desensor® handpiece (Electrodent®, Fig. 353). An anesthetic effect is purported to occur as a result of the action of a small generator built within the handpiece. The current is from .5 to .7 volts and 10 kc at a handpiece speed of 300,000 RPM. Preliminary studies have shown that no pulpal injury occurs. The theoretical cause of the tooth desensitization is a depolarization of pulpal nerve fibers by the electric current traveling through the dentinal tubules. The instrument has been promoted for use in endodontic procedures where local anesthetics are ineffective because of inflammation. It is premature to state definitely whether this instrument is effective in causing desensitization without pulpal injury. Its use in endodontics requires further testing.

TOPICAL ANESTHESIA

This is a method of obtaining anesthesia of surface tissues (skin and mu-

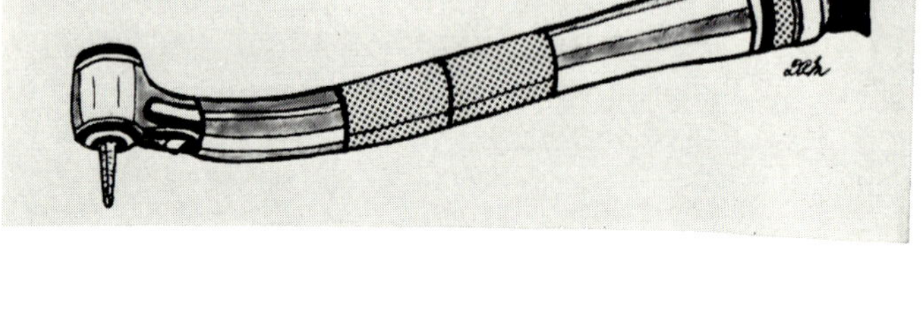

Figure 353. Desensor handpiece (Electrodent, Inc.).

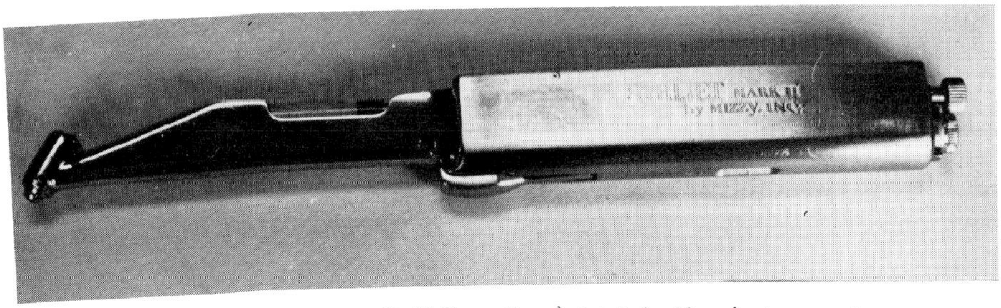

Figure 354. Syrijet® (Mizzy Inc.) jet injection instrument.

cous membranes). In endodontics, it is used prior to local anesthetic injections, to anesthetize the labial (buccal) and lingual (palatal) gingiva before the application of rubber dam clamps, to temporarily relieve the pain of ulcers, cuts, and abrasions, and to aid in the taking of periapical radiographs. The forms include sprays and ointments. It is dangerous to use a spray-type topical anesthetic. The anesthetic can get into the highly vascular mucous membrane of the throat from where it can be easily absorbed. Most of the sprays contain tetracaine which can produce serious toxic manifestations if absorbed, as well as allergic manifestations, including dangerous laryngoedema. The newest spray dispensers have metered valves with detachable spray nozzles, which help localize the spray (Cetylite® spray topical anesthetic with tetracaine HCl, 2%, benzocaine, 14%, butyl aminobenzoate, 2%, benzalkonium chloride, 0.5%, and cetyl dimethyl ethyl ammonium bromide, 0.005%; Topical Anesthetic Aerosol Spray with benzocaine, 12%, tetracaine HCl, 2%, chlorobutanol, 2%, benzalkonium chloride, 0.5%; Topicale Spray® with benzocaine 10%, tetracaine HCl, 2%, and benzalkonium chloride 0.5%). A favorite and effective topical anesthetic ointment is Xylocaine ointment 5%. A topical anesthetic that is unrelated to the previous ones and therefore can be used for individuals who are allergic to any of them, is dyclonine hydrochloride (Dyclone® solution 0.5%). Ethyl chloride spray can cause anesthesia by refrigeration. It is rarely used for this purpose in endodontics.

JET INJECTION ANESTHESIA

This is a method of obtaining intramucosal anesthesia to a depth of 4 to 6 mm (depending upon the density of the tissue), by the use of a jet injection instrument with standard anesthetic solutions (Fig. 354). The instrument produces an anesthetic jet stream that permeates relatively painlessly through the mucosa and produces a circumscribed wheal of about 5 to 7 mm. Manufacturers instructions should be followed. In order to prevent tissue trauma, the instrument must be used perpendicular to the tissues, and the tissues must have alveolar bone support. There is a *popping sound* that is heard at the moment of release of one jet injection instrument, and the patient should be forewarned. Its primary use in endodontics is to allow for a painless hypodermic local anesthetic injection. The local anesthetic is injected into the wheal area formed by the jet injection. Jet injection anesthesia can be used alone for mucous membrane anesthesia prior to clamp insertion, for incision and drainage, for suture removal, and for removal of small bony spicules.

BIBLIOGRAPHY

General

American Dental Association: *Accepted Dental Therapeutics 1973/1974.* 35th ed. Chicago, American Dental Association, 1973.

Gurney, B. F.: Anesthesiology and pharmacology in endodontics. *Dent Clin North Am, 11:*615, 1967.

Ingle, J. I.: *Endodontics.* Philadelphia, Lea & Febiger, 1965.

Quinn, T. W. (Ed.): Symposium on anesthesia and analgesia. *Dent Clin North Am, 17,* April 1973.

Weine, F. S.: *Endodontic Therapy,* St. Louis, Mosby, 1972.

Nitrous Oxide Analgesia

Langa, H.: *Relative Analgesia in Dental Practice: Inhalation Analgesia with Nitrous Oxide.* Philadelphia, Saunders, 1968.

Monheim, L.: Analgesia in dentistry, now and in the future. *Anesth Progr, 18:*100, 1971.

Morse, D. R.: Analgesia and endodontics. *J Am Anal Soc, 6:*4, 1968.

Morse, D. R.: Nitrous oxide analgesia and endodontic practice. *J Natl Anal Soc, 1:*55, 1972.

Pleasants, J. E.: The case against relative analgesia. *Dent Clin North Am, 15:*839, 1971.

Chemanalgesia and General Anesthesia

Baird, E. S., and Flowerdew, G. D.: Intravenous diazepam in conservative dentistry: a clinical trial. *Br Dent J, 128:*11, 1970.

Best, E. J., Bragman, R. D., and Gurney, B. F.: Utilization of general anesthesia and hospital facilities in surgical endodontics. *Oral Surg, 17:*779, 1964.

Foreman, P. A.: Pain control and patient management in dentistry—a review of current intravenous technics. *JADA, 80:*101, 1970.

Monheim, L. M.: General anesthesia in dental practice. *Dent Clin North Am, 14:*805, 1970.

Sachs, A. S.: A survey of neuroleptanalgesia. *Anesth Progr, 16:*105, 1969.

Acupuncture and Electroanesthesia

Alexander, R. E.: Acupuncture: Ancient art, modern enigma. *JADA, 86:*813, 1973.

Brooks, B., Reiss, R., and Umans, R.: Local electroanesthesia in dentistry. *J Dent Res, 49:*298, 1970.

Fields, R. W., Sen Savara, B., and Tacke, R.: Regional electroanalgesia and its potentialities in control of oralfacial pain. *Oral Surg, 34:*693, 1972.

Rubin, M., and Chie-Ling-Teng, P.: Acupuncture: Its Application to Dentistry. Presented at the Greater L. I. Dent. Meeting, Mar. 1973, Hempstead, New York.

Local and Topical Anesthesia

Epstein, S.: Clinical study of prilocaine with varying concentrations of epinephrine. *JADA, 78:*85, 1969.

Gidden, D. B.: Current research in local anesthesia. *Anesth Progr, 16:*201, 1969.

Gurney, B. F.: Chemotherapy in dental practice: topical anesthetics; oil soluble. *Dent Dig, 72:*513, 1966.

Gurney, B. F.: Chemotherapy in dental practice: topical anesthetics; water soluble. *Dent Dig, 72:*558, 1966.

Gurney, B. F.: Chemotherapy in dental practice: compound topical anesthetics. *Dent Dig, 74:*129, 1968.

Jorgensen, N. B.: Local anesthesia and intravenous premedication. *Anesth Progr, 13:* 168, 1966.

Kronman, J. H.: Anatomical Principles in the Successful Application of Local Anesthetics. Presented at the Annual Meeting of the Amer. Assoc. of Endodontists, April, 1973, Dallas, Texas.

Reeve, L. W.: Modern pharmacodynamic concepts of local anesthesia. *Dent Clin North Am, 14*:783, 1970.

Schacher, V., Iranpour, B., and Mills, J.: The local anesthetic efficacy of tripellennamine hydrochloride. *J Oral Ther Pharm, 3*:308, 1967.

Walton, J. G., and Thompson, J. W.: Pharmacology for the dental practitioner. 12—Local anaesthetics (local analgesics). *Br Dent J, 127*:567, 1969.

Welborn, J. F., and Kane, J. D.: Conduction anesthesia using diphenhydramine hydrochloride. *JADA, 69*:706, 1964.

CHAPTER 6

STERILIZATION PROCEDURES AND RUBBER DAM USE

STERILIZATION PROCEDURES

In order to help insure an aseptic technique, it is essential that all materials brought to the field of operation are sterile. As dental practitioners do not work either in a vacuum, under ultra-violet radiation, or in a room with laminar-air flow, it is not possible to insure that absolute air contamination will not occur. However, it is important to try and keep contamination to an absolute minimum. Prior to sterilization, instruments should be washed and for cleaning small instruments the ultra-sonic cleaner is a definite asset (Fig. 355). Tray set-ups should be used, with sep-

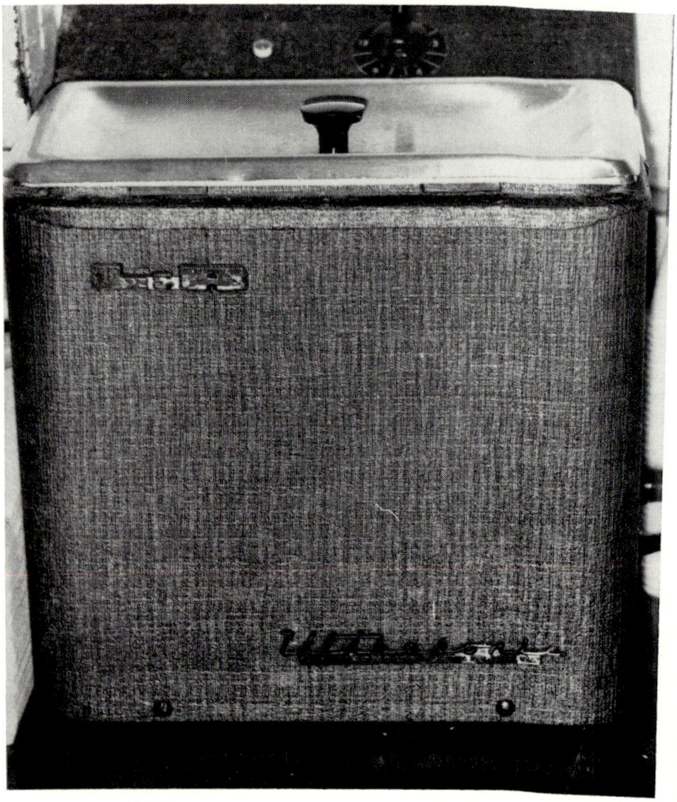

Figure 355. Ultrasonic cleaner (L. and R. Mfg. Co.)

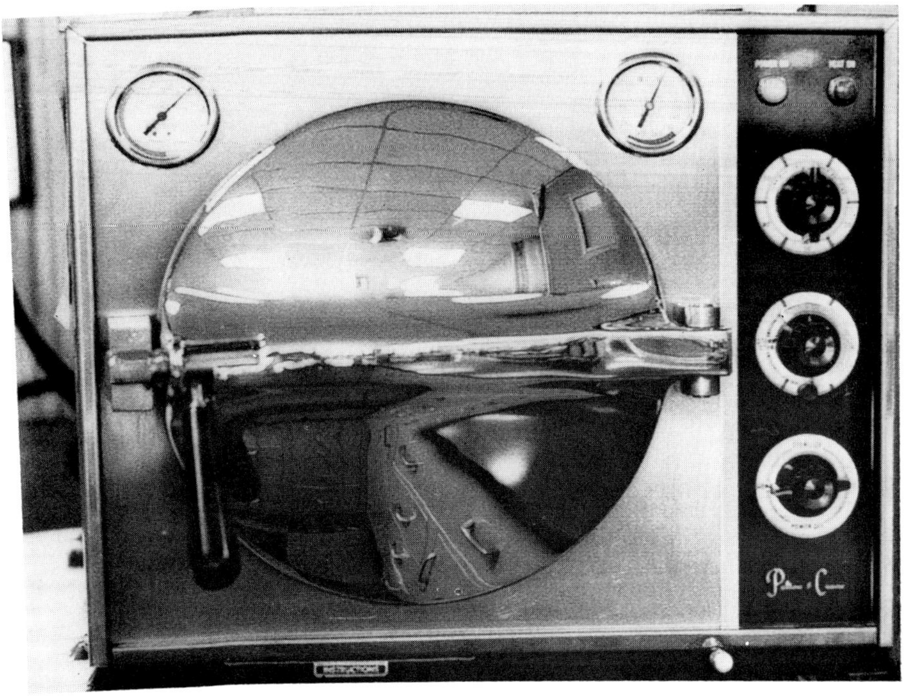

Figure 356. Autoclave (Pelton and Crane).

arate trays for instrumentation, obturation, endodontic surgical procedures, emergency periodontal treatment, bleaching, and splinting. The majority of trays are of the first three types, which are for the more usual endodontic procedures. Each tray set-up can be sterilized separately in an autoclave at 120°C (250°F), for 20 minutes (Fig. 356). The instruments are placed in one towel and covered with another. After sterilization, the set-up is placed on a tray and put in a rack with the remaining trays for the day. To prevent air contamination, it is preferable to sterilize surgical tray set-ups as close as possible to the time that they are to be used. Scalpels, suture needles, and injection needles should be of the disposable pre-sterilized type. It is preferable to sterilize small root canal instruments (which could rust in an autoclave), as well as cotton rolls, gauze, cotton pellets, and absorbent points, in the dry heat oven at 160°C (320°F) for one hour (Fig. 357). Some dentists find it convenient to sterilize all their root canal instruments, large as well as small in a large metal tray in the dry heat oven. Other dentists keep small root canal instruments in bottles of cold disinfectant solution, such as Zephiran® chloride, Metaphen® solution, Cidex®, or Cetylcide®. Regardless of what method is used initially, it is good practice to resterilize immediately before use, all files, reamers, broaches, and burs, in the hot salt (or glass bead) sterilizer (Fig. 358). If absorbent points and cotton pellets were not initially sterilized or in

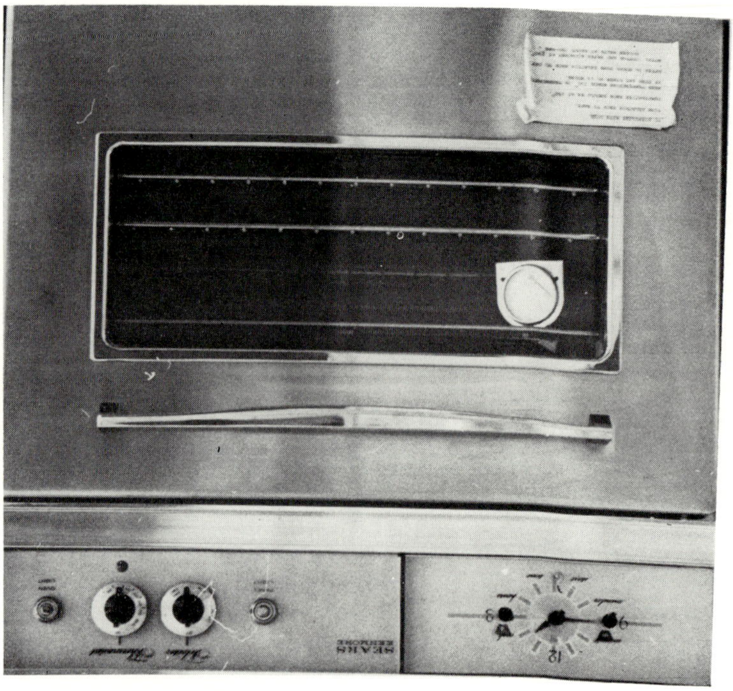

Figure 357. Dry heat oven (Sears-Kenmore).

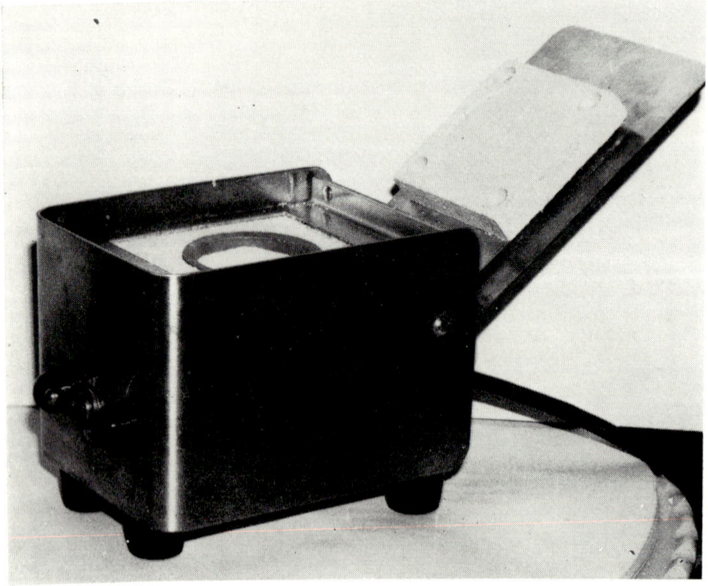

Figure 358. Hot salt sterilizer (B.D.M.® Sterilizer-Buffalo Dental Mfg. Co.).

sterile packs, they can be sterilized in the salt sterilizer. In using this instrument, it is mandatory that a thermommeter be kept in the salt, because differences in temperature can occur at different levels of the sterilizer. To be effective the temperature should be between 225 to 250°C (437-482°F). Small root canal instruments are sterilized in approximately five seconds, and absorbent points and cotton pellets require ten seconds. Irrigating syringes (with the plunger and barrel separated) are sterilized by autoclaving. Endodontic implants should be sterilized immediately before use by immersion in the salt sterilizer for 5 seconds. Gutta-percha cones can be disinfected by placement in a cold disinfectant solution such as Betadine® solution, Zephiran chloride, tincture of metaphen, 70% alcohol, or Cidex. Studies have shown that Cidex is the most efficient sporocide and Betadine is more effective than tincture of iodine. A recently reported study indicates that gutta-percha cones may be sterilized by the use of propylene oxide (six hour period is necessary). Cement slabs and dappen dishes can be disinfected with one of the aforementioned chemical disinfectants. Recently two new methods have been introduced into dentistry for sterilization of instruments. These are ethylene oxide and ultra-violet radiation. Ethylene oxide is being used to sterilize pharmaceuticals, biological products, and disposable instruments. Its chief drawback is the long time period necessary to achieve sterilization (up to 48 hours). However, there are new types being developed which may decrease the time factor greatly, and then this method may come into wider use. Ultra-violet radiation has been used to disinfect operating rooms. Recently, small units (Steril-Lite®) have been developed which are supposed to sterilize dental instruments. Whether complete sterilization occurs is debatable and further research is necessary.

RUBBER DAM

The use of the rubber dam is mandatory in endodontic practice for several reasons: It allows for better visualization of the tooth, it helps in the maintenance of an aseptic field, it prevents the aspiration or swallowing of root canal instruments, it discourages interference by the tongue, it decreases the chance of bur injury to oral mucous membranes, it collects debris (prevents particles and solutions from going down the throat or injuring adjacent soft tissues), it disallows conversation by the patient, which can distract the dentist from doing the procedures, if nitrous oxide-relative analgesia is being used, it generally discourages mouth breathing and thereby enhances the analgesic effect, and it causes less irritation and nausea than absorbent cotton rolls or gauze packs.

Technique

Time should never be a factor in preventing a dentist from using the rubber dam. In most cases, a rubber dam can be placed on a tooth in thirty seconds or less. For badly broken down teeth, the gingiva can be anesthetized on both the labial (buccal) and lingual (palatal) surfaces, and if necessary the clamp can be placed directly on the gingiva. The usual after-effect is slight soreness for a day or so. It may be necessary to perform a gingivectomy, using a scalpel, or electrosurgery to expose a badly broken down tooth or root so that a rubber dam clamp can be placed. This is also done for a fracture beneath the gingiva. The fractured portion is removed and then the overlying gingiva is removed either by a scalpel or electrosurgery. Electrosurgery has the advantage of minimizing bleeding which enables definitive endodontic therapy to be performed at the same visit. However, it is still possible to proceed with treatment at the same visit after using a scalpel to remove gingival tissue. Approximately 2 to 3 mm of tissue is removed, and bleeding can usually be controlled with gauze. In other cases that are not severely broken down, a copper band, aluminum band (or crown) or a stainless steel crown can be festooned and cemented in position to allow for rubber dam placement (Fig. 359). It is also possible to insert amalgam or zinc phosphate cement when only one wall is missing. In anterior teeth, acrylic or polycarbonate crown forms can be used (Fig. 360). In the extremely rare case where a clamp cannot be placed on the tooth for anatomical reasons, the tooth should be isolated with cotton rolls and the throat should be packed with gauze. The root canal file or reamer that is to be used is attached to an Endodontic Safety Chain (Ransom and Randolph). This instrument is designed to prevent the accidental dropping of the file or reamer (Fig. 361). However, there is still the problem of contamination, tongue interference, etc., and if these factors cannot be controlled, then consideration

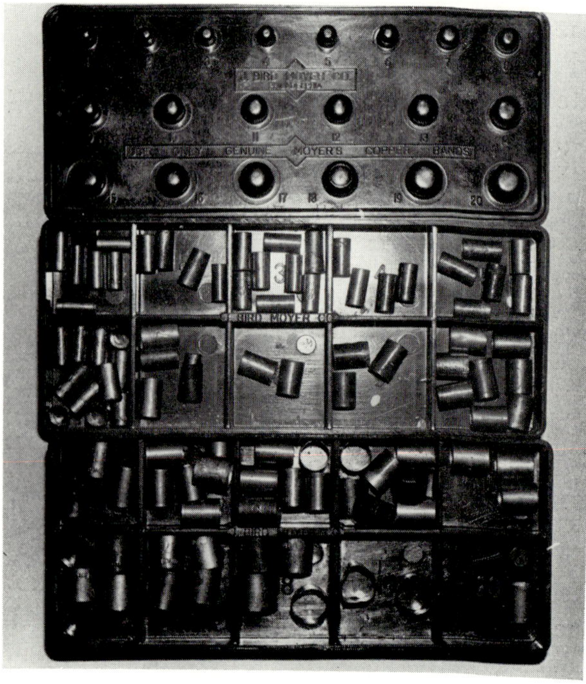

Figure 359. Copper band selection kit (J. Bird Moyer Co.); for use with broken down posterior teeth in order to allow for rubber dam placement.

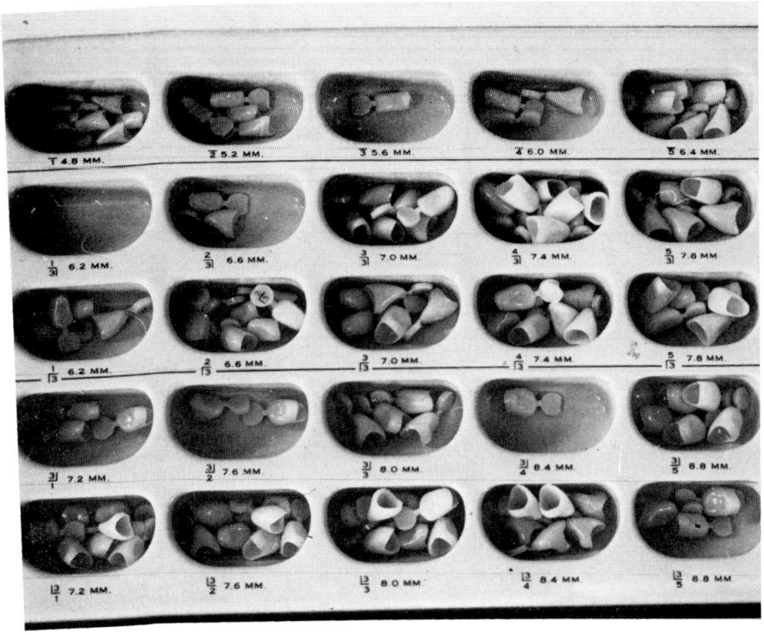

Figure 360. Polycarbonate selection kit; for use with broken down anterior teeth in order to allow for rubber dam placement.

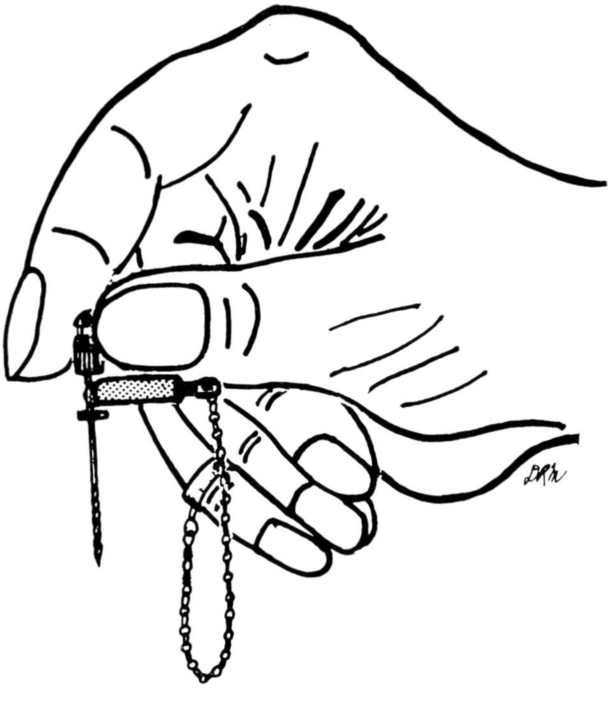

Figure 361. Endodontic Safety Chain® (Ransom and Randolph).

should be given to a retrograde filling. If this is not feasible, then an intentional replant should be done. In endodontics, unlike the use of the rubber dam in restorative dentistry, only the tooth being worked on is clamped. The practitioner also does not have to worry about keeping a large supply of clamps on hand. With only four winged clamps, any tooth in the mouth can be clamped (under most circumstances). These are Ivory No. 0 for upper centrals, Ivory No. 00 for upper laterals and lower centrals and laterals, Ivory No. 2A for upper and lower canines and premolars (occasionally No. 0 clamps can be used for canines), and either Ivory No. 4, 14, or 14A for molars (permanent or primary). Other clamps that can be used are Ivory No. 9 for anterior teeth, S.S.W. No. 211 for upper laterals and lower incisors, S.S.W. No. 26 for molars, and S.S.W. No. 27 for premolars (Fig. 362). Winged clamps are generally used because they spread the dam out to give better visualization. The rubber dam that is recommended is medium (dark or light) 6 inches by 6 inches (Hygienic) (Figure 363). The Young's rubber dam frame is serviceable, but for taking of radiographs with the dam in position, a plastic type is preferable (Fig. 363). A good rubber dam punch is the Ivory model and the Ivory rubber dam forceps is recommended (Fig. 363). A procedure for hole determination is the following. Punch a hole in the rubber dam at the appropriate place. In selecting the location for the hole to be

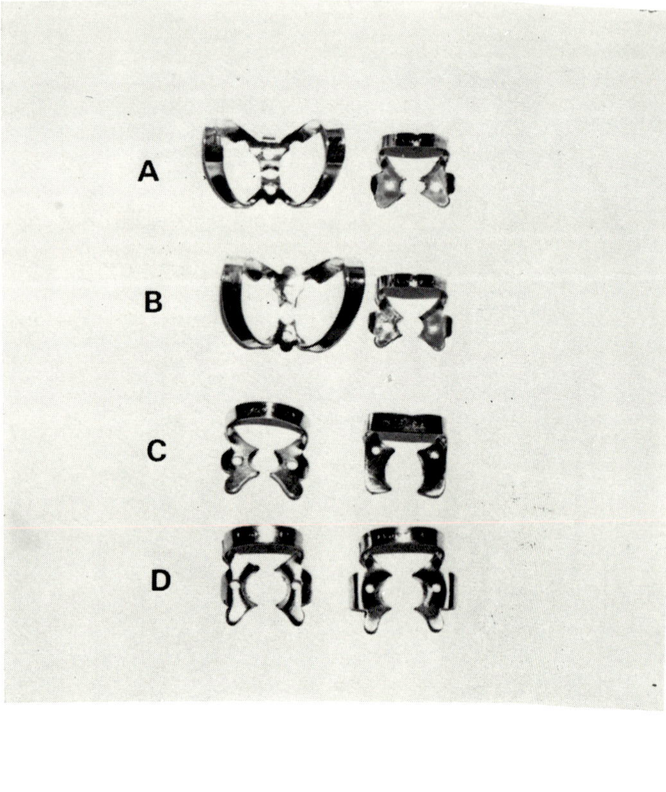

Figure 362. Rubber dam clamp selection; from left to right. A. Ivory No. 9—Ivory No. 00—upper laterals and lower anteriors. B. SSW No. 211—Ivory No. 0—upper centrals. C. Ivory No. 2A—SSW No. 27—premolars. D. Ivory No. 14—Ivory No. 4—molars.

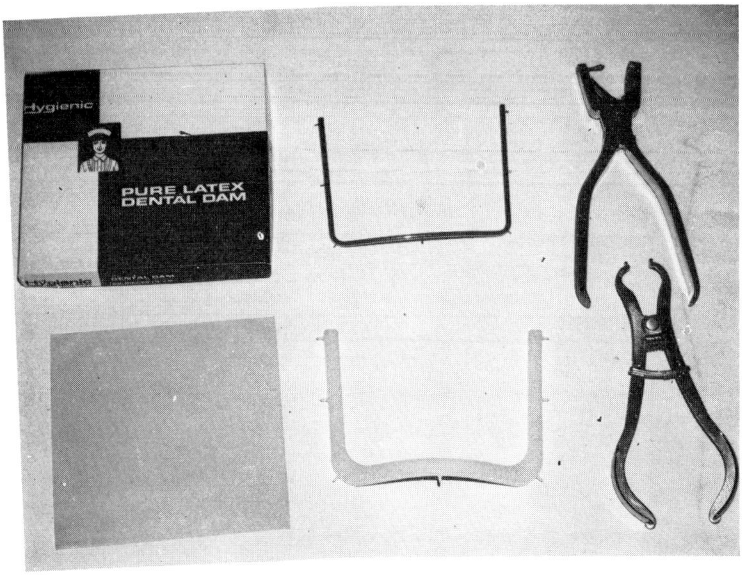

Figure 363. Rubber dam armamentarium; left to right. 1st row—Box of rubber dam (Hygienic); Young's frame, Ivory rubber dam punch. 2nd row—Sheet of rubber dam; plastic frame (Star Lite Visi Frame®); Ivory rubber dam forceps.

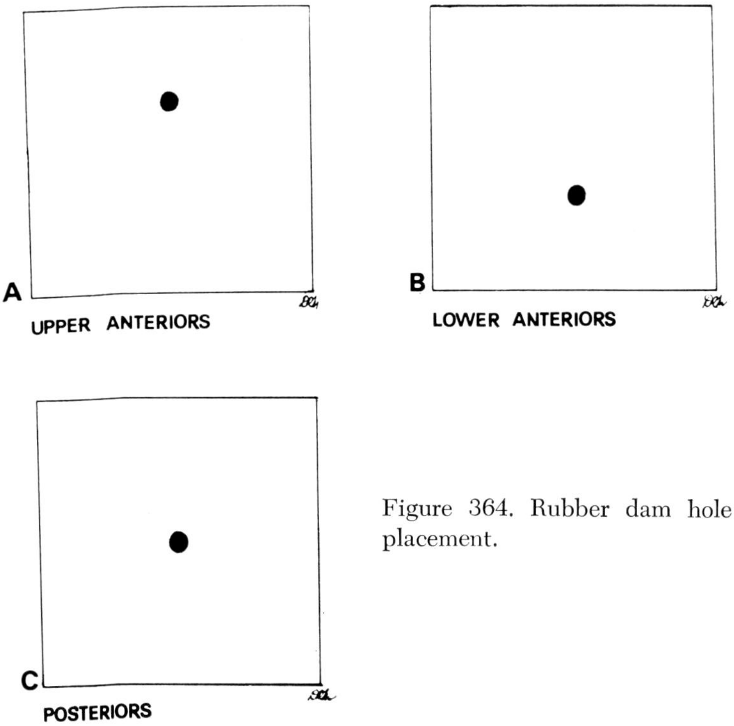

Figure 364. Rubber dam hole placement.

punched, choose a central site from right to left. The top of the rubber dam should be beneath the patient's nose to allow for proper breathing. Therefore, for an upper anterior tooth, the centered hole should be placed near the top of the rubber dam, approximately ⅓ down. For a lower anterior tooth, the hole should be centered, ⅓ up from the bottom. For a posterior tooth, the hole should be placed in the center of the rubber dam (Fig. 364). There are three possible ways to put the dam on the tooth. These are (1) dam first, (2) clamp first, and (3) clamp and dam together. If the dentist has a chair-

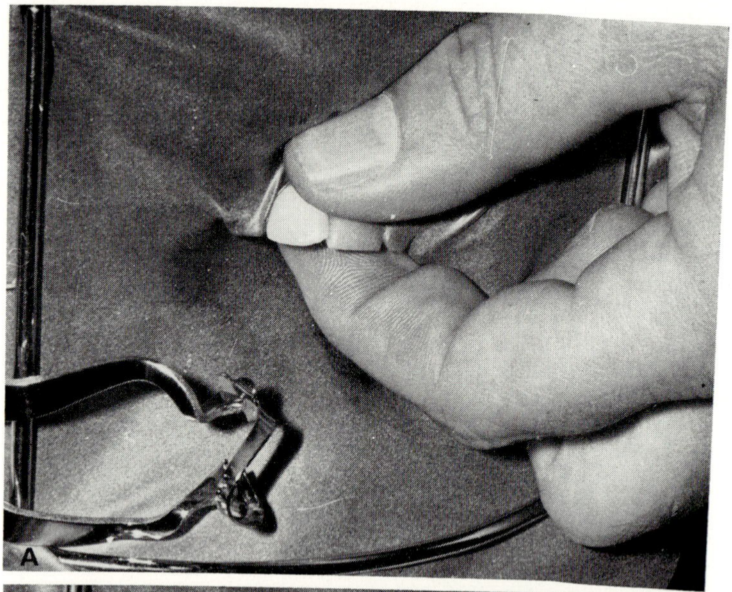

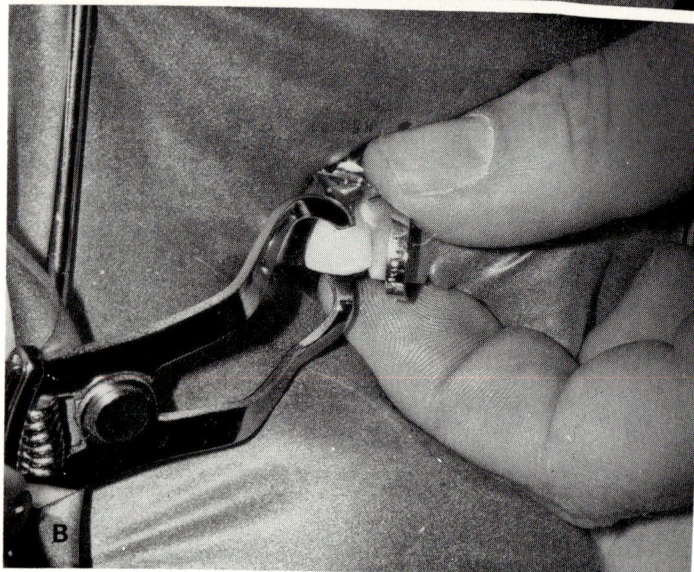

Figure 365. Rubber dam placement. 1. Dam first; doctor alone. A. Dam held over tooth, while clamp is being brought to the tooth. B. Clamp placed on tooth.

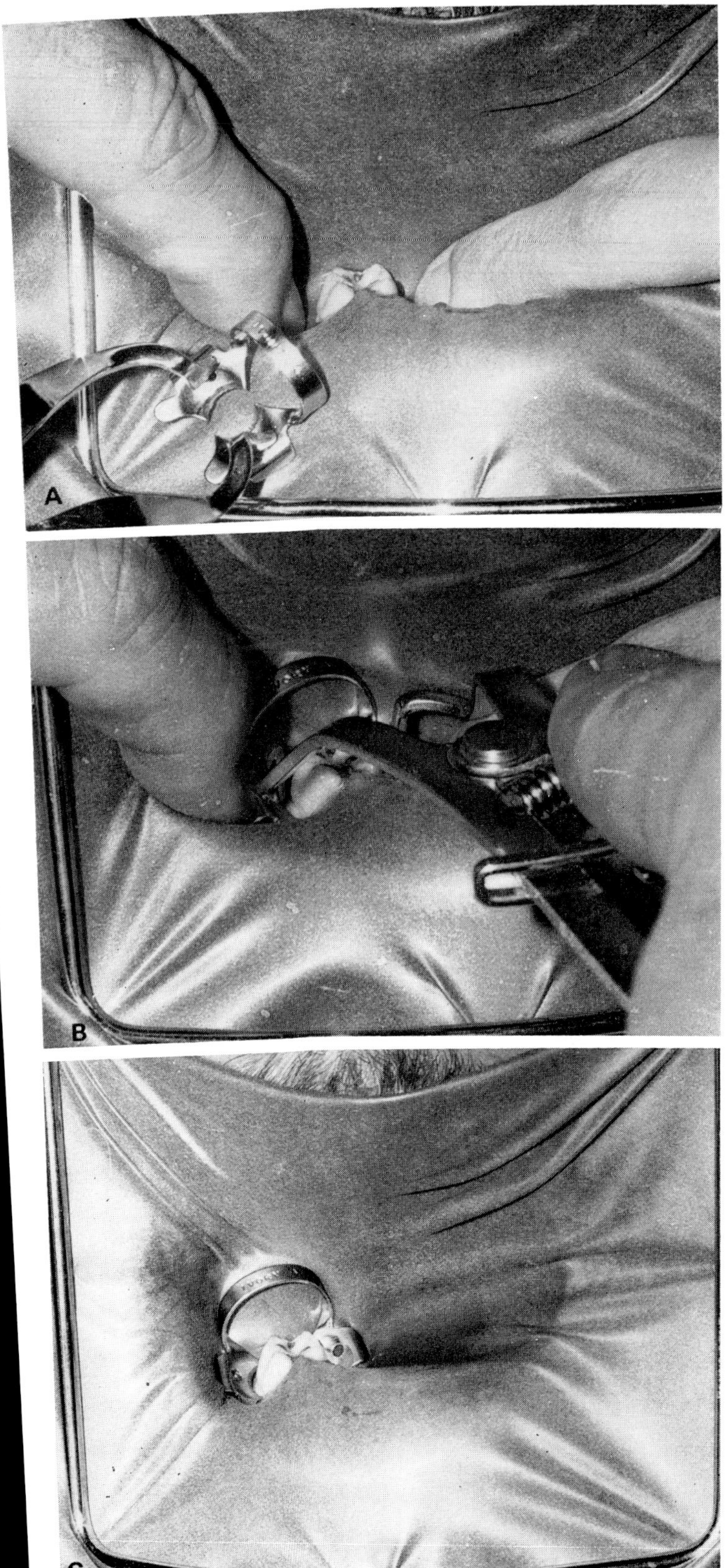

Figure 366. Rubber dam placement. 2. Dam first; assistant aided. A. Assistant holds the dam over the lingual aspect of the tooth, while the doctor holds it down over the buccal aspect; the clamp is being brought over to the tooth. B. Clamp being placed on tooth. C. Clamp in position.

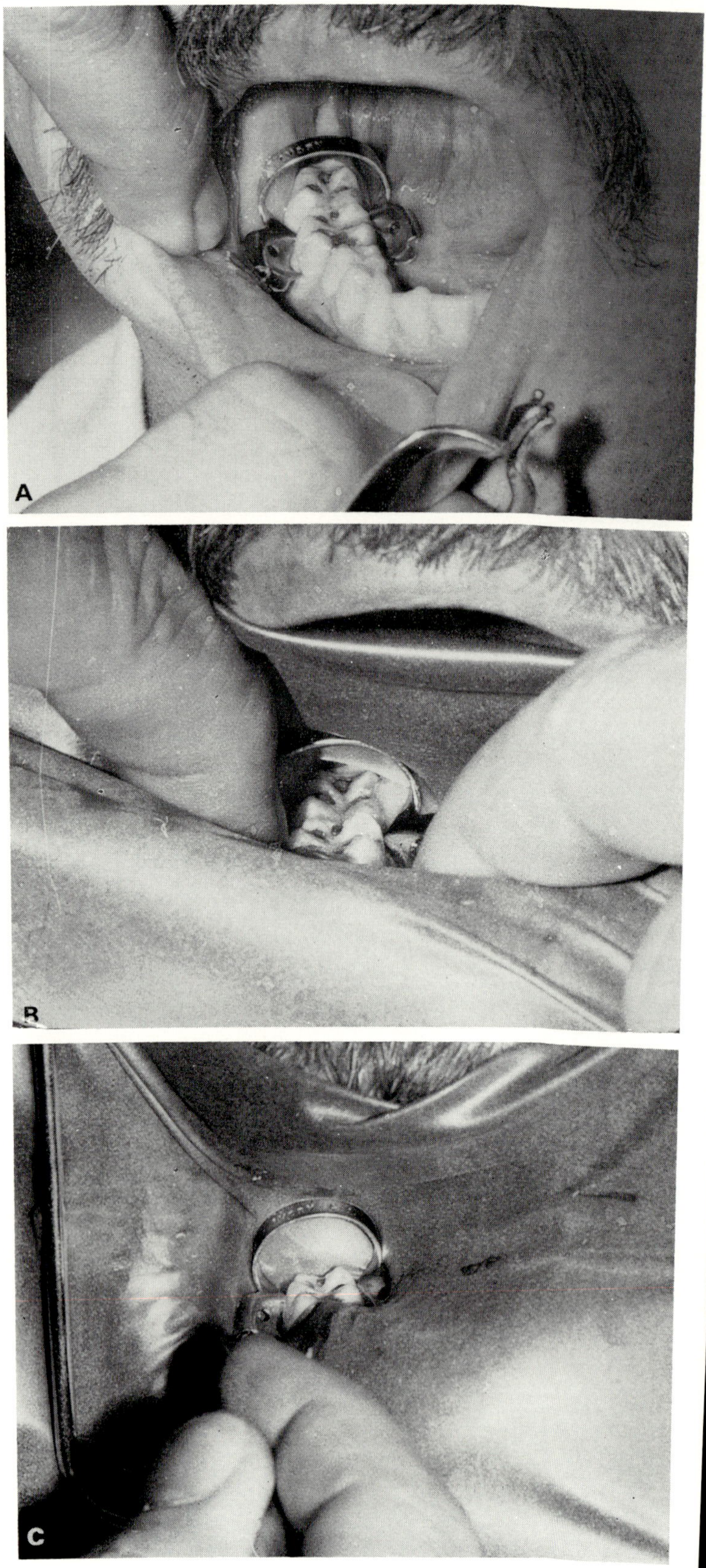

Figure 367. Rubber dam placement. 3. Clamp first. A. Clamp placed on tooth. B. Rubber slipped over wings of clamp. C. Frame attached to rubber dam.

side assistant, then the fastest method is to place the rubber dam with attached frame on first. For all teeth except lower posteriors, it is easy for the dentist to put the dam on himself. For lower posterior teeth, it is easier for the assistant to hold down the dam on the tooth while the dentist applies the clamp. The dam with the attached frame is placed with the punched hole going over the crown of the tooth, and resting on the cervix. The dam is then held in this position by the dentist with his left hand (if he is right handed), while he places the clamp (held in the rubber clamp forceps), over the tooth (Fig. 365A). For lower posterior teeth, the assistant holds the rubber dam in position, because the tongue interferes with the dentist holding down both buccal and lingual aspects of the dam with one hand (Fig. 366A). The dentist then places the clamp in position (Figs. 365B, 366B, C).

In some cases it is difficult to place the dam on in this manner and it is easier to first place the clamp on the tooth (Fig. 367A). The hole in the rubber dam is then placed over the involved tooth and the rubber is slipped under the wings of the clamp (Fig. 367B). The frame is then attached to the rubber dam (Fig. 367C). A dentist who practices without chairside assistance could use the method of placement of dam and clamp together. The clamp is placed in the hole with the rubber covering the wings (Fig. 368A). The attached clamp-dam-frame is then placed over the tooth (Fig. 368B, C). With a flat ended plastic instrument, the rubber is then slipped under the wings of the clamp (Fig. 368D).

Rubber Dam Aids

If while the rubber dam is in position, there is some leakage present around the tooth and removal of the dam would cause contamination, then the leak should be sealed. Methods that have been used in the past include placement of warmed compound around the tooth, sealing the leak with cold-cure acrylic, zinc oxide-eugenol cement around the tooth, and the use of Cavit (Premier®) around the tooth. However, very good results can be obtained with the use of Orahesive® (Squibb) placed with a cotton applicator around the circumference of the tooth cervix. If there is a bad leak and the rubber dam must be changed, then cotton is placed in the chamber. This is then covered with Cavit, in order to prevent salivary contamination when the dam is removed. There is no need to remove the frame while taking radiographs. Removal of the frame allows for salivary contamination, especially during measurement x-rays, when Cavit cannot be placed in the occlusal (incisal) opening. With the plastic frame, there is no radiopaque image from the frame on the radiograph. If the metal frame is used, it is necessary to turn it so that the path of the x-ray beam will not penetrate the metal and produce a radiographic image (Fig. 369). Use of liquid soap over the opening in the dam allows it to slip more easily over the tooth and helps prevent tears. Untinted tincture of metaphen can be sprayed

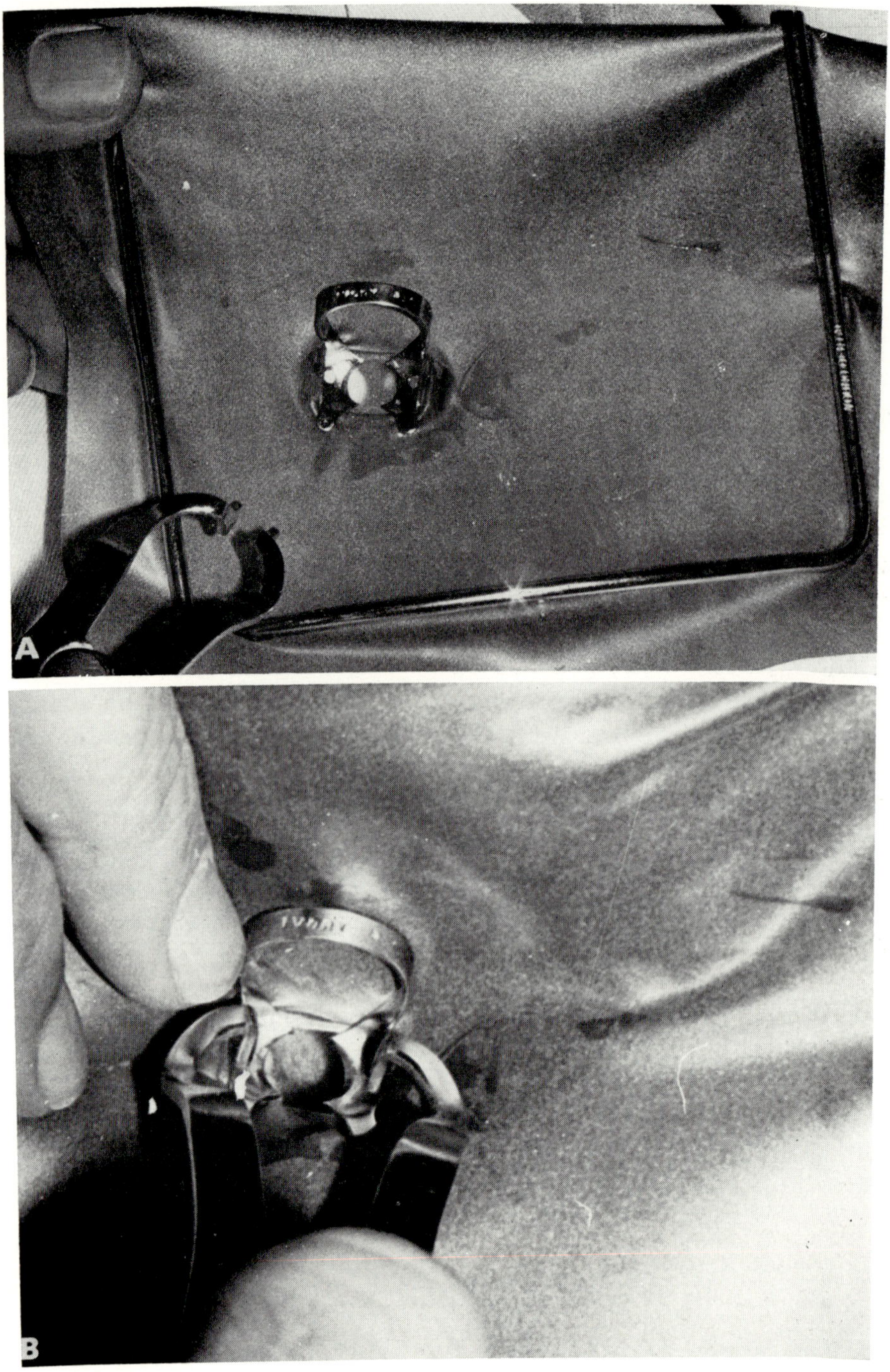

Figure 368. Rubber dam placement. 4. Dam, clamp, and frame together. A. Clamp placed in dam with attached frame. B. Forceps is placed into clamp. C. Dam-clamp-

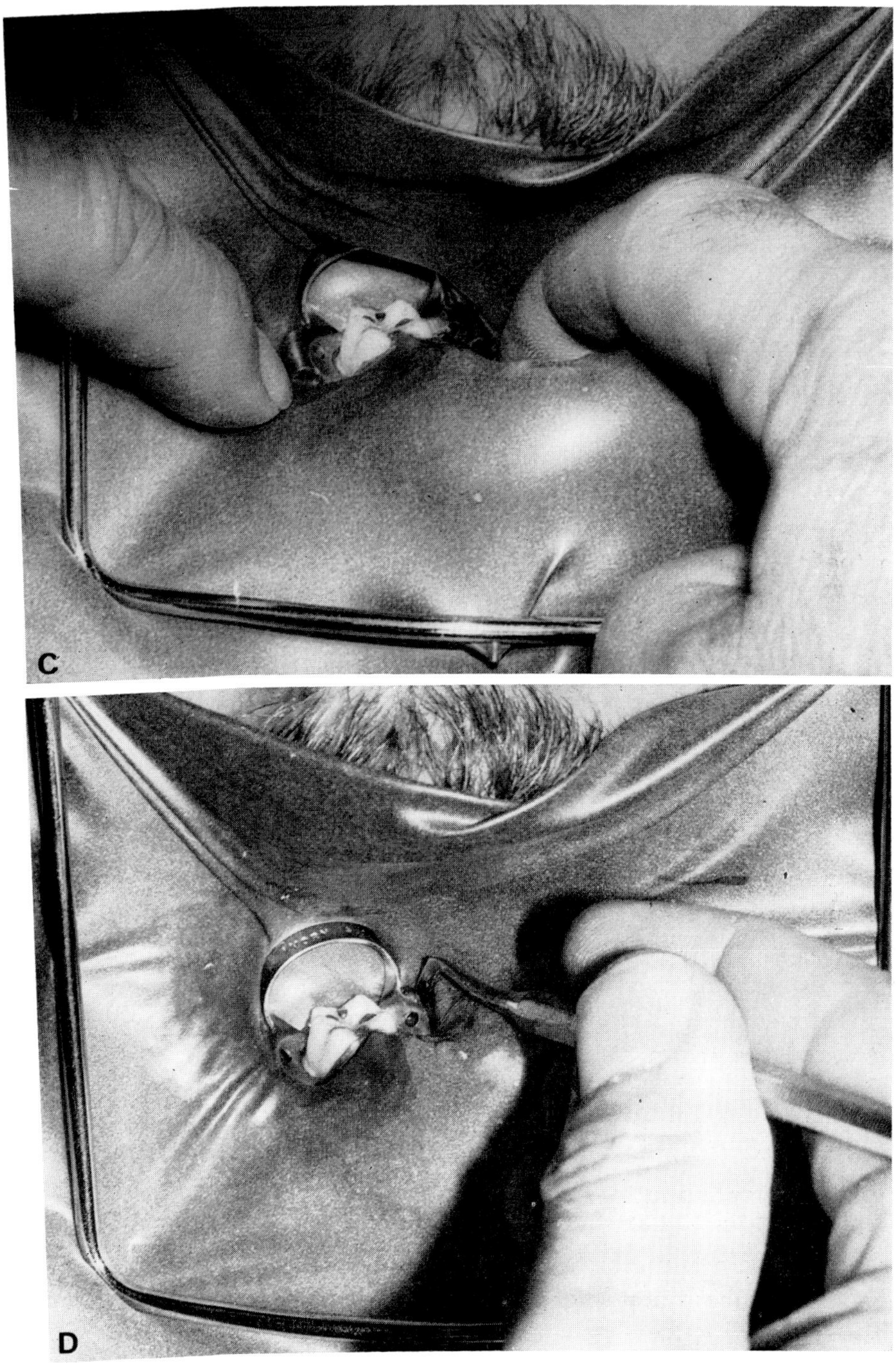

frame is placed on tooth. D. Flat ended plastic instrument used to slip dam under wings of clamp.

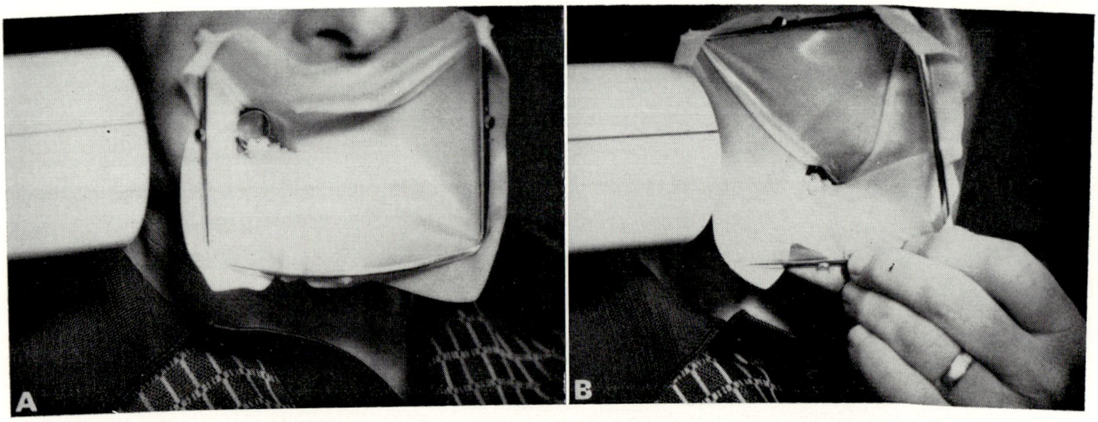

Figure 369. Avoiding radiopaque image from rubber dam frame. A. Normal angulation. B. Turning the frame so that the metal will not appear on the radiograph.

(or placed with a cotton applicator) over the tooth, clamp, and dam. This does not insure sterility, but as the objective is asepsis, antiseptic use does decrease microbial contamination. Before beginning access, all caries are removed and a cement filling is inserted. Cavit is usually satisfactory, but if there is a great amount of decay, an amalgam filling is inserted. In anterior teeth, plastic or silicate fillings are used. Caries removal is important for two reasons: (1) decay can continue in pulpless teeth, and (2) the restoration prevents seepage under the rubber dam. The patient is allowed to hold the saliva ejector with his (or her) hand and move it if it presses against the cheek or floor of the mouth. Suction should be adequate, but not too powerful, as the latter type can cause excessive drying and pain. The dentist should have a tissue or towel in his hand as he removes the rubber dam. Usually saliva comes out with the dam, and it is a nice gesture to wipe the patient's cheek as soon as the dam is removed.

BIBLIOGRAPHY

General

Abramson, I. I., and Norris, J. P.: *Atlas of Endodontic Technique: A Clinical Guide.* Saint Louis, Mosby, 1966.

American Dental Association: *Accepted Dental Therapeutics 1973/1974,* 35th ed. Chicago, American Dental Association, 1973.

Grossman, L. I.: *Endodontic Practice,* 7th ed. Philadelphia, Lea & Febiger, 1970.

Ingle, J. I.: *Endodontics.* Philadelphia, Lea & Febiger, 1965.

Sommer, R. F., Ostrander, F. D., and Crowley, M. C.: *Clinical Endodontics: A Manual of Scientific Endodontics,* 3rd ed. Philadelphia, Saunders, 1966.

Weine, F. S.: *Endodontic Therapy.* St. Louis, Mosby, 1972.

Sterilization

Blair, H. A.: Effectiveness of gas sterilization of endodontic materials. *J Ky Dent Assoc,* 23:22, 1971.

Ehrmann, E. H.: Four handed sit-down endodontics. Presented at the Fifth International Conference on Endodontics, Sept. 1973, Philadelphia, Pennsylvania.

Gillette, W. B.: Ethylene oxide sterilization in dentistry. *J Oral Ther Pharm,* 2:440, 1966.

Ham, J. W., Patterson, S. S., and Healey, H. J.: An evaluation of handpiece sterilization for periapical surgery. *J Oral Surg, 28*:353, 1970.

Malveaux, F. J., Whitehurst, V. E., and Magerman, L. A.: Relative effectiveness of certain chemosterilizers on selected microbial species. *J Dent Res, 51*:62, 1972.

Miller, C. H., Lu, D. P., and Crimmel, J. E.: Bactericidal efficiency of some antimicrobial chemicals. *J Dent Res, 52*:184, 1973.

Montgomery, S.: Chemical decontamination of gutta-percha cones with polyvinylpyrrolidone-iodine. *Oral Surg, 31*:258, 1971.

Trachtenberg, D. I.: On methods of instrument sterilization—An opinion. *Penn Dent J, 40*:15, 1973.

Walsh, R. F., and Ames, M. I.: Reinforcing the aseptic chain in hospital dental practice. *J Hosp Dent Pract, 6*:57, 1972.

Rubber Dam Use

Cragg, T. K.: Cases and comments: the use of rubber dam in endodontics. *J Can Dent Assoc, 10*:376, 1972.

Glick, D. H.: Use of a protective emollient as an endodontic aid. *Oral Surg, 24*:250, 1967.

Going, R. E., and Sawinski, V. J.: Parameters related to the use of the rubber dam. *JADA, 77*:597, 1968.

Nazif, M.: A rubber dam clamp in the nasal cavity: report of case. *JADA, 82*:1099, 1971.

CHAPTER 7

PULP CONSERVATION TREATMENTS

THE PULP CONSERVATION treatments discussed are indirect pulp capping, direct pulp capping, pulpotomy for permanent teeth, and pulpotomy for primary teeth.

INDIRECT PULP CAPPING

Armamentarium is shown in Figure 370. The superficial and middle layers of caries are removed using a No. 4, 5, or 6 round bur in a slow speed contra-angle. A spoon excavator may be used but it should not be used for the deeper caries as it can easily cause a pulp exposure. The deepest layer of stained or leathery decay is not removed. A calcium hydroxide paste is then inserted over the caries. This is followed by a thick mixture of zinc oxide and eugenol (with zinc acetate crystals incorporated to accelerate the set). This is then covered with a permanent type amalgam or synthetic restoration (Fig. 277). The tooth should be checked at three month intervals (Fig. 371). If there is any sign of pulpal or periapical disease occurring, then complete endodontic therapy should be performed.

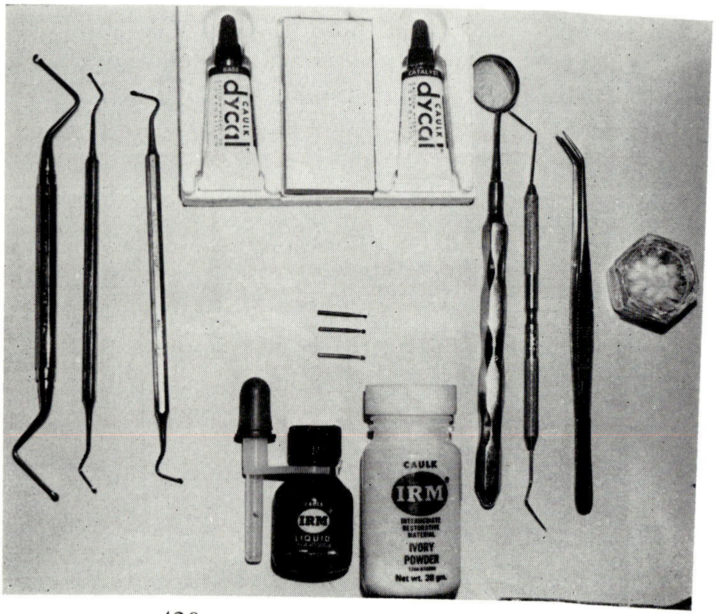

Figure 370. Armamentarium for direct or indirect pulp capping; left-endodontic spoon excavators, plugger; top—calcium hydroxide (Dycal®-Caulk); middle—round burs; bottom—temporary cement (IRM®-Caulk); right—mirror, explorer, cotton pliers, cotton pellets; not shown is the permanent restorative material.

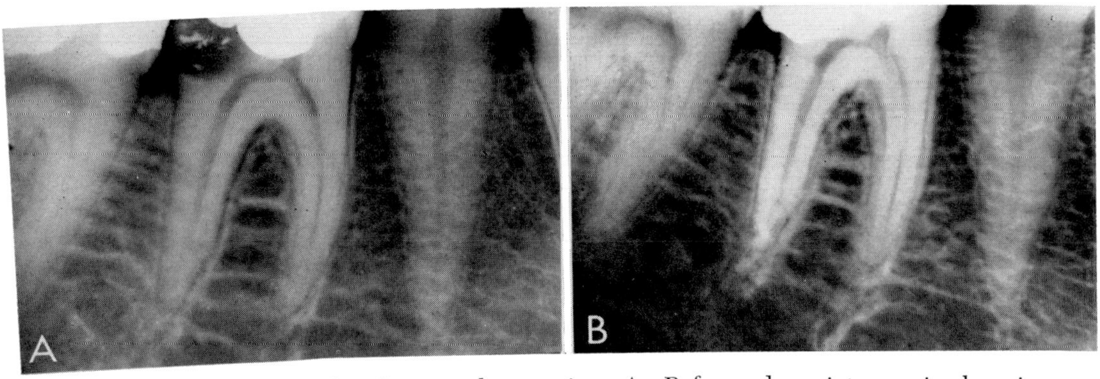

Figure 371. Successful indirect pulp capping. A. Before; deep interproximal caries; gross caries was removed and a ZOE dressing was placed. B. Six months later; the tooth is asymptomatic; the pulp is vital. (From S. Seltzer and I. B. Bender, *The Dental Pulp*, J. P. Lippincott Co., 1965. Used with permission of J. P. Lippincott Company.)

DIRECT PULP CAPPING

Armamentarium is shown in Figure 370. The exposure is visualized as a small pinkish spot, or a slight amount of bleeding is seen. The first sign of an exposure may be a twinge of pain felt by the patient, when an explorer touches a pulp horn. If there is bleeding, the surface is blotted with a cotton pellet impregnated with sterile saline. A calcium hydroxide paste is placed directly over the exposure and is made of sufficient thickness so that it covers it well. Then a thick mix of zinc oxide-eugenol with zinc acetate crystals is placed over the calcium hydroxide. As is the case with the indirect pulp capping cases, it is suggested that the permanent restoration be placed at the same visit (Fig. 277). The tooth should be checked at least every six months (Fig. 372). If any clinical or radiographic sign of endodontic disease occurs, then complete endodontic therapy should be performed.

PULPOTOMY FOR PERMANENT TOOTH

Armamentarium is shown in Figure 373. After local anesthesia is obtained, the tooth is isolated under the rubber dam. Caries is removed using a No. 4, 5, or 6 round bur, in an ultra-high speed contra-angle, with copious water spray. Spoon excavators can also be used. After all the caries are removed, access is prepared (described in Chapter 9) using a 701 bur with an effective water spray. Using long shanked spoon excavators, the pulp is removed to the levels of the orifice(s). Bleeding is controlled with sterile saline irrigation, followed by drying with sterile cotton pellets. A calcium hydroxide paste is then inserted over the floor of the chamber. After it sets, a thick mix of zinc oxide-eugenol with zinc acetate crystals is placed over the calcium hydroxide. Once the cement sets, a preparation is made and a permanent-type restoration is inserted (Fig. 277). The tooth is checked at six month

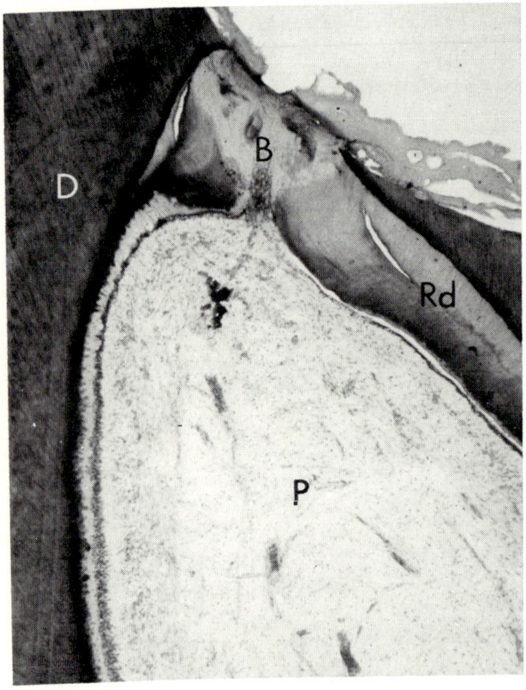

Figure 372. Successful pulp capping with a calcium hydroxide paste; B = "bridge," D = dentin, R = reparative dentin, P = pulp (×54). (From S. Seltzer and I. B. Bender, *The Dental Pulp*, J. P. Lippincott Co., 1965. Used with permission of J. P. Lippincott Company.)

intervals and when root development is complete, nonsurgical endodontics is performed (Fig. 374).

PULPOTOMY FOR PRIMARY TOOTH

Armamentarium is shown in Figure 375. The treatment is almost the same for vital or pulpless teeth. After good local anesthesia is present, the rubber dam is placed over the involved tooth. Local anesthesia should also be used for pulpless teeth, as there may still be some vital tissue remaining. Caries is removed and access is made as described for a pulpotomy of a permanent tooth. It must be realized that the pulp chamber is smaller in primary teeth; hence penetration to the pulp chamber occurs sooner than is the case for permanent teeth. In vital cases, the pulp is removed and the bleeding is controlled (as has been described in the previous section). In pulpless cases, the necrotic debris is removed with long shanked spoon excavators. Irrigation is performed with sterile saline, after which the floor of

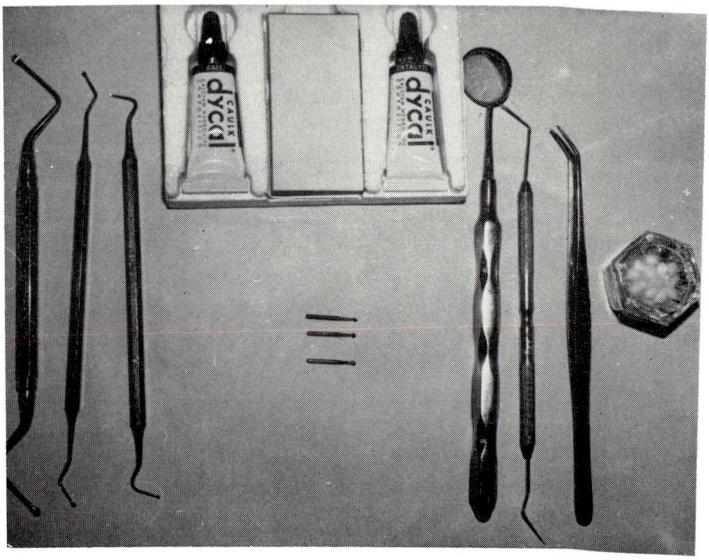

Figure 373. Armamentarium for pulpotomy. Left to right; endodontic spoon excavators and pluggers, round burs, mirror, explorer, cotton pliers, dappen dish with cotton pellets, top; calcium hydroxide paste (Dycal®-Caulk); not shown is the ZOE cement and the permanent restorative material.

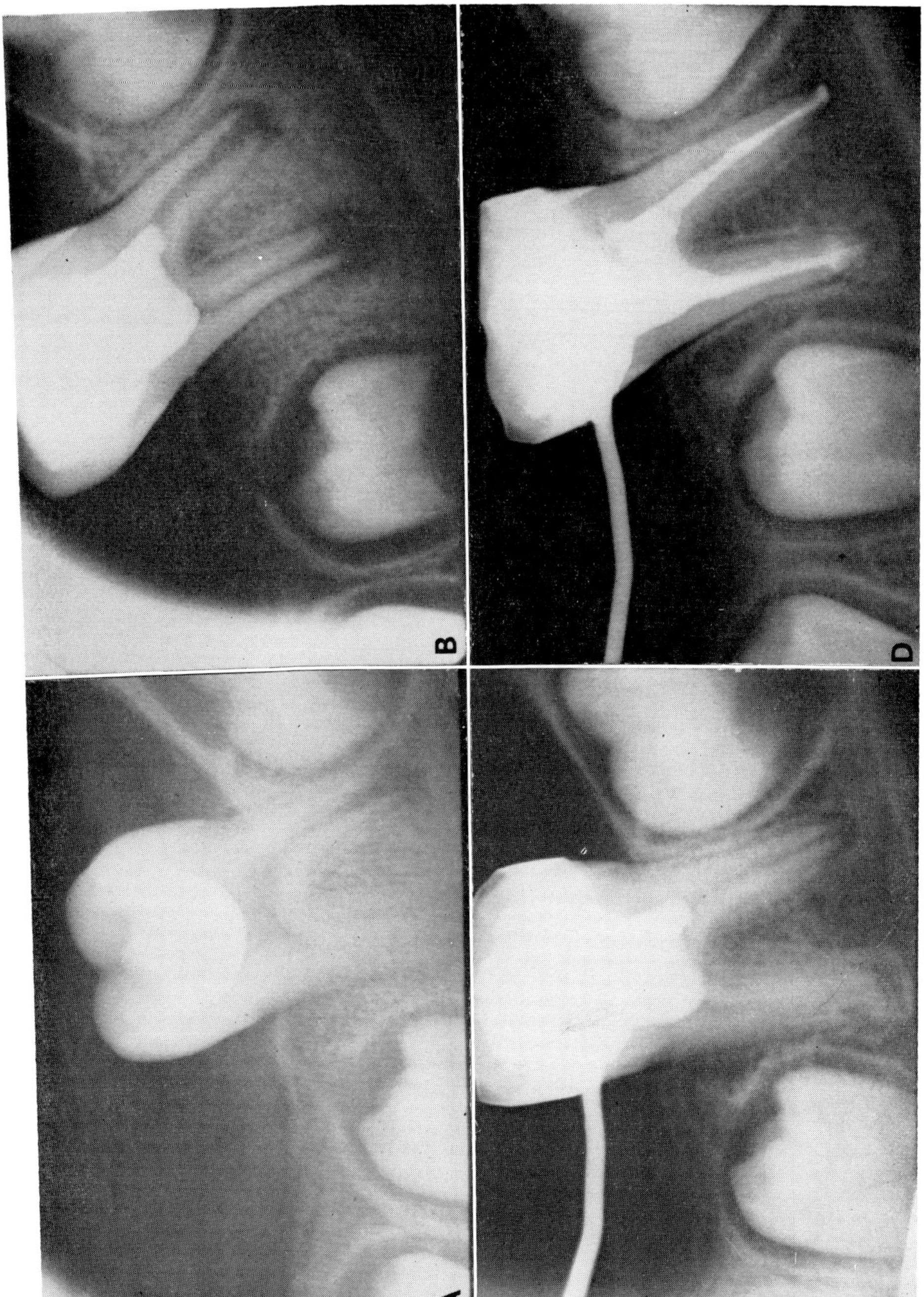

Figure 374. Pulpotomy for a lower molar. A. Large exposure in a vital, immature lower molar. B. After calcium hydroxide pulpotomy. C. One year later, root development is complete; space maintainer is in position. D. Nonsurgical endodontic therapy with gutta-percha-chloropercha completed. (From D. R. Morse, "The Management of Endodontic Problem Cases," *JDA South Africa, 27*:387, 1972)

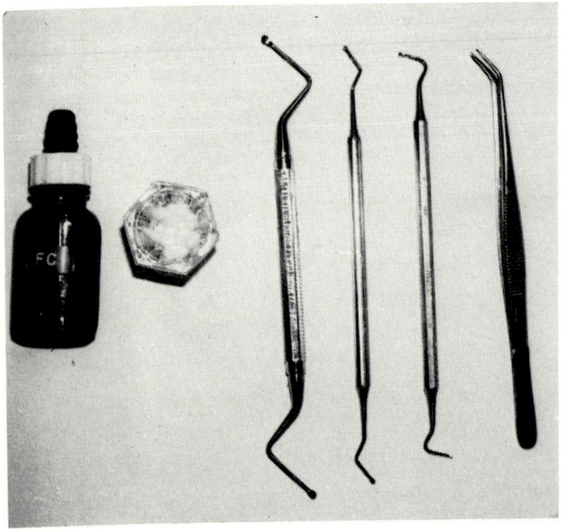

Figure 375. Armamentarium for pulpotomy for a primary tooth. Left to right; bottle of formocresol, dappen dish with cotton pellets, endodontic spoon excavators, plugger, cotton pliers; not shown are round burs, mirror, explorer ZOE temporary cement, and a permanent restorative material.

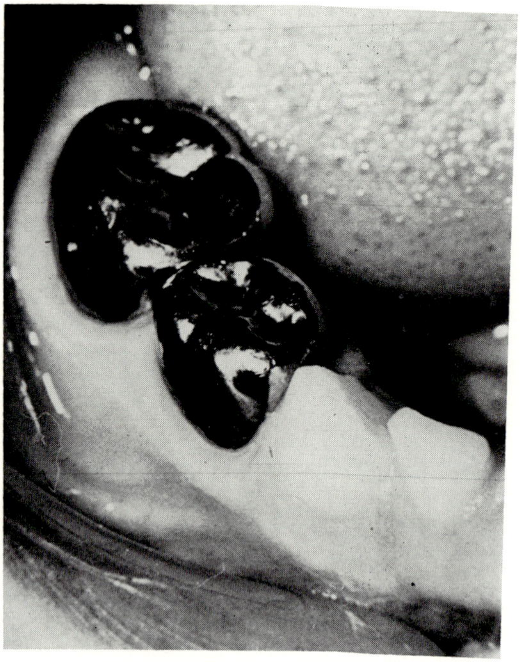

Figure 376. Stainless steel crowns for badly broken down lower primary molars. (Courtesy of Dr. K. Bomze, Cherry Hill, N. J.)

the chamber is blotted dry with sterile paper points. The remaining procedures are the same for both type cases. Formocresol is dropped on a large cotton pellet, placed in the floor of the chamber, and is then blotted to remove the excess. The tooth is then left alone for about five minutes, after which the cotton pellet is removed. A thick mix of zinc oxide-eugenol (with zinc acetate crystals) plus one drop of formocresol is prepared and inserted into the floor of the chamber.* Once it is set, a permanent type restoration is placed (Fig. 277). For teeth that have to last more than one year, a stainless steel crown is advisable (Fig. 376).

* Although clinical studies have shown a greater success rate for formocresol primary pulpotomies as compared to calcium hydroxide pulpotomies, further clinical research may reinforce the possibility that the use of a formaldehyde-type preparation can lead to hypersensitivity reactions, and therefore should be avoided.

BIBLIOGRAPHY

Berger, J. E.: A review of the erroneously labeled "mummification" techniques of pulp therapy. *Oral Surg, 34:*131, 1972.

Canby, C. P., and Burnett, G. W.: Clinical management of deep carious lesions. *Oral Surg, 16:*999, 1963.

Fisher, F. J.: The effect of a calcium hydroxide/water paste on micro-organisms in carious dentine. *Br. Dent J, 133:*19, 1972.

Jordan, R. E., and Suzuki, M.: Conservative treatment of deep carious lesions. *J Can Dent Assoc, 37:*337, 1971.

Nishida, O., Okada, H., Kawagoe, K., Tokunaga, A., Tanihata, H., Aono, M., and Yokomizo, I.: Investigation of homologous antibodies to an extract of rabbit dental pulp. *Arch Oral Biol, 16:*739, 1971.

Shovelton, D. S., Friend, L. A., Kirk, E. E. J., and Rowe, A. H. R.: The efficacy of pulp capping materials: a comparative trial. *Br Dent J, 130*:385, 1971.

Shröder, U.: Evaluation of healing following experimental pulpotomy of intact human teeth and capping with calcium hydroxide. *Odontol Revy, 23*:329, 1972.

CHAPTER 8

ACUTE SITUATION TREATMENTS

THESE ARE THE ENDODONTIC emergency procedures. Treatment of the following conditions are discussed: hypersensitive dentin, acute apical periodontitis, acute exacerbation of chronic pulpitis, acute apical abscess, acute exacerbation of chronic periapical condition, cellulitis, localized fluctuant abscess, tooth fractures, odontalgia following root canal obturation, acute periodontal abscess, luxation, and avulsion. Acute flare-ups that occur during nonsurgical endodontic therapy, and acute reactions such as hemorrhage and infection that may follow surgical procedures, are discussed in later chapters. Also, medical emergencies or reactions to endodontic drugs or treatment procedures are described in Chapter 16. For all of these cases, if pain and/or infectious disease is present appropriate analgesics and antibiotics should be used (see Chapter 4) along with the treatment described.

OCCLUSAL ADJUSTMENT

A simple, uncomplicated acute apical periodontitis in a vital tooth only requires occlusal adjustment. With the diagnostic aid of articulating paper, or bite tabs, the interfering *high* spots are taken out of occlusal contact. This is done with a diamond stone in an ultra-high speed handpiece, and copious water spray. The area is then gently polished with a rubber wheel in a slow speed contra-angle. The latter treatment is also used for a tooth fracture that only involves the enamel (Fig. 275A).

SEDATIVE RESTORATION

If a patient had experienced a solitary, short-lived toothache, it is probable that it was dentinal pain rather than pulpal pain. The treatment required for this type case is caries and/or restoration removal by the use of No. 4 or 5 round bur in an ultra-high speed contra-angle with copious water spray. Provided that there is no chance of a pulpal exposure, all the caries are removed. A zinc oxide and eugenol sedative dressing is then placed (Fig. 277). If there is a chance of pulpal exposure, indirect pulp capping (described in Chapter 7) should be performed. The use of a zinc oxide and eugenol sedative dressing is also indicated for crown fractures in which both the enamel and dentin are involved. If the fracture is extensive, but without a pulp exposure, then a celluloid crown form should be fitted for the tooth. After proper festooning, it is cemented on the tooth with a zinc oxide and eugenol paste. An alternative is the use of an acid-etch technique (Figs. 275B, 276).

PULPOTOMY OR PULPECTOMY

If a patient has a severe toothache (acute pulpalgia) and according to the history and diagnostic tests, the underlying condition is an acute exacerbation of a chronic pulpitis, then the treatment is immediate pulp extirpation.

First anesthesia is obtained and the rubber dam is applied (as described previously). Access is gained with a 701 bur in an ultra-high speed contra-angle, and the complete pulp is removed with a broach (if possible) in single rooted teeth. In posterior teeth, it has been found from clinical experience that only a pulpotomy has to be performed (see Chapter 7). If time permits, partial extirpation of the pulp in the canals can also be performed. With cotton pellets and absorbent points, the hemorrhage is controlled. A cotton pellet is moistened with either Cresatin® (must be fresh, as old solutions can form acetic acid) or eugenol. This pledget is then placed in the pulp chamber and blotted with a second pledget to absorb the excess. If there are no systemic complications (see Chapter 1), a corticosteroid paste can also be used. A temporary restoration of Cavit or zinc oxide and eugenol is placed. When the tooth is symptomless, endodontic therapy should be continued (a complete description of all stages of treatment from access through obturation is given in Chapter 9). The same treatment (pulpotomy or pulpectomy) is performed for teeth with crown fractures in which there is a pulp exposure. As described under the sedative restoration section, if there is a large fracture, a crown form is cemented into place. For those patients in which it is not possible or advisable to perform pulp extirpation, a mummification procedure can be employed (see Chapter 5).

EMERGENCY ENDODONTIC THERAPY

If the patient has an acute apical abscess or an acute exacerbation of a chronic periapical condition, drainage should be attempted through the root canal. As local anesthesia is difficult to

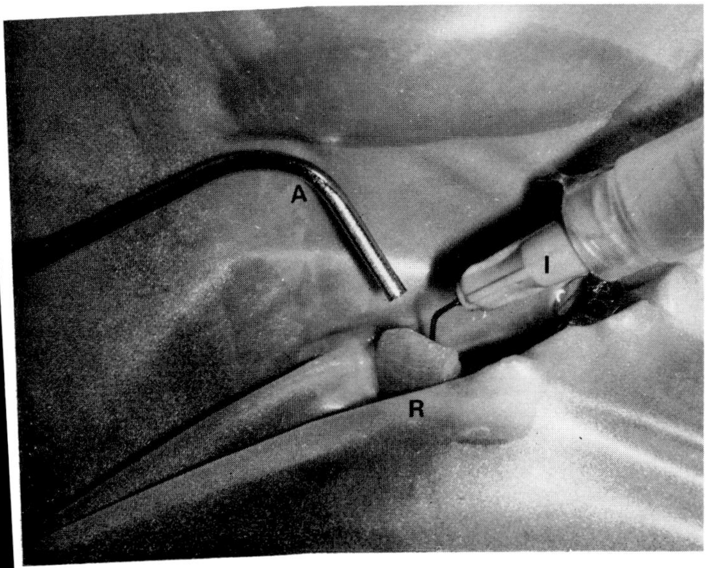

Figure 377. Use of suction tip to either aspirate fluid drainage or following irrigation; A = aspirating tip, R = rubber dam, I = irrigating syringe.

obtain, nitrous oxide analgesia is a good adjunct. Access is performed using a 701 bur in an ultra-high speed contra-angle. If there is a purulent or sanguineous exudate that does not cease, then the tooth should be left open for drainage. Use of an aspirating tip with a suction device aids in the evacuation of fluid (Fig. 377). The patient should be advised to rinse his (or her) mouth with warm saline (especially after eating) until the next appointment. The patient should be further counseled to keep the opening patent by the use of a toothpick, interdental stimulator, or rubber tip. Endodontic therapy should be continued when symptoms have abated.

If the patient has an acute periapical condition, and there is no drainage, then a rubber dam should be inserted. After access is completed, a root canal file should be placed through the apex into the periapical area. This may cause the occurrence of fluid flow. If the drainage can be controlled or if no fluid is withdrawn, then partial instrumentation should be performed short of the apex. This causes removal of some necrotic material. Irrigation is with 5% sodium hypochlorite solution, with care being taken not to express it periapically. The canal(s) is then dried with cotton pellets and absorbent points. Although there is controversy about the efficacy or necessity of intracanal medicaments, it may be useful to use an intracanal medicament in these acute cases. Formocresol (1:50) can be used if it is dropped on a cotton blotter to remove the excess, and then placed on the floor of the pulp chamber. It is important not to use formocresol on an absorbent point that may contact periapical tissues or to have it touch skin or mucous membranes, as a severe burn can result (Fig. 297) (See note at end of Chapter 7). Other intracanal medicaments that may be used on cotton pellets are camphorated monochlorophenol and Cresatin®. After the cotton pellet is placed in the chamber (with or without medication), a temporary restoration of zinc oxide-eugenol

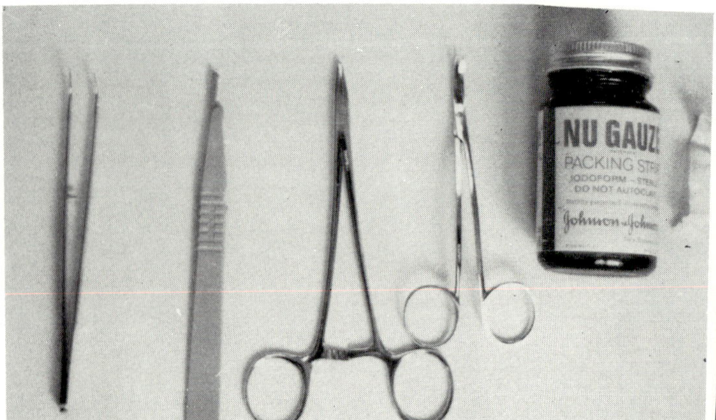

Figure 378. Armamentarium for incision and drainage. Left to right; cotton pliers, disposable scalpel (Bard-Parker No. 15), hemostat, scissors, bottle of iodoform gauze (Nu Gauze®—J & J), gauze strip.

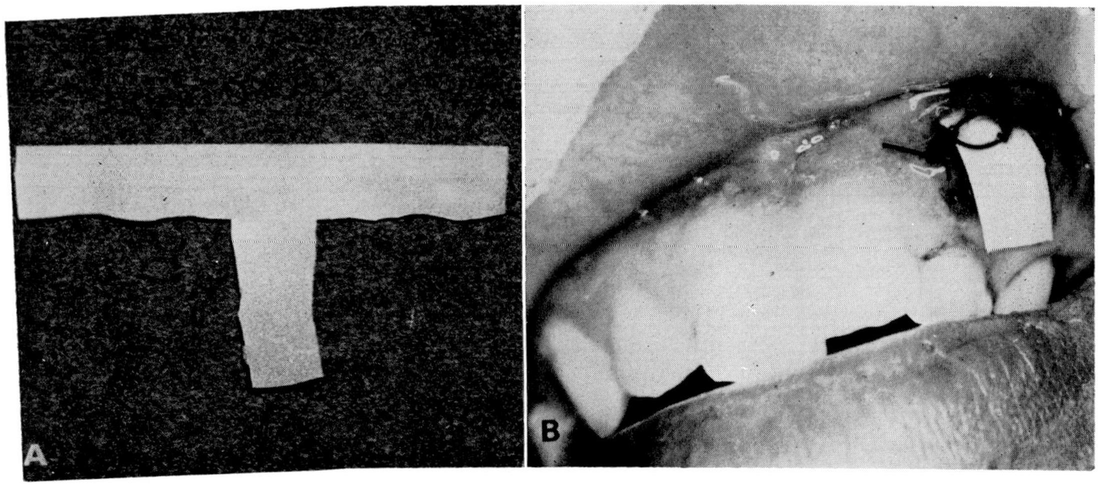

Figure 379. Rubber dam wick for incision and drainage. A. Rubber dam drain in shape of T. B. Rubber dam T drain inserted into incised area; held in position with one suture. (Courtesy of Dr. M. Gross, Philadelphia, Pa.)

or Cavit is placed. When the tooth is calm, endodontic therapy is continued (complete description is in Chapter 9).

INCISION AND DRAINAGE

If there is a diffuse cellulitis present, then antibiotic therapy should be instituted (see Chapter 4). If the drug is effective, after a few days, the swelling either may be completely resolved or a localized fluctuant abscess may develop. When the latter condition is present, an incision and drainage (I&D) is done (Fig. 320A, B). The necessary armamentarium is shown in Figure 378. Nitrous oxide analgesia or chemanalgesia are helpful adjuncts, as local anesthesia is difficult to obtain. When injecting a local anesthetic, the solution is first deposited around the circumference of the swelling. It is injected very slowly and gradually it infiltrates toward the center of the mass (Fig. 320C). The patient must be forewarned of some pain, even with the use of *nitrous* or IV sedation. It is important that the incision is made rapidly (to decrease the pain) at the most dependent part of the swelling and into bone (if possible) (Fig. 320D). The assistant should have the aspirating tip ready with the suction apparatus turned on as soon as the doctor is ready to make the incision. Once the fluid comes out, it is aspirated immediately (Fig. 320F). With the beaks of a hemostat, the opening is spread to enhance the fluid evacuation (Fig. 320E). After the evacuation appears complete, a drain of iodoform gauze is inserted with a few mms left protruding into the mouth (Fig. 320G). A rubber dam wick can also be used (Fig. 379). Another method that can be used to perform drainage is electrosurgical treatment. A fine needle electrode is applied to the fluctuant area with the current turned on. This is less painful than a

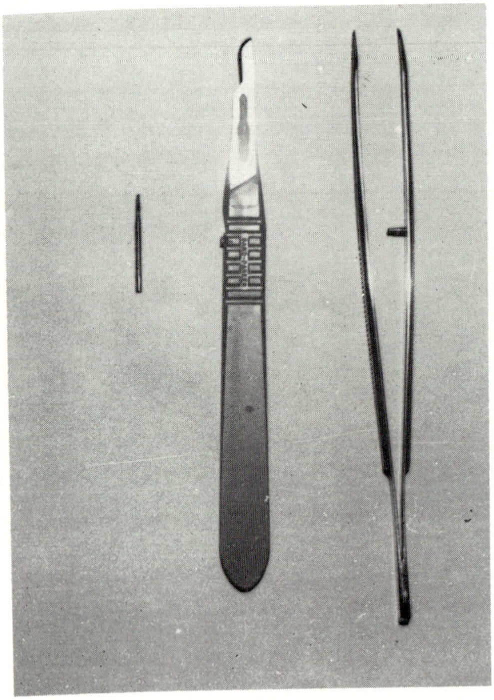

Figure 380. Armamentarium for trephination. Left to right; surgical friction grip 701 bur, disposable scalpel (Bard-Parker No. 15), cotton pliers.

local anesthetic injection and it causes rapid drainage. The electrode can also be used to scarify the margins of the opening. This allows the opening to remain patent for several days. It is important that the current is only applied for a few seconds or else healing will be unduly prolonged. The patient is advised to rinse his (or her) mouth as often as possible for the next few days. In about three days, the patient is asked to return, at which time the drain is removed. Once the swelling is noticeably decreased, endodontic therapy is begun.

TREPHINATION

For those acute cases (acute exacerbation of chronic pulpitis, acute apical abscess, acute exacerbation of chronic periapical condition) in which the root canal is clinically calcified or a post, instrument, or silver cone cannot be dislodged, trephination should be attempted. Armamentarium is shown in Figure 380. First, local anesthesia is obtained. Then a small incision is made in the region of the apex with a No. 11 or 15 scalpel. A 701 bur in an ultra-high speed contra-angle is used with copious water spray and penetration is made to the vicinity of the apex (Fig. 322). The use of the Sargenti Fistulator is shown in Figure 323. A radiograph is taken with an explorer held in position by the patient at the estimated site of the apex. This aids in the localization of the apex and is especially helpful in posterior teeth. The patient is told to rinse with warm saline as often as possible. When the acute situation is under control, definitive endodontic therapy is begun. This treatment can also be used for unbearable pain following root canal obturation. If pain relief is not obtainable, then periapical surgery or intentional replantation may be necessary.

PERIODONTAL CURETTAGE

If there is a periapical condition in which there is arrested drainage through the gingival sulcus (or periodontal pocket), it may be necessary to perform curettage of the sulcus (or pocket). The purpose is to stimulate drainage, and relieve the pain. The curette is placed to the depths of the sulcus (or pocket) and curettage is performed until fluid flow begins (Fig. 321). The patient is advised to rinse with warm saline. When the acute symptoms have

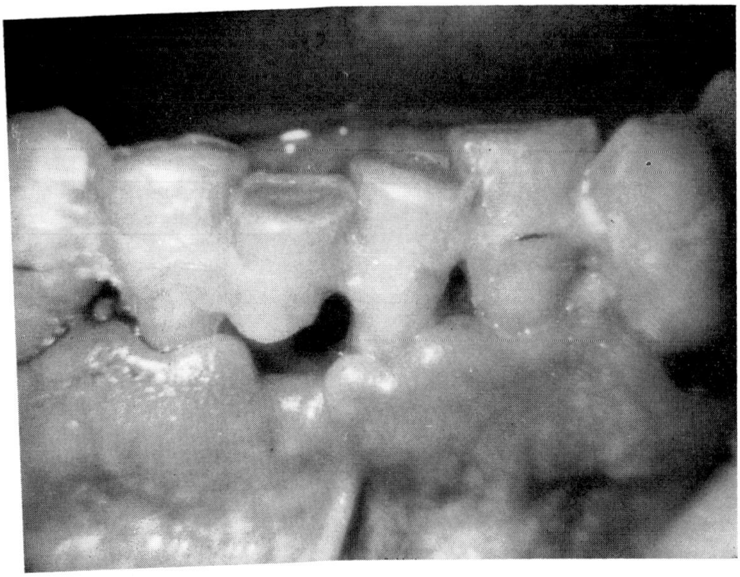

Figure 381. Wire acrylic splint. (Courtesy of Dr. K. Bomze, Cherry Hill, N. J.)

lessened (usually in a few days), the patient returns for definitive treatment.

ROOT FRACTURE TREATMENTS

Treatment depends upon location of the fracture, extent of the fracture, vitality of the pulp, and degree of mobility (Fig. 275).

No Treatment

If the only sign of a fracture is the radiographic image, and the tooth is symptomless, not mobile, and tests vital, then it should be left alone. Periodic check-ups are indicated.

Splinting

If a tooth has radiographic indications of a fracture, and it is also mobile, then it should be splinted. The splint should be removed in six weeks, at which time mobility should be tested, another periapical radiograph taken, and vitality checked. Splints are also usually used for cases requiring repositioning, replantation, transplantation, hemisection, and implantation (all described in later chapters). In Figure 381, the wire-acrylic method is shown. Armamentarium is shown in Figure 382. The disadvantage of this method is lingual interference with access by the wire. A good method for anterior teeth is the use of heavy gauge rectangular orthodontic wire (.0215 by .028 inch) that is cemented onto the labial surfaces of the involved tooth and at least two teeth on either side (Fig. 317). The cement used is the strongly adhesive zinc polycarboxylate cement (Duralon®, Poly-C®). It should be mixed and applied according to the manufacturers directions. Using the same cement, orthodontic brackets can be attached and then a wire can be inserted (Fig. 312). For posterior splinting of teeth in which there are restorations on the occlusal and proximal surfaces, an excellent splint is the amalgam A-splint (Fig. 314). This type splint (using acrylic

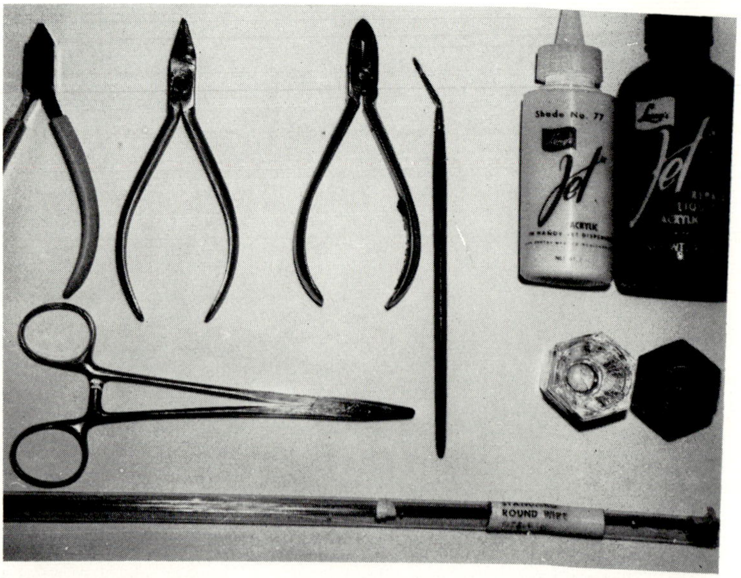

Figure 382. Armamentarium for wire acrylic splint insertion. Left to right: top row—orthodontic pliers, acrylic (Lang's); middle row—hemostat, fine brush, dappen dishes for mixing the acrylic; bottom row—orthodontic round wire.

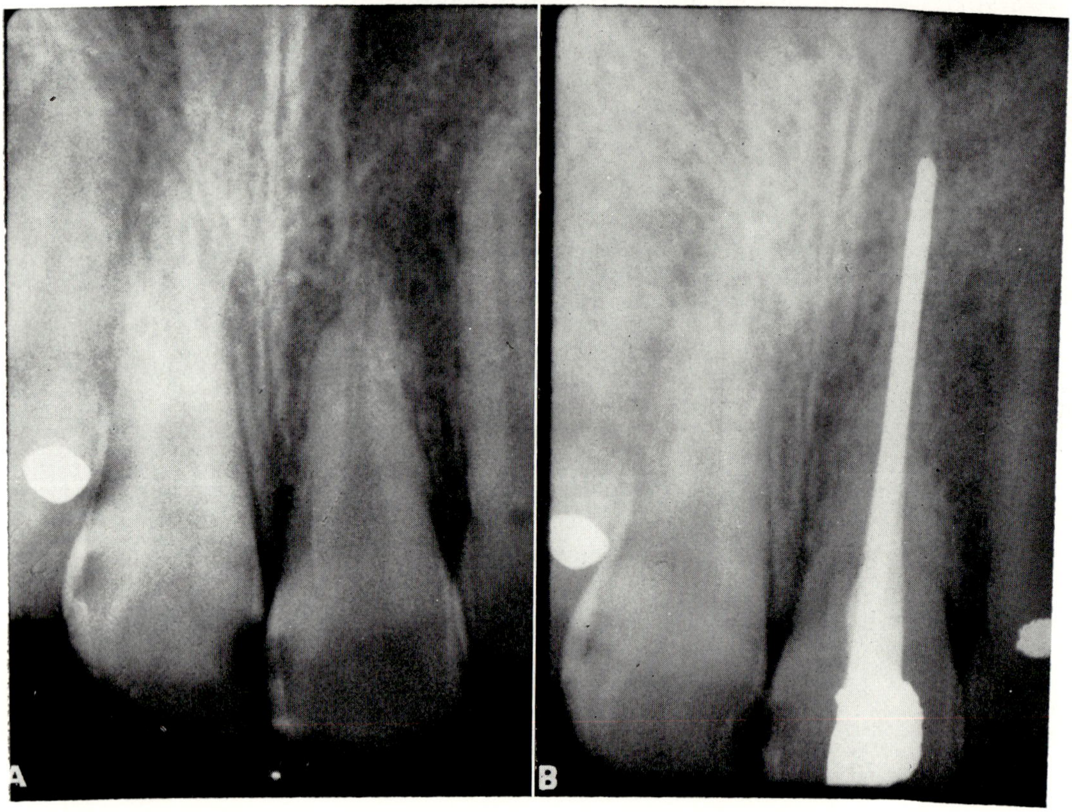

Figure 383. Stabilizing a mobile, replanted tooth with an endodontic implant. A. Nine months after replantation, mobility and root resorption is present. B. Over two years following insertion of an endodontic implant (Vitallium), there is no evidence of pathosis; tooth is firm and symptomless. (From D. R. Morse, "The Significance of Endodontics in Plantation Procedures," *JDA South Africa*, 26:263, 1971)

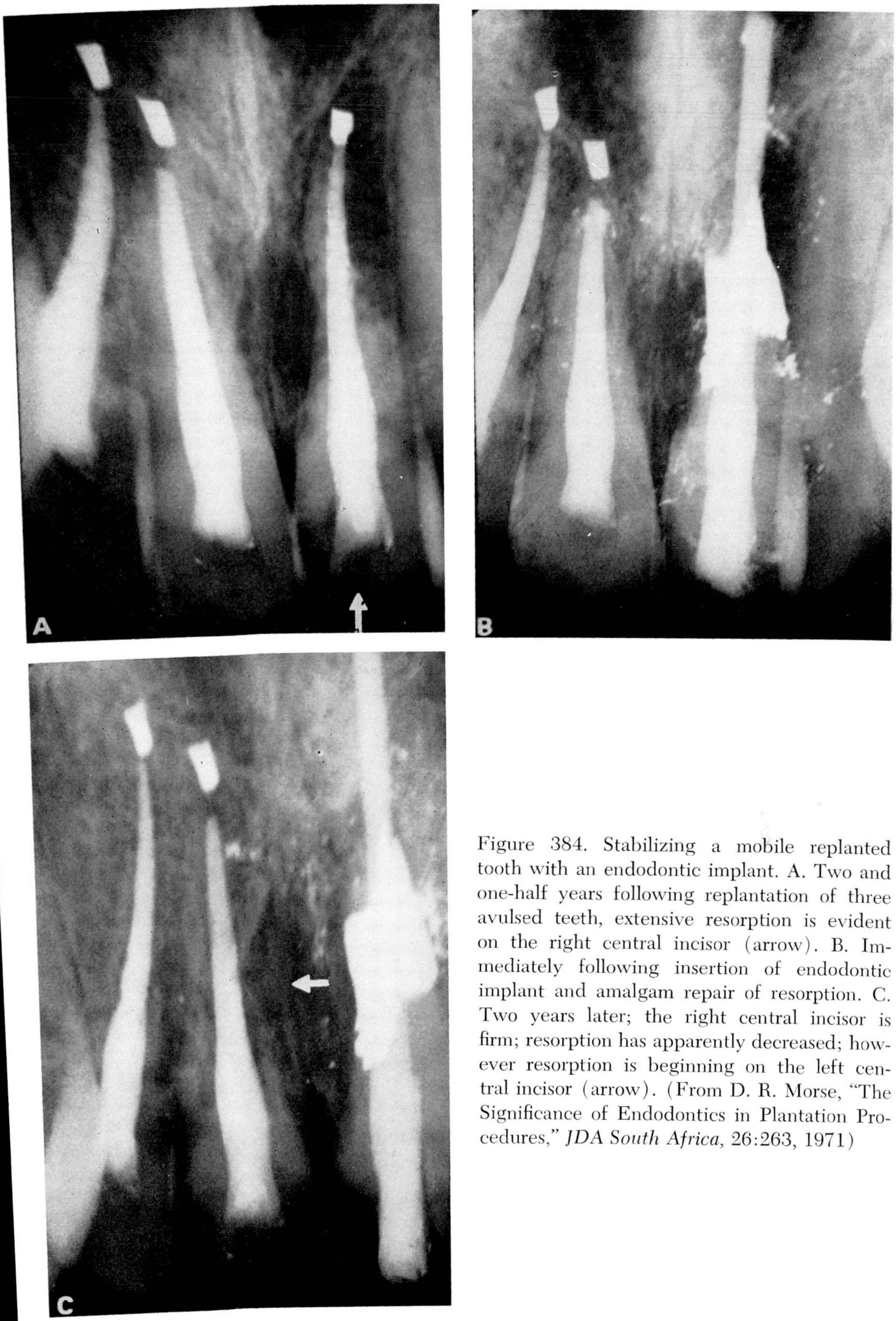

Figure 384. Stabilizing a mobile replanted tooth with an endodontic implant. A. Two and one-half years following replantation of three avulsed teeth, extensive resorption is evident on the right central incisor (arrow). B. Immediately following insertion of endodontic implant and amalgam repair of resorption. C. Two years later; the right central incisor is firm; resorption has apparently decreased; however resorption is beginning on the left central incisor (arrow). (From D. R. Morse, "The Significance of Endodontics in Plantation Procedures," *JDA South Africa*, 26:263, 1971)

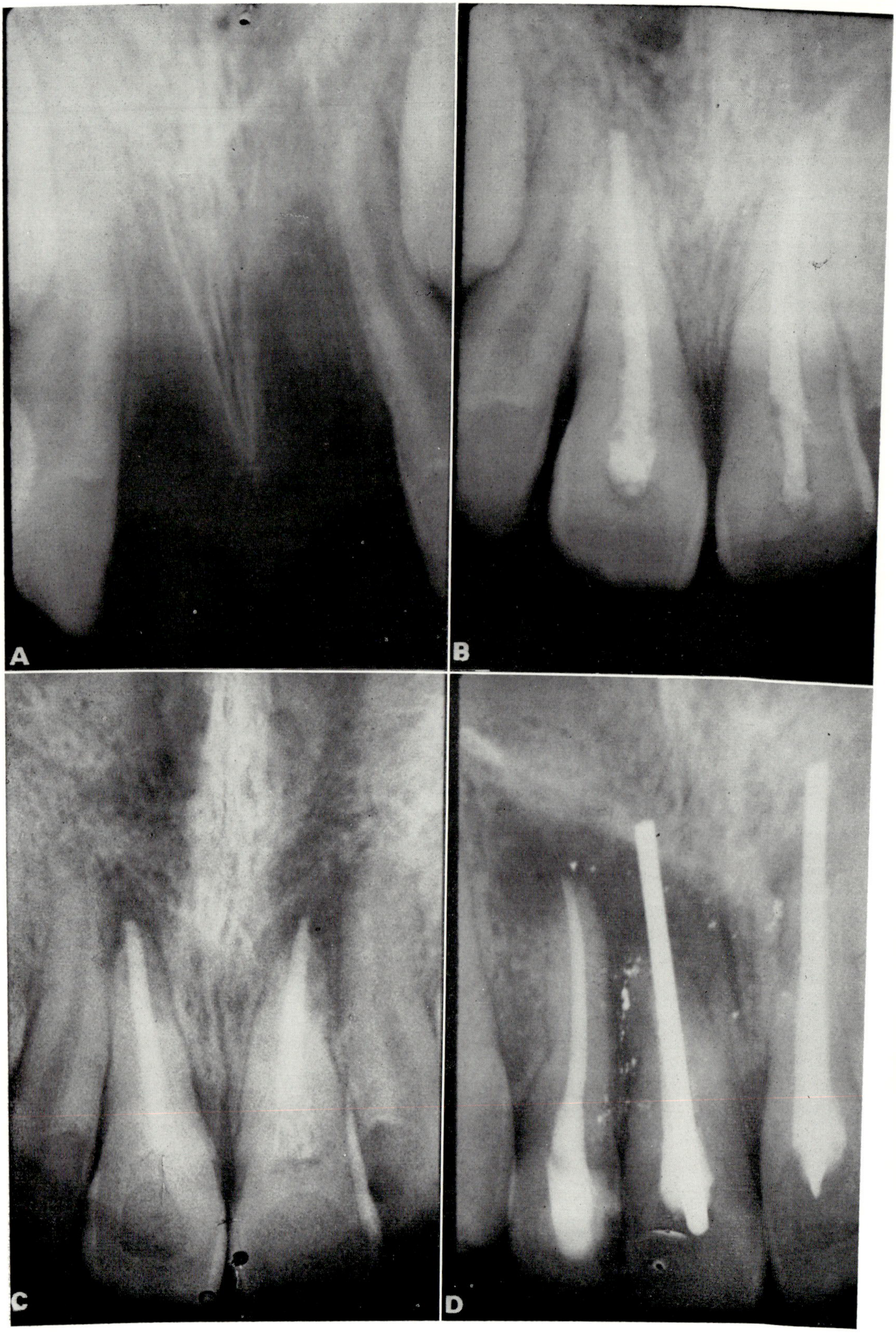
A
B
C
D

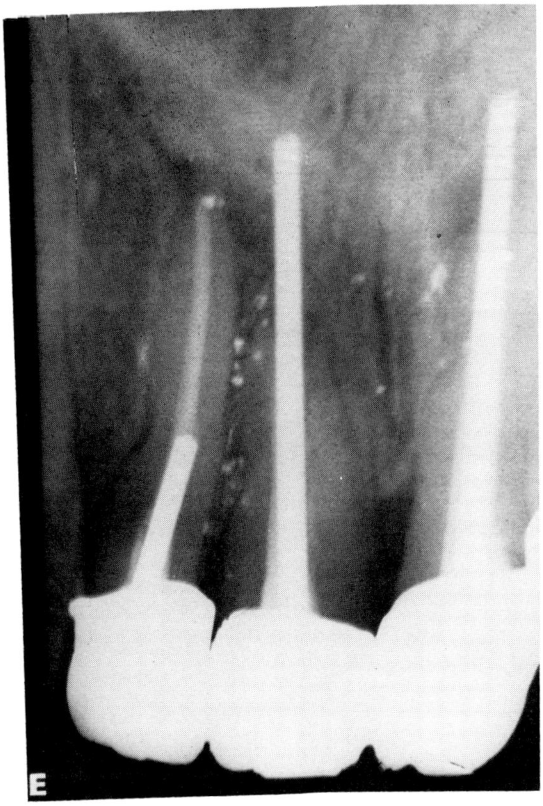

Figure 385. Stabilizing mobile replanted teeth with endodontic implants. A. Two upper central incisors had been avulsed as a result of trauma. B. After three hours extra-oral duration, the teeth were replanted and the canals were obturated (extra-orally) with gutta-percha. C. Four years later, the teeth showed evidence of root resorption and periapical pathosis; they were very mobile, and the upper right lateral incisor developed a necrotic pulp. D. A periapical curettage was performed; the lateral incisor canal was obturated with gutta-percha-chloropercha, and endodontic implants were inserted into the central incisors. E. Two years later, a fixed splint was made; periapical healing is evident; the teeth are firm and symptomless. (From D. R. Morse, "The Significance of Endodontics in Plantation Procedures," *JDA South Africa,* 26:263, 1971)

instead of amalgam) can also be used to attach a mobile, isolated anterior tooth to teeth that have been previously splinted with fixed restorations (Fig. 315).

Surgical Treatments

The treatments for cases of root fracture with wide separation of parts (immediate surgical endodontics) and mobility (endodontic implants) are described in later chapters.

REPOSITIONING AND SPLINTING

If a tooth has been displaced labially (buccally), or lingually (palatally), or intruded or extruded, an attempt should be made to reposition it. The tooth should be manually replaced to as close an approximation as possible of its previous position. For an intruded tooth, it may be necessary to use a forceps to gently bring the tooth into its former position (Fig. 343). Before initiating treatment, local anesthesia and analgesia (*nitrous* or *IV*) is used. After the tooth has been repositioned, an external splint is placed. The tooth should then be checked periodically by radiographs and other diagnostic tests. If the pulp becomes necrotic, nonsurgical endodontic therapy is performed. After six weeks, the splint is removed.

REPLANTATION AND SPLINTING

Armamentarium is shown in Figure 382. When the patient arrives, periapical radiographs are taken of the socket and teeth in the immediate area and opposite jaw. While the radiographs are being developed, the patient is draped, and the blood (if present) is washed off from the face. Nitrous oxide analgesia or chemanalgesia is administered followed by local anesthesia. Meanwhile, the dentist puts on sterile rubber gloves, takes the tooth, washes it to remove the debris, and wraps it in saline-moistened gauze. After the radiograph is read, the socket is probed with a surgical curette to remove root fragments (if present), debris or any blood clot. As discussed previously in the treatment planning chapter, the time element is crucial. Teeth that have been out of the mouth for one-half hour or less are replanted without any endodontic therapy or tooth alteration. The tooth should be placed as close to its normal anatomic site as possible. This should be verified by an x-ray. No endodontic therapy should be performed at this time. A splint is then placed but undue pressure should not be used. If the tooth *snaps* into position, a splint is not necessary. The tooth should be checked periodically by radiographs and clinical tests. If the pulp becomes necrotic, endodontic therapy is performed. The splint is removed after six weeks. If mobility hasn't ceased, an endodontic implant is inserted (Fig. 344A).

For the tooth that has been extraoral for more than one-half hour, the following procedures are performed (Fig. 344B). After the tooth is washed, access is completed by the use of a 701 bur in an ultra-high speed contra-angle. The pulp is removed, and instrumentation is completed, along with copious sodium hypochlorite irrigation. This should be done over a basin to prevent irritation to the hands or clothes. The lingual access is left open. The periodontal ligament is then scraped off with a curette. The tooth is soaked in an enzyme solu-

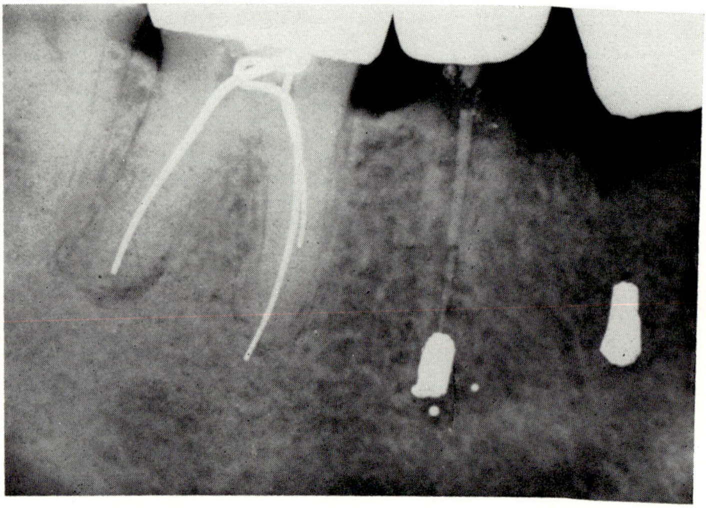

Figure 386. Complete resorption of replanted teeth; the lower left premolars had been avulsed as a result of an accident eight years previously; the teeth were extra-oral for eight hours; the canals were obturated with gutta-percha and retrograde amalgams extra-orally; the teeth are now completely resorbed, with only traces of gutta-percha and amalgam remaining in the bone. (From D. R. Morse, "The Significance of Endodontics in Plantation Procedures," *JDA South Africa*, 26:263, 1971)

tion for about twenty minutes. A method* that may be used is to place the tooth inside a test tube filled with pronase solution. This is then placed in a water bath at 50°C in an ultrasonic dental cleaner for approximately twenty minutes. The tooth is then placed in a 2.4% phosphate-sodium fluoride solution (Luride® phosphate topical solution) that has been buffered to pH 5.5 by the addition of 7.0 ml of 10.0 N.NAOH to the 250 ml bottle of the fluoride solution. The access may be left open or the root canal is sealed with a laterally condensed gutta-percha filling. The tooth is then replaced back into its socket and splinted. When the root canal has been sealed pain may occur and an analgesic should be prescribed. However, if the pain lasts for more than twenty-four hours, and it is severe, then a trephination should be done (see section on trephination). If the access was left open, then the obturation is completed one to two weeks later (provided that there are no untoward clinical manifestations). Typical cases are shown in Figures 82, 167, 383-386.

* This treatment method is based on recent findings by Dr. Leonard B. Shulman at Harvard University School of Dental Medicine.

BIBLIOGRAPHY

Auslander, W. P.: The acute apical abscess. *NY State Dent J, 36:*623, 1970.

Ehrmann, E. H.: The endodontic management of the acute pulpal or periapical lesion. *Aust Dent J, 17:*279, 1972.

Lance, J. R., and Marshall, F. J.: Emergency endodontic therapy: report of case. *JADA, 85:*1119, 1972.

Shulman, L. B.: Allogeneic tooth transplantation. *J Oral Surg, 30:*395, 1972.

Siskind, M.: Endodontic Implants and Transplants. Presented at the Annual Meeting of the A.D.A., Oct. 1971, Atlantic City, New Jersey.

CHAPTER 9

APEXIFICATION AND NONSURGICAL ENDODONTIC THERAPY

SUBJECTS INCLUDED in this chapter are apexification, nonsurgical endodontic therapy for permanent teeth, and nonsurgical endodontic therapy for primary teeth.

APEXIFICATION

Armamentarium is shown in Figure 387. Local anesthesia is useful as vital tissue shreds may be present and *nitrous oxide* is a helpful aid. The rubber dam is positioned on the appropriate tooth and access is gained with a 701 bur in an ultra-high speed contra-angle. The use of water spray for apexification or nonsurgical endodontic therapy is questionable. Some authorities state that it is not necessary as the pulp is either necrotic or will be removed anyway. However, others state that aside from injury to the pulp, the heat generated by the bur can cause burns of the dentin and possible dessication of the enamel and dentin (Fig. 388). These latter two factors may cause an increase in caries development and fractures, which could conceivably be a future problem. Instrumentation and irrigation are performed next (discussed fully in the following section). One modification is that the use of large Hedström files allow for better instrumentation of the wide open apex (Fig. 389C). After irrigation, the canal is dried with absorbent points and an

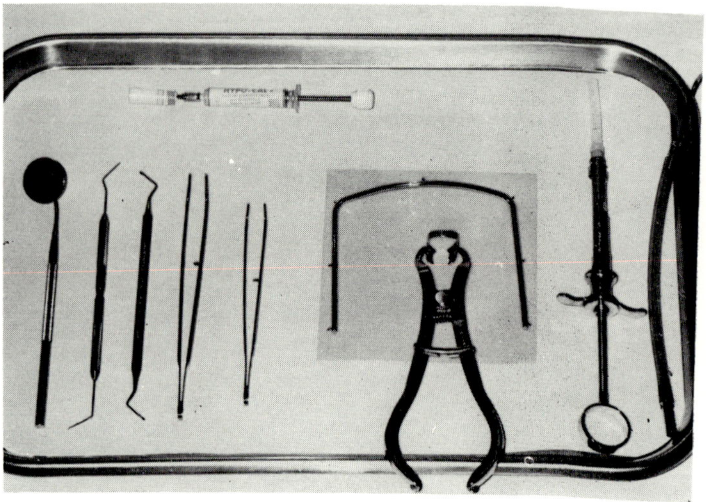

Figure 387. Armamentarium for apexification. Top—calcium hydroxide, injectable form (Hypo-Cal®-Ellman), left to right; mirror, explorer, plugger, cotton pliers, rubber dam set-up, injection syringe, aspirating tip; not shown is the 701 bur and Hedström files.

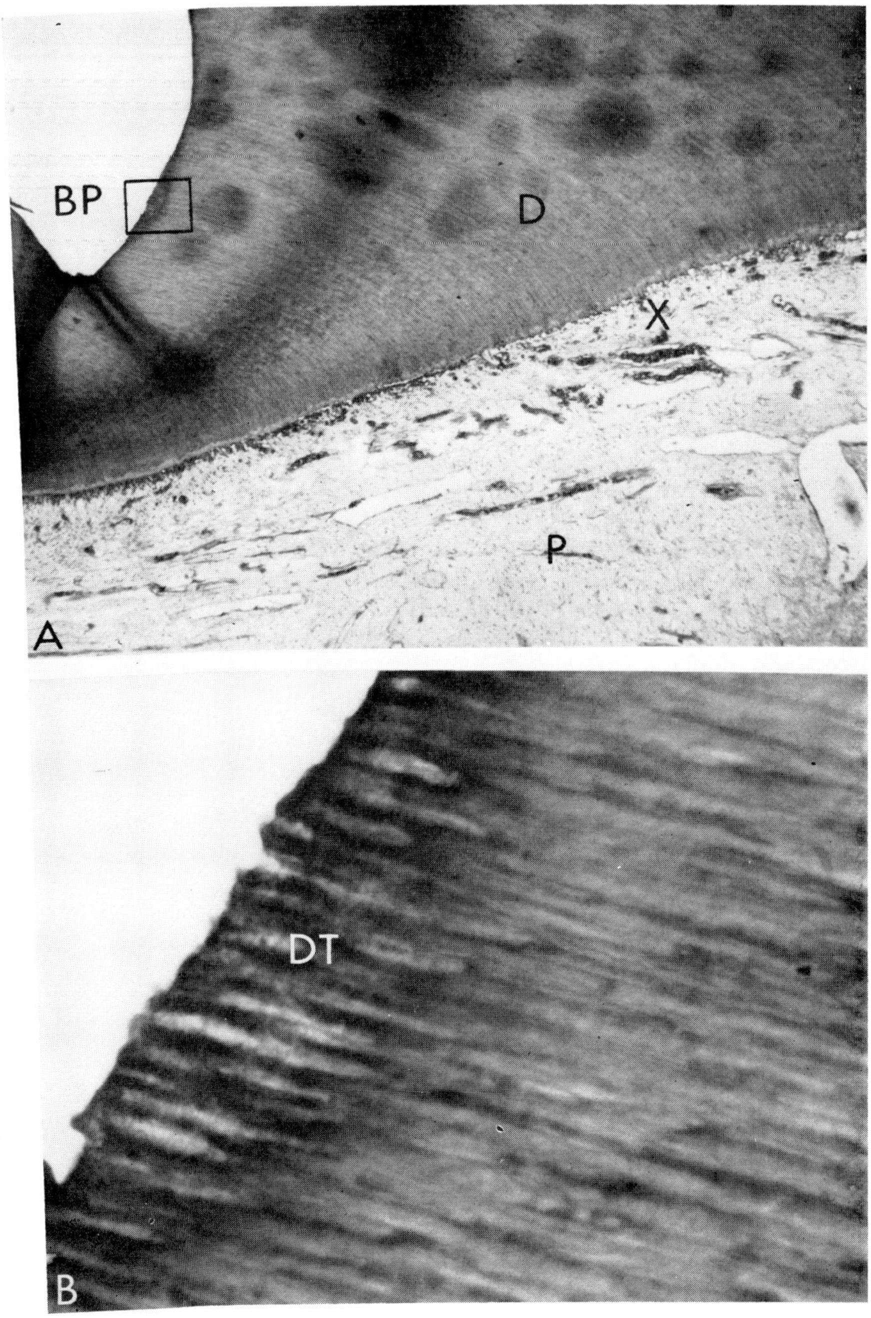

Figure 388. Burn lesion of the dentin caused by high-speed preparation; histologic section. (From S. Seltzer and I. B. Bender, *The Dental Pulp*, J. P. Lippincott Co., 1965. Used with permission of J. P. Lippincott Co.) A. D = dentin, P = pulp, BP = region of bur preparation. X = region of odontoblastic layer of the pulp that is damaged (×54). B. Higher magnification of section included in square; DT = charred dentinal tubules which are more vulnerable to subsequent decay.

intracanal medicament on a cotton pellet (CMCP or formocresol) is placed in the chamber. This phase of the treatment is debatable, as no medication may be just as effective. The access opening is then sealed with Cavit or ZOE. Provided that there are no symptoms, after a few days, the tooth is reopened under rubber dam. The dressing or plain cotton is removed. A paste of calcium hydroxide and water (or CMCP) is inserted about two-thirds the way up the root canal, using a root canal plugger or injected from a syringe. However, this phase of the treatment is also debatable as some studies have shown clinical success using no cement in the root canal. The next step is to place a sterile cotton pellet in the chamber followed by a ZOE or Cavit seal of the access opening (Fig. 277). The tooth is then checked every six months for up to two years (Fig. 277). Once apexification occurs, complete nonsurgical endodontic therapy is performed (Fig. 390). If apexification doesn't occur, the treatment may be repeated. However it is usually necessary to perform periapical surgery (described in Chapter 10).

NONSURGICAL ENDODONTIC THERAPY*

Nonsurgical endodontic therapy is the primary treatment performed in endodontic practice. It is the first type of complete endodontic therapy that is attempted. Only if nonsurgical endodontic therapy cannot be performed are surgical procedures used. Nonsurgical

* The preparation of this section was aided by Dr. George Biron, Clinical Assistant Professor and Director Undergraduate Clinic, Department of Endodontology at Temple University School of Dentistry, Philadelphia, Pa.

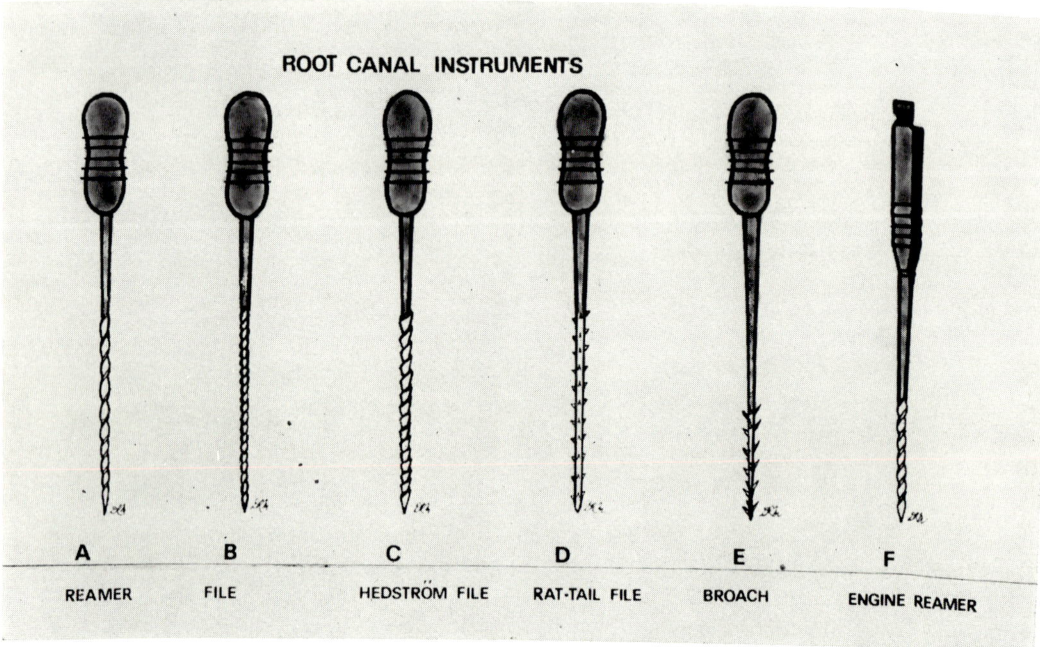

Figure 389

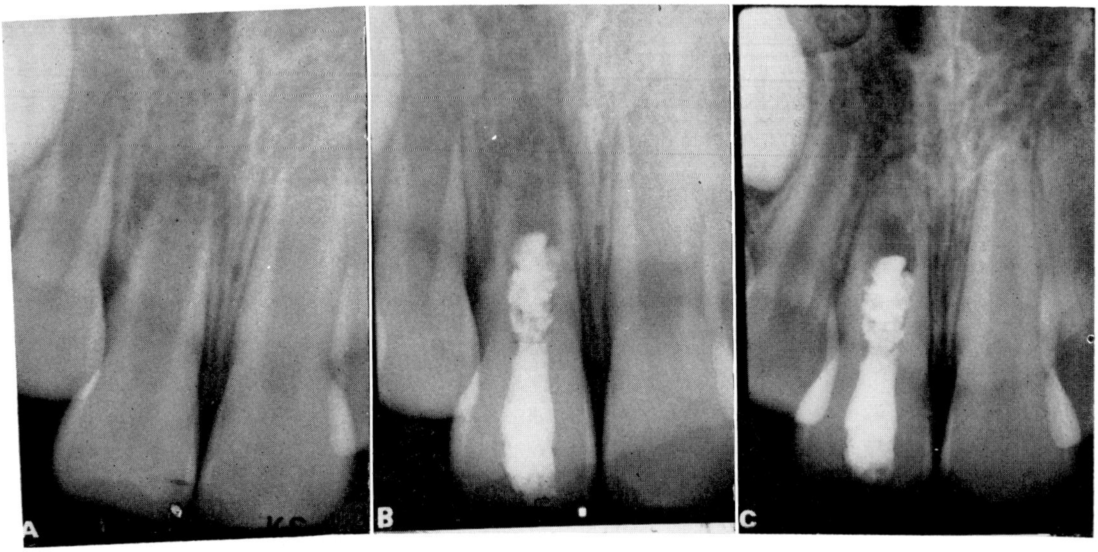

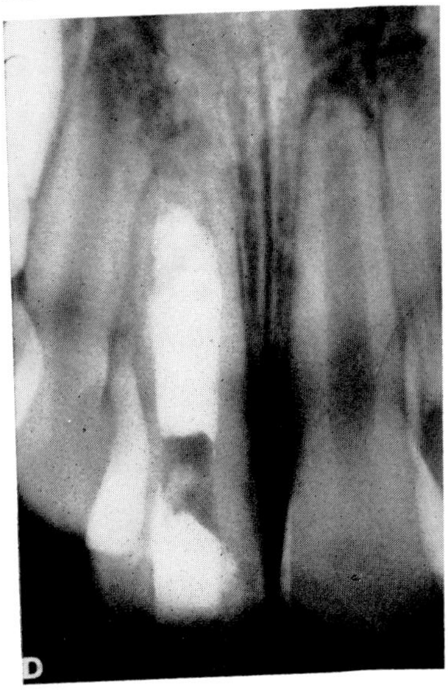

Figure 390. Apexification. A. Upper left central incisor with a necrotic pulp and an open apex. B. Apexification performed, using calcium hydroxide and water. C. One year later; apical portion of root has calcified irregularly. D. Canal obturated with gutta-percha-chloropercha. (From D. R. Morse, "The Management of Endodontic Problem Cases," *JDA South Africa*, 27:387, 1972)

therapy is performed on vital (or partially vital) and pulpless (nonvital) teeth. The latter teeth may or may not have periapical areas of pathosis present. The treatment for the two cases (vital and pulpless) is generally similar. However, there are some important differences which are discussed below. Access preparation is the same for both cases, but instrumentation and obturation show certain variations. The armamentarium for nonsurgical endodontic therapy is shown in Figure 391.

Access

After anesthesia and analgesia is obtained, a rubber dam is inserted (see Chapter 6). Access preparation is made with a 701 fissure bur in a water-cooled ultra-high speed contra-angle. If the

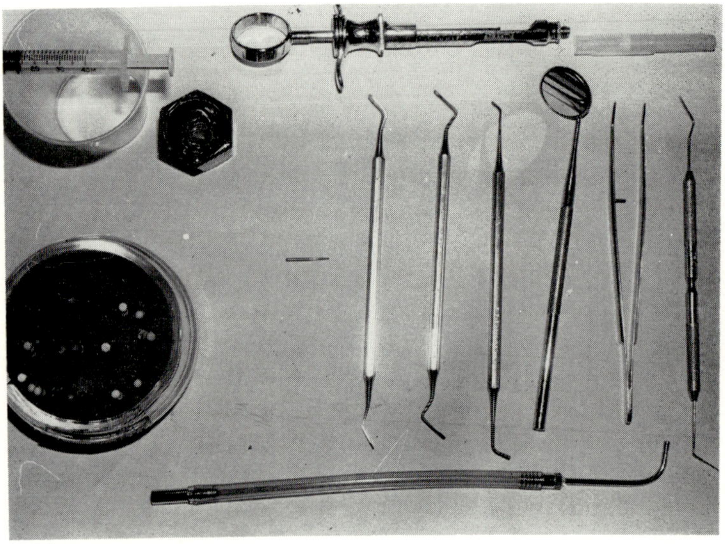

Figure 391. Armamentarium for nonsurgical endodontic therapy (access, pulp extirpation, instrumentation, irrigation); left to right; top row; irrigation syringe and cup, dappen dish, anesthetic syringe and disposable needle. Middle row; sponge containing cold disinfecting solution and root canal instruments (files, reamers, rat-tail files, Hedström files, broaches), friction grip 701 bur, plastic instrument, endodontic spoon excavators, plugger, mirror, cotton pliers, and DG-16 explorer (Star), bottom row; aspirating tip; not shown is the rubber dam set-up.

tooth is mobile, it should be stabilized with firm finger pressure during the access preparation and should be taken out of occlusal contact. If the mobility is not the result of endodontic disease, then external splinting should be done (e.g. wire and acrylic). Diagrams of access preparation for the various teeth are shown in Figure 392. As lower anteriors look similar, to avoid treating the wrong tooth, the lingual access preparation should be begun before inserting the rubber dam. Penetration is only into the dentin. Another method of identification is to mark the indicated tooth with a crayon before beginning treatment. For teeth with canals that are only patent in the apical portion, a long shank bur (No. 701, 3 or 4 round bur) is used to gain access. A DG-16 (Star®) explorer is used to probe the access openings for orifice location. In gaining access to fine curved molar canals, it may be very difficult to insert a file or reamer. The file or reamer can be guided into the orifice if it is held by either a lock tweezer, hemostat, or silver cone forceps.

Vital Case

A description is given of exact measurement, instrumentation, irrigation, intracanal medication, and obturation.

Exact Measurement

A reamer with an attached rubber stop is the first instrument used in the canal (Fig. 389A). The size is dependent upon the diameter of the canal. In fine molar canals, often a No. 15 reamer is the first one used. In anteriors a No. 35 or 40 reamer may be the first instrument used. The instrument should go in with some slight pressure felt, but it should not feel tight in the canal. Using a cotton pliers, a slight bend is placed at the apical end of the instrument. Then with a gentle back and forth wiggling motion, the instrument is advanced into the canal until it meets with resistance. The pretreatment radiograph is used as a guide for apical penetration. When it appears that the apex is reached, a periapical radiograph is taken with the rubber stop resting against the incisal (occlusal) edge. With the use of the formula (shown in Chapter 1, section on treatment periapical radiographs), the exact measurement is determined and entered on the patient's chart. All subsequent instruments that are used have rubber stops placed on them to the determined measurement.

Instrumentation and Irrigation

In patent canals, a suitable size broach (one that loosely fits the mesial-distal diameter of the canal) is used to remove the pulp (Fig. 389E). Quite often, the pulp does not come out with one penetration. Use of several broaches is advantageous. As one is being used, the assistant is sterilizing the others in the salt sterilizer. She can then immediately hand the dentist another broach as he withdraws the previous one. With large pulps, the simultaneous use of two broaches allows for pulp removal in one piece. In fine canals, files are used rather than broaches, as the latter can readily snap within the canal. Bleeding is controlled by irrigation with sterile saline followed by drying with absorbent points. If this is not satisfactory, then the use of the local anesthetic solution as an irrigant usually controls hemorrhage. Excessive bleeding may indicate that some pulp tissue is still remaining in the canal, as pulpal blood vessels enlarge as they descend (or ascend in lower teeth) coronally. If broaching indicates that the bleeding is occurring from periapical blood vessels and it cannot be controlled by the previously described methods, then the use of a small amount of formocresol placed on the tip of an absorbent point is usually very effective. The point is placed in the canal up to the apex and left there for approximately 30 seconds, after which it is withdrawn. The bleeding usually stops. The procedure may be repeated once. The slight amount of formocresol used does not cause any apparent clinical problems. However, it is essential that excess formocresol is not used as it is highly irritating and caustic and has been shown to cause injury to the periodontal ligament with subsequent ankylosis (See note at end of Chapter 7).

After the broaching of the canal is completed, the use of files is begun (Fig. 389B). I do not find any advantage in the use of a reamer, except as the previously described pathfinder. A reamer does not cut as efficiently as a file, and if a file is used as is to be de-

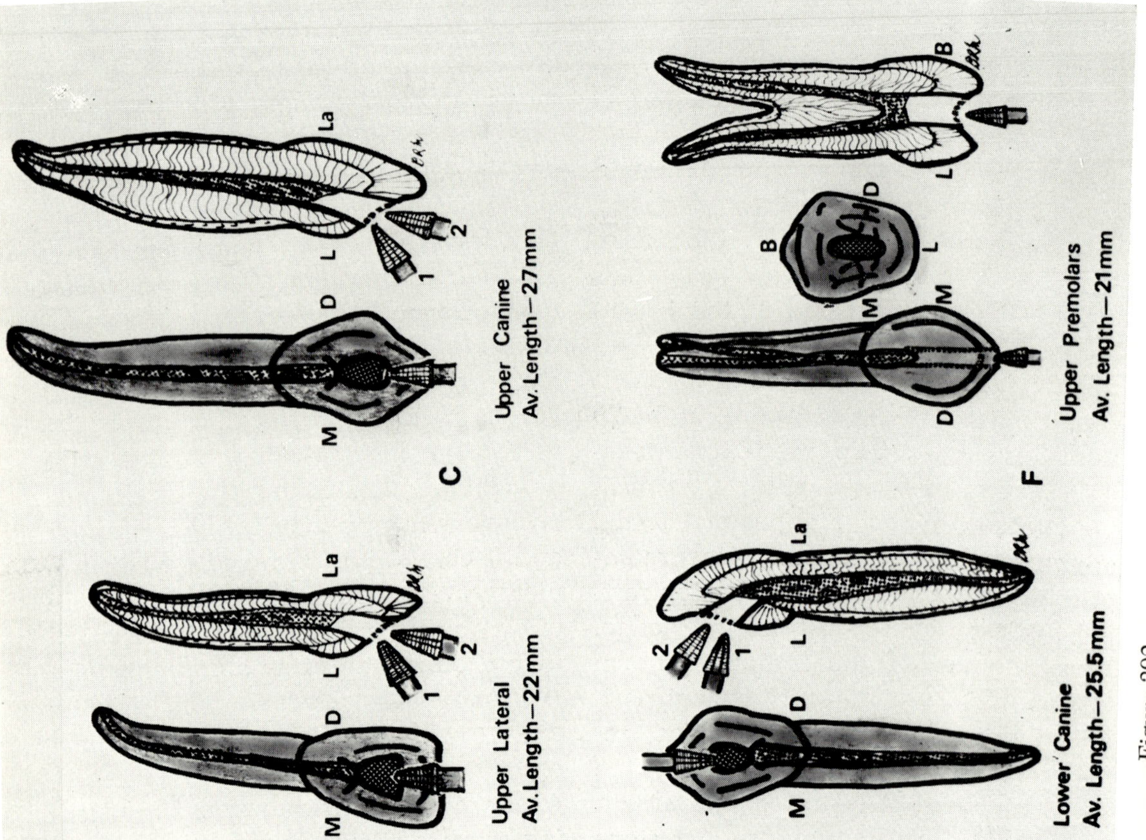
A
Upper Central
Av. Length—22 mm
B
Upper Lateral
Av. Length—22mm
C
Upper Canine
Av. Length—27mm
D
Lower Incisors
Av. Length—22 mm
E
Lower Canine
Av. Length—25.5mm
F
Upper Premolars
Av. Length—21mm
M
D
L
La
B
1
2

Figure 392

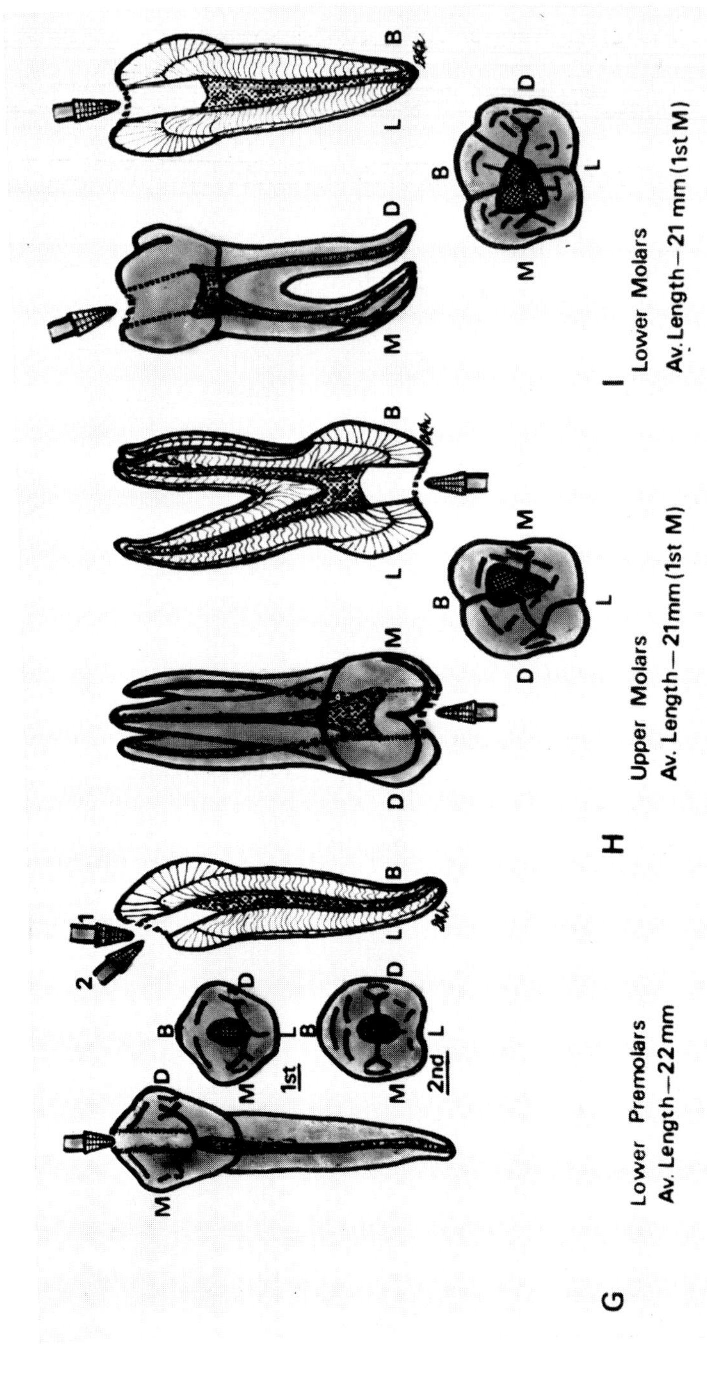

Figure 392 A-I. Access preparation for various teeth.

scribed, it does not cause the canal to be clogged. The first file used is one that goes securely into the canal. This is usually the same numbered file as the reamer that was used for determination of exact measurement. As with the reamer, a slight apical bend is placed, and penetration is made slowly as the instrument is gently rotated. Once the apex is reached (as judged by the instrument stop), the file is withdrawn against the wall by a pull-stroke. This is continued along all walls of the canal (Fig. 393B). Sterile saline irrigation is then used. Sodium hypochlorite is not used. As a pulp tissue solvent, it might cause necrosis of tissue in lateral and accessory canals. The necrotic tissue could then become a nidus for periapical irritation. Recent *in vitro* findings have shown that 5% sodium hypochlorite (usual clinical concentration) is more damaging to tissues than it is to microbes, while .5% sodium hypochlorite dissolves necrotic tissue and not vital tissue. If this latter finding is verified by clinical studies, then .5% sodium hypochlorite could be recommended for clinical application.

After the first file used is loose within the canal, the next numbered instrument is used in the same manner. Again, liberal amounts of saline irrigation are used. There is no definite numbered instrument to which a canal should be filed.

The instrumentation is continued until the walls of the canal feel smooth, and clean, white shavings are removed. The removal of white shavings is merely an indication that the canal walls are clean. Current scanning electron microscope studies at Temple University show that apparently well instrumented and irrigated root canals *(in vitro)* still contain organic debris, pulpal tissue, and microorganisms. Nevertheless, clinical results have shown that even if the canal is not completely instrumented (as judged by scanning *scope* pictures), if it is well obturated, clinical success can be achieved. After the filing is completed, the canal(s) is irrigated again, and dried with absorbent points. There are certain precautions to follow in this stage of treatment.

(1) After the use of a higher numbered instrument, the previously used instrument should be reinserted to insure that no blockage occurred.

(2) Each file used should receive the same type apical bend.

(3) Irrigation should be used after instrumentation with each numbered file. It is better to over-irrigate than under-irrigate.

(4) In fine canals (mesials of lower molars, buccals of upper molars), it is rarely necessary to instrument beyond a No. 35 file. If larger instruments are used, there is a much greater chance of perforation.

(5) Use of EDTA or R-C Prep® (Premier®) helps in the instrumentation of fine or partially calcified canals. EDTA is placed in an irrigating syringe and a few drops are withdrawn into the canal. It can be replenished as it is needed. At this writing, EDTA has not been approved by the F.D.A.,

hence R-C Prep should be used. R-C Prep is placed within the canal on a file and is replaced as it is needed. It is an excellent lubricant.

(6) Do not overuse instruments. If a file or reamer is bent, rusted, has separated flutes, or is twisted, it should be discarded.

(7) In large canals, Hedström files can be used to obtain smooth walls in a relatively rapid manner (Fig. 389C).

(8) In fine canals, once the curvature has been straightened out (if this can be done), then rattail files can be used to obtain more efficient cutting (Fig. 389D).

Intracanal Medication

Obviously, if a case is completed in one visit, no intracanal medication is used. Otherwise, a sedative-type dressing such as eugenol, Cresatin, or Ledermix® can be used. Many cases have been treated using no intracanal medicaments, with excellent results. Any pain between visits was controlled with oral analgesics and/or by temporarily opening the tooth (see Chapter 15). When using a medicament, it is placed on a sterile cotton pellet, which is then inserted into the chamber. A second pellet is pressed down on the first to remove the excess medicament and the former is then removed. Medicaments are not placed on absorbent points because the medication can come in contact with periapical tissues and cause irritation, and absorbent points can imbibe tissue fluid and then become extremely difficult to remove. The access opening is sealed with Cavit or ZOE. A double seal of gutta-percha and ZOE is not essential. The rationale of the double seal is that gutta-percha prevents the particles of cement from occluding the orifice, and helps cushion the tooth against masticatory forces. At Temple University, no differences in clinical results have been found as far as fracture or orifice occlusion is concerned, with the use of a single or a double seal.

Obturation

Obturation is done when the tooth is symptomless, the canal is dry or can be dried with absorbent points, and the walls are tapered and smooth. This may be the first, second, or third visit. Armamentarium for obturation is shown in Figure 394. At this visit, it is a good idea to use nitrous oxide analgesia alone so that rubber dam insertion and obturation will not cause discomfort. The temporary seal and cotton pellet are removed. The canal is reinstrumented with the same size file as was last used, in order to remove any dentin debris that may have accumulated between visits. The canal is then irrigated and dried with sterile absorbent points. At this point, the case is ready for the fitting of the master cone.

MASTER CONE FIT. A master gutta-percha cone is chosen and placed in Betadine®, Cidex®, or similar type solution or a presterilized cone can be chosen from a sterile tray. Using cold disinfectants, various sized cones can be

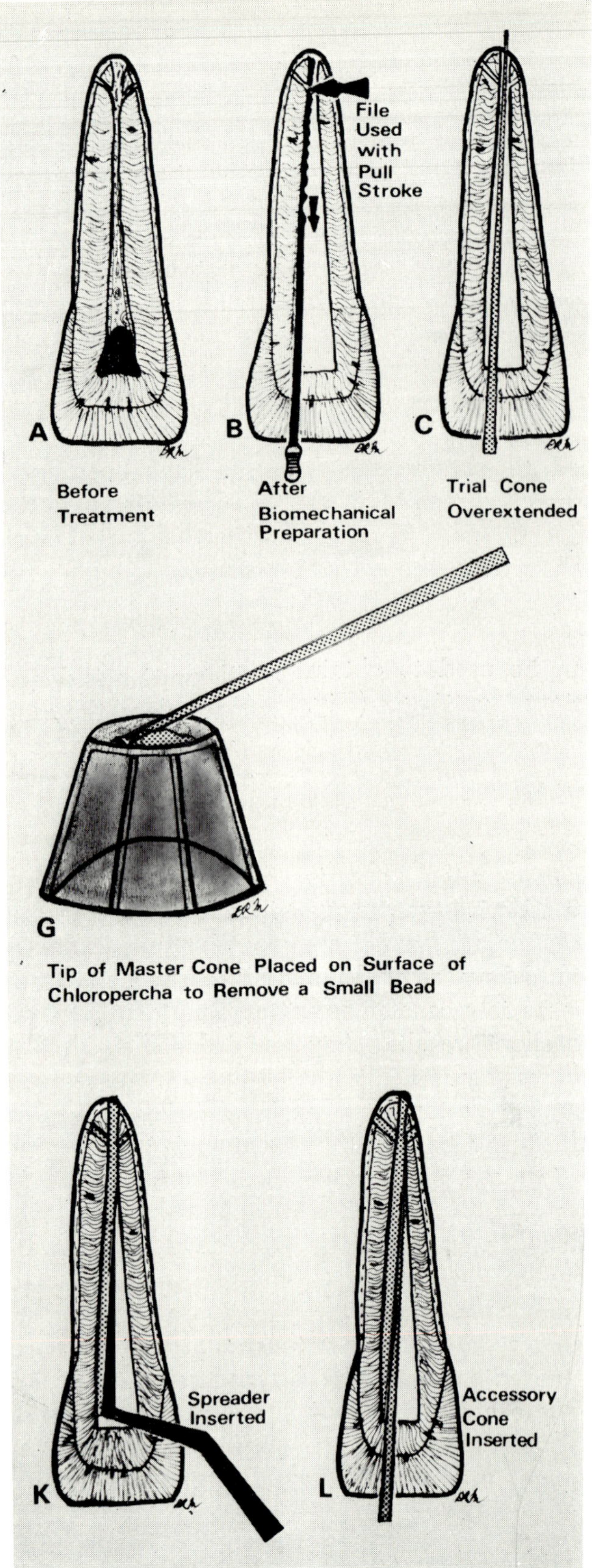
File Used with Pull Stroke
A
B
C
Before Treatment
After Biomechanical Preparation
Trial Cone Overextended
G
Tip of Master Cone Placed on Surface of Chloropercha to Remove a Small Bead
Spreader Inserted
Accessory Cone Inserted
K
L

Figure 393

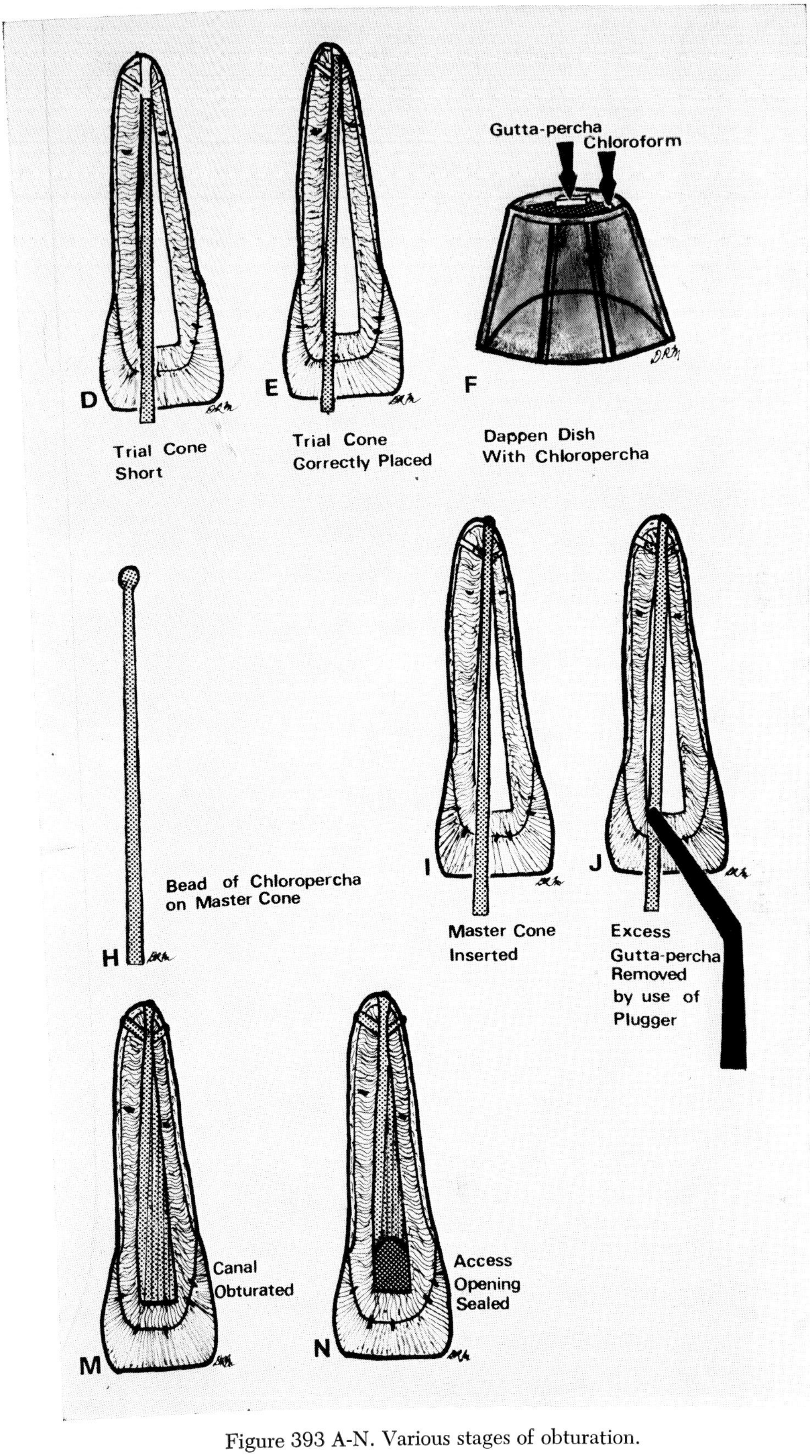

Figure 393 A-N. Various stages of obturation.

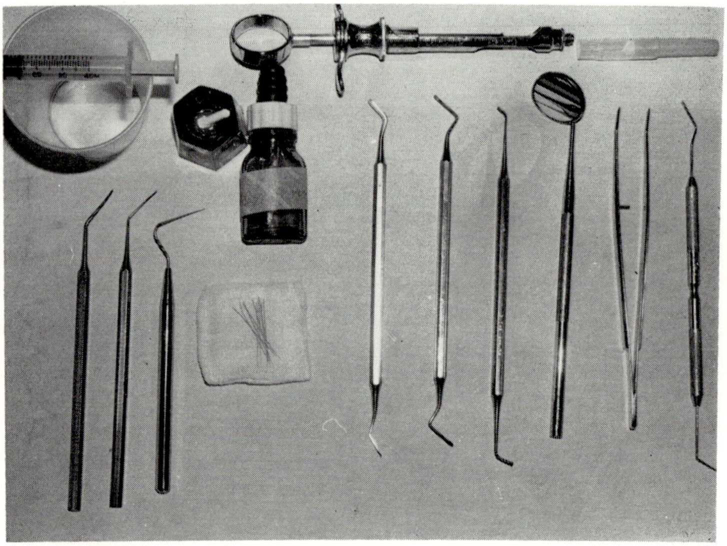

Figure 394. Armamentarium for obturation. Top row—irrigating syringe and cup, anesthetic syringe and disposable needle. Middle row—chloropercha (gutta-percha dissolved in chloroform) in a dappen dish, bottle of chloroform. Bottom row—Luk's pluggers (Star), 4X spreader (20th Century), gutta-percha cones, plastic instrument, endodontic spoon excavator, plugger, mirror, cotton pliers, DG-16 (Star) explorer.

kept in different vials. The size of the last file used is taken as a guide to the number of the gutta-percha cone that it is to be tried in. The gutta-percha cone should fulfill certain requirements. It should go into the root canal to its entire length, as determined by the exact measurement. The cone should bind in the apical third of the canal. Resistance should be felt as the cone is withdrawn *(tug back)*. Figure 393E shows the proper fit of a master cone. If the cone is loose in the canal, although it reaches the estimated apex, the next larger size cone is used, until the *tug back* is felt. An alternative method is to cut back the loose cone by one mm sections until *tug back* is achieved. Once all three requirements are met (correct length, apical bind, and *tug back*), a periapical radiograph of the fitted cone is taken. The periapical radiograph will show either of three possibilities: (1) the cone goes right to the radiographic apex, (2) the cone goes beyond the radiographic apex, and (3) the cone is short of the radiographic apex. If the cone goes to the radiographic apex, it is cut back approximately one and one-half mm. This is to compensate for the fact that the clinical apex is usually shy of the radiographic apex, and the condensation procedure should push the filling to the clinical apex. If the cone goes beyond the radiographic apex, it must be cut back the number of excess millimeters plus an additional one and one-half mm. If the cone appears short on the radiograph, and it is within the one and one-half mm limits, it can be used as is. If the cone is too short, another cone must be selected and refitted.

CONDENSATION. The master cone is removed and placed on sterile gauze. If it has to be adjusted, it is done at this time. A small square of gutta-percha is placed on the top well of a dappen dish, and chloroform is dropped in to form a loose paste (Fig. 393F). The master cone is then inserted into the paste to form a bead of chloropercha on the apex of the cone (Fig. 393G, H). The cone is then inserted with a cotton pliers up to its previously determined level in the canal (Fig. 393I). A radiograph is taken to ascertain that the cone is seated to the apex. If inadvertently, it has gone beyond the apex, the cone is not removed because the chances are good that the cone would stretch and break upon removal. From clinical experience, it has been found that a well condensed canal case is generally successful, even if there is some filling material protruding beyond the apex. If the cone appears short, it probably bent back on itself during the insertion. If it cannot be removed, then chloroform is placed in the canal to soften the cone. With a small file, the cone is either removed or bypassed. Once the apex is cleared, the canal is irrigated, dried and another point is fitted and inserted. A No. 9 or 11 root canal plugger is then heated in the flame of a bunsen burner and inserted into the orifice to remove the excess gutta-percha (Fig. 393J). Then, a No. 4X spreader (Twentieth Century Broach Co.®), or a similar fine spreader) is inserted adjacent to the cone as far as it can go. The handle of the spreader is rotated through 180° several times, after which it is removed with a quick, downward (upward in lower teeth) motion in line with the long axis of the tooth (Fig. 393K). A fine-fine gutta-percha cone is then inserted into the space created by the spreader (Fig. 393L). In large canals, a medium fine or even fine cone can be used. It is important that the cone goes up into the full extent of the created space, or else voids in the filling will occur. After the first auxiliary cone is inserted, the excess beyond the orifice is also removed with a heated No. 9 or 11 root canal plugger. The reason that the cones are not allowed to protrude until the end of the filling procedure, is that removing the excess from each cone after its insertion, greatly improves the visibility for spreading and cone insertion. The procedures of spreading, insertion of fine-fine cones, and removal of the excess, is continued until no other cones can be introduced. Then, a fine plugger (No. 4), is placed into the orifice and pressed apically (Fig. 393M). Another radiograph is taken to check on the completeness of the filling. If there are any voids, then more cones are added until the filling is well condensed. The access opening is then sealed with Cavit or ZOE cement (Fig. 393N). If the patient will not be receiving a *permanent* restoration for two weeks or more, then a zinc oxyphosphate cement, or a reinforced ZOE cement (e.g. IRM; Caulk) should be used. Routine vital cases filled with this technique are shown in Figures 97, 283, 395, 396.

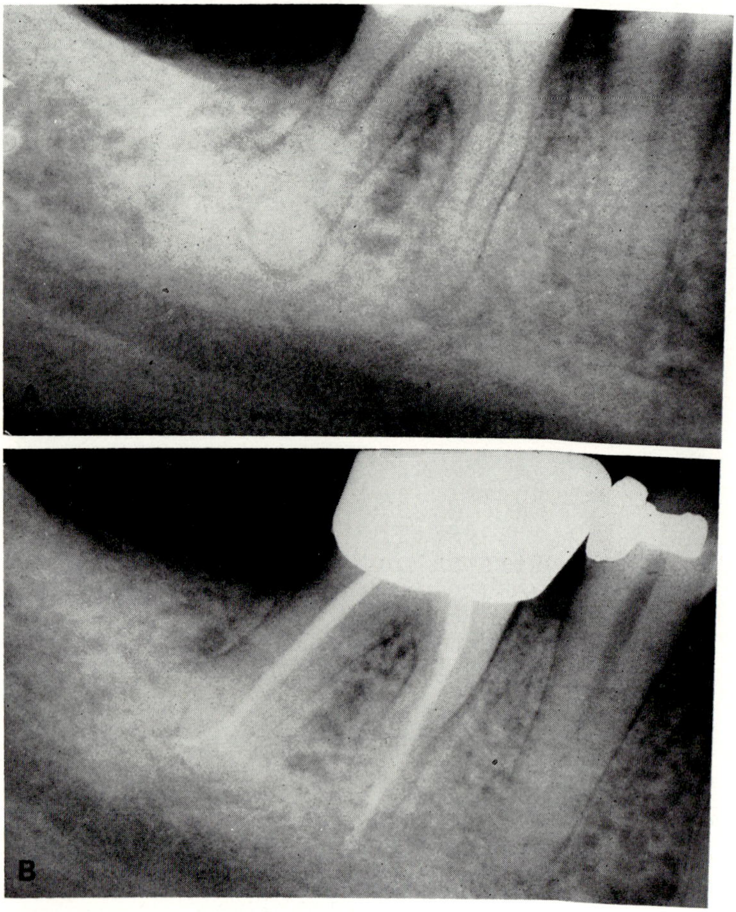

Figure 395. A case with hypercementosis; canals obturated with gutta-percha-chloropercha. A. Before. B. After; canal obturated as far as it went; lateral branch is evident.

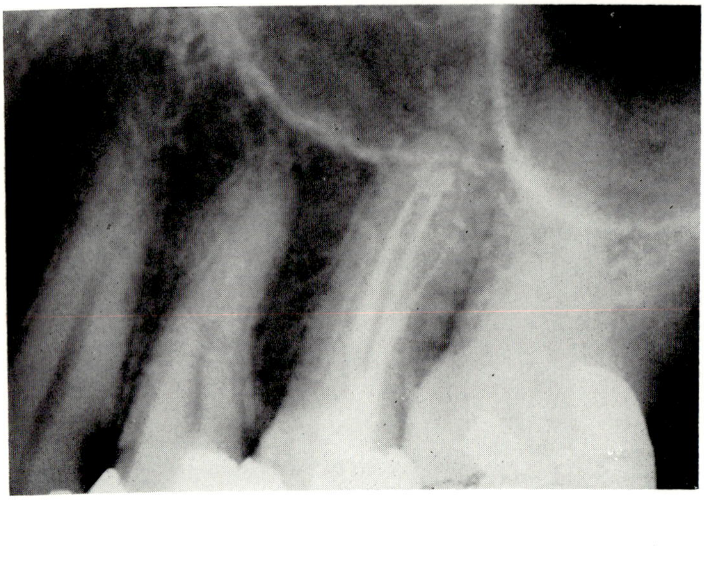

Figure 396. Upper second premolar with three canals obturated with gutta-percha-chloropercha.

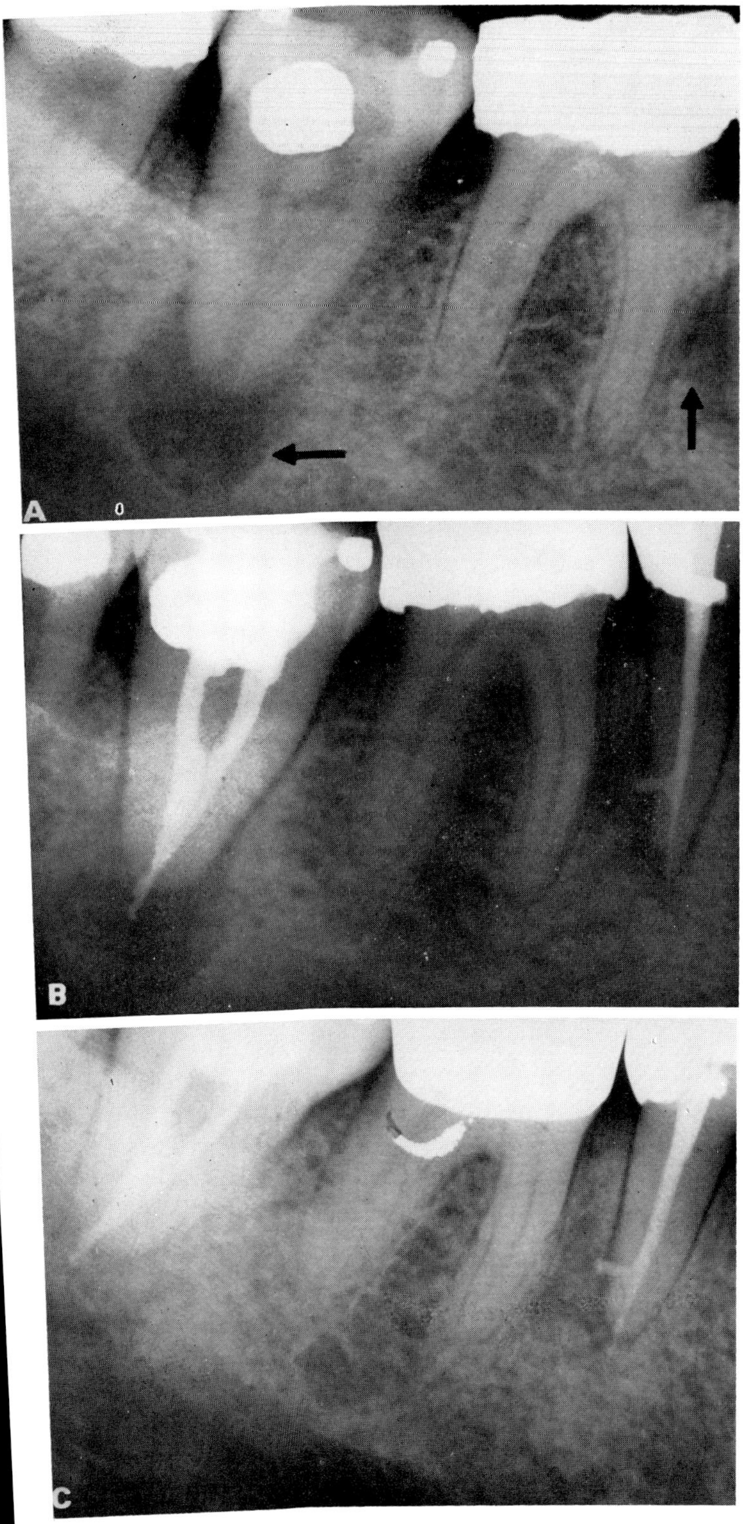

Figure 397. Periapical and lateral areas of pathosis; healing evident after obturation with gutta-percha-chloropercha. A. Periapical and lateral *areas* are evident (arrows). B. After obturation, some excess expressed beyond the apex and into the lateral *area*. C. Over one year later; repair is evident.

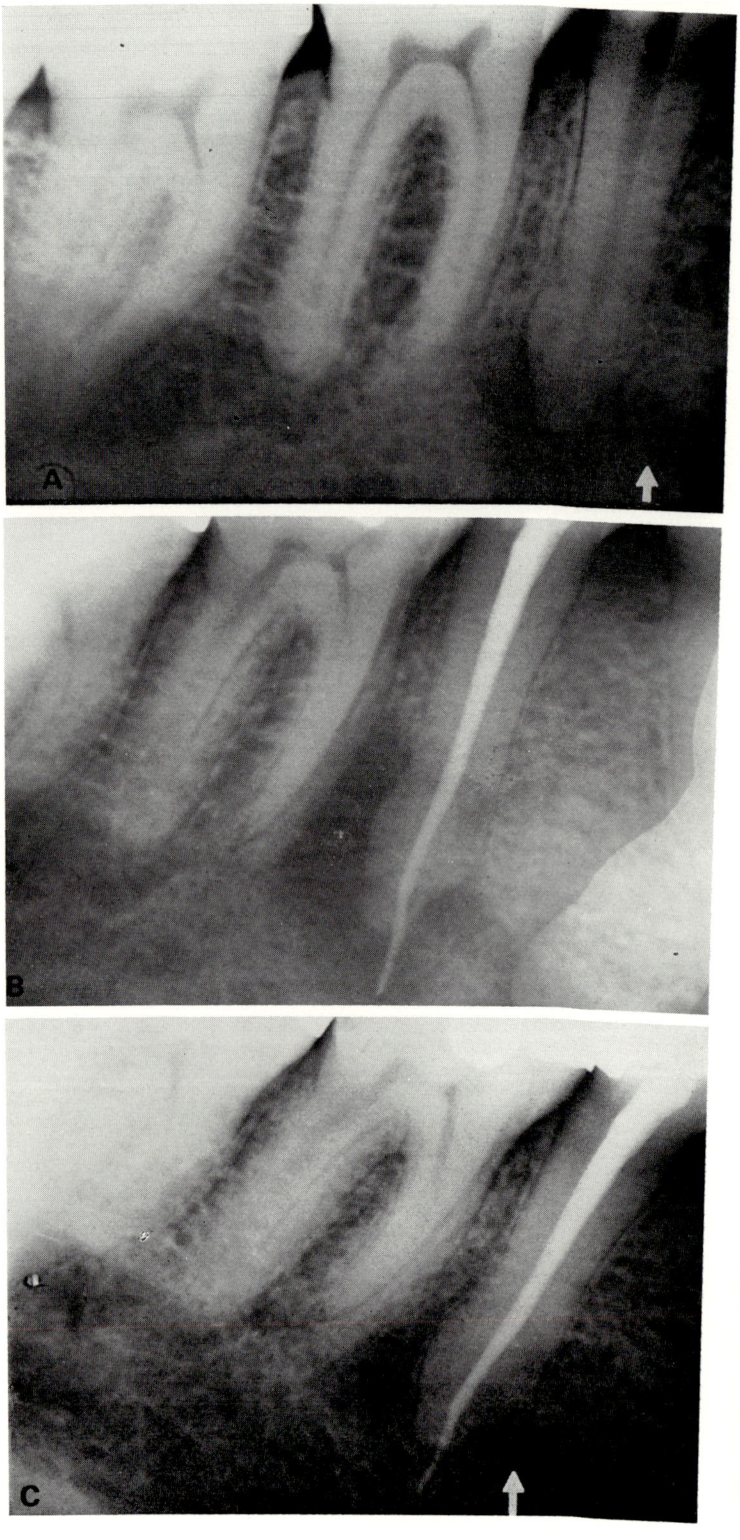

Figure 398. Unintentional overfilling of a lower premolar using gutta-percha-chloropercha technique. A. Before treatment; large periapical *area* is evident; note proximity of mental foramen (arrow). B. Obturation; excess into periapical *area*. C. Three years later; in spite of overfilling, periapical repair is evident; note mental foramen (arrow).

Pulpless Case

Included are descriptions of exact measurement, instrumentation and irrigation, intracanal medication, and obturation.

Exact Measurement

This is taken in the same manner as the vital case, except instrumentation goes beyond the determined measurement.

Instrumentation and Irrigation

Instrumentation is the same as described for vital cases, except that all instrumentation goes into the periapical area. As there may be necrotic tissue present in lateral and accessory canals, irrigation is done with sodium hypochlorite solution (5%), which is a good necrotic tissue solvent. Care must be exercised to insure that no solution is forcibly expressed beyond the apex, as pain and swelling may result. Also, it is important not to spill the solution on the patient's or doctor's clothes as bleaching and irritation can occur.

Intracanal Medication

If medicaments are used, application is as discussed for a vital case.

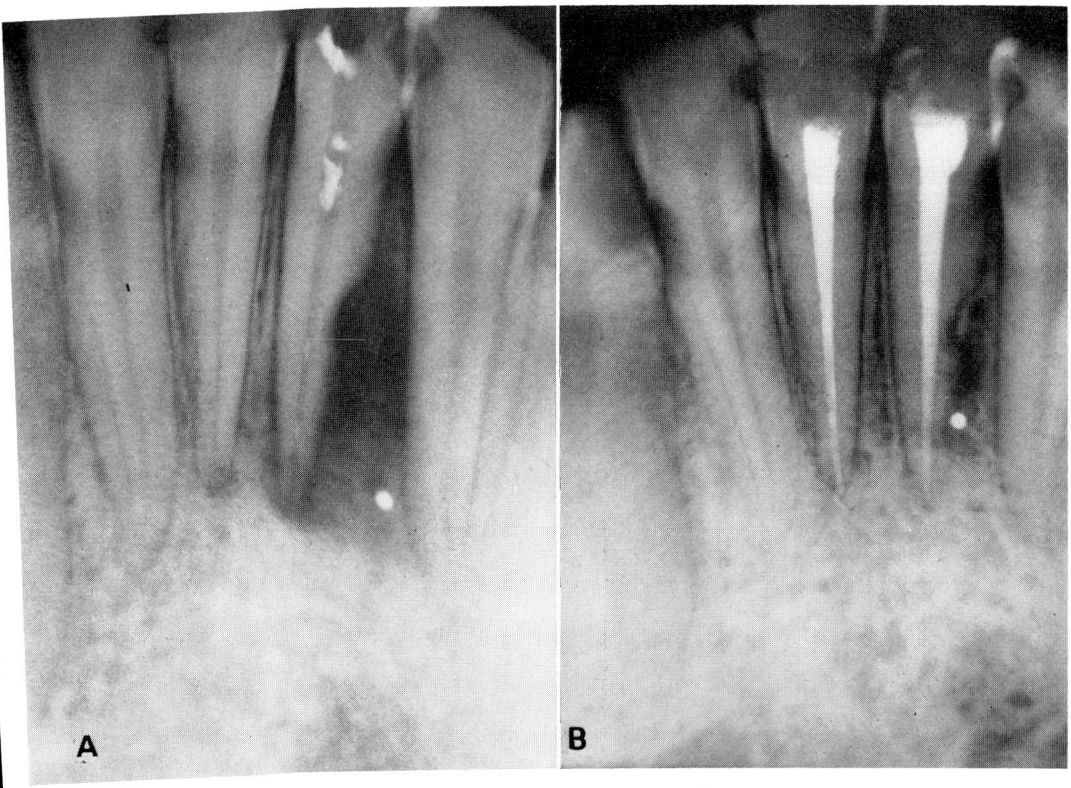

Figure 399. Case of external resorption of unknown origin being treated by non-surgical endodontic therapy. A. Both lower centrals are pulpless; external resorption and bone destruction can be seen on the right central incisor. B. Two years after obturation with gutta-percha-chloropercha, bony repair is evident; resorption apparently has stopped.

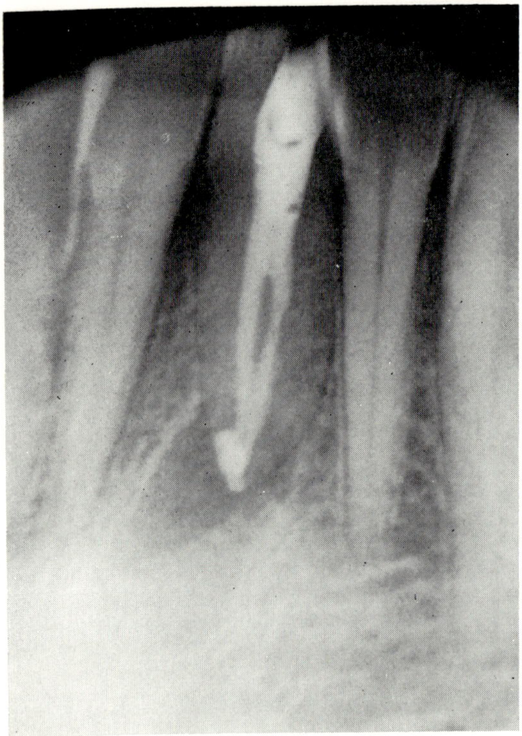

Figure 400. Lower central incisor with two canals and a periapical area of pathosis; obturated by gutta-percha-chloropercha technique.

Obturation

Once the canals are clean, smooth, tapered, and dry and the tooth is symptomless, then obturation can be done. This may be the first, second, third or fourth visit.

The technique is the same as for a vital case, except there is a better chance to fill lateral and accessory canals, especially, if the necrotic material has been dissolved out by the irrigating solution. Whether these branches have to be filled is debatable, but there is more logic in trying to fill them in cases with lateral canals and lateral *areas* present (Figs. 180, 397). Routine pulpless cases filled by nonsurgical endodontics are shown in Figures 71, 72, 80, 96A, 128, 179, 298-303, 310, 311, 398-400.

NONSURGICAL ENDODONTIC THERAPY FOR PRIMARY TEETH USING A ZINC OXIDE EUGENOL PASTE*

Access is gained as is the case with a permanent molar, except consideration must be taken for the smaller size of the primary tooth pulp chamber. The canals are instrumented with 18 mm files until clean shavings are removed. As primary roots are much shorter than permanent roots, care must be exercised to prevent over-instrumentation with possible damage to the underlying permanent successor. The canals are irrigated and dried with absorbent points. A creamy mix of zinc oxide and eugenol is made. It is then placed into a pressure syringe (Fig. 401). This material is then injected into each canal (Fig. 402). Any excess into the periapical tissues tends to be absorbed. A reinforced ZOE cement (e.g. IRM) restoration is placed in the access opening

* The preparation of this section was aided by Dr. Kurt Bomze of Haddonfield, N. J., a Diplimate of the American Board of Pedodontics.

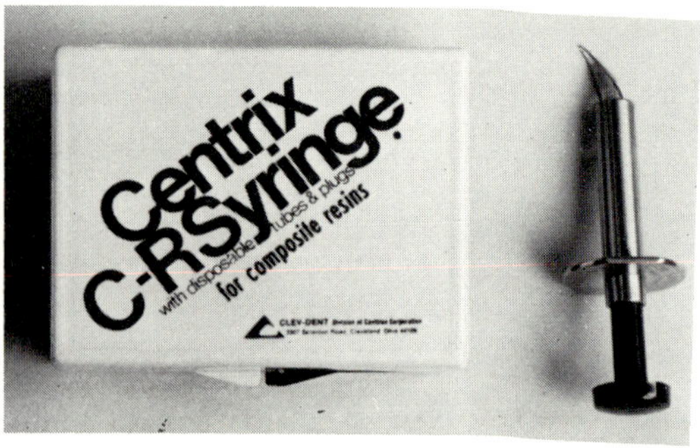

Figure 401. One type of pressure syringe (Centrix-C-R®-Clev-Dent.); another type is the Pulpdent Pressure syringe (Figs. 280, 402).

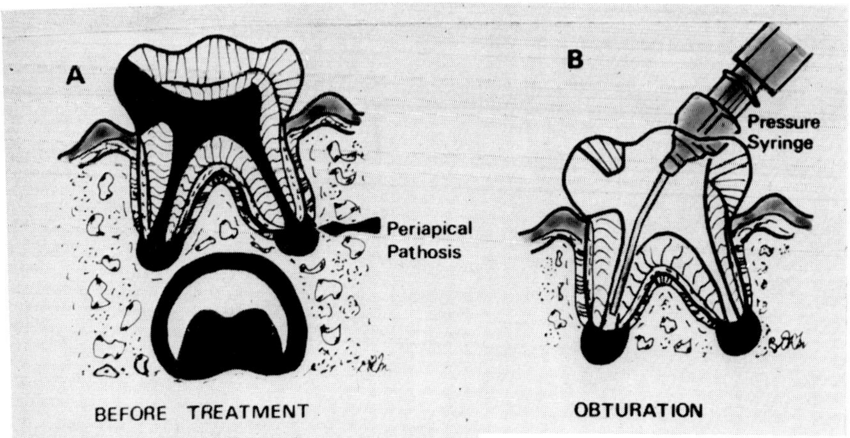

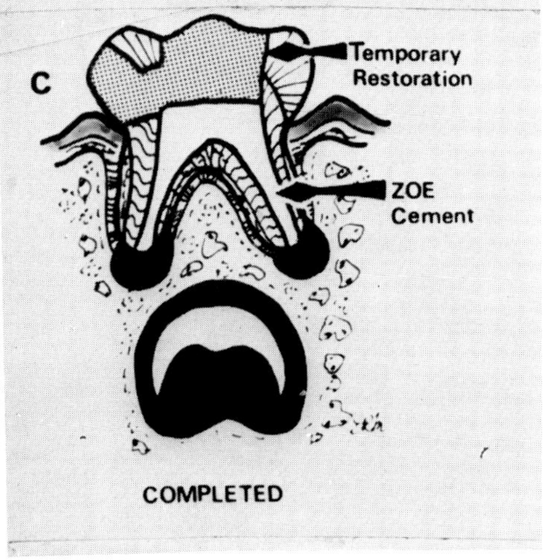

Figure 402 A-C. Three stages of non-surgical endodontic therapy for a primary tooth.

and a permanent restoration (preferably a stainless steel crown) can be placed as soon as the tooth is symptomless.

Some pedodontists advocate the use of a zinc oxide-eugenol paste with paraformaldehyde added (e.g. Oxpara®-Ransom and Randolph) for the following reasons:

(1) As a result of the antimicrobial action, the paste should take care of any residual infected tissue.

(2) The consistency of the paste allows for adequate working time and

(3) Clinical results have shown no deleterious effects to the permanent tooth from the added paraformaldehyde.

A possible alternative to the Oxpara is to mix in an equal proportion of formocresol to the eugenol in the zinc oxide-eugenol paste mixture (See note at end of Chapter 7).

BIBLIOGRAPHY

Krakow, A. A., and Berk, H.: Efficient endodontic procedures with the use of the pressure syringe. *Dent Clin North Am,* 9:387, 1965.

Langeland, K.: Pulp reactions to cavity preparation and to burns in the dentin. *Odont T, 68:*463, 1960.

Seltzer, S.: A scanning electron microscope examination of root canals following instrumentation and irrigation. In preparation.

Senia, E. S., Marshall, F. J., and Rosen, S.: The solvent action of sodium hypochlorite on pulp tissue of extracted teeth. *Oral Surg, 31:*96, 1971.

Spangeberg, L.: Cellular reactions to intracanal medicaments. Presented at the Fifth International Conference on Endodontics, September 1973, Philadelphia, Pennsylvania.

CHAPTER 10

PERIAPICAL SURGERY

In this chapter, the techniques of periapical curettage, apiocoectomy and retrograde seal are detailed. There are sections on preparation for surgery, flap designs, suturing technique, post-surgical instructions and treatments, management of complications, and treatment of posterior teeth.

If the patient has acute signs or symptoms these must first be controlled with either analgesics, antibiotics, incision and drainage, trephination, drainage through the root canal or some combination of these procedures (see appropriate chapter for these procedures).

PREPARATION FOR SURGERY

Very apprehensive patients should be premedicated (see Chapter 4). Two sterile towels should be placed over the apron covering the patient's chest. The patient's hair should be covered with a towel from the front to the back of the head. This will keep the hair well clear of the operator's hands, thus eliminating one source of contamination.

A two by two gauze sponge is folded twice and placed between the two arches. The patient is instructed to close on the gauze sponges, thus enabling both lips and cheeks to be retracted farther than if the mouth were open. The dentist should remove watches, rings or any other jewelry and the patient's glasses (if present). Although absolute sterility is not obtainable when working in the oral cavity, it is important for the operator to avoid introducing contamination. Therefore, the use of sterile rubber gloves is good practice.

When performing immediate surgical endodontics, it is not necessary to use chemical disinfectants, such as phenol, or ionization to disinfect the root canal prior to obturation and surgery. Any irritating products (microbial or tissue) are removed during the periapical surgery, and complete instrumentation should insure that the vast majority of the microbes are removed. There are two methods of performing immediate surgical endodontics: one is to do the instrumentation and obturation first; the second is to do the periapical surgery first. There are advantages and disadvantages to each method. If the canal treatment is performed first, there is less hemorrhage and exudation into the canal. There is also a visible marker (the excess filling material) for the root

---

The preparation of this chapter was aided by Dr. Marvin Gross, Clinical Associate Professor and Director, Graduate Clinic, Department of Endodontology, Temple University School of Dentistry, Philadelphia, Pa.

apex localization, when the periapical surgery is being performed. The disadvantage is that irritants are being pushed into the periapical tissues and there could conceivably be dissemination of infectious material. The advantages of the surgery first technique are visualization of the entire instrumentation and obturation procedure and prevention of dissemination of debris. The disadvantage is that it is difficult to prevent seepage from going into the root canal. This makes drying of the root canal more difficult and time consuming. Another disadvantage is that the surgical flap has to be retracted for a longer period of time, thereby increasing the possibility for post-operative swelling. Most often cases are managed by the canal treatment first method.

Nitrous oxide analgesia is a good adjunct to use during surgery. It helps keep the patient's mind off the procedure. Profound anesthesia is an important factor in the endodontic surgical technique. Infiltration injections for maxillary teeth are usually effective. This type injection also produces local vasoconstriction, thus reducing hemorrhage during surgery. Care should be taken to obtain complete anesthesia both labially (buccally) and palatally (lingually). For treatment of anterior teeth, a supplementary nasopalatine injection is necessary if anesthesia is not complete, and occasionally an infraor-

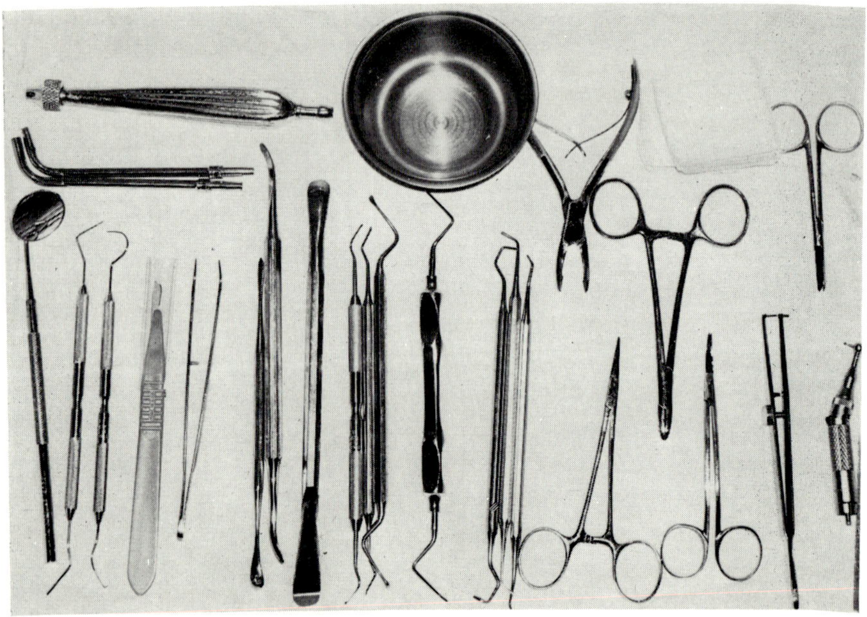

Figure 403. Armamentarium for periapical surgery; left to right. First row—surgical aspirating tips and holder, pan with sterile saline, Rongeur bone forceps, sterile gauze, suture scissors. Second row—mirror, explorers, sterile disposable scalpel (Bard-Parker No. 15), cotton pliers, retractors, curettes, pluggers, hemostats, scissors, retrograde amalgam carrier, miniature contra-angle.

bital injection is necessary. For posterior teeth, a posterior-superior alveolar injection may be necessary. Subperiosteal injections may also be needed (see Chapter 5). For periapical surgery in the mandible, an inferior alveolar injection is given, along with a long buccal injection. Supplemental subperiosteal injections are administered in the same way as in the maxilla. When the operative field is close to the midline, local infiltration into the labial and lingual (palatal) region on both sides of the midline is necessary to allow for possible cross innervation.

ARMAMENTARIUM

The basic instruments and supplies necessary for periapical surgery are shown in Figure 403.

FLAP DESIGNS—PRINCIPLES

The requirements for flap design in endodontic surgery are the same as in oral surgery or periodontal surgery. Errors in flap design caused by inadequate pre-operative preparation can be prevented. The following is a list of basic principles that should be followed when designing a flap for periapical surgery.

(1) If periodontal disease is present, it is important to have a periodontal consultation. This is for correct design of the flap for both periapical and periodontal consideration, and also for the possibility of combined endodontic-periodontic treatment at the same visit. If during periapical surgery, a periodontal defect is discovered, it should be treated. All endodontic practitioners should have a background in the diagnosis and treatment of periodontal diseases.

(2) The base of the flap should be the widest point of the design. This is to allow for sufficient circulation to the raised portion of the flap. Before any incision is made with a scalpel, the entire flap design should be outlined either by using a sterilized indelible pencil or the point of an explorer to penetrate the mucosa.

(3) The full extent of the pathosis should be included in the flap design. If a large periapical area of rarefaction is present, or if a considerable amount of bone must be removed in order to gain access to the lesion, the vertical (or oblique) incision should be placed two teeth over from the involved tooth.

(4) Incision should not be made over bony defects. This is true for any bony defect that existed preoperatively or which might occur during the surgical procedure. Therefore, if in doubt, the flap should be extended proximally.

(5) Sharp corners should be avoided in the prepared flap. When a sharp cornered flap is made, there is a tendency for the corners to become ischemic. Ischemia may result in sloughing of the edges with retarded healing, and possible scar formation.

(6) In the presence of a possible fenestration or dehiscence, a split

thickness flap should be used. A fenestration is a localized area over the root in which the facial bone has been lost. A dehiscence is a cleft in the bone over the root in which the bone is lost up to the level of the alveolar crest. These defects occur most often with canine roots, and buccal roots of upper molars and first premolars. It is difficult to diagnose these conditions, as periapical radiographs do not show facial bone levels. A possible diagnostic method is the following. After giving a local anesthetic (infiltration), using a needle or fine probe (Michigan 00 Explorer®), the bone can be probed. If a defect is present, it can usually be felt. If a full-thickness flap is raised in such an area, with the elevation of the periosteum and mucosa, there is a very strong possibility that the tissue will not reattach properly after surgery. What occurs is a clefting of the marginal gingiva or the formation of a periodontal pocket. If a fenestration in the gingival portion of the root or a dehiscence is suspected, a split thickness flap should be used at the gingival half of the flap. The periosteum is left attached to the root in that region by carefully separating the flap with a sharp scalpel. A full thickness flap is used to expose the bone over the apex of the tooth being treated (Fig. 404G, H). An alternative flap is a semilunar type near the apex (Fig. 404A). However, the latter type has certain disadvantages which will be discussed later. It has been reported in a recent paper that these defects may be the cause of recalcitrant post-endodontic pain. The pain was relieved following apicoectomies.

(7) Once the flap is elevated, it should be kept away from the surgical site. The retractor is placed under the tissue and allowed to rest on bone, in order to hold the tissue firmly. Care should be taken so that the retraction does not injure the soft tissue. Failure to follow this basic principle will result in interference of the blood supply to the tissues with resultant ischemia and delayed healing.

FLAP DESIGNS—TECHNIQUES

There are numerous types of flaps that can be utilized in endodontic surgery. The flaps considered here are semilunar, modified semilunar, triangular, trapezoidal, full flap, and split thickness.

Semilunar Flap

This is the oldest and probably the most commonly used flap in endodontic surgery. The curved incision is made completely through the gingival tissue (usually alveolar mucosa) and periosteum. The convexity of the curve is down in the maxilla and up in the mandible. The proximal extension of the flap should include at least one tooth on either side of the involved tooth (Fig.

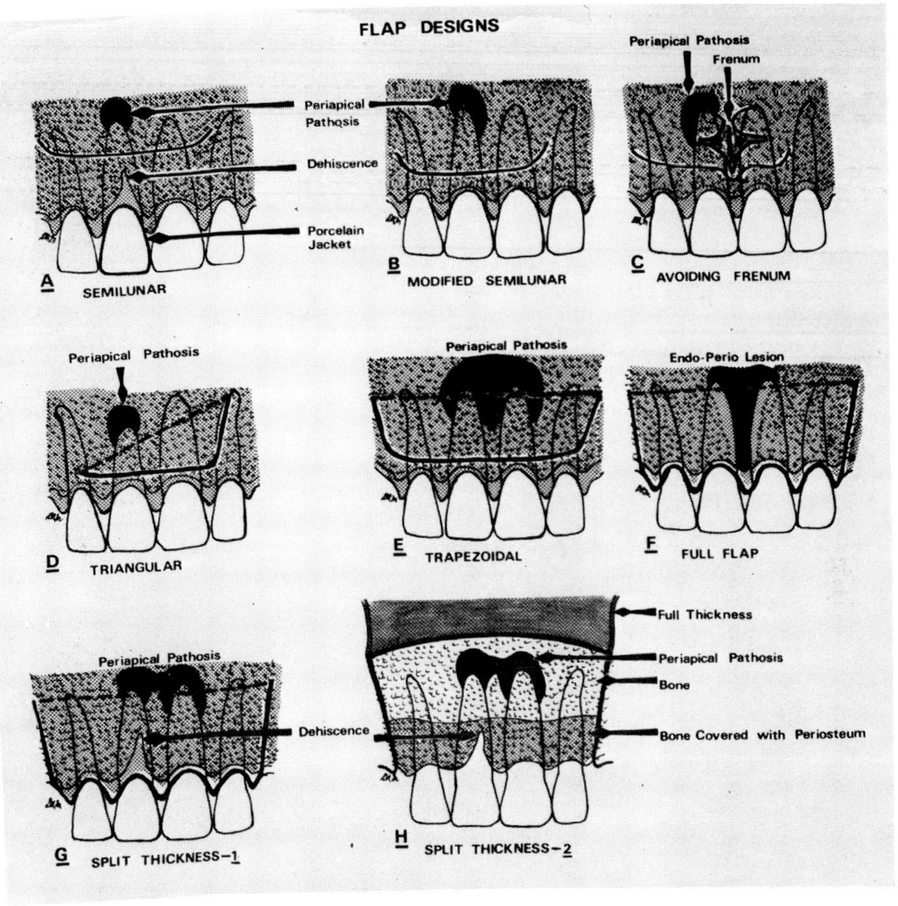

Figure 404

404A). When the labial frenum is involved, the incision should follow the outline of the frenum and not extend across the middle of the attachment (Fig. 404C). One of the advantages of this flap is that it allows for broad tissue retraction and easy accessibility to the periapical area. It also is easy to do, requiring only one incision. It is advantageous in cases of porcelain jackets, in which it is desirous to maintain the shape and contour of the gingival margins. The incision should not be used where one suspects the buccal or labial cortical plate to be missing. The use of the curved flap in these situations will result in the possible formation of a fenestration or dehiscence. The semilunar near the apex can be used for suspected fenestration cases, but semilunar flaps have a greater tendency toward separation and scar formation. A modification of the semilunar flap is to make the horizontal portion of the flap in the attached gingiva (a minimum of 2 mm from the depth of the gingival sulcus).

The horizontal extent of the flap can be continued as far as necessary for accessibility (Fig. 404B). This flap is easily done, does not interfere with the marginal gingiva, and has a lesser chance for separation than the normal semi-lunar because it is less movable during mouth movements. Another modification of the semilunar is to make the incision V shaped, rather than U shaped. The former type is easier to reposition and suture.

Triangular Flap

The principal indication for this flap is for teeth with short roots. The horizontal incision is made along the attached gingiva with one vertical (or oblique) incision made on one tooth over from the involved tooth (Fig. 404D). This flap should not be used when performing surgery on teeth with long roots. The use of the flap in those cases would necessitate a long relaxing incision that would extend far into the alveolar mucosa and would result in excessive traumatic stretching of the tissue.

Vertical or Oblique Flaps

The horizontal incision includes the separation of the marginal gingiva in cases of endodontic-periodontic involvement, or where a root is to be removed (Fig. 404F). In other cases, the horizontal incision is in the attached gingiva (Fig. 404E). When the marginal gingiva are separated, the relaxing incisions are made on the distal aspect of the interdental papilla one tooth away from the involved site (with large areas of destruction two teeth away) (Fig. 404F). In posterior surgery, it is ex-

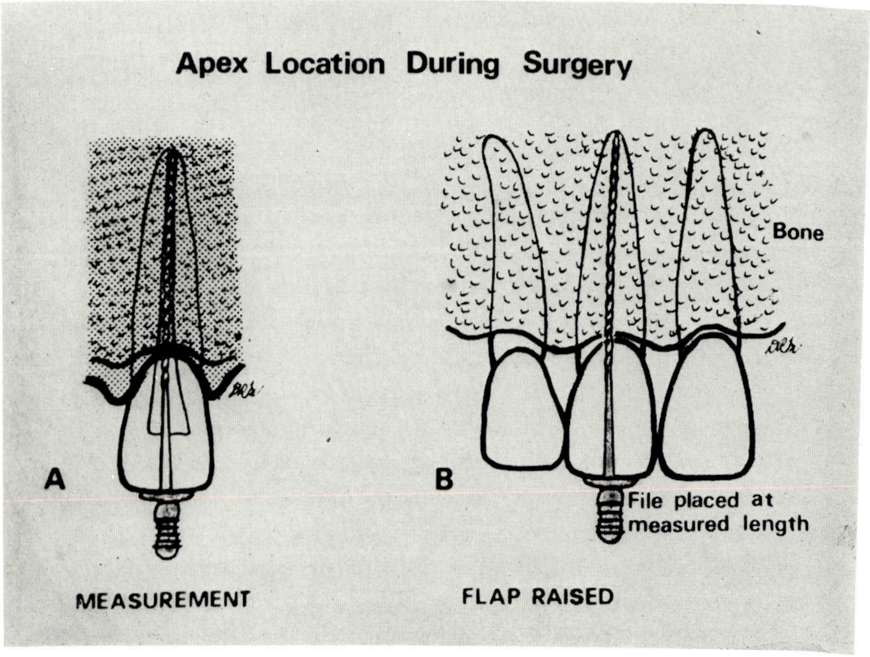

Figure 405

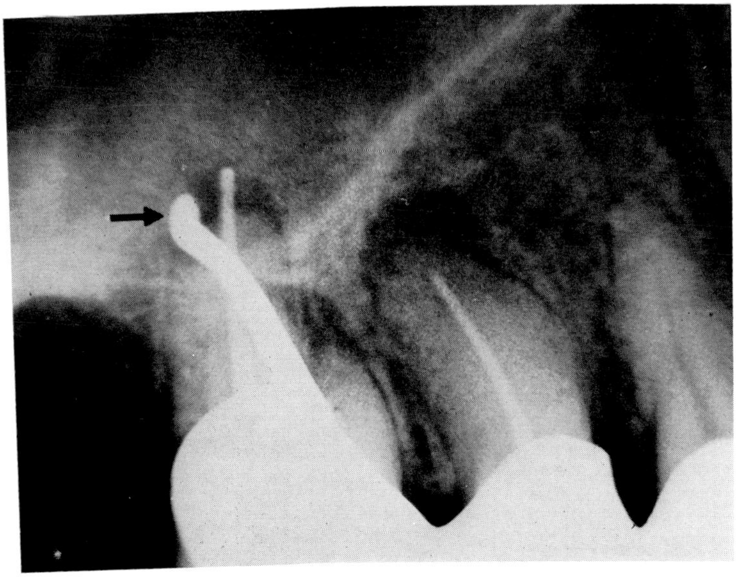

Figure 406. Apex location during surgery by use of an explorer (arrow) followed by a periapical radiograph.

tremely difficult to have two relaxing incisions. A single relaxing incision is made toward the mesial and has to be continued deep into the alveolar mucosa in order for adequate visibility to be maintained.

PERIAPICAL CURETTAGE

Once the flap is retracted, the alveolar bone overlying the root is visible. Often the bone is destroyed on the facial aspect, and there is no problem in gaining access to the root apex. If there is any doubt about location of the root apex, there are two methods to help in the localization. One is to place a file with a stop indicating the predetermined tooth length, along the alveolar bone from the incisal edge of the involved tooth (Fig. 405). A second method is to place an explorer, or heated gutta-percha square in the alveolar bone in the approximated region of the apex. A periapical radiograph is then taken to see how close the marker is to the apex (Fig. 406). With the use of a 701 surgical length bur in an ultra-high speed contra-angle and sterile saline irrigation, the bone overlying the apex is removed. Enough bone should be removed in order to have good visibility, but it is important that the adjoining roots should not be impinged upon. Also, the facial bone should not be removed toward the incisal (occlusal) to such an extent that there would be no alveolar bone remaining over the entire root. There is some clinical evidence to show that rather than removing the bone, healing is facilitated if the bone is kept attached to the undersurface of the flap. The bone is then replaced with the flap at the conclusion of the surgical procedure. The bone acts as a nidus for new bone formation, and it maintains the alveolar contour giving support to the flap. Once the granulomatous tissue is visible, it should be dissected from the bony compartment with

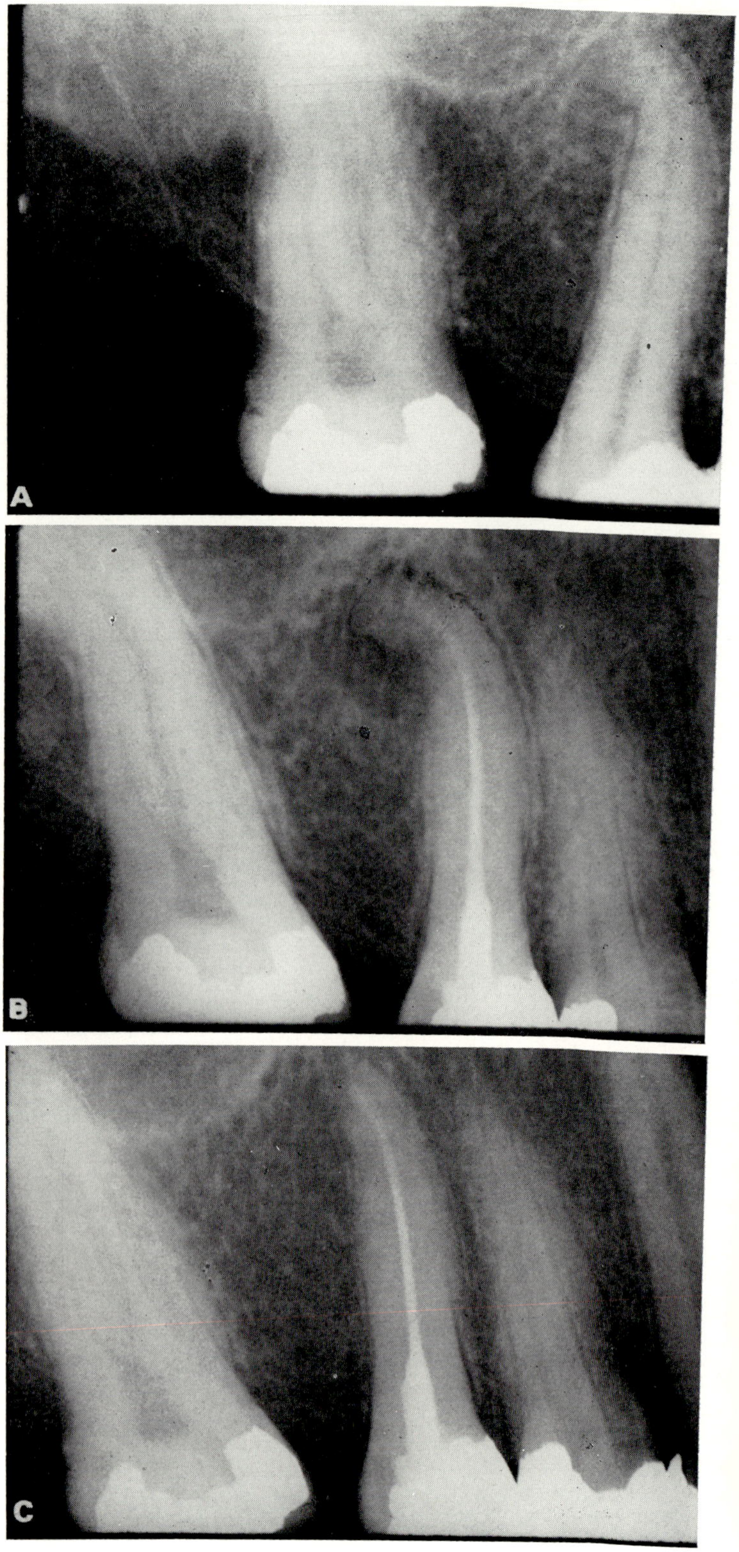

Figure 407. Apicoectomy on an upper premolar with a dilacerated root. A. Root apex of premolar that is apparently calcified. B. One year following obturation with gutta-percha-chloropercha, periapical area of pathosis developed, and an apicoectomy was done. C. Two years following apicoectomy, complete repair is evident.

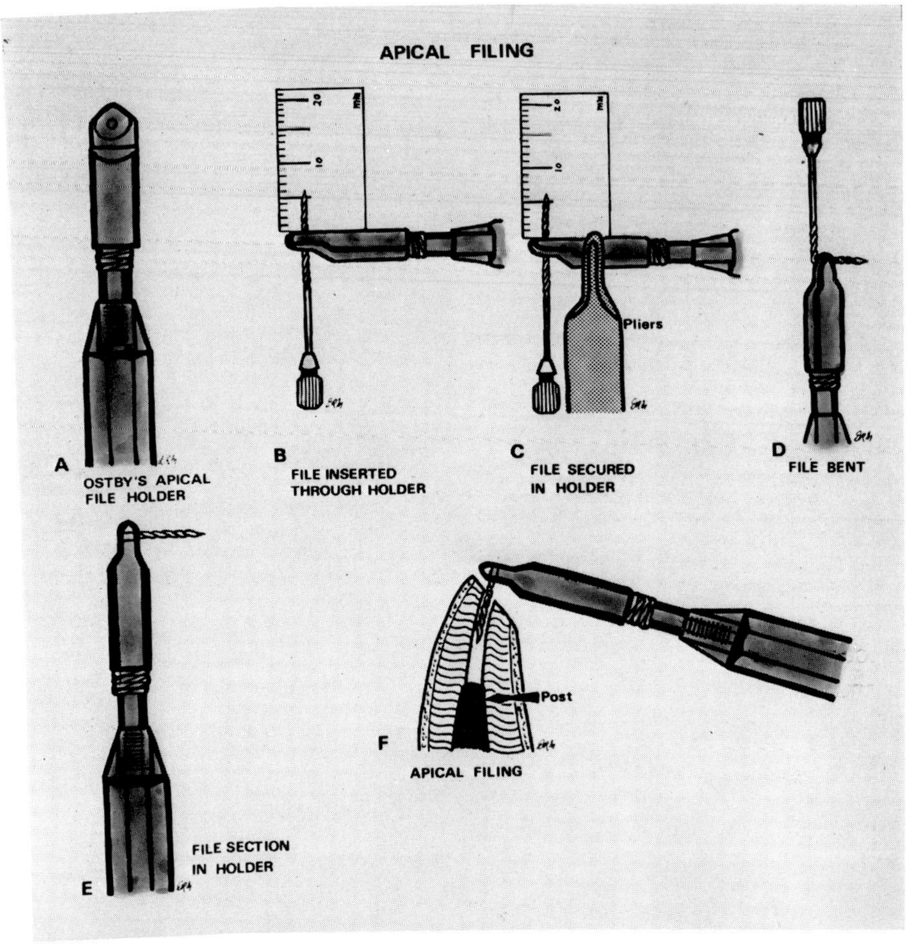

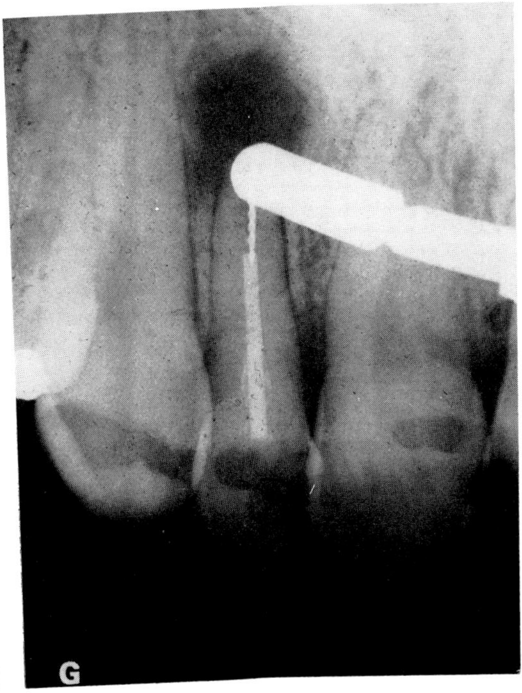

Figure 408. Apical filing; A-F—Various stages in the filing procedure. G—Radiograph of a clinical case in which apical filing is being done. (From W. Soltanoff, "Apical Sealing Procedures," *Journal of the New Jersey Dental Association*, 44:36, 1973.)

the use of double ended curettes. This tissue is usually very adherent and it is necessary that the curettes are kept sharp, in order to aid in the removal. The back of the curette is placed between the bony wall and the tissue and pressure is applied to break the attachment (Fig. 304). Once the tissue is removed (in one piece or in sections), it is placed into a bottle of 10% formalin, which is then sent to a pathology laboratory for tissue analysis. As much of the granulomatous material as possible should be removed, but it is not essential that every piece be withdrawn.

Once the apex is exposed, the root tip is freshened with the bur. The gutta-percha is smoothed against the root. Use of a hot instrument might cause shrinkage, and is therefore not recommended. The flap is then repositioned and sutured (see section on suturing). Typical cases are shown in Figures 73 and 303.

APICOECTOMY

In the indicated cases (see endodontic-periodontic section, Chapter 3) the root tip is removed with a 701 bur (Fig. 305). In fractured root tip cases, the root is cut at the point of fracture. In cases where the apex is to be removed because of accessibility for tissue removal, only as much of the root should be removed as is necessary to allow for the use of the curette. The root apex should not be cut to the base of the lesion, as this would unnecessarily sacrifice tooth support for visibility. The exposed gutta-percha is treated as discussed under periapical curettage. Figure 407 shows a representative case.

RETROGRADE SEAL

In this procedure, the root tip is cut at an oblique angle while maintaining the palatal (lingual) length of the root (Fig. 306A). With the use of a 33½ inverted cone bur in an ultra-high speed contra-angle, a small Class I preparation is made at the apical foramen (Fig. 306B). If adequate access is possible, actual instrumentation of the apex can be performed with an Ostby® apical file holder (Fig. 408). In working in the posterior part of the mouth or in areas where the contra-angle cannot be placed, a miniature contra-angle can be used (Fig. 409). A dry field is maintained with a piece of gauze, or cotton placed into the defect surrounding the root (Fig. 306C). With a large root, a small piece of rubber dam with a small opening can be slipped over the apex. Using a retrograde carrier (Union Broach®), a piece of amalgam is placed into the opening (Fig. 306C). It is then condensed with a small plugger. Excess is removed (verified by a periapical ra-

Figure 409. Miniature contra angle.

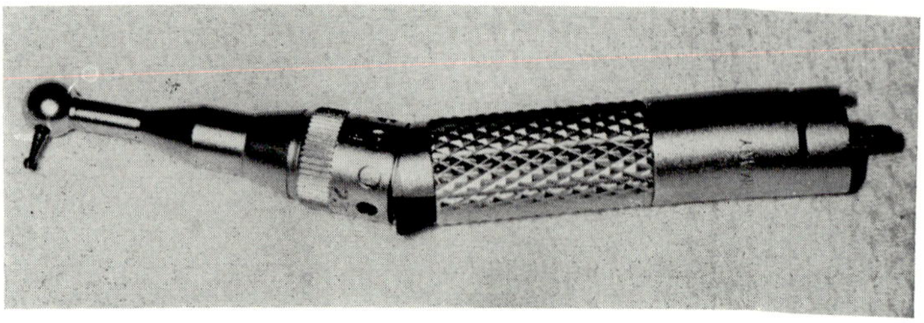

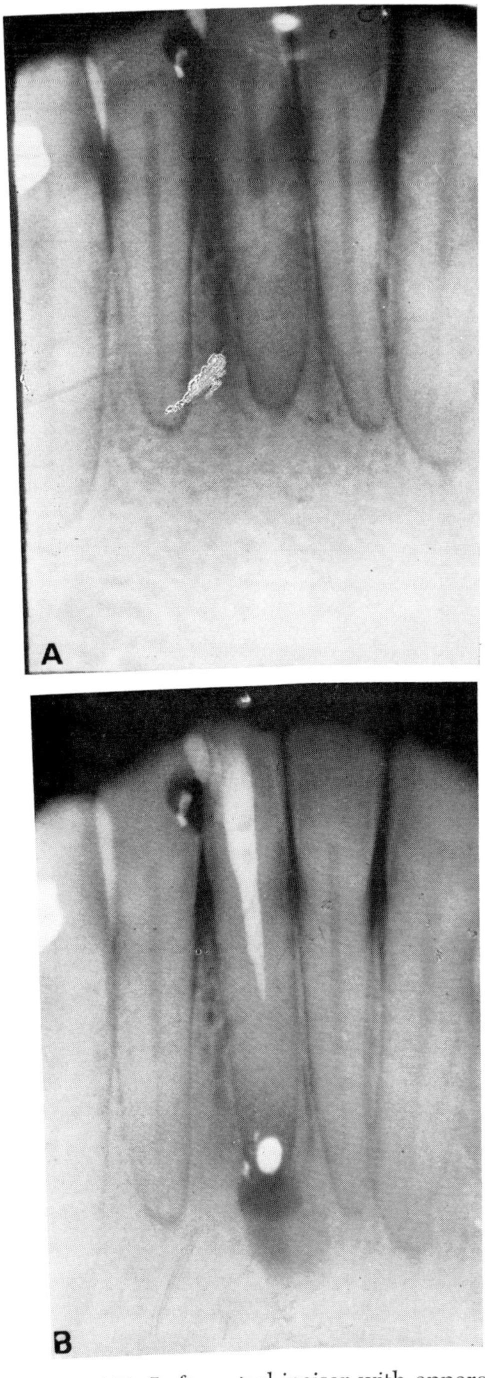

A

B

Figure 410. Left central incisor with apparently calcified apical half of the root canal; treated by obturation with gutta-percha as far as the canal went; followed by a retrograde amalgam seal. A. Before. B. After. (From D. R. Morse, "The Management of Endodontic Problem Cases," *JDA South Africa,* 27:387, 1972.)

diograph), and the amalgam root interface is smoothed with moist cotton (Fig. 306D). Typical cases are shown in Figures 307, 326, 328-330, 332, 337-339, and 410. Recently, new techniques have been introduced. One technique is to use gold foil. It is placed in with a gold foil carrier and condensed with a plugger. Typical cases are shown in Figures 308, 340, and 411. A recent technique is a retrograde seal with polycarboxylate cement. It is usually mixed in a one to one ratio of liquid to powder. The cement is inserted with a special pressure syringe (Fig. 401). The results so far appear promising (Fig. 309).

UPPER POSTERIOR TEETH

There are certain considerations in the management of upper posterior teeth.

(1) In upper two rooted premolars, the palatal root is usually deep within the palatal bone. It is often necessary to obliquely cut the buccal root apex in order to be able to gain access to the palatal root (Fig. 412). To get at the palatal root, a great amount of facial bone must be removed.

(2) Doing periapical surgery on the buccal roots of upper molars is rarely more difficult than upper anterior periapical surgery. Often there is little or no facial bone covering the root apexes and this simplifies visualization

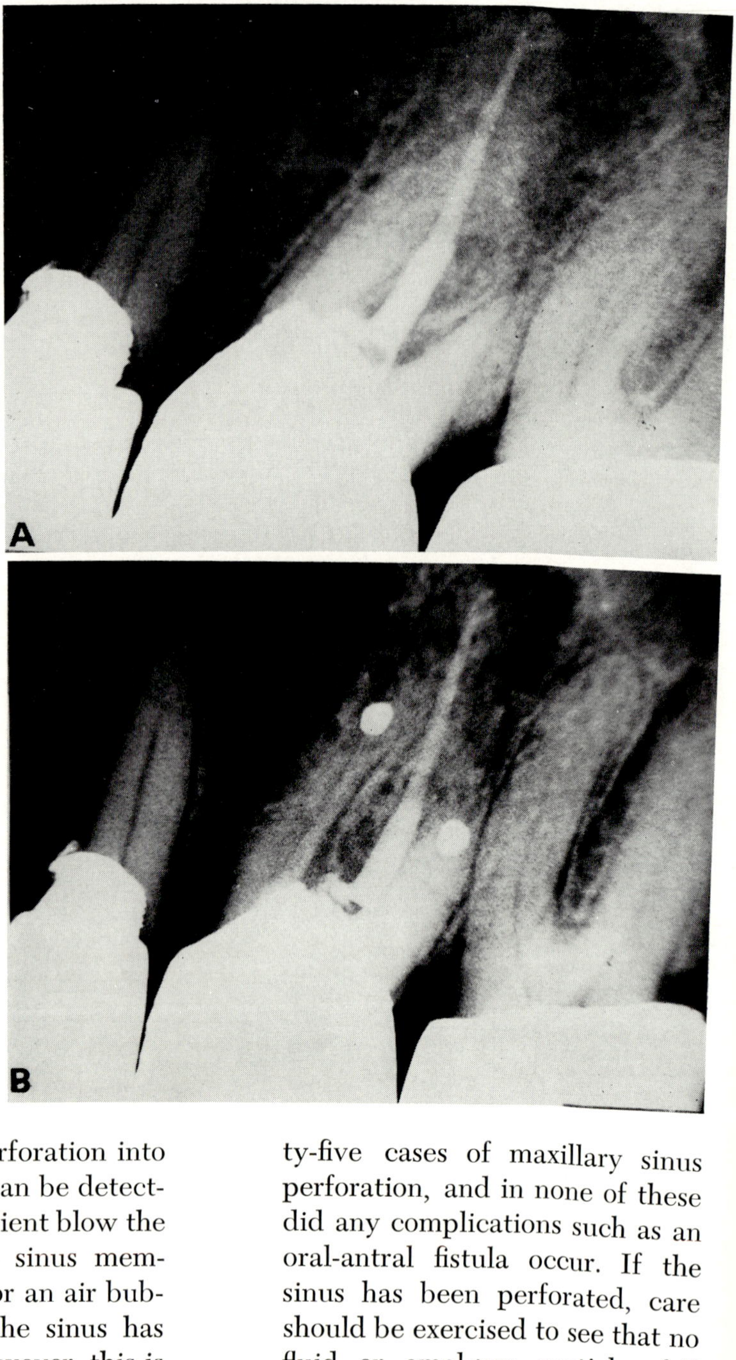

Figure 411. An upper molar with clinically calcified buccal canals sealed with retrograde gold foils. A. Before; palatal root had been obturated with gutta-percha. B. After; buccal canal apexes sealed with gold foil. (From W. K. Kopp and H. Kresberg, "Apioectomy with Retrograde Gold Foil: A New Technique," *New York State Dental Journal*, 39:8, 1973.)

(Figs. 411, 413). Perforation into the maxillary sinus can be detected by having the patient blow the nose gently. If the sinus membrane vibrates and/or an air bubble appears, then the sinus has been perforated. However, this is usually no problem. The author has treated approximately seventy-five cases of maxillary sinus perforation, and in none of these did any complications such as an oral-antral fistula occur. If the sinus has been perforated, care should be exercised to see that no fluid or amalgam particles fall into the opening. The flap should be sutured tightly, a periodontal

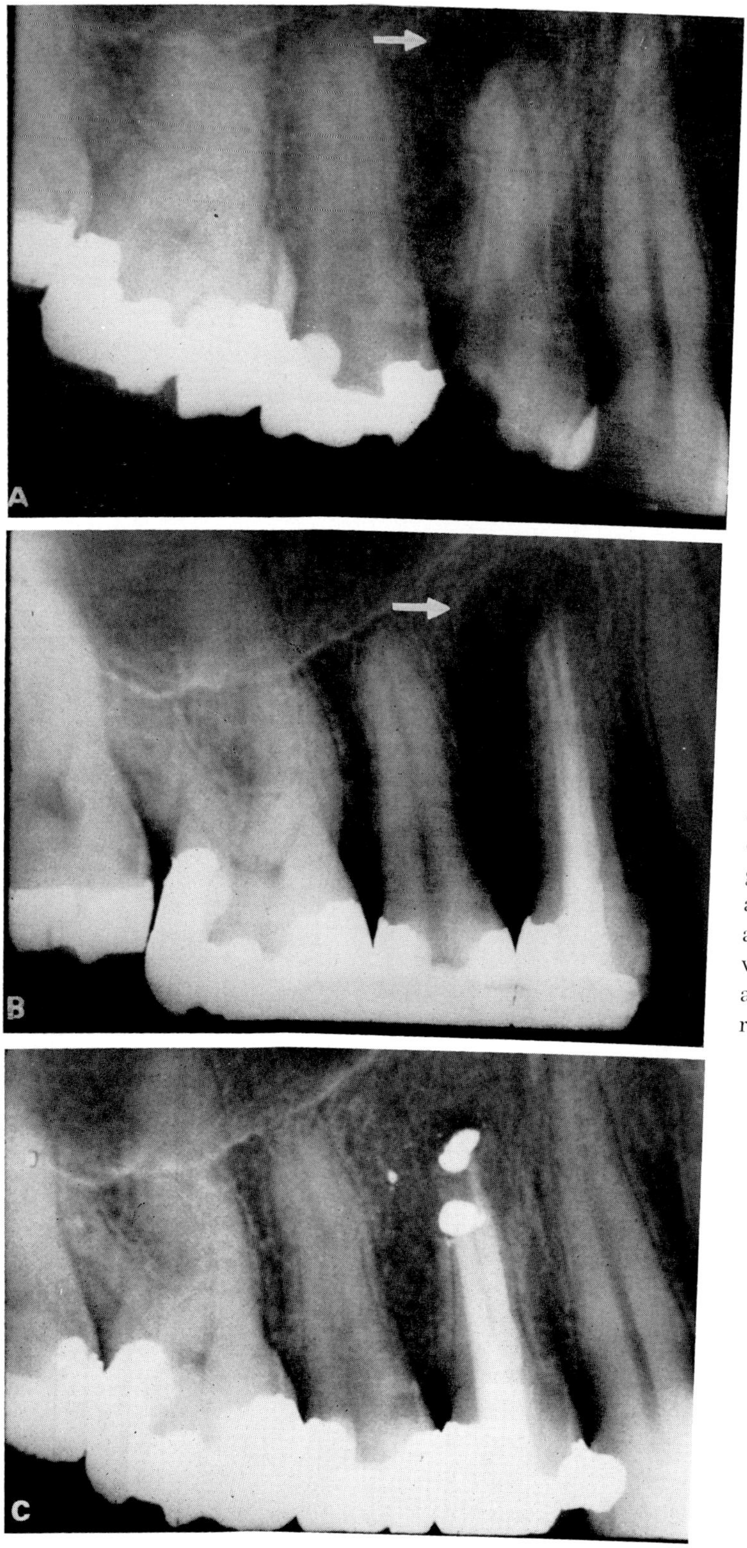

Figure 412. Surgical retreatment of a two-rooted upper premolar. A. Periapical area present on the upper first premolar. B. One year following an apparently good obturation with gutta-percha-chloropercha, the periapical *area* became larger; the buccal root was cut obliquely to gain access to the palatal root and a periapical curettage and retrograde amalgams were placed. C. Two years after the surgery, periapical repair is evident.

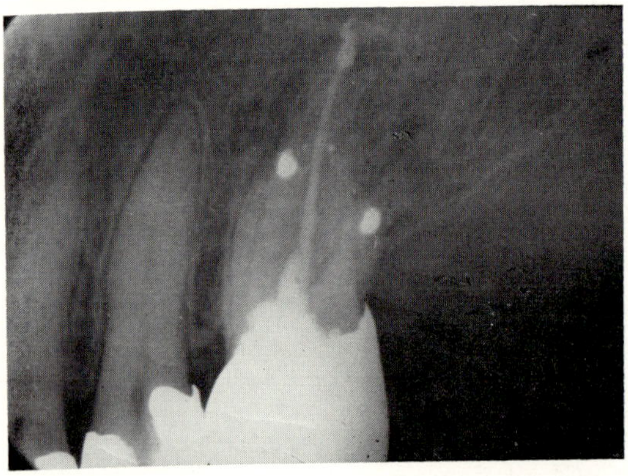

Figure 413. Retrograde amalgam seals of buccal root apexes of an upper molar with clinically calified buccal root canals; palatal root canal was obturated with gutta-percha-chloropercha. (From D .R. Morse, "The Significance of Endodontics in Plantation Procedures," *JDA South Africa,* 26:263, 1971.)

pack placed, and the patient given the following instructions:

(a) Do not blow your nose; wipe it gently.

(b) Try not to sneeze (the latter two instructions are given in order to try and prevent displacement of the sutures with a possible development of an oral-antral fistula).

(c) Take Neo-Synephrine nose drops or spray (this tends to keep the ostium open, as the vasoconstrictor shrinks the nasal membranes).

(d) Bleeding may occur through the nose, into the throat, or through the incision (the vasoconstrictor also helps control the bleeding).

(e) Take penicillin for seven days or erythromycin if an allergy exists to penicillin (if the patient has a history of sinisitis). In routine cases, antibiotics are not necessary.

(3) Performing periapical surgery on upper molar palatal roots can be difficult. The flap must be carefully prepared. The incision is made around the gingival margins to a distance of two teeth to the mesial and distal of the tooth in question. The vertical incision is placed between the canine and first premolar, in order to avoid the large palatine vessels. Because of the thickness of the flap, to improve accessibility, the flap is retracted and sutured over to the opposite side (Fig. 414).

Once the procedure is completed, the suture is cut and the flap is repositioned and sutured normally. A typical case is shown in Figure 415.

LOWER POSTERIOR TEETH

There are precautions and special considerations in treating these teeth. Before treatment is begun, the patient should be advised about the possibility

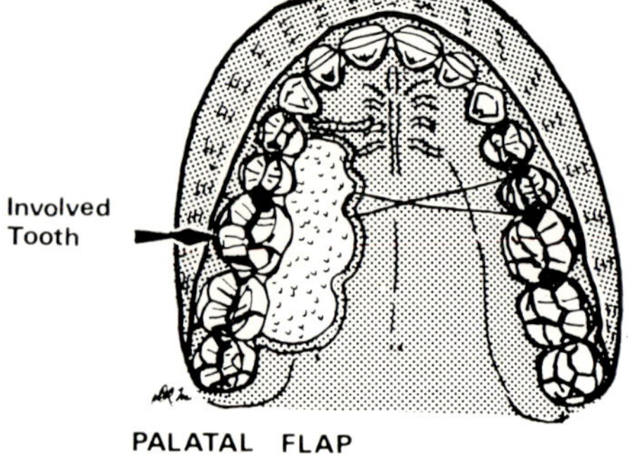

Figure 414

of paresthesia. Paresthesia is usually transient, but it may last for months or even more than a year. In performing surgery in lower premolars or molars these steps should be followed:

(1) The buccal cortex is usually thick in lower posterior teeth and a great amount of bone must be removed to get to the vicinity of the roots.
(2) Localization is helped with the use of an instrument and a periapical radiograph (Fig. 416C).
(3) The apex is cut from above at a severe oblique angle. The tip is then removed with an elevator or Stieglitz® forceps. This is done in order to avoid impingement on the inferior alveolar canal or mental foramen. A typical case is shown in Figure 416.

SUTURING AND PACKS

Suturing is performed with a No. 000 suture and a No. X-1 needle (Ethicon®-J & J) or a comparable type set-up. The needle is placed from the movable flap to the attached tissue. The technique of interrupted suturing is shown in Figure 417. A folded two by two gauze is placed over the sutures to control the hemorrhage. When there is exposed cementum or a gingivoplasty has been performed, a periodontal pack is placed to protect the exposed surfaces. A thick mix of the zinc oxide-eugenol resin pack (Ward Wonder Pack®) is tacked into the area. Orahesive bandage (Squibb®) is another method of protection that can be used. Cyanoacrylates have been used experimentally and appear to be very successful in controlling hemorrhage and protecting the area. They should be available shortly for clinical use.

POST-SURGICAL INSTRUCTIONS

The following written instructions are given to the patient.

(1) Don't lift up your lip or have excessive mouth movements.
(2) Don't touch the sutures.
(3) For the remainder of the day of the procedure, put an ice pack over the involved area for twenty minutes on, ten minutes off.
(4) Starting tomorrow, rinse the area with a warm salt solution several times a day for at least one week.
(5) Take analgesics for pain according to instructions (if necessary).
(6) Take antibiotics for infection (if prescribed).
(7) Drink plenty of fluids.
(8) Eat a soft diet and take nutritional supplements (if prescribed).
(9) If bleeding occurs, place a piece of sterile gauze that you received, over the sutured area.
(10) If you have severe pain, swelling, bleeding, or other problems, call the office.
(11) Return in four to five days (as per your appointment) to have the sutures removed.

POST-SURGICAL TREATMENTS

The only routine post-surgical treatment is to remove sutures in four to five days. Although this is a relatively

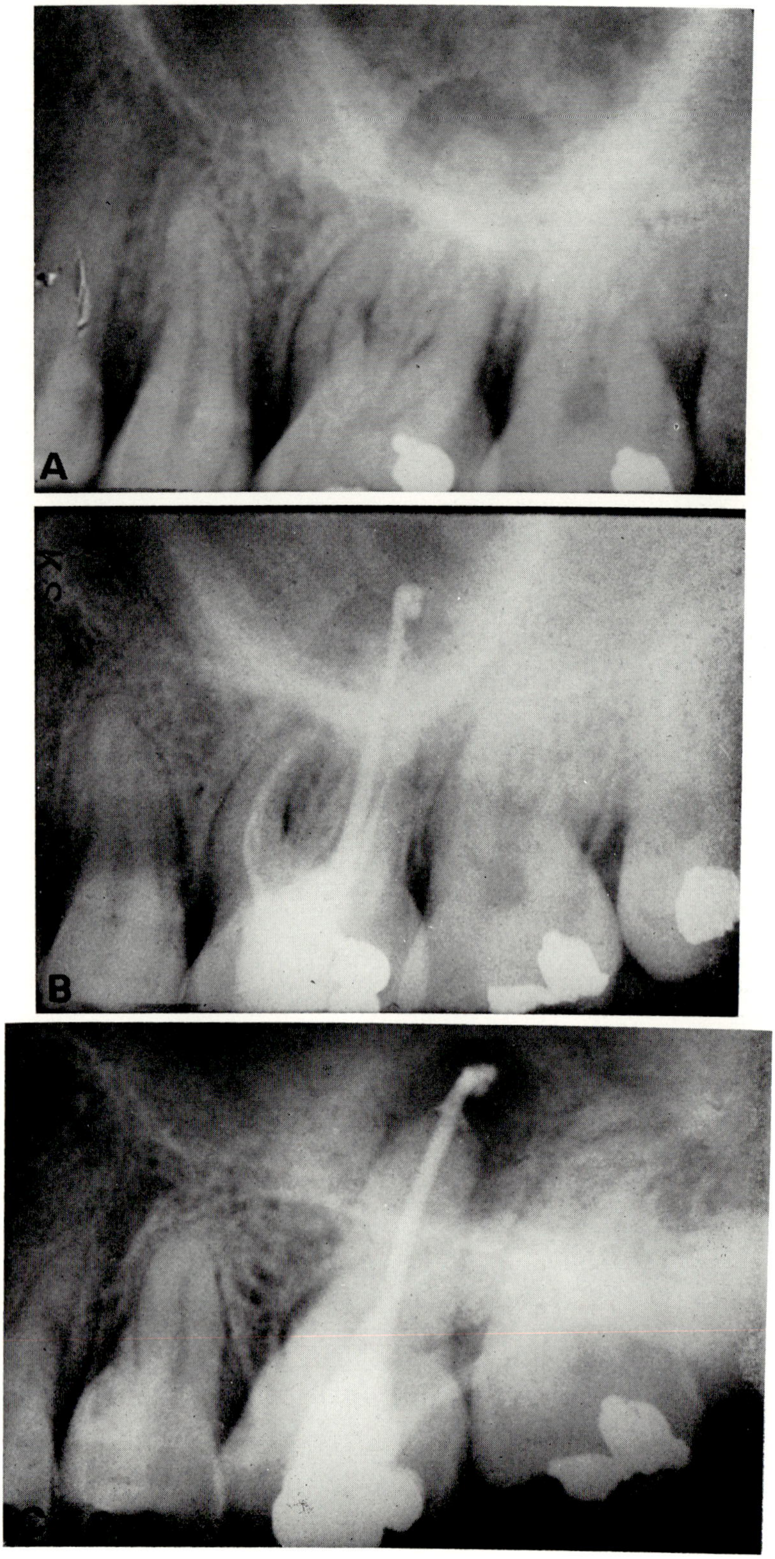
A
B
C

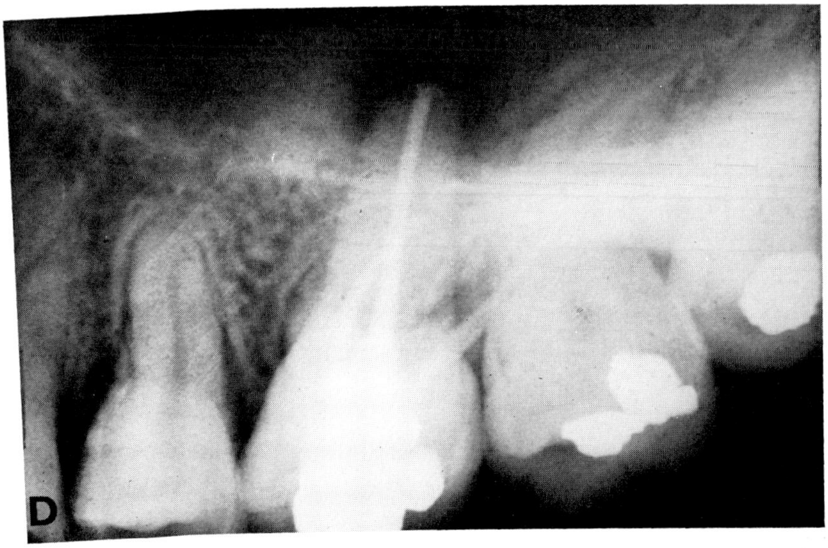

Figure 415. Periapical curettage of the palatal root of an upper molar. A. Upper first molar with periodontal and periapical breakdown of palatal root. B. Three canals were obturated with gutta-percha-chloropercha; palatal root canal was inadvertently overfilled; periodontal surgery was performed on the palatal root (the pocket had reached the apex). C. One month later; periapical bone destruction continued on palatal root. D. A periapical curettage was performed; if healing does not occur, the palatal root will be resected.

simple procedure, to the patient, it still may be painful. Therefore, nitrous oxide analgesia is a helpful adjunct. If the sutures have become buried, local anesthesia should be used. If a pack has been inserted, it is removed at the time of suture removal.

TREATMENT COMPLICATIONS

Severe complications are discussed in Chapter 16. Minor complications are discussed in this section.

Hematoma

This is a tumor-like collection of blood in the soft tissues that results from trauma (Fig. 42). It generally breaks down and is resorbed, but the process may take a few weeks. The patient should be reassured.

Ecchymosis

This is due to extravasation of blood into the soft tissues and is also related to trauma. The appearance is *black and blue.* This also resolves by itself and the patient should be so informed. Proteolytic enzymes are sometimes effective in hastening the resolution (see Chapter 4).

Trismus

This results from trauma to the jaw musculature, with the clinical manifestation being difficulty in opening the jaw. It usually takes more than one

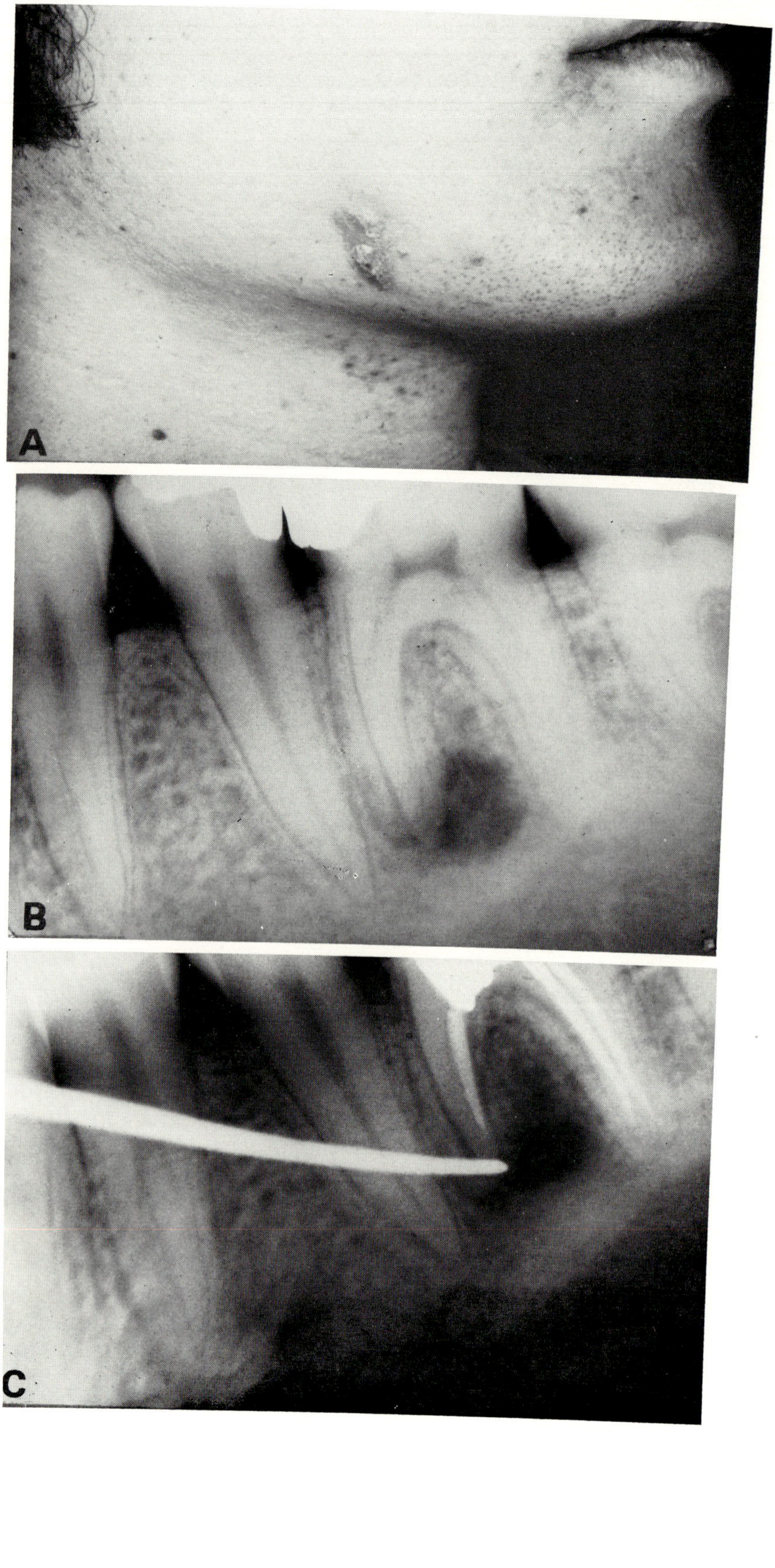
A
B
C

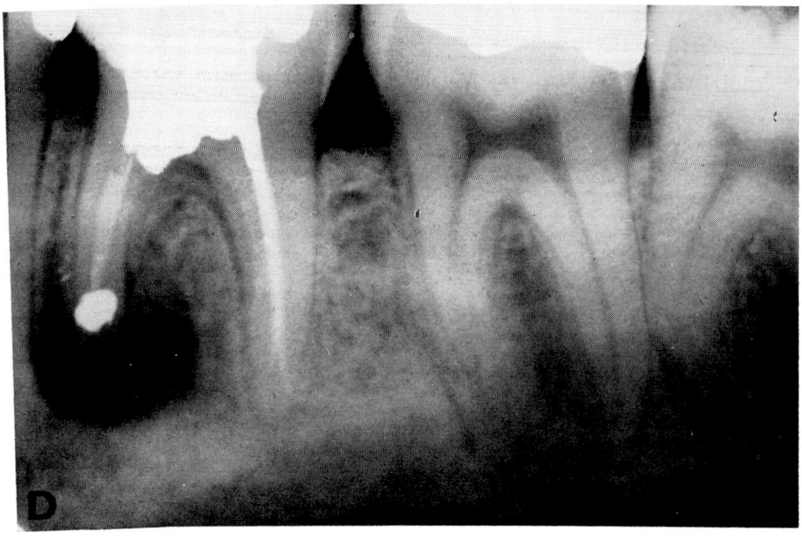

Figure 416. Periapical surgery in a lower molar. A. Skin sinus tract related to an infectious process in the mesial root of a lower first molar. B. Periapical x-ray showing the periapical area of pathosis around the mesial root of the first molar. C. Explorer used to aid in apical localization; the canals were sealed with gutta-percha-chloropercha; the mesial canals were sealed as far as possible. D. An apicoectomy and a retrograde seal was performed on the mesial root.

week for a return to normalcy. Use of chewing gum and chewing exercises may help in alleviating the condition.

Hemorrhage

If the bleeding is slight, the patient can control it by the use of gauze or by the use of a moist tea bag (contains hemostatic tannic acid) pressed to the area. If these measures do not work, then the patient should be seen in the office. The clots are removed, and the area is irrigated with warm saline. If the bleeding originated from bone, then pressure is applied by means of an instrument in order to crush the bleeding vessels. Oxidized cellulose with thrombin can be placed into the area to act as a matrix. Loose sutures are removed and the flap is repositioned and resutured. If the wound is raw, a periodontal pack is placed in the area. Severe hemorrhage is discussed in Chapter 16.

Fenestration with Loss of Mucosal Covering

At times, following periapical surgery, the alveolar mucosa fails to cover a portion of the root (Fig. 418). This may occur when a fenestration has been previously present and/or when a retroseal has been placed. If the retroseal does not appear to be deficient and there are no clinical signs of a root fracture, then it is possible to repair the soft tissue defect with a laterally repositioned split-thickness pedicle flap graft.* A horizontal incision is made

* This section is based on a technique discussed by Drs. C. M. Holman and F. J. Marshall, Ohio State University, College of Dentistry, Columbus, Ohio.

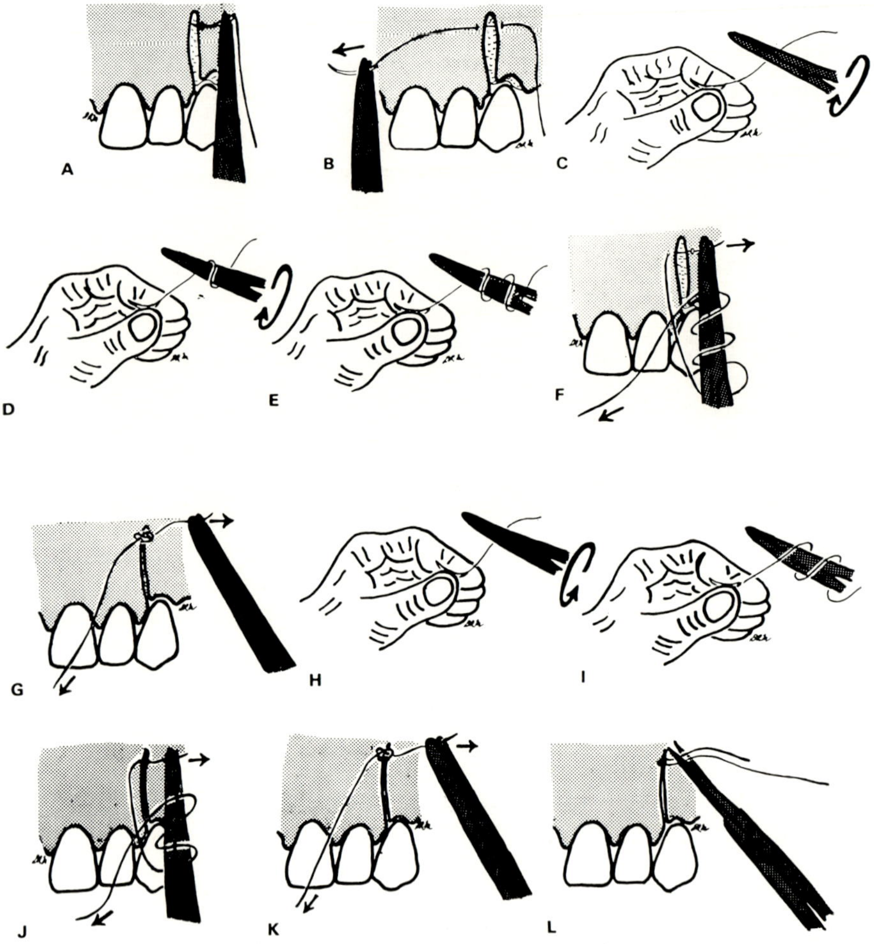

Figure 417 A-L. Various stages of suturing.

approximately 2 mm above the marginal gingiva and two vertical relaxing incisions are made. The soft tissue defect is curetted out completely and the root is planed. The epithelium is removed from the area surrounding the defect but the periosteum is left intact. A split-thickness pedicle flap is made, leaving the periosteum on the donor site. Blood clots are removed from the recipient site and the flap is repositioned to cover the recipient site, leaving the donor area, covered only by periosteum. The repositioned pedicle flap is then sutured to its new position (Fig. 419). The entire area is covered with a periodontal pack. The patient is cautioned to try and not move the mouth. Four to five days later, the sutures are removed and the pack is replaced. At this point, the donor site should begin to granulate in. After one week, the second pack is removed and the patient is advised to take care during eating and not to irritate

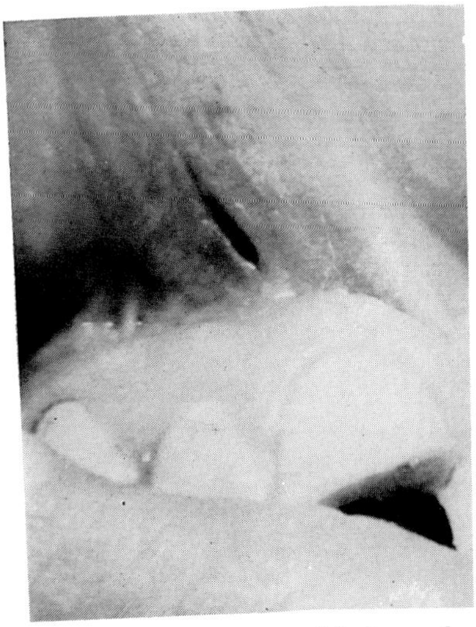

Figure 418. Fenestration with loss of mucosal covering.

the area. Within a few weeks, epithelialization should be complete.

BIBLIOGRAPHY

Best, E. J., and Grothaus, B.: A clinical evaluation of an intra-oral bandage in endodontic surgery. *JSCDA, 38:*884, 1970.

Bhaskar, S. N., Frisch, J., Margetis, P. M., and Leonard, P.: Application of a new chemical adhesive in periodontics and oral surgery. *Oral Surg, 22:*526, 1966.

Chivian, N.: Surgical endodontics: a conservative approach. *J NJ Dent Assoc, 40:*234, 1969.

Grossman, L. I.: *Endodontic Practice,* 7th ed. Philadelphia, Lea & Febiger, 1970.

Holman, C. M., and Marshall, F. J.: Pedicle graft repair of an endodontic defect: report of case. *JADA, 85:*1362, 1972.

Ingle, J. I.: *Endodontics.* Philadelphia, Lea & Febiger, 1965.

Kopp, W. K., and Kresberg, H.: Apicoectomy with retrograde gold foil: a new technique. *NY State Dent J, 39:*8, 1973.

Selden, H. S.: A pedicle bone flap for periapical surgery. *Oral Surg, 31:*654, 1971.

Sommer, R. F., Ostrander, F. D., and Crowley, M. C.: *Clinical Endodontics: A Manual of Scientific Endodontics,* 3rd ed. Philadelphia, Saunders, 1966.

Spasser, H. F., and Wendt, R.: Apical fenestration; a cause for recalcitrant post endodontic pain. *NY State Dent J, 39:*25, 1973.

Tarsitano, J. J.: The use of antibiotics in dental practice. *Dent Clin North Am, 14:*697, 1970.

Weine, F. S.: *Endodontic Therapy.* St. Louis, Mosby, 1972.

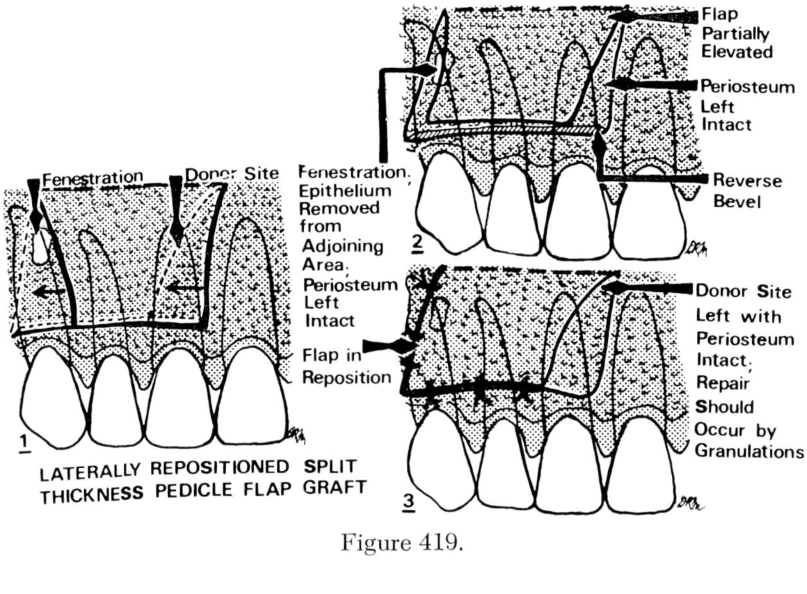

Figure 419.

CHAPTER 11

RADISECTOMY AND HEMISECTION

In this chapter, the surgical techniques of radisectomy and hemisection are discussed.

RADISECTOMY (ROOT AMPUTATION)

Armamentarium is the same as described for periapical surgery (Fig. 403). The case is handled in a routine manner except that the root to be amputated only needs partial instrumentation. At the obturation visit all three canals are sealed with gutta-percha (Fig. 420A). An alternative method is to make a partial post-type preparation into the root to be amputated and fill that preparation with amalgam (Fig. 420B). The patient is then given local anesthesia, with inhalation or IV sedation being a useful adjunct. A full flap is made (see Chapter 10) and the root

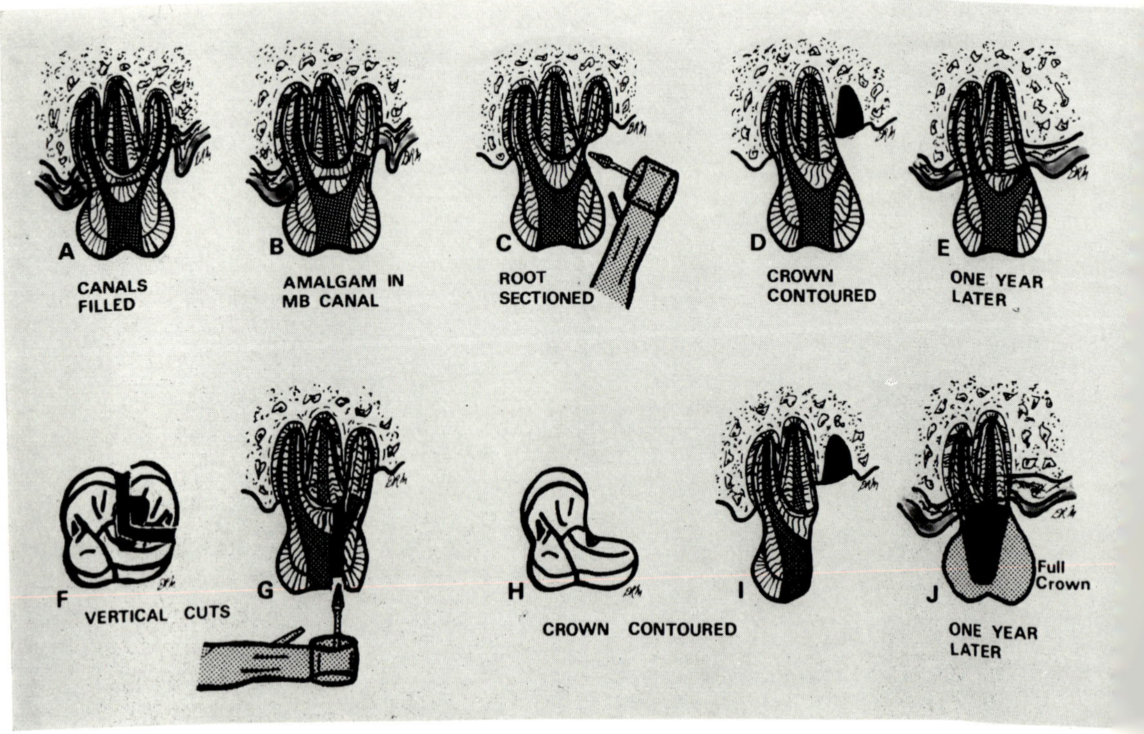

Figure 420 A-J. Various stages in the procedure of radisectomy.

to be removed is examined. Although it is possible to perform a radisectomy without first making a surgical flap, it is preferable to utilize a flap in order to have better visualization of the procedure. There are three basic methods to remove the root. The first is by mallet and chisel, which is not advocated because of the possible trauma to the patient. A second method is by the use of a 701 surgical bur in an ultra-high speed contra-angle with water spray (Fig. 420C). The crown is contoured as the root is being removed (Fig. 420D). In this technique, the crown is kept basically intact, with only the root being removed. The disadvantage is that occlusal forces may tend to be destructive on the remaining roots. The third method uses the same 701 bur to make two intersecting vertical cuts to the furcation area, followed by crown contouring (Fig. 420F-J). In this technique, the coronal portion of the tooth overlying the involved root is removed, necessitating a full crown restoration. In this case, occlusal forces tend to be in the long axis of the remaining roots. The vertical-cut method is generally the easiest to do and causes the least possibility of debris falling into the socket. In the vertical-cut method, the initial vertical cut (for buccal root removal) is made through the buccal groove to the furcation. The second cut is made from the proximal about two thirds the buccal-lingual distance (from the buccal) until it intersects the other cut (Fig. 420F, G). It is also made into the furcation area. Before the root is completely severed, the crown should be contoured (Fig. 420H). This will help prevent debris from falling into the socket. After the crown is contoured, the root is severed by the use of the bur cuts aided by a straight elevator. The root is then removed with an upper forceps. If the root does not come out, then additional bone is removed and an angled elevator is used to loosen the root. The socket is irrigated with sterile saline and the flap is sutured. After-effects are generally minimal and sutures are removed within four to seven days (see Chapter 10). If upon removal of the resected root, a maxillary sinus perforation is evident, then the patient should be treated as is discussed in the section on complications of periapical surgery in Chapter 10. Figures 310 and 421 show radisectomy cases.

HEMISECTION

The armamentarium is the same as described for periapical surgery (Fig. 403). After anesthesia and analgesia is obtained, a full flap is made. As with root amputations, it is preferable to raise a flap prior to performing the hemisection procedure. Although mallet and chisel may be used to perform a hemisection, the use of a 701 surgical bur in an ultra-high speed contra-angle, with water spray is less traumatic and very effective. The cut is made vertically through the crown into the furcation area (Fig. 422B). If one root is to be removed, a lower universal forceps can be used. It is important not to injure the root that is to remain. Before the root is removed, the crown portion of

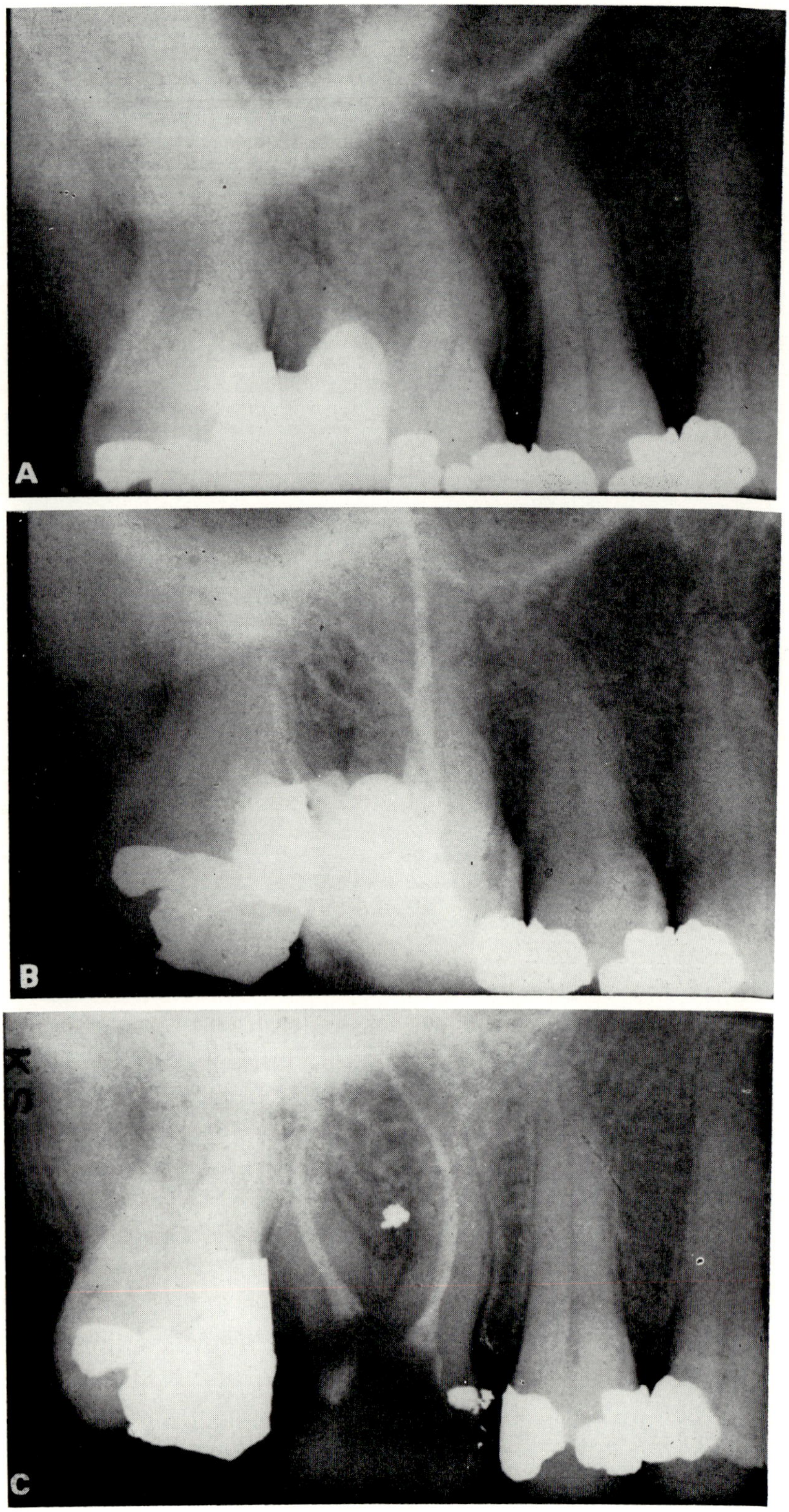
A
B
C

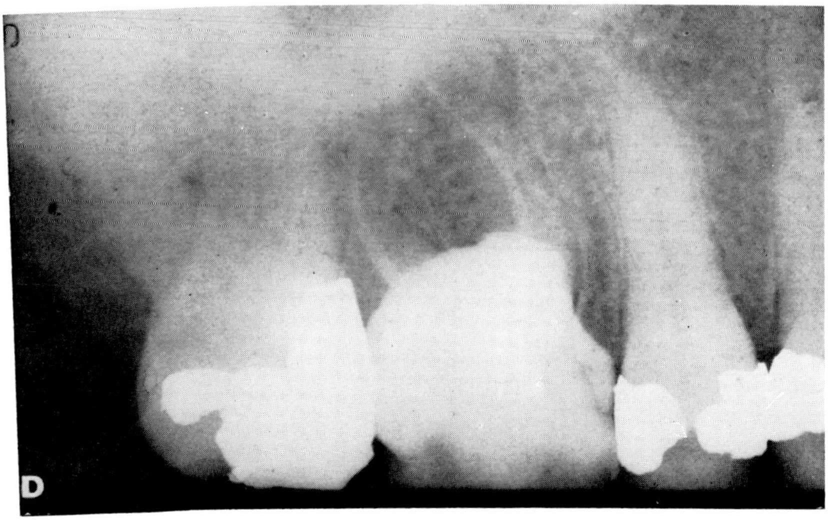

Figure 421. Radisectomy of a fractured palatal root of an upper first molar. A. Before treatment. B. Three canals obturated with gutta-percha-chloropercha. C. Palatal root fractured during mastication; root was amputated. D. Three months later; healing is evident and a permanent crown is being fabricated. (From D. R. Morse, "The Significance of Endodontics in Plantation Procedures," *JDA South Africa*, 26:263, 1971.)

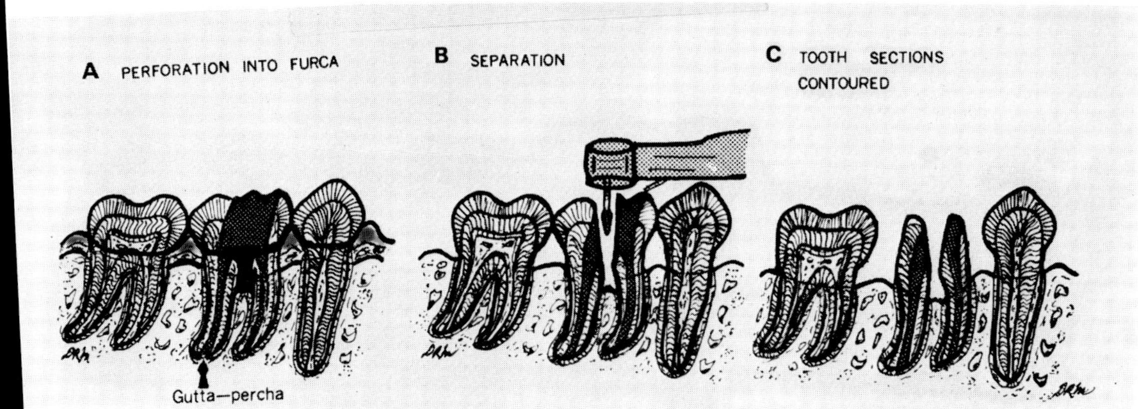

Figure 422 A-E. Various stages in the procedure of hemisection.

the remaining root should be contoured to help prevent debris from falling into the socket. After the root is removed, the flap is sutured and a temporary splint is inserted. If both roots are to remain, then the crowns are contoured, the flap is sutured, and a temporary splint uniting the two sections is made (Fig. 422C, D). The postoperative results and treatment are similar to those described for radisectomy. A typical case is shown in Figure 311.

BIBLIOGRAPHY

Kirchoff, D. A., and Gerstein, H. G.: Presurgical crown contouring for root amputation procedures. *Oral Surg, 27*:379, 1969.

Ingle, J. I.: *Endodontics.* Philadelphia, Lea & Febiger, 1965.

Weine, F. S. *Endodontic Therapy.* St. Louis, Mosby, 1972.

CHAPTER 12

PLANTATION PROCEDURES

In this chapter, a discussion is given of endodontic implants (apical and lateral root endosteal), tooth transplants (autologus and allogeneic) and intentional replants (for primary and permanent teeth).

ENDODONTIC IMPLANTS

Endodontic implants can be inserted through the apex (apical) or through the side of the root (lateral root endosteal). There are also two approaches, nonsurgical and surgical. Each of these methods are now to be discussed.

Nonsurgical Apical Endodontic Implants

Representative implants and accessories are shown in Figure 423. In a vital case, the first visit is similar to a routine case with pulp extirpation and instrumentation being performed. The main difference is that access is incisal rather than lingual to allow for penetration into bone rather than into the alveolar mucosa (Fig. 424.1A). In connection with an incisal approach, it should be noted that crowns are usually indicated after treatment. This is because of the possibility of incisal fracture and the visualization of the implant through the thin incisal tooth structure.

In the second visit, instrumentation is completed within the canal to approximately a No. 70 reamer. The size depends on the mesial-distal diameter of the tooth. The implant to be inserted should not be wider than one-third the mesial-distal diameter of the root or else root fracture may take place. The bone should next be penetrated several mm beyond the apex with a No. 70, 40 mm reamer (Kerr®, Star®, Union Broach). In an average case of a mobile (CL II) upper central incisor, reaming is continued up to a No. 100 to 130 reamer approximately 10 to 15

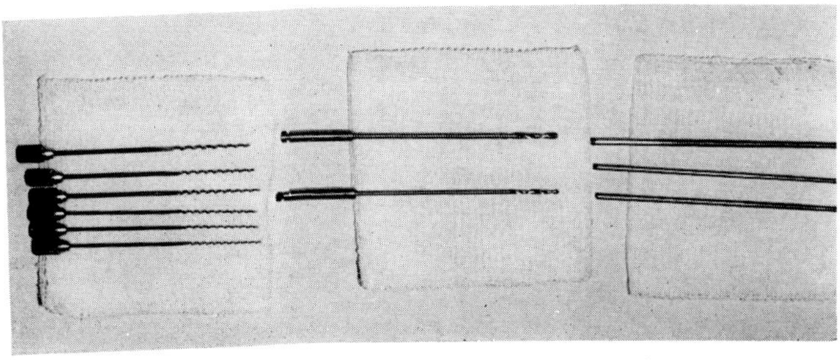

Figure 423. Endodontic implants and reamers; left to right, 40 mm hand reamers, engine reamers, smoooth endodontic implants.

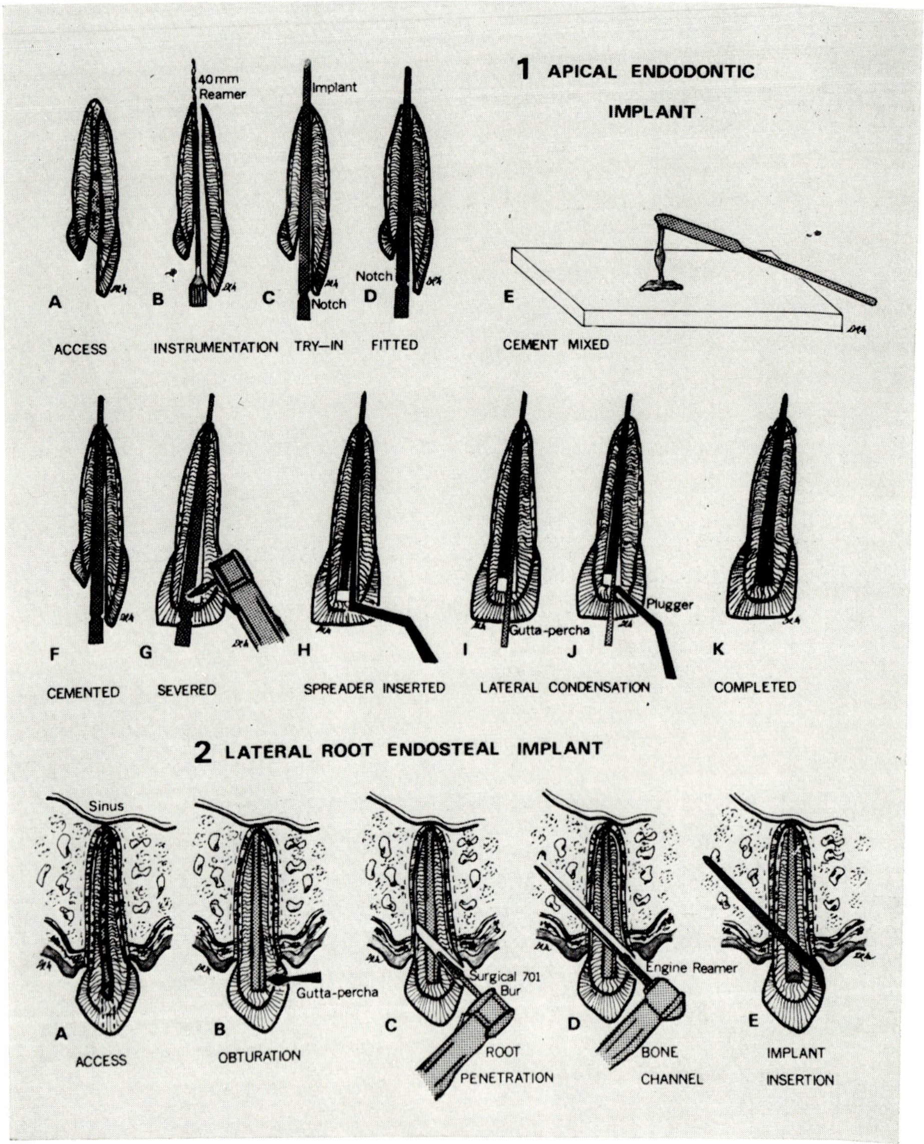

Figure 424

mm beyond the apex (Fig. 424.1B). This is checked by a radiograph. Irrigation is with sterile saline. Hemorrhage is usually controllable with this irrigant and the use of absorbent points. A sedative dressing such an eugenol or Cresatin on a cotton pellet may be inserted followed by a temporary seal of Cavit or ZOE. Generally, post-operative pain is minimal. At the third visit, instrumentation is completed (if it was not at the previous session). It may be necessary to use engine reamers (Fig. 423). These are used in a slow speed contra-angle with sterile saline irrigation. Engine reamers should be used only after the apex has been penetrated or else a perforation may occur. Also, one size smaller engine reamer than the last hand reamer should be first used to prevent binding and possibly breakage within the canal. It is essential that the direction the reamer is traveling is definitely known, and in this regard radiographs may be deceptive. In an upper central incisor, the apex is closer to the labial surface, and it is quite possible to penetrate the alveolar mucosa rather than the bone. Keeping the access toward the incisal helps to prevent this occurrence. If the practitioner has doubt about the penetration of the reamer, he (or she) should hold the index finger along the alveolar mucosa, as the reaming is taking place. The instrument can be felt with the finger if penetration occurs. If, because of the axial inclination of the tooth, penetration is unavoidable, then the root canal is obturated with gutta-percha and an intentional perforation is made. This is followed by the insertion of a lateral root endosteal implant (discussed later). With the normal case, after the instrumentation is completed, an endodontic implant of the corresponding size is tried and the tooth stability is checked. If the previously mobile tooth is now stable, a radiograph is taken. There is no definite distance beyond the apex that the implant must penetrate. The implant should feel as if it binds well at the apex as well as within bone.

Once the implant is judged to be satisfactory, it is notched at the incisal edge with a bur, and then withdrawn (Figure 424.1C). It is not possible to know definitely that the apex has a tight seal. Therefore, just before cementation, approximately 1 mm is removed from the apical end of the implant, to help insure that the binding will be at the apex (Figure 424.1D). The tooth should be held with one hand as the implant is being removed. A mix is made of any standard root canal cement and it is placed on the endodontic part of the implant and inserted in the canal up to the previously notched level (Fig. 424.1 E, F). With the use of a mallet and a small vertical instrument (a mirror handle will do), the implant is gently tapped into its final seat. The jaw beneath the implant should be held firmly during the tapping. The assistant then holds the intraoral part of the implant with a hemostat, and the operator severs the implant with a bur within the chamber (Fig. 424.1G). If a post is anticipated in the tooth, there are two possible alternatives. One is to notch the implant at the desired level within the canal prior to cementation. After cementation, the implant is twisted until it breaks at the notched area. A second method is to serrate the exposed part of the implant and fuse acrylic to that part. This would then be used as part of the crown preparation. After the implant is cemented in position, a second radiograph is taken. Lateral condensation with fine-fine gutta-percha points is then performed in order to help insure that the apex and any possible lat-

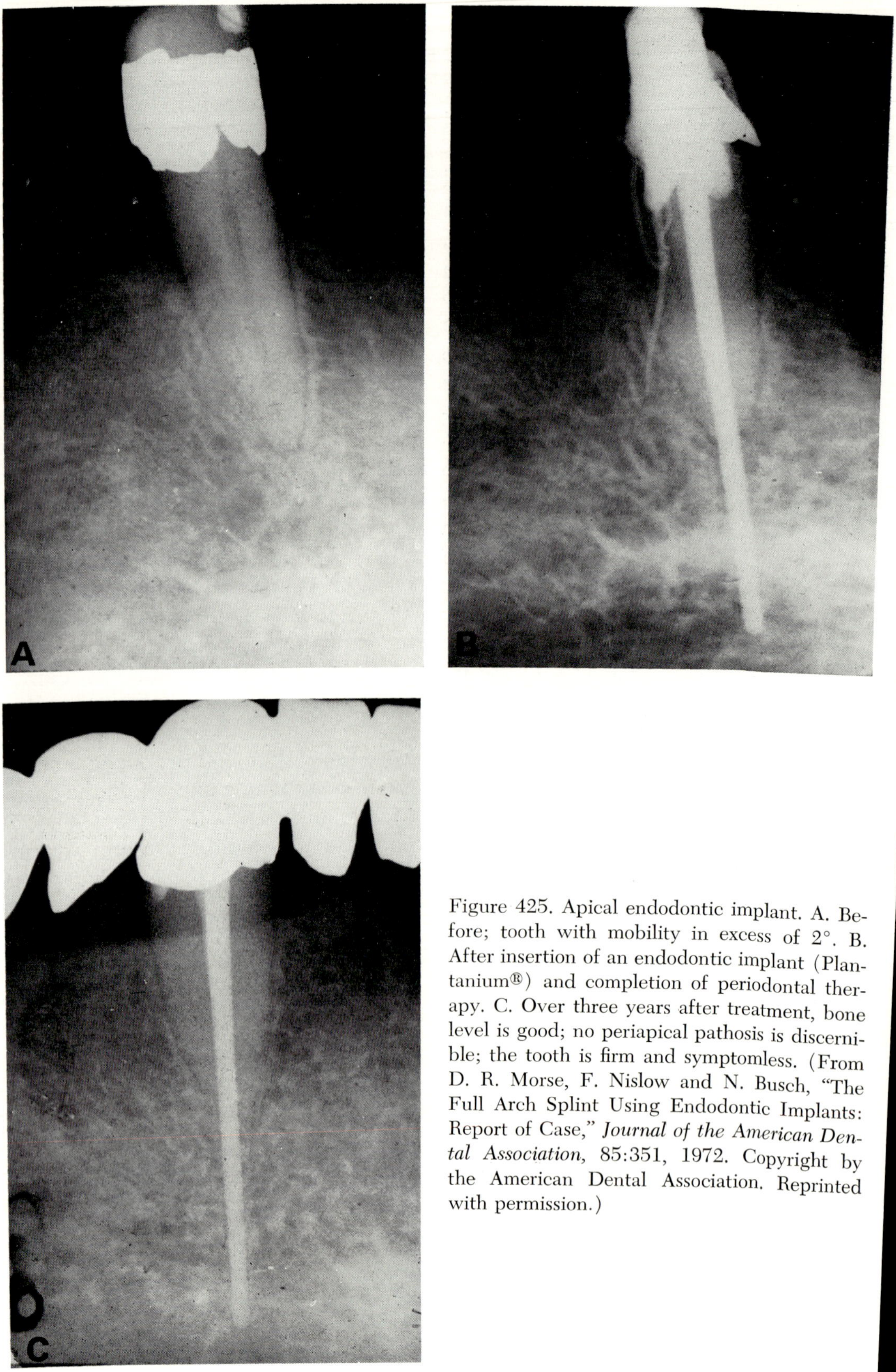

Figure 425. Apical endodontic implant. A. Before; tooth with mobility in excess of 2°. B. After insertion of an endodontic implant (Plantanium®) and completion of periodontal therapy. C. Over three years after treatment, bone level is good; no periapical pathosis is discernible; the tooth is firm and symptomless. (From D. R. Morse, F. Nislow and N. Busch, "The Full Arch Splint Using Endodontic Implants: Report of Case," *Journal of the American Dental Association*, 85:351, 1972. Copyright by the American Dental Association. Reprinted with permission.)

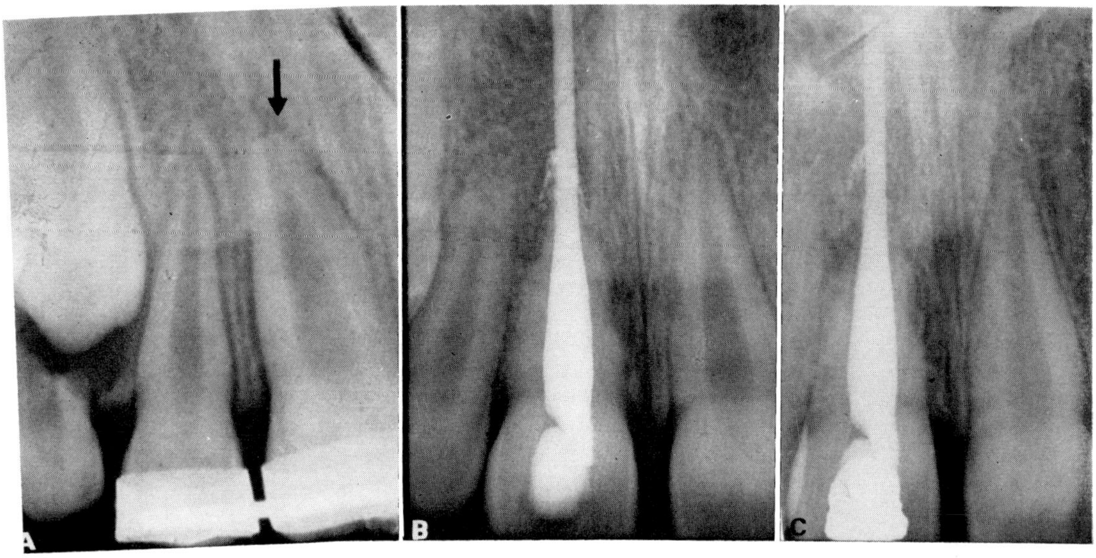

Figure 426. Apical endodontic implant for a replanted tooth. A. Upper left central incisor had been avulsed and was replanted after several hours extra-oral duration. B. Endodontic implant cemented in place. C. One and one-half years later; tooth is firm and slight apical resorption is present. (From D. R. Morse, "The Management of Endodontic Problem Cases," *JDA South Africa*, 27:387, 1972.)

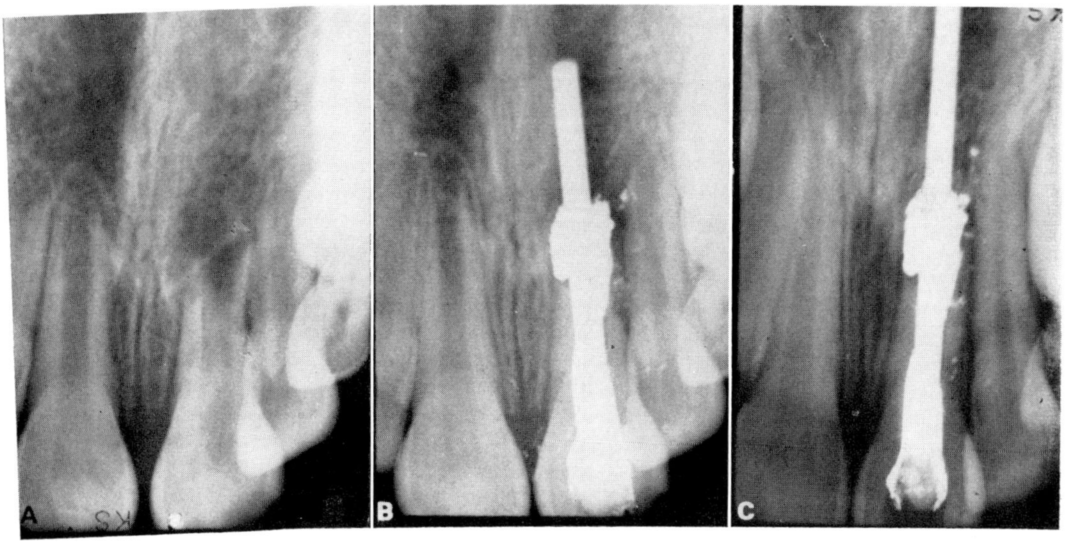

Figure 427. Apical endodontic implant for a tooth with a wide open apex. A. Upper right central incisor with a necrotic pulp, an open apex, and excessive mobility. B. Endodontic implant inserted (Vitallium®); retrograde amalgam seal placed. C. Two and one-half years later; tooth is firm and symptomless; no pathosis is evident. (From D. R. Morse, "The Management of Endodontic Problem Cases," *JDA South Africa*, 27:387, 1972.)

eral canals are sealed (Fig. 424.1H-J). The chamber and the access opening is closed off with Cavit or a ZOE cement (Fig. 424.1K). At a subsequent visit, when the tooth is symptomless, a permanent restoration is inserted. Generally post-implant insertion symptoms are minimal and similar to those after routine nonsurgical endodontic therapy. Routine cases are shown in Figures 87, 96B, D, 318, 319A, 336, 425, and 426.

Surgical Apical Endodontic Implant

The surgical approach has the advantage of allowing for visualization of bone penetration both during instrumentation and implant insertion. A full

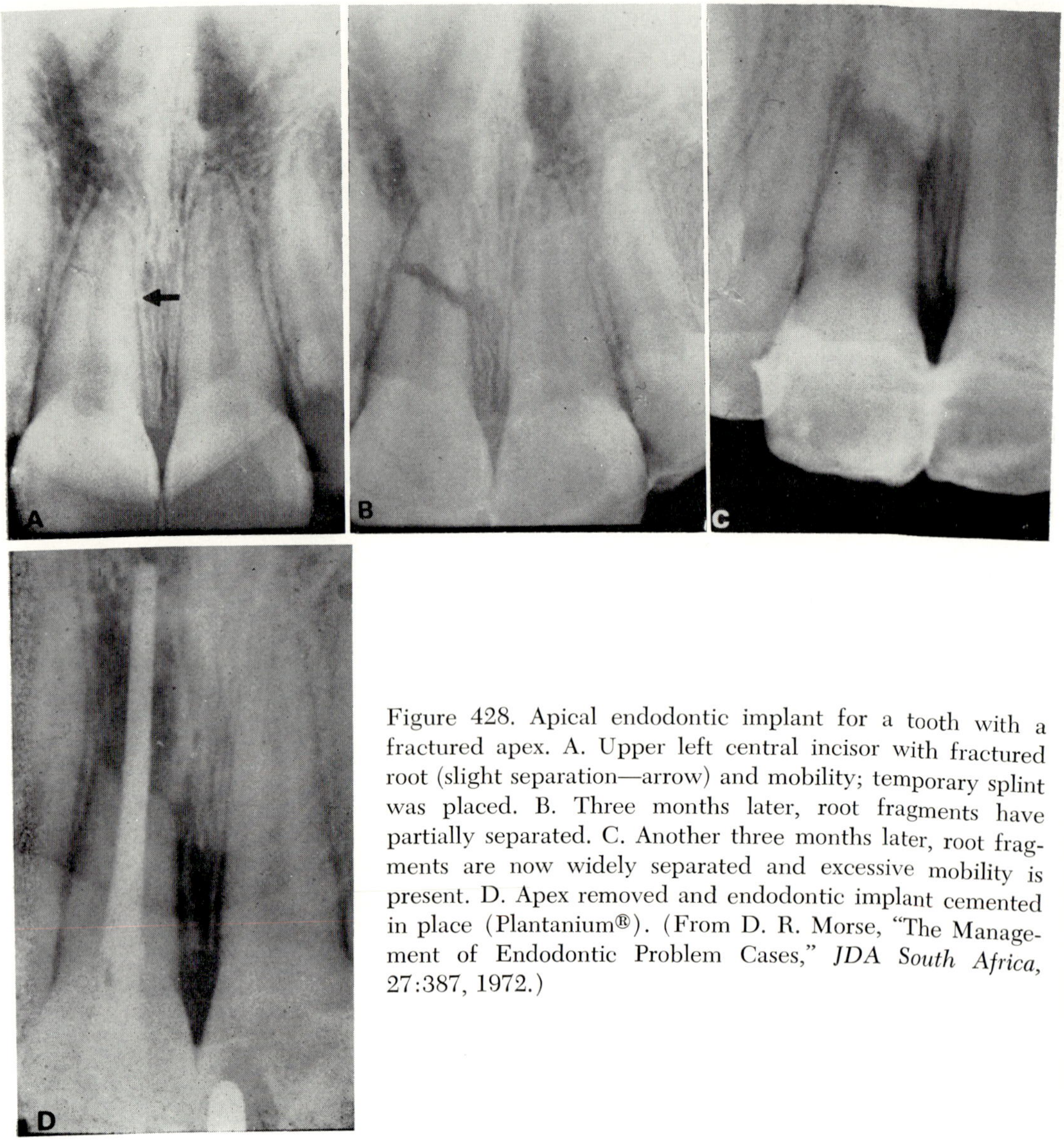

Figure 428. Apical endodontic implant for a tooth with a fractured apex. A. Upper left central incisor with fractured root (slight separation—arrow) and mobility; temporary splint was placed. B. Three months later, root fragments have partially separated. C. Another three months later, root fragments are now widely separated and excessive mobility is present. D. Apex removed and endodontic implant cemented in place (Plantanium®). (From D. R. Morse, "The Management of Endodontic Problem Cases," *JDA South Africa*, 27:387, 1972.)

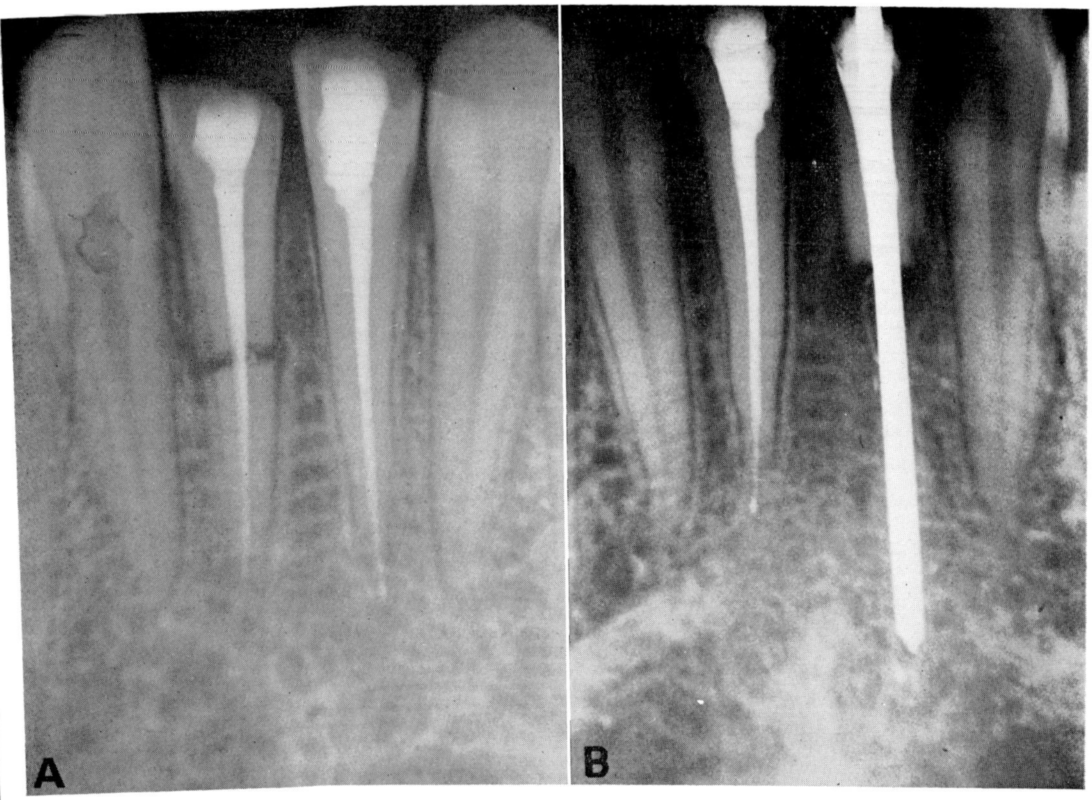

Figure 429. Apical endodontic implant following root fracture which occurred after completion of endodontic therapy. (From D. R. Morse "Endodontic Implants: A Review and New Approach," *New York State Dental Journal,* 35:5, 1969.) A. Root fracture in left central incisor, tooth is mobile and sinus tract is present. B. One and one-fourth years after apical section had been removed and an endodontic implant (Vitallium®) had been inserted; bone repair is evident, but it is not complete.

flap is made and the surgical phase is completed (see Chapter 10). Then instrumentation and implant insertion is performed (as described previously). If the apex is not sealed (usually results from case with a wide open apex), then a retrograde seal is inserted. Amalgam had previously been used (Fig. 427), but because of the possible deleterious effects of the interactions of dissimilar metals, it is preferable to use a nonmetal. Recently I have used a thick mix of zinc polycarboxylate cement for this purpose (Fig. 334). Before suturing the flap into position, a radiograph is taken to check the seal and possible presence of foreign particles. The post-operative effects are similar to those described for periapical surgery (see Chapter 10). Typical cases are shown in Figures 314B, 315, 334, 335, 427-429.

Lateral Root Endosteal Implant

Cases are performed surgically or nonsurgically. The basis for the decision is the same as for the apical endodontic implant. Armamentarium is the same as for the apical endodontic implant. The technique is as follows: Endodontic therapy with gutta-percha is completed in the usual manner (Fig. 424.2A, B). From an examination of the radiographs and the alveolar mucosa, the area of root perforation and direction of insertion is determined. With the use of a 701 L bur in a water-cooled ultra-high speed contra-angle, an opening is made through the desired root into the bone (Fig. 424.2C). Penetration is completed through the bone using 40 mm hand reamers or engine reamers (with the same precautions as described previously) (Fig. 424.2D). It is important that the point of emergence of the implant into the bone must be below the level of attached bone (for lower teeth; above the bone level for upper teeth). This is essential in order to avoid the creation of a periodontal involvement (Fig. 424.2E). If the original path chosen does not allow for adequate bone penetration and tooth stabilization, then the opening must be sealed with amalgam and another path has to be chosen (Fig. 430). After the instrumentation is completed, the implant is cemented into position (as has been described for the apical implant). The opening through the root is then sealed. Formerly amalgam was used (Fig. 431), but currently zinc polycarboxylate cement is advocated to prevent interaction between metals. A representative case is shown in Figure 432. All implant cases should be checked periodically. Several implants that were inserted have been clinically successful for over eight years, but failures may occur as is possible with other forms of endodontic therapy.

TOOTH TRANSPLANTS

Tooth transplants are of two types, autogenous and allogeneic. Each type is now discussed.

Autogenous Tooth Transplantation

Necessary armamentarium is shown in Figure 433. Local anesthesia and analgesia are used. For lower molar transplants, in addition to an inferior alveolar injection, infiltration must be given in the buccal and lingual mucosa overlying the partially developed lower third molar. A small amount of anesthetic should also be placed in the buccal and lingual alveolar mucosa surrounding the lower first molar. Flap design is shown for the lower third molar in Figure 346.1B. With the use of a lower molar forceps or elevator, the first molar is extracted, the interradicular bone is removed, and sterile gauze is placed in the socket (Figure 346.1C). Then, with the use of an elevator and/or a lower molar forceps, the third molar is removed. The gauze and any debris is removed from the first molar socket, and the third molar is carefully positioned in the first molar socket (Fig. 346.1D). The flap is then closed with interrupted sutures (Fig. 346.1E). It is important that the tooth is positioned so that it is in good alignment and is in infraocclusion (Fig. 346.1D). Thumb pressure and slight biting pressure is used to align the tooth. It may be necessary to

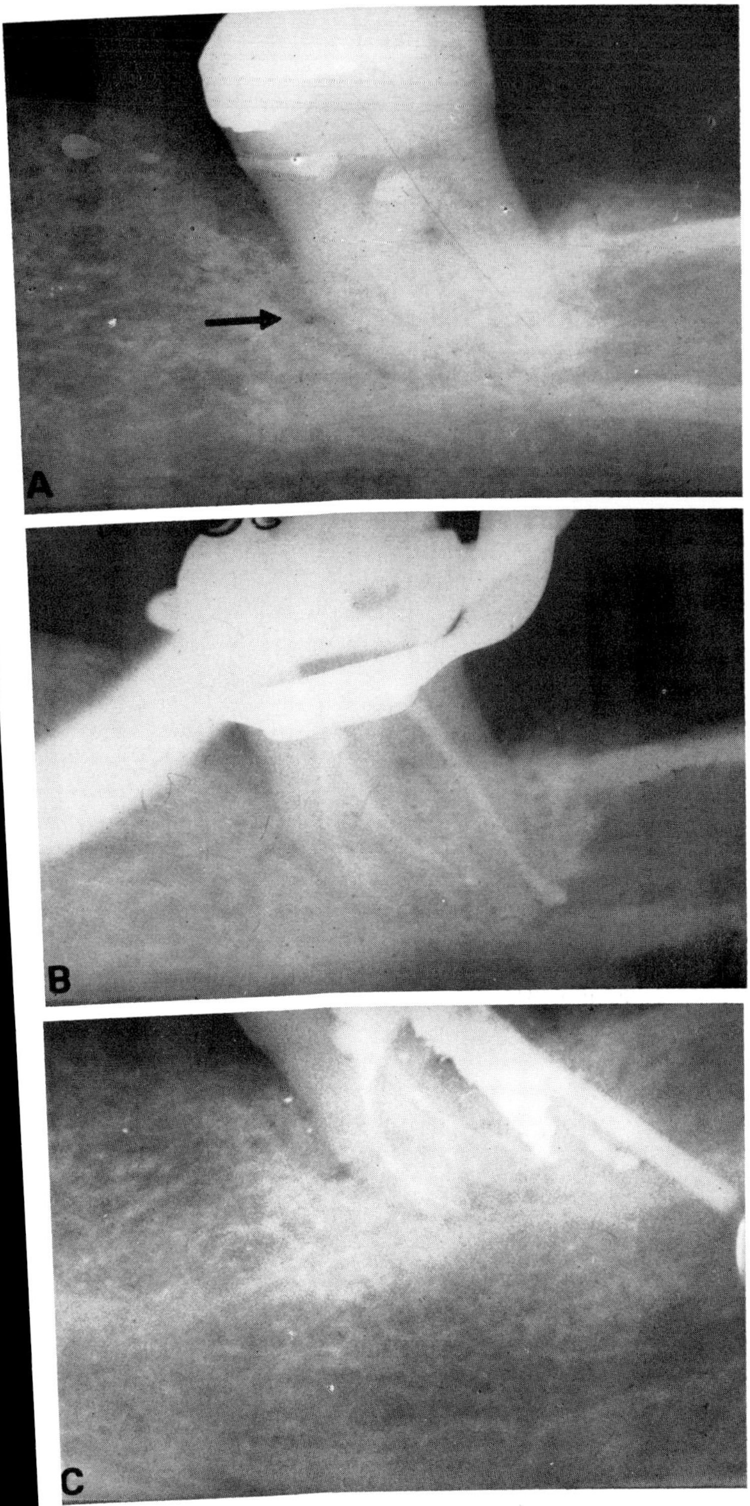

Figure 430. Lateral root endosteal implant; change in direction. A. Before; note severe bone defect on mesial aspect (arrow). B. Root canals obturated with gutta-percha-chloropercha. C. Lateral root endosteal implant cemented into position; original opening in distal aspect sealed with amalgam. (From D. R. Morse, F. Nislow, and N. Busch, "The Full Arch Splint Using Endodontic Implants; Report of Case," *Journal of the American Dental Association,* 85:351, 1972. Copyright by The American Dental Association. Reprinted by permission.)

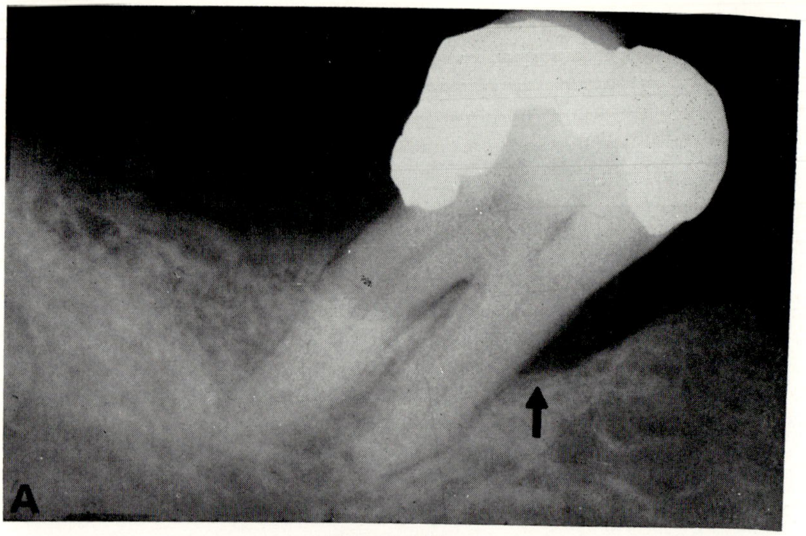

Figure 431

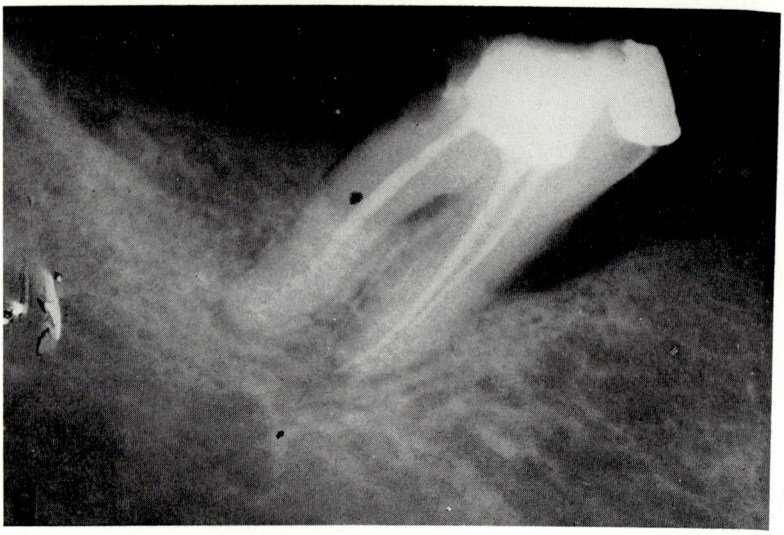

Figure 431

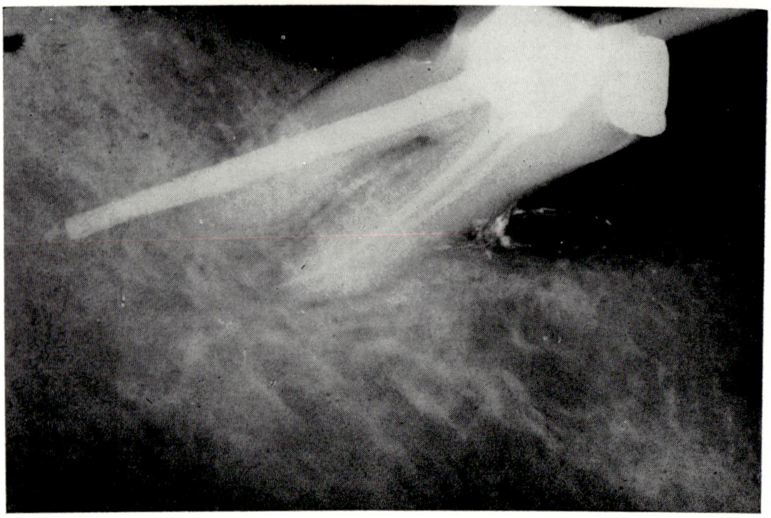

Figure 431

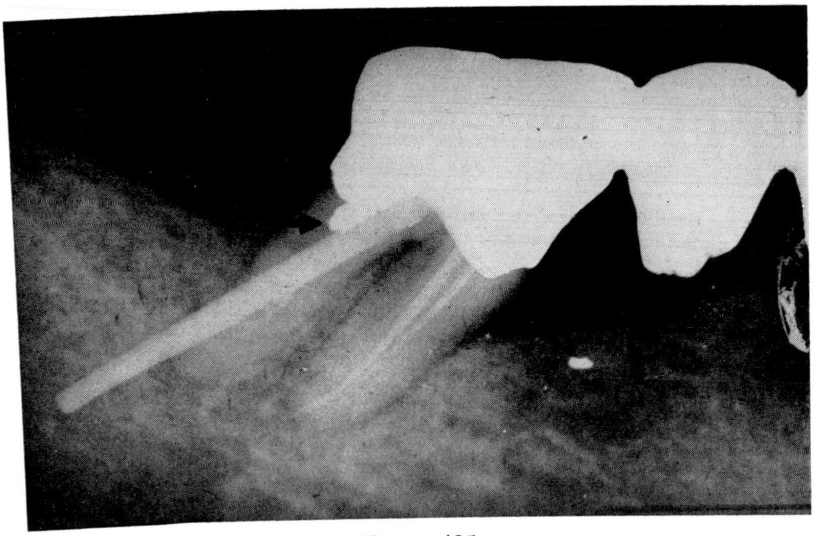

Figure 431

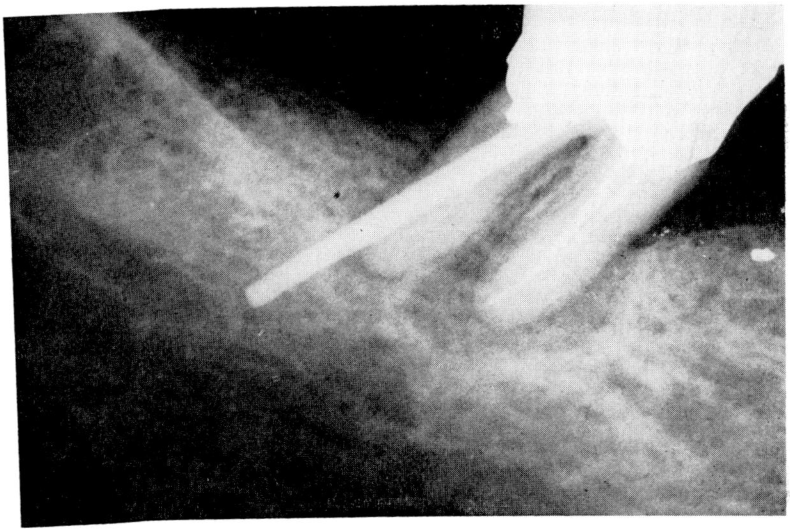

Figure 431

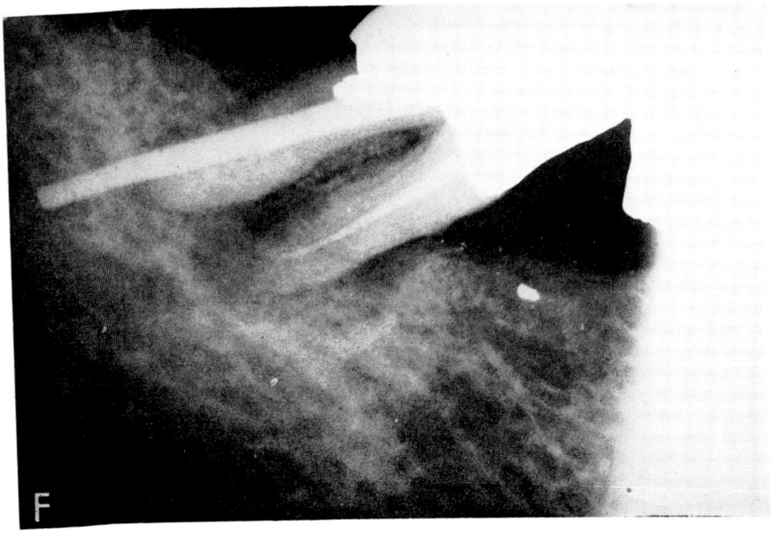

Figure 431

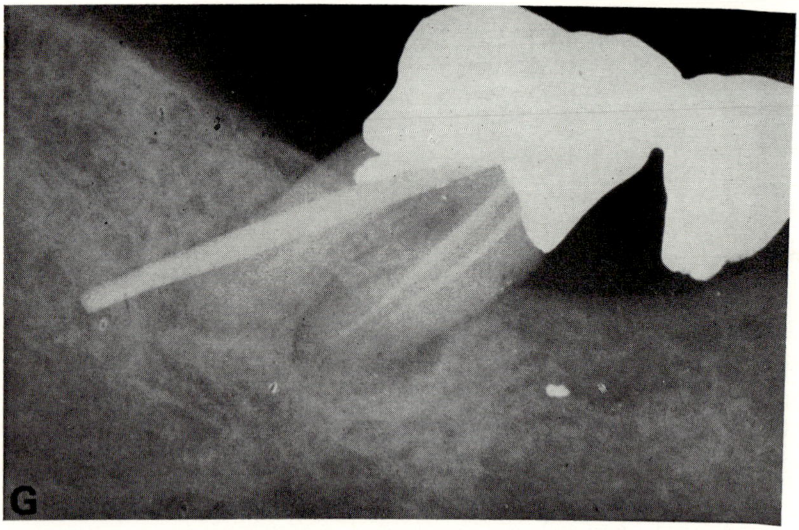

Figure 431. Lateral root endosteal implant; salvaging a failure. A. Before, note severe bone defect on mesial aspect (arrow). B. Root canals obturated with gutta-percha-chloropercha. C. Lateral root endosteal implant cemented in position. D. Over one year later; no clinical problems or radiographic changes evident; occlusal seal is with amalgam (arrow). E. Two years after treatment, definite radiolucency envelopes the mesial root. F. Periapical curettage and apicoectomy performed on mesial root. G. 39 months after initial treatment, bone defect on mesial appears to be healing well. (From D. R. Morse, F. Nislow, and N. Busch, "The Full Arch Splint Using Endodontic Implants: Report of Case," *Journal of the American Dental Association,* 85:351, 1972. Copyright by the American Dental Association. Reprinted by permission.)

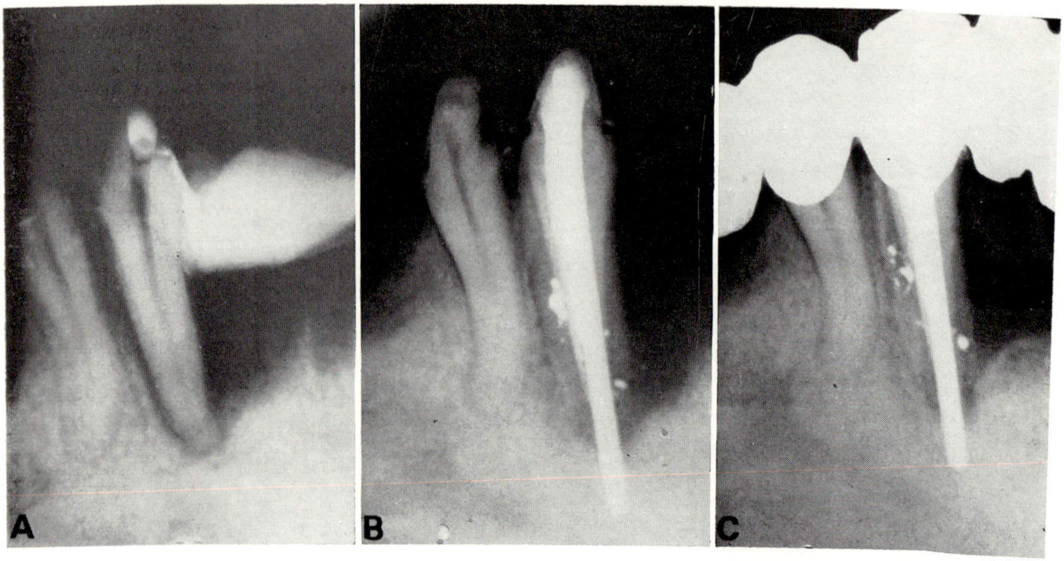

Figure 432. Lateral root endosteal implant for a severely periodontally involved tooth. A. Lower left canine with periodontal involvement and excess mobility; periodontal pack and temporary splint is in position. B. Canal obturated with gutta-percha-chloropercha; *lateral* implant cemented in place. C. One and one-half years later; some bone repair is evident. (From D. R. Morse, "The Management of Endodontic Problem Cases," *JDA South Africa,* 27:387, 1972.)

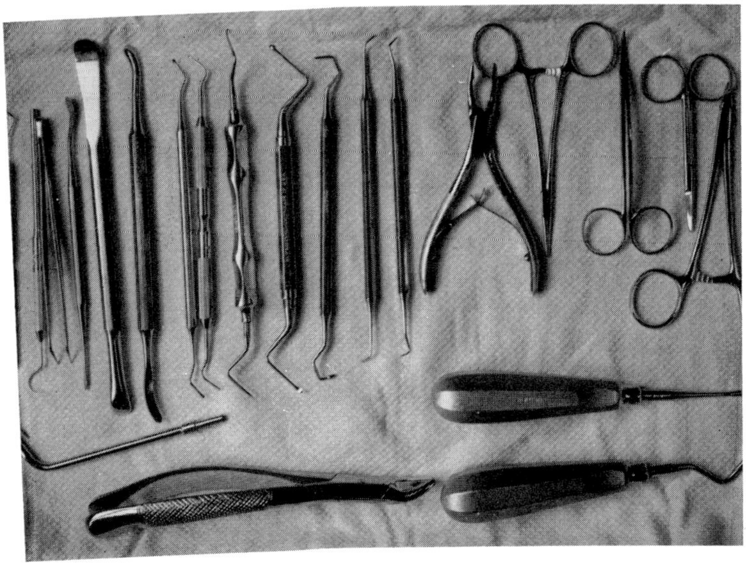

Figure 433. Armamentarium for autogenous tooth transplantation or intentional replantation; left to right. First row; explorers, cotton pliers, retractors, curettes, pluggers, bone forceps, hemostats and scissors (tissue and suture). Second row; aspirating tip, forceps, elevators.

spot grind the tooth in order to maintain it in infraocclusion. For lower molars, no splint is usually necessary. For upper molars, one of the previously described splints can be used. Sutures should be removed in five to seven days, at which time pulp vitality is tested. The tooth may test nonvital at this time, but no endodontic therapy should be performed unless there are cardinal signs of pulpal-periapical disease. If a splint was used, it should be removed in six weeks. The tooth should be pulp tested and a periapical radiograph taken. If at that time, or any subsequent time, the pulp becomes endodontically-involved, then nonsurgical endodontic therapy should be performed. If the tooth is mobile because of the short roots, endodontic implants can be inserted. However, careful consideration must be given to the direction of insertion because of the proximity of the inferior alveolar canal (for lower molars).

Allogeneic Tooth Transplantation*

Armamentarium is shown in Figure 434. As it is difficult to have immediately available the correct size tooth for a potential transplant, it is preferable to have fully formed teeth kept in a *tooth bank*. Teeth can be stored in a refrigerated balanced salt solution. One such solution is refrigerated Gey's balanced salt solution. It contains neomycin, polymyxin and lincomycin along with necessary salts. The mesial-distal and buccal-lingual diameters of the tooth socket and the tooth to be transplanted must be determined in order to obtain as good a fit as possible. Prior to placing the tooth in the storage medium, the periodontal ligament should be removed as described in the section on replantation and splinting. Once a usable tooth is found, root canal instrumentation

* The present treatment method discussed is based on recent findings by Dr. Leonard B. Schulman at Harvard University School of Dental Medicine.

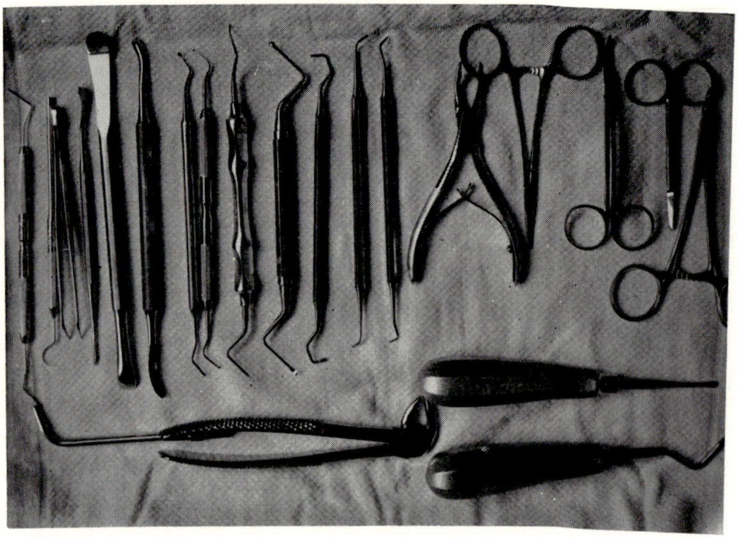

Figure 434. Armamentarium for allogeneic tooth transplantation (e.g. upper premolar); left to right. First row; explorers, cotton pliers, retractors, curettes, pluggers, bone forceps, hemostats and scissors (tissue and suture). Second row; aspirating tip, upper forceps, elevators.

should be completed and the fluoride solution applied (see replantation of avulsed teeth in Chapter 8). The canal(s) are then sealed with gutta-percha (lateral condensation) and the tooth is ready for transplantation. Local anesthesia is used to obtain anesthesia for the socket. It is also possible to create a socket for the reception of a transplant, although this procedure has not had much clinical verification. After anesthesia is obtained, the tooth is inserted into the socket and the occlusion is checked. It should be in slight occlusal contact (Fig. 346.2). A splint is then placed in position. This is removed in six weeks. If mobility occurs at that or any subsequent time, an endodontic implant can be inserted. The use of the endodontic implant can give added retention. If signs of apparent rejection occur (ankylosis with the crown appearing to submerge, and root resorption), then a treatment that has been advocated is the performance of a periapical curettage. This procedure may delay, but it will not prevent the resorption process.

INTENTIONAL REPLANTS

Intentional replantation can be performed for primary molars and permanent teeth.

Intentional Replantation For Primary Molars*

Armamentarium is shown in Figure 433. After anesthesia and analgesia is given, the molar is extracted using a lower forceps. The buccal-lingual luxation should be very gentle, with little force applied to prevent fracture. The socket is packed with sterile gauze. The extracted tooth is then placed in sterile saline-moistened gauze and complete instrumentation of the canals is performed. The canals are filled with a zinc-oxide eugenol paste, and the apexes are removed (approximately 2 mm). The orifice is sealed with Cavit and the

* This section is based on a technique devised by Dr. I. B. Bender of Philadelphia, Pa.

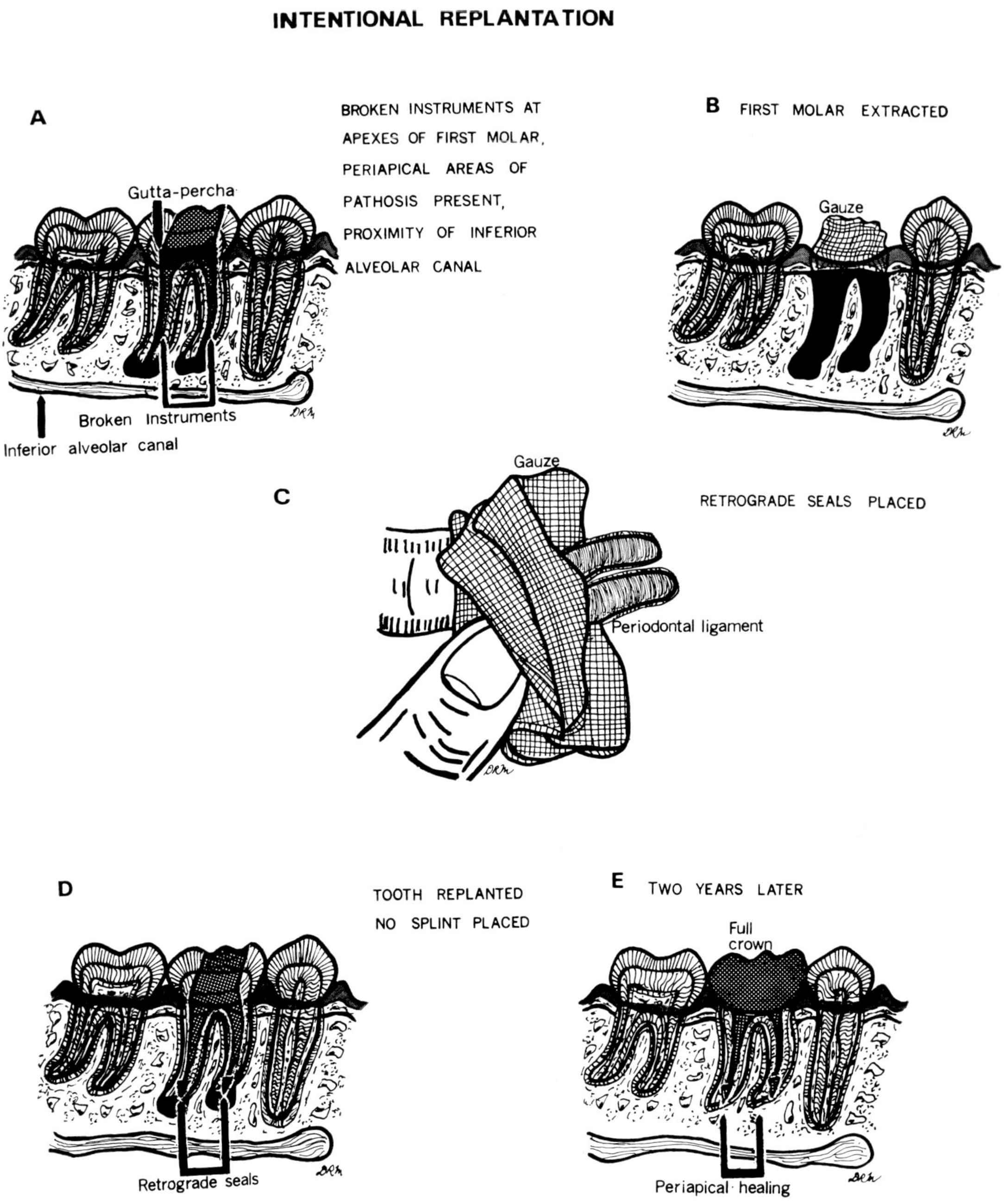

Figure 435 A-E. Various stages of intentional replantation.

tooth is reinserted gently into the socket (Fig. 280). No splinting is used.

Intentional Replantation For Permanent Teeth

The necessary tray set-up is shown in Figure 433. After anesthesia and analgesia, the canals are instrumented and obturated with gutta-percha as far as is possible. This is usually performed at a previous visit, but can be done at the surgical visit, if time permits. The tooth is cautiously extracted with a lower forceps (as described in the previous section). Gauze is placed in the socket, and the extracted tooth is held in a piece of sterile saline-moistened gauze.

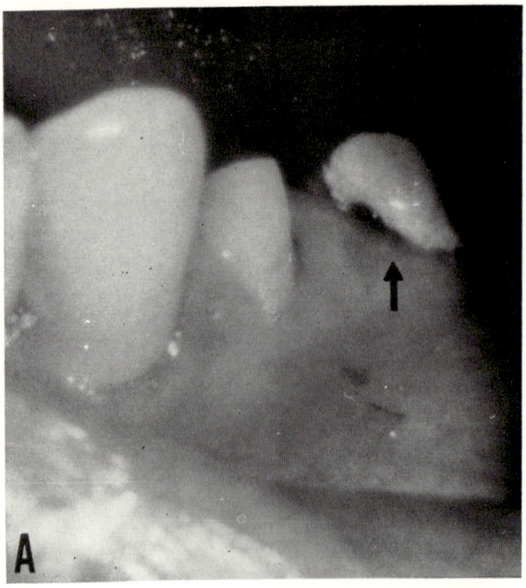

Figure 436

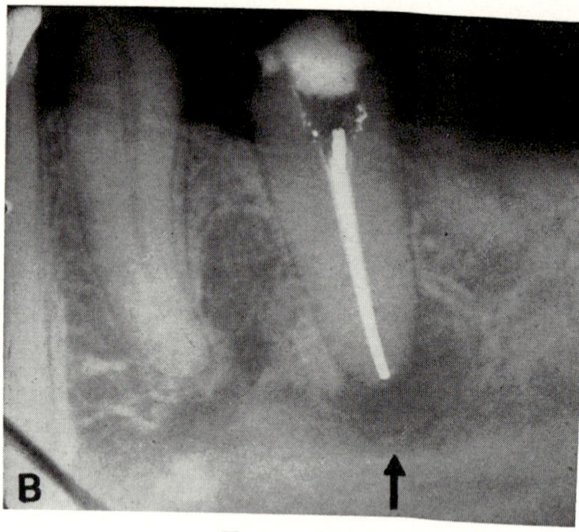

Figure 436

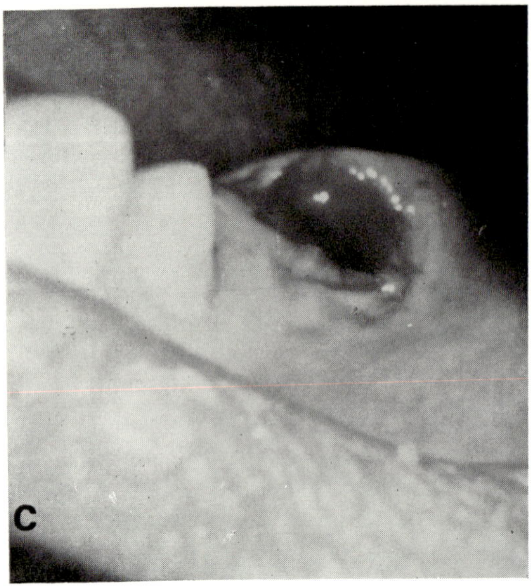

Figure 436

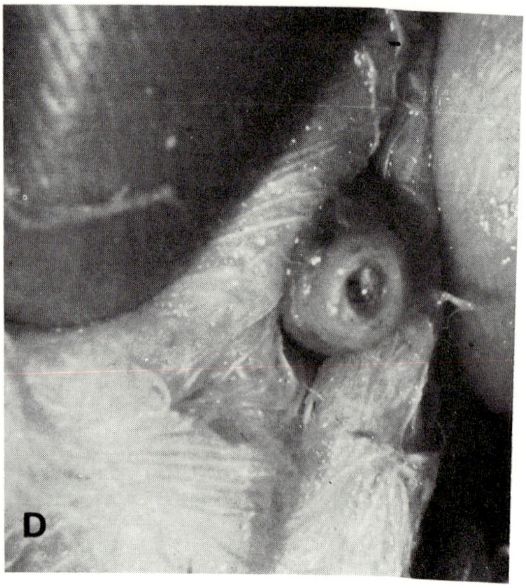

Figure 436

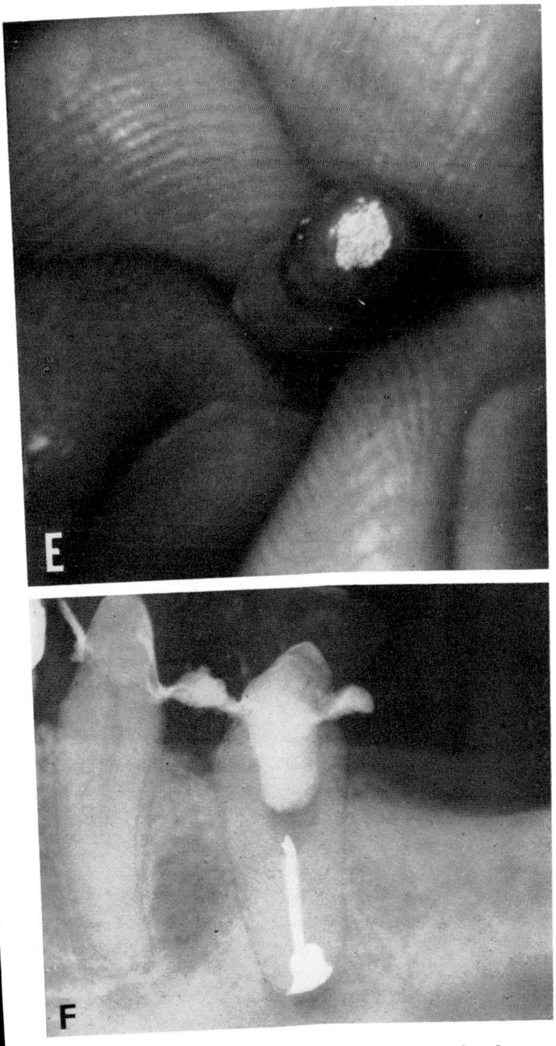

Figure 436. Intentional replantation of a lower premolar. A. Clinical appearance of a lower premolar. B. Radiographic appearance showing irretrievable silver cone, periapical area of pathosis, and proximity of inferior alveolar canal (arrow). C. Tooth was extracted. D. Apex prepared with a No. 35 inverted cone bur. E. Amalgam seal in place. F. Radiographic appearance of replanted tooth; temporary splint in position. (Courtesy of Dr. R. Wollard, Philadelphia, Pa.)

The tooth is carefully checked for fractures, and if it is satisfactory (no vertical fractures), then the apical 2 mm (or so) are removed with a No. 701 bur. A class I cavity preparation is made at the apexes with a No. 35 inverted cone bur, and the opening is sealed with amalgam, gold foil, or polycarboxylate cement. The tooth is then reinserted into the socket (Fig. 435). If the retention is good, no external splinting is necessary. If additional stabilization is necessary, then one of the previously described posterior splints can be used. A satisfactory splinting action can be accomplished using a periodontal pack. Radiographs and photographs of a completed case are shown in Figure 436.

BIBLIOGRAPHY

Anthony, A. J.: Vital tooth transplant into a surgically created socket: report of a case, *Oral Surg, 27:*293, 1969.

Baer, P. N., and Gamble, J. W.: Autogenous dental transplants as a method of treating the osseous defect in periodontosis. *Oral Surg, 22:*405, 1966.

Grossman, L. I., and Ship, I. I.: Survival rate of replanted teeth. *Oral Surg, 29:*899, 1970.

Marano, P. D.: Dental transplantation, simplified. *Oral Surg, 24:*567, 1967.

Morse, D. R.: Endodontic implants: a review and new approach. *NY State Dent J, 35:*5, 1969.

Shulman, L. B.: Allogeneic tooth transplantation. *J Oral Surg, 30:*395, 1972.

Siskind, M.: Endodontic Implants and Transplants. Presented at the Annual Meeting of the A.D.A., Oct., 1971, Atlantic City, New Jersey.

CHAPTER 13

BLEACHING

In this chapter, bleaching of pulpless teeth and tetracycline-stained vital teeth are discussed.

BLEACHING OF PULPLESS TEETH

This procedure involves two phases, one is preventative and the second is treatment. Armamentarium for both phases is shown in Figure 437.

Preventative

There are six factors in preventative tooth bleaching. (1) During the access preparation, the pulp horns are completely cleaned out. (2) Copious irrigation aids in removing necrotic debris. The oxygenating irrigants (3% hydrogen peroxide, 5% sodium hypochlorite, urea peroxide, RC-Prep) may begin the

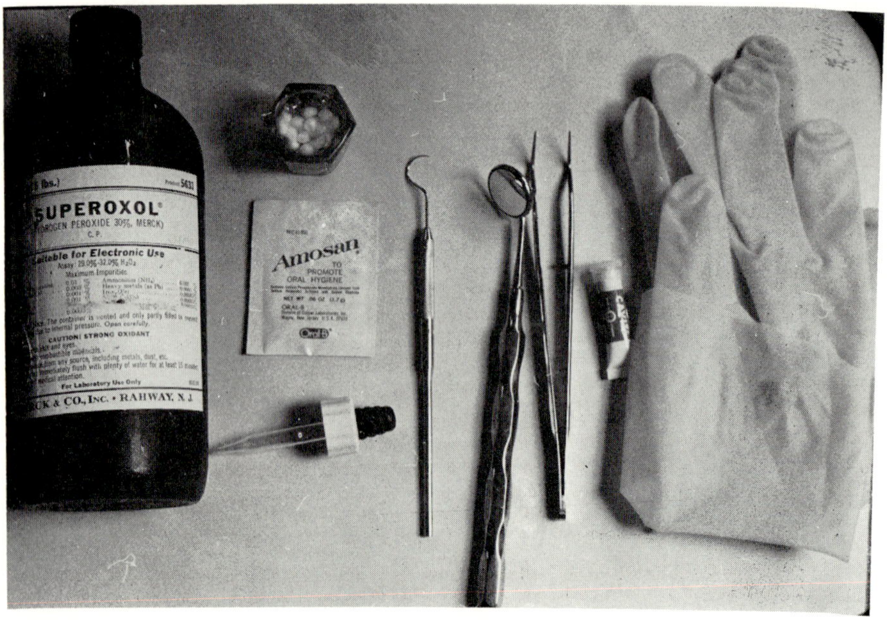

Figure 437. Armamentarium for bleaching; left to right. Superoxol (some studies have shown water to be almost as effective), Amosan® (any sodium perborate preparation can be used). Top; dappen dish with cotton pellets. Bottom; medicine dropper, explorer, mirror, cotton pliers, Cavit (or other temporary restorative material), sterile gloves; not shown, rubber dam set-up.

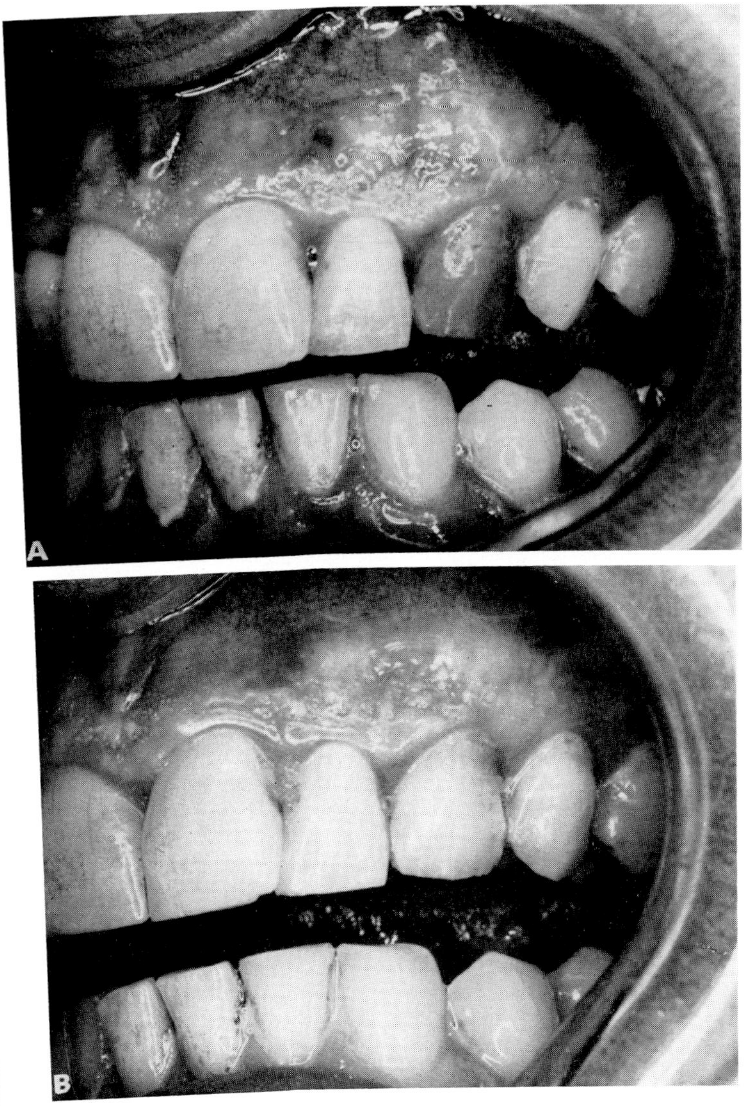

Figure 438. Bleaching case using sodium perborate and water. A. Before. B. After. (Courtesy of Dr. H. Spasser, New York.)

bleaching process. (3) The dentist should not use intracanal medicaments or fillings that are capable of staining the dentinal tubules. These include azochloramid, silver nitrate, iodoform, formocresol, root canal cements containing silver, tetracyclines, and silver amalgam. (4) The root canal filling is removed to a level approximately 2 mm below the cervical line. (5) A plastic or silicate restoration is placed in the access opening. (6) At the completion of endodontic therapy, if there is any evidence of discoloration, sodium perborate is mixed with water to make a thick paste (Amosan or Vince can be used). This is then placed on cotton and sealed in the chamber for about

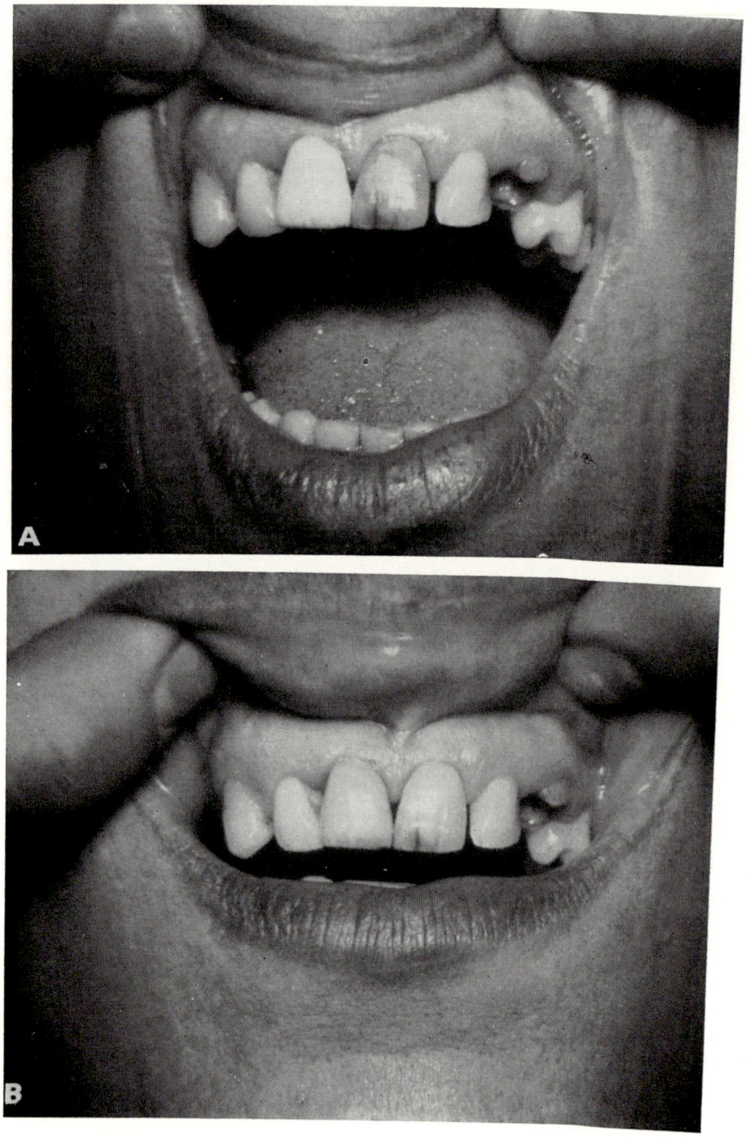

Figure 439. Another bleaching case using sodium perborate and water. A. Before. B. After. (Courtesy of Dr. H. Spasser, New York.)

one week. Cavit or zinc phosphate cement is used to seal the access opening. At the end of that time, the cotton is removed and a permanent restoration is placed.

Treatment

The tooth is isolated under rubber dam. Access is gained. All stained or discolored dentin is removed with a round bur (No. 3 or 4) in a slow speed contra-angle. The root canal filling is removed to 2 mm below the cervical line. A thick mix of sodium perborate and Superoxol (or water) is made. Only the amount of Superoxol that is needed is removed from the bottle and placed in a dappen dish. The remainder is tightly stoppered and placed back in the refrigerator. The mixed paste is placed inside the chamber. Also with a cotton pliers, a few wisps of cotton are dipped into the Superoxol and placed on the labial aspect of the tooth. Then a hot burnisher is placed over the labial surface spreading the cotton over the entire surface. The cotton is then removed and the access opening is sealed with Cavit or zinc phosphate cement (Fig. 349). The patient is seen again about one week later. If the tooth shade is satisfactory, then the paste is removed with a spoon excavator and a silicate or plastic restoration is inserted. If the shade is still too dark, the process can be repeated one or two more times. If after a few attempts, the results are still not satisfactory, then the fabrication of a porcelain jacket crown should be suggested to the patient. Representative cases are shown in Figures 438 and 439.

BLEACHING OF TETRACYCLINE-STAINED TEETH*

Recent results have shown that non-endodontically treated tetracycline-stained teeth can be successfully bleached. The tooth is isolated under the rubber dam; the gingiva is lubricated with petroleum jelly (Vaseline®) and cotton pledgets saturated with Superoxol are placed on the labial and lingual surface of the involved tooth. A special heating instrument (Union Broach-Indiana U. bleaching instrument®) is applied to both surfaces for twenty minutes. The temperature is set 10°F. less than the reading at which the patient first responds clinically, when the heat generating unit is applied to the surface of the tooth. After twenty minutes, the area is washed with alcohol and warm water, and the rubber dam is removed. The procedure is repeated at weekly intervals for two more visits. The results appear to be good. At this time, there have not been any reports of deleterious effects occurring to the pulp from the heat application, but this remains a possibility.

* This discussion is based on a technique devised at Indiana University School of Dentistry by Drs. Donald E. Arens, Jeffrey J. Rich, and Harry J. Healey.

BIBLIOGRAPHY

Arens, D. E., Rich, J. J., and Healey, H. J.: A practical method of bleaching tetracycline-stained teeth. *Oral Surg, 34:*812, 1972.

Grossman, L. I.: *Endodontic Practice,* 7th ed. Philadelphia, Lea & Febiger, 1970.

Ingle, J. I.: *Endodontics.* Philadelphia, Lea & Febiger, 1965.

Nutting, E. B., and Poe, G. S.: A new combination for bleaching teeth. *JSCDA, 31:* 289, 1963.

Spasser, H. F.: A simple bleaching technique using sodium perborate. *NY State Dent J, 27:*332, 1961.

CHAPTER 14

RESTORATIONS

The management of endodontically-involved teeth requires four phases: endodontic therapy, periodontal therapy (if necessary), occlusal equilibration, and restoration of the endodontically-treated tooth. In this chapter, the restorative aspect is considered. As this is not a textbook of restorative dentistry or fixed partial prosthesis, only a general outline of the restorative procedures is presented.

Some patients have the erroneous concept that once the *nerve* is gone, the tooth can no longer decay. Figure 440 shows an example of how rapidly caries can occur in an endodontically-treated tooth. Another problem relative to restorations, is that some dentists like to wait and see if the endodontic therapy is successful. However, this period of *watchful waiting* with a temporary restoration in place can allow for periodontal disease to occur (Fig. 441), recurrent caries to take place (Fig. 440), and root fracture to occur (Fig. 442). Therefore, it is preferable to place a final restoration within two weeks following the completion of the endodontic therapy.

It has been a clinical impression that endodontically-treated teeth are more brittle than teeth with vital pulps. However, scientific verification of this concept has been lacking. Recently a study has shown that pulpless teeth have a decreased water content as compared to vital teeth. This indicates that the clinical impression of brittleness is true. Nevertheless, not all endodontically-treated teeth require posts (dowels), cores, and crowns.

Traumatized teeth (with no, or only enamel fractures) that have no restorations, require that the access opening and pulp chamber be sealed. In anterior teeth, a silicate or plastic restoration is used; in posterior teeth an amalgam restoration is sufficient. Anterior teeth with small synthetic restorations generally do not require a post and crown, although some authorities advocate the latter procedure for these teeth. Anterior teeth with either large synthetic restorations, fractures involving considerable enamel and dentin, or evidence of a vertical fracture that doesn't go through the root, require a post and crown. It is not necessary or desirable to reduce the crown entirely and make a complete post and core. As much sound tooth as possible should be retained for the crown preparation (Fig. 443A-3). The post is prepared so that its length is approximately equal to the length of the restored crown (Figs. 443A-4, 444).

Any canal that requires a post should

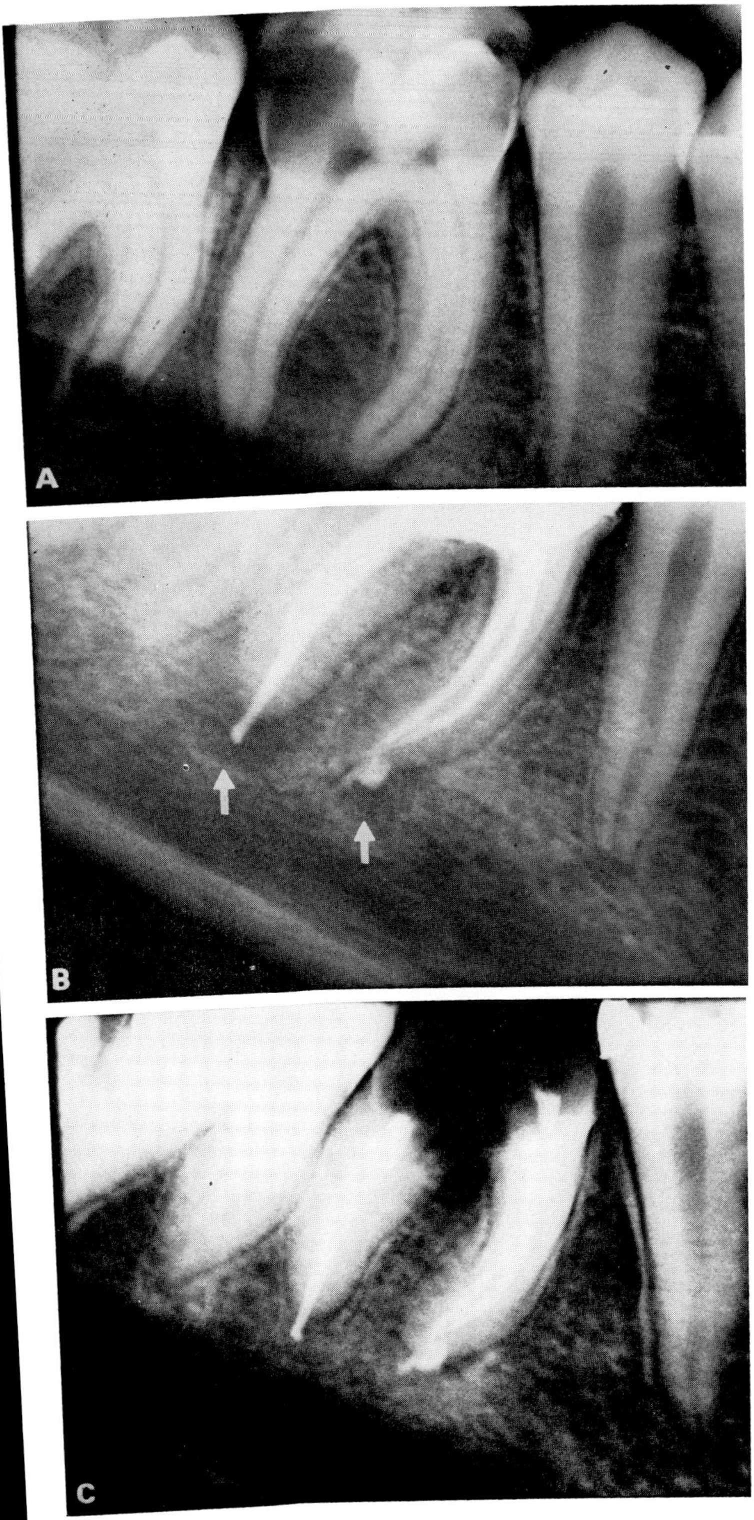

Figure 440. The importance of restoration. A. Carious pulpal exposure in a lower left first molar. B. Endodontic therapy completed with gutta-percha-chloro-percha; there is unintentional overfilling, periapical breakdown is visible (arrows). C. Two years later; although patient was informed about the necessity of having a permanent restoration, he failed to return to his family dentist and as a result carious process continued and destroyed the entire crown. It is interesting to note that in spite of the overfilling, periapical repair is evident; this again reemphasizes the importance of as complete obturation as possible.

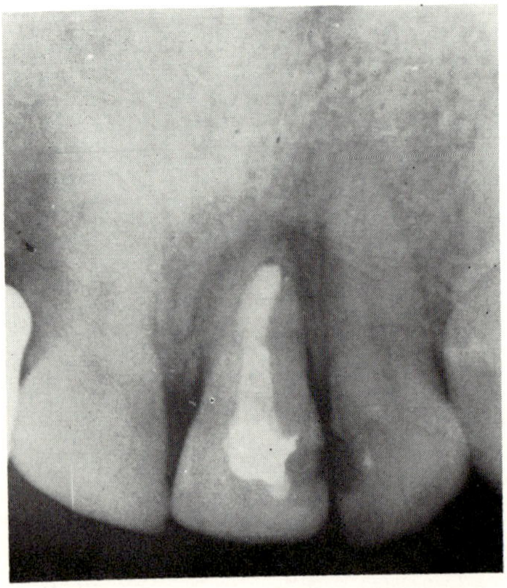

Figure 441. Periodontal disease occurred during period of *watchful waiting,* possibly as a result of trauma of temporary restoration in supraocclusion. (From D. R. Morse, "The Significance of Endodontics in Plantation Procedures," *JDA South Africa,* 26:263, 1971.)

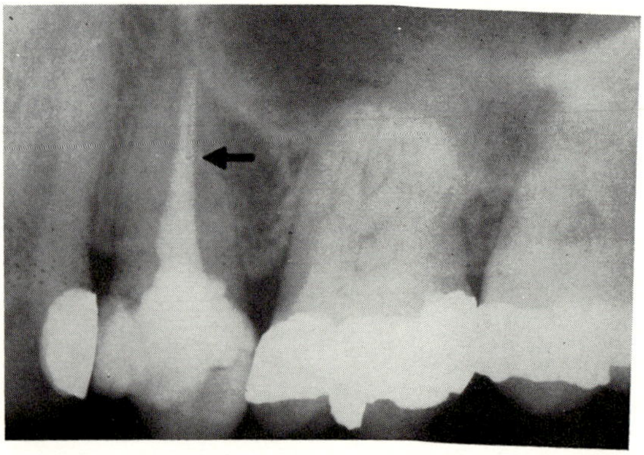

Figure 442. Root fracture occurred as a result of biting pressure into temporary restoration. (From D. R. Morse, "The Management of Endodontic Problem Cases," *JDA South Africa,* 27:387, 1972.)

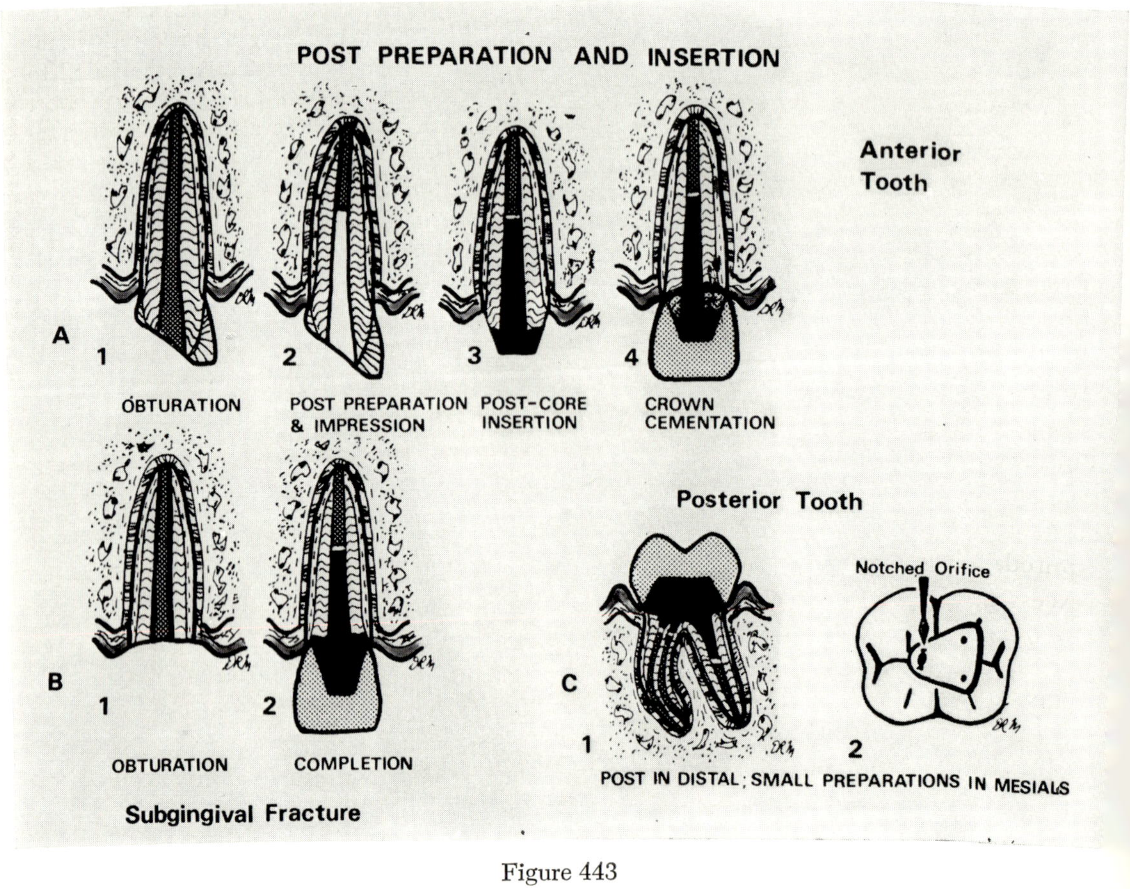

Figure 443

be prepared to a sufficient diameter so that it would not be necessary to use a bur for post preparation. A case of a deleterious result from a bur preparation for a post is shown in Figure 445. As the minimum width of the Endo-post® (Kerr) is size 70 and the Endowel® (Star) is size 80, root canals requiring a post of these types must be open to at least those diameters (Fig. 446.3). There is some evidence to show that posts made of stainless steel, and various alloys can corrode. The corrosion products may lead to root fractures in some cases. Posts should not be used if they are discolored or if the surface appears defective. The portion that goes into the root canal should not be ground or cut as the latter procedures would increase corrosion. As gold posts corrode only slightly, they may be advantageous. However, other metal posts can be used if the aforementioned conditions are followed (e.g. Dentatus Screw Post System®—Schweb®; Fig. 446.2; Kurer Crown Anchor System®—Union Broach). A step by step procedure for post preparation and insertion is shown in Figure 443A. A tooth that is fractured to the gingival margin or below requires a gold post, a core (coping) and a crown (Fig. 443B). If the root is partially or completely submerged, then a gingivectomy and/or ostectomy is required. With the use of a scalpel, the excess gingiva is removed and the bone is contoured using a 701 bur in a water-cooled ultra-high speed contra-angle. This can also be accomplished by the use of electrocautery, which has the advantage of minimizing bleeding. Epinephrine (8% racemic) should not be used to expose roots. It can readily get into the systemic circulation and cause a serious hypotension. Several submerged teeth can be used for overlay dentures, once they are uncovered and restored. A specific type of attachment for these teeth is a Zest Anchor® (American Precision Metals). It is attached to the denture and fits into a receptacle within the root (Fig. 447). In posterior teeth, crowns are not always necessary. In lower posteriors and upper molars, if one, or no, proximal walls are involved by caries or restorations, then an

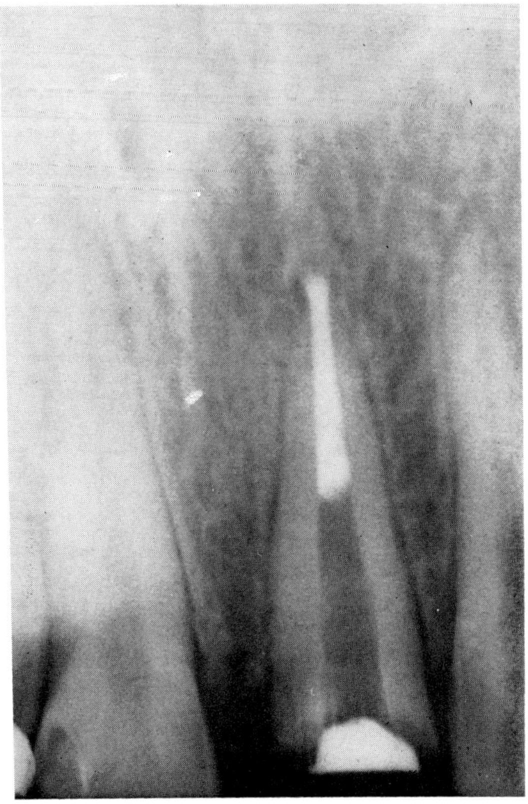

Figure 444. Post preparation in an anterior tooth.

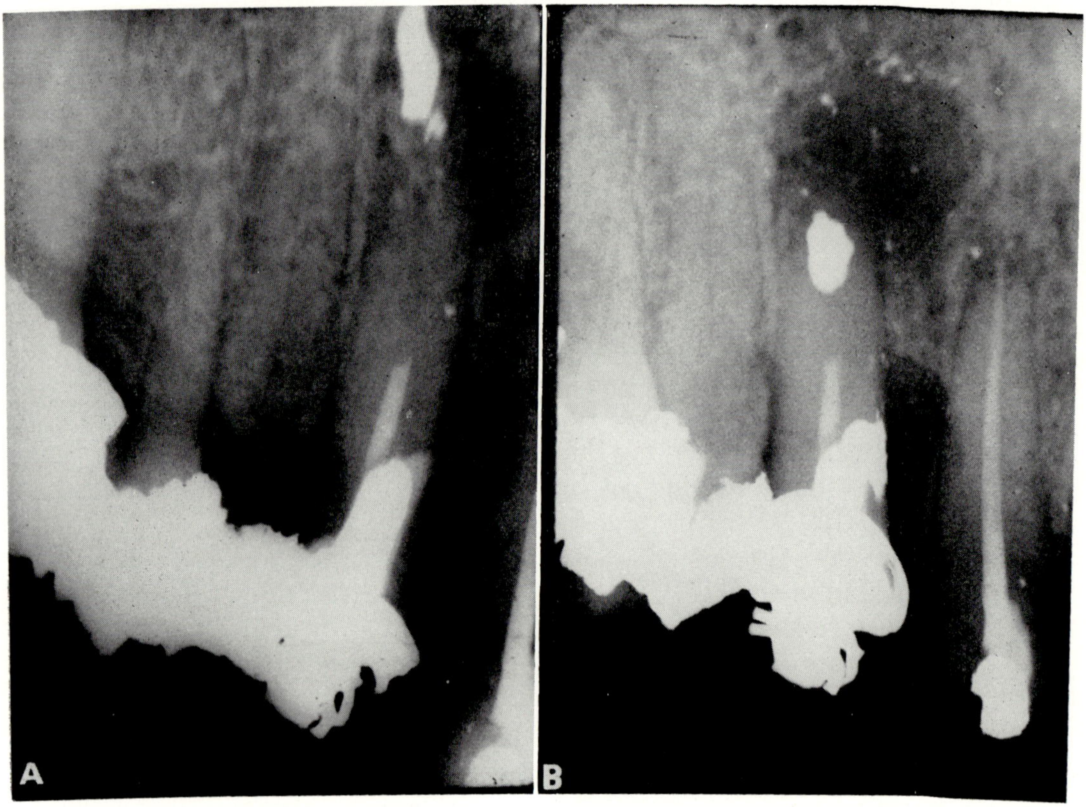

Figure 445. Post preparation causing a lateral perforation; sealed by a surgical repair with amalgam. A. Before; note rarefaction near the perforation and further up along the root. B. Immediately after periapical and lateral surgery; an amalgam seal was placed at the perforation and the apex.

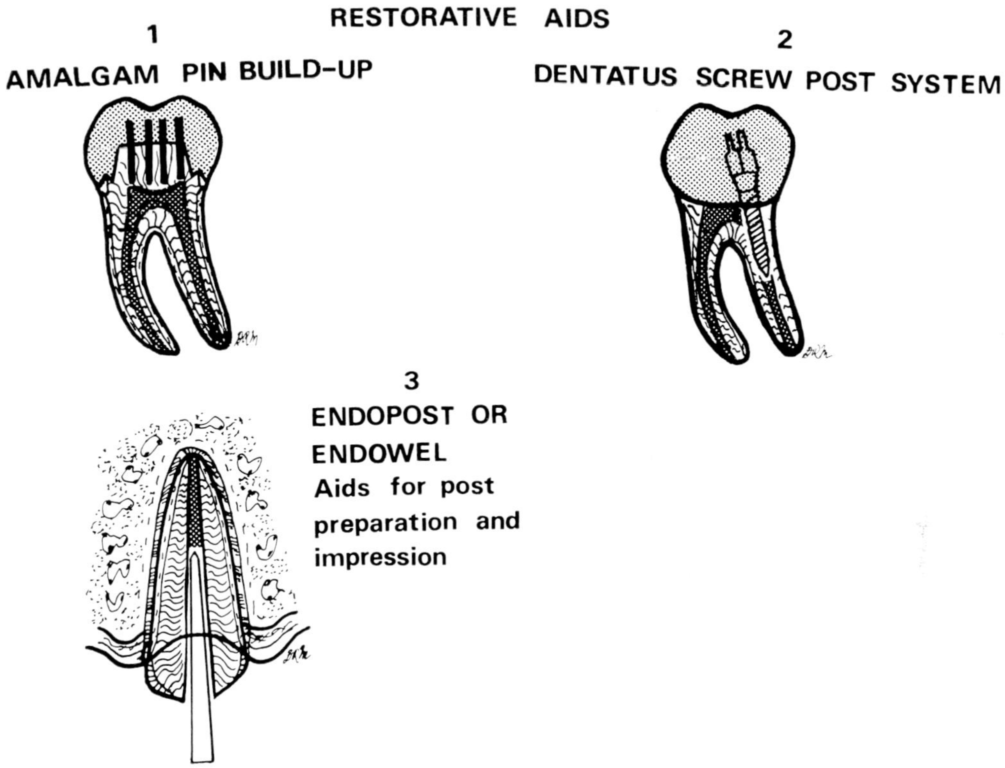

Figure 446

amalgam restoration is sufficient. If the mesial and distal marginal ridges are no longer intact, but the rest of the tooth is structurally sound, then a MOD gold onlay is a good approach (Fig. 448). It is also possible to build up these teeth by means of threaded, cemented, or friction-lock pins followed by amalgam restorations. Many clinicians have had clinical success with these methods (Figs. 446.1, 449) although the long range reliability is not yet known. There is some evidence that threaded pins may cause fractures if improperly placed; while cemented pins do not cause fractures but have less retention. Badly broken down posterior teeth and all upper premolars should have posts and crowns. The reason upper premolars should have full coverage is that the access preparation for these teeth undermines the buccal and lingual walls. If full coverage is not used, vertical fractures may occur and then extraction is often the only alternative (Fig. 442). In post preparations for posterior teeth, only the largest canal is needed for the post. This is the palatal canal of upper molars, the distal canal of lower molars, and usually the lingual canal of upper premolars. Small notches are made with a No. 35 inverted cone bur into sections

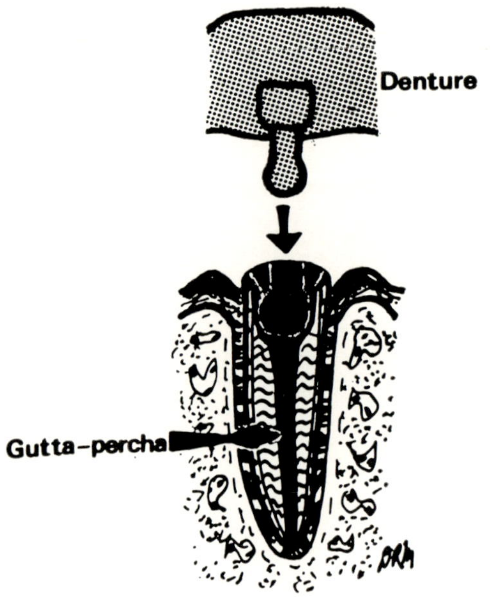

Figure 447. Zest® anchor (American Precision Metals).

of the orifice for the post preparation. Small grooves are made into the other canals (approximately 2-3 mm) for added retention (Fig. 443C).

Another adjunctive method is to use both a post and pins. An example is the Para-Post system® (Whaledent®, Inc., Fig. 450). As with anterior teeth, as much sound tooth as possible should be used as part of the crown preparation. A full core is used when no or little sound tooth remains (Fig. 443C). If possible, the crown preparation should finish on sound tooth rather than on gold.

An Endopost or serrated wire clip with a temporary crown form and cold-cure acrylic can be used to make a

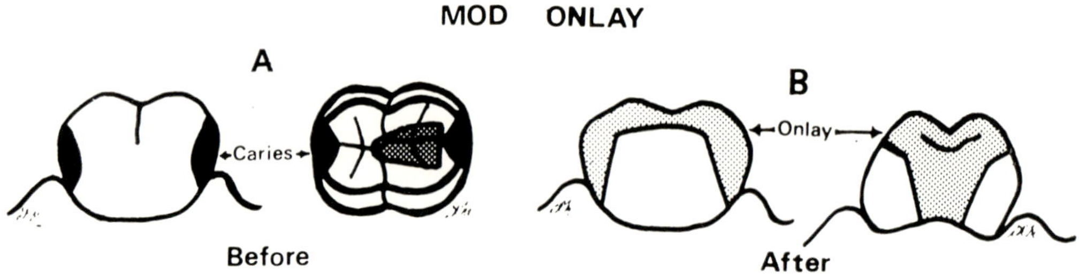

Figure 448

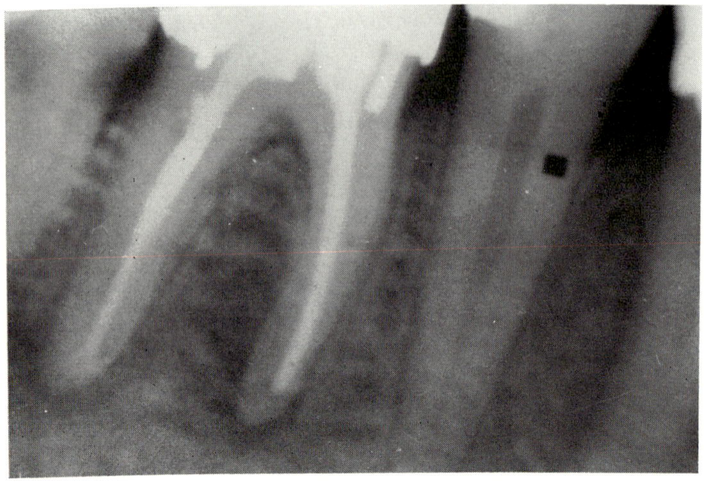

Figure 449. Lower molar restored with pins and amalgam, following endodontic therapy.

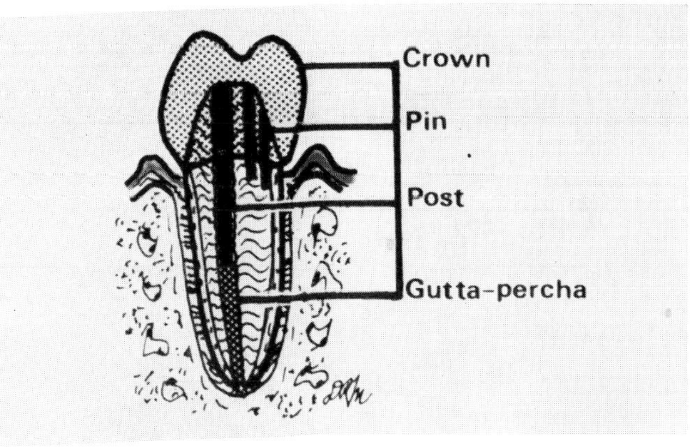

Figure 450. Para-Post system (Whaledent, Inc.).

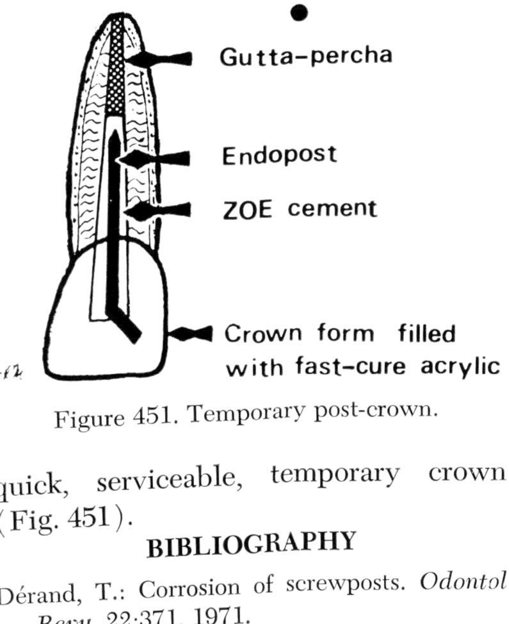

Figure 451. Temporary post-crown.

quick, serviceable, temporary crown (Fig. 451).

BIBLIOGRAPHY

Dérand, T.: Corrosion of screwposts. *Odontol Revy, 22:*371, 1971.

Frank, A. L.: Protective coronal coverage of the pulpless tooth. *JADA, 59:*895, 1959.

Helfer, A. R., Melnick, S., and Schilder, H.: Determination of the moisture content of vital and pulpless teeth. *Oral Surg, 34:*661, 1972.

Ingle, J. I.: *Endodontics.* Philadelphia, Lea & Febiger, 1965.

Lerner, T. R., Symons, B., and Schlagel, E.: Restoring and rebuilding the endodontically treated teeth. *NY State Dent J, 32:*107, 1966.

Markley, M. R.: Pin-retained and pin-reinforced amalgam. *JADA, 73:*1295, 1966.

Neagley, R. L.: The effect of dowel preparation on the apical seal of endodontically treated teeth. *Oral Surg, 28:*739, 1969.

Pameijer, C. H., and Stallard, R. E.: Effect of self-threading pins. *JADA, 85:*895, 1972.

Perel, M. L., and Muroff, F. I.: Clinical criteria for posts and cores. *J Prosthet Dent, 28:*405, 1972.

Rosenberg, P. A., and Antonoff, S. J.: Gold posts: common problems in preparation and technique for fabrication. *NY State Dent J, 37:*601, 1971.

Sapone, J.: Endodontic abutment prosthesis. *J Prosthet Dent, 29:*210, 1973.

Spasser, H. F.: Proper protection and restoration of endodontically treated teeth. *NY State Dent J, 29:*247, 1963.

Weine, F. S.: *Endodontic Therapy.* St. Louis, Mosby, 1972.

CHAPTER 15

ENDODONTIC AIDS

THIS CHAPTER is divided into sections dealing with diagnostic aids, treatment planning aids, treatment aids, recall procedures, case presentation, use of auxiliaries, and dentist-endodontist interrelationship.

DIAGNOSTIC AIDS

Treatment Periapical Pathosis

Periapical bone breakdown can occur or increase during treatment of an endodontic case. This is the result of inflammatory products released during the treatment and is not indicative of a failure. Quite often the *area* heals within a few months after the treatment is completed (Fig. 452).

Fiber Optics

With the use of fiber optics illumination, it is possible to look up (or down) a root canal. This may help in detecting obstructions, dilacerations, broken instruments, etc. (Fig. 129).

Paresthesia

In rare cases, after the pulp has been removed, the patient may develop a paresthesia that is located in the gingiva and/or alveolar mucosa of the involved tooth. This rarely lasts more than a few days. It probably results from injury to the alveolar nerves. Overfilling of a

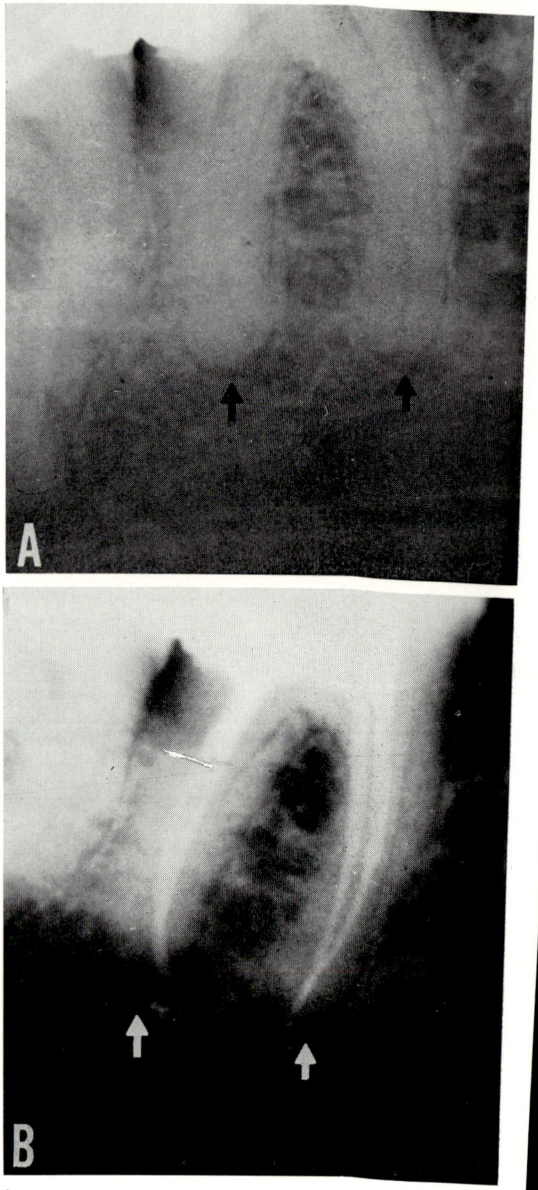

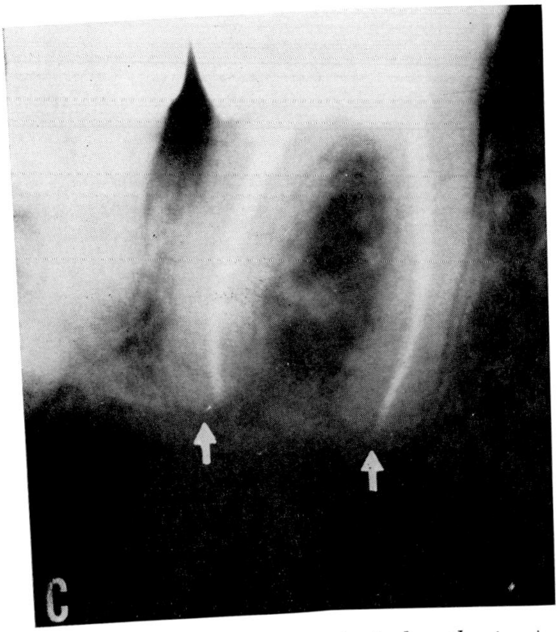

Figure 452. Treatment periapical pathosis. A. Before; slight periapical areas of rarefaction are present. B. Immediately after obturation, periapical *areas* have enlarged; also notice the unintentional gutta-percha overfill. C. Two years later; the excess gutta-percha has been absorbed, and the periapical *areas* have healed.

lower molar that lies in proximity to the inferior alveolar nerve can result in the development of a paresthesia of the involved side up to the lip. It may last for several months (Fig. 453). The inflammatory response causes pressure on the nerve bundle that probably results in injury to the nerve. If the paresthesia does not subside, then it is necessary to perform an apicoectomy (see Chapter 10). If an apicoectomy is not possible, then the tooth must be extracted and if possible the apex could be cut off for several millimeters. Then a retrograde amalgam can be placed and the tooth replanted (see Chapter 12). If no further injury occurs to the nerve during either of the latter two procedures, then the paresthesia should gradually disappear. If not, it may persist for a year or longer.

TREATMENT PLANNING AIDS

Doubtful Multirooted Cases

In doubtful multirooted cases, treat the most difficult canal first. If it is successful, continue the case; if not, do periapical surgery, intentional replantation, or extraction. In upper molars, if the palatal root can be treated nonsurgically, then if the buccal roots cannot be treated nonsurgically, it is still feasible to treat them surgically (Figs. 308, 411, 413). Palatal periapical surgery is much more difficult (Fig. 415).

Apical Blockage

In cases where the apical portion of the canal is either very curved, very fine, or partially blocked, a gutta-percha-chloropercha diffusion technique can be used. After the canal is instrumented, the master cone is inserted into the canal as far as it can go. The excess past the orifice is removed with heat. With an irrigating syringe, chloroform is deposited into the chamber. Using a file with a pumping motion the mass is softened and pushed apically. This process (chloroform-deposition and pumping) is continued until a periapical radiograph reveals that the apical canal appears to be sealed. Then, with the use of absorbent points, the canal is dried and lateral condensation with gutta-percha is completed (Fig. 288).

Retreatments

The first decision on retreatments is whether to retreat. The second decision

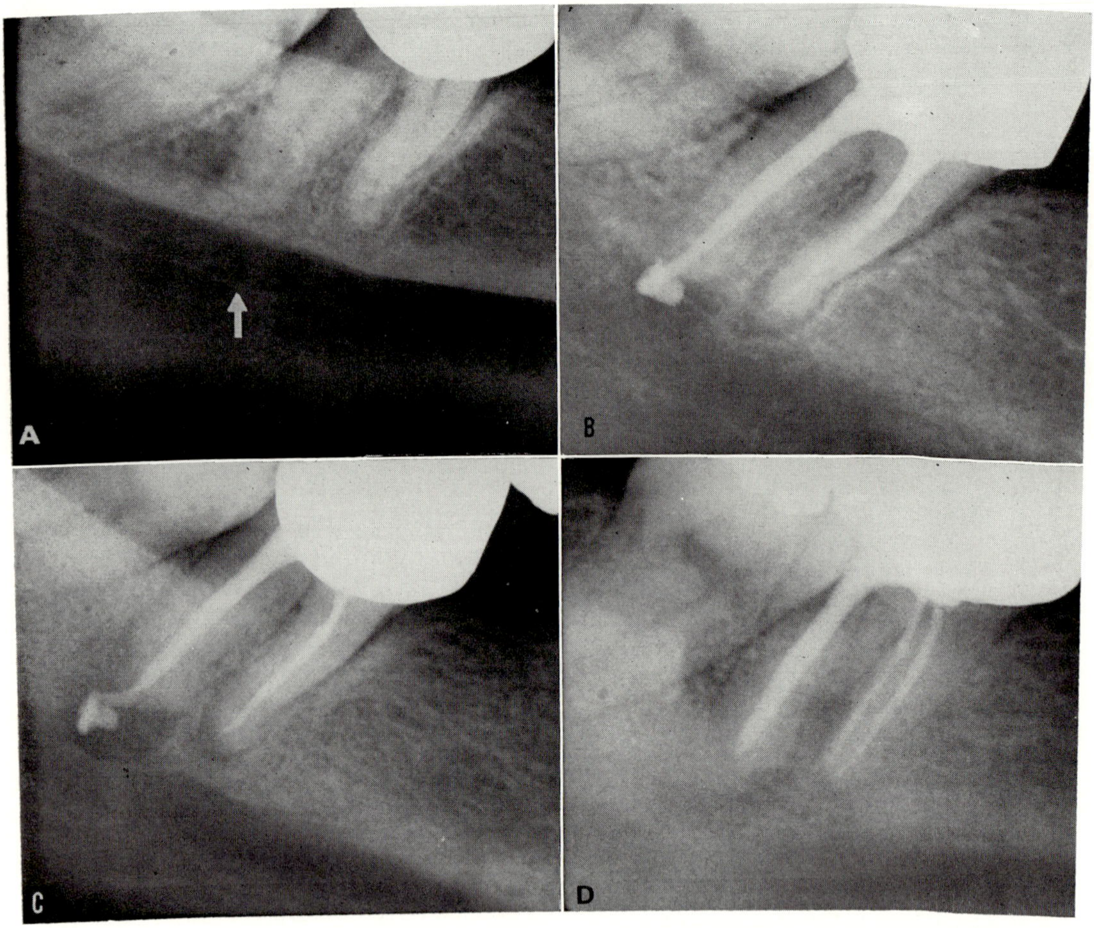

Figure 453. Deleterious result of overfilling, and the treatment of the mal-effect. A. Lower molar requiring endodontic therapy; note the proximity of the inferior alveolar canal (arrow). B. After obturation with gutta-percha-chloropercha, inadvertently a *puff* went beyond the apex. Undoubtedly this case was overinstrumented, which is not indicated for a vital case. However, because of the patient's extreme gagging it was not possible to take treatment radiographs with the rubber dam in position. C. Periapical area of pathosis developed soon afterward causing an inflammation and deflection of the inferior alveolar canal with a resultant paresthesia; this is one example when overfilling, even with gutta-percha, is definitely detrimental. D. Approximately one year after an apicoectomy (performed at a severe oblique angle from above to avoid impingement on the inferior alveolar canal), periapical healing is evident. Paresthesia stopped soon after the surgery.

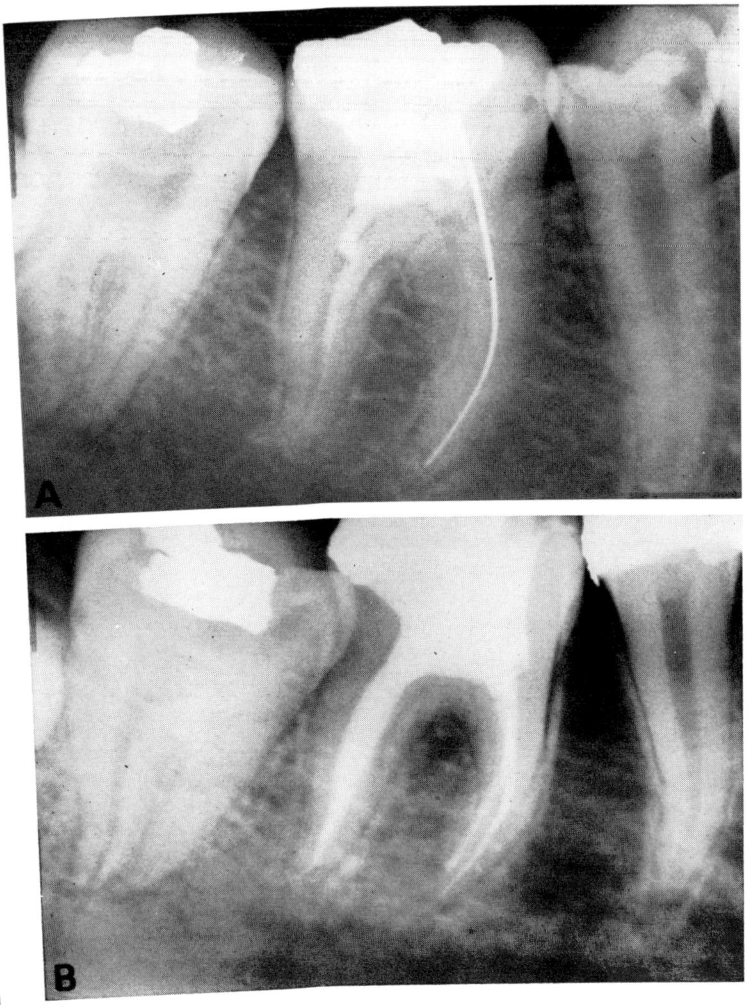

Figure 454. Retreatment of a poorly obturated root canal. A. Canals had been *filled* with a silver cone and gutta-percha; patient had pain. B. Canals reinstrumented and obturated with gutta-percha-chloropercha; tooth is symptomless.

is should the retreatment be nonsurgical or surgical. If the previous root canal filling appears to be deficient (incomplete obturation, failure to fill lateral or accessory canals, perforation) and the filling can be removed or bypassed, then nonsurgical endodontic therapy should be done (Figs. 454-456). If the filling cannot be removed or bypassed, if there is a perforation or root fracture, or if there is an overfilling with untoward clinical manifestations, then periapical surgery should be done (Figs. 328, 332, 337, 338, 340, 407, 412, 457, 458). If there is a perforation or lateral canal, that opens onto the lingual (or palatal) surface, then retreatment cannot be done. Cases of possible treatment of vertical fracture are described in a later section. If the tooth becomes nonrestorable, then retreatment is not possible (Fig. 440).

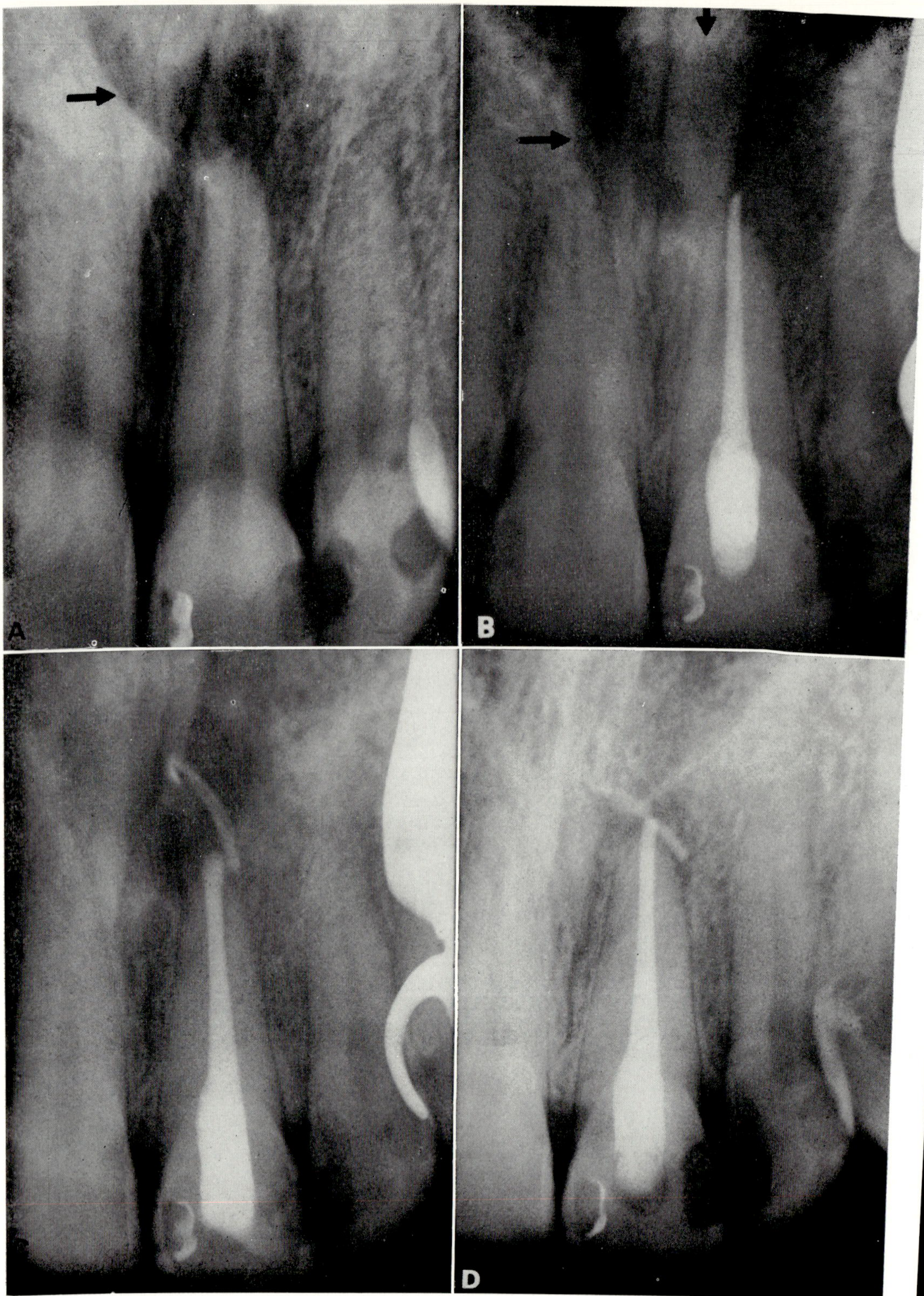

Figure 455. Retreatment; nonsurgical. A. Upper right central incisor has a large periapical area of pathosis (arrow). B. One year after obturation with gutta-percha and root canal cement, periapical *area* had enlarged; root canal filling was overextended, but poorly obturated. C. Retreatment; canal was reinstrumented and obturated with gutta-percha-chloropercha; some excess was extruded beyond the apex. D. Over one year later; excess gutta-percha is being absorbed and periapical repair is almost complete.

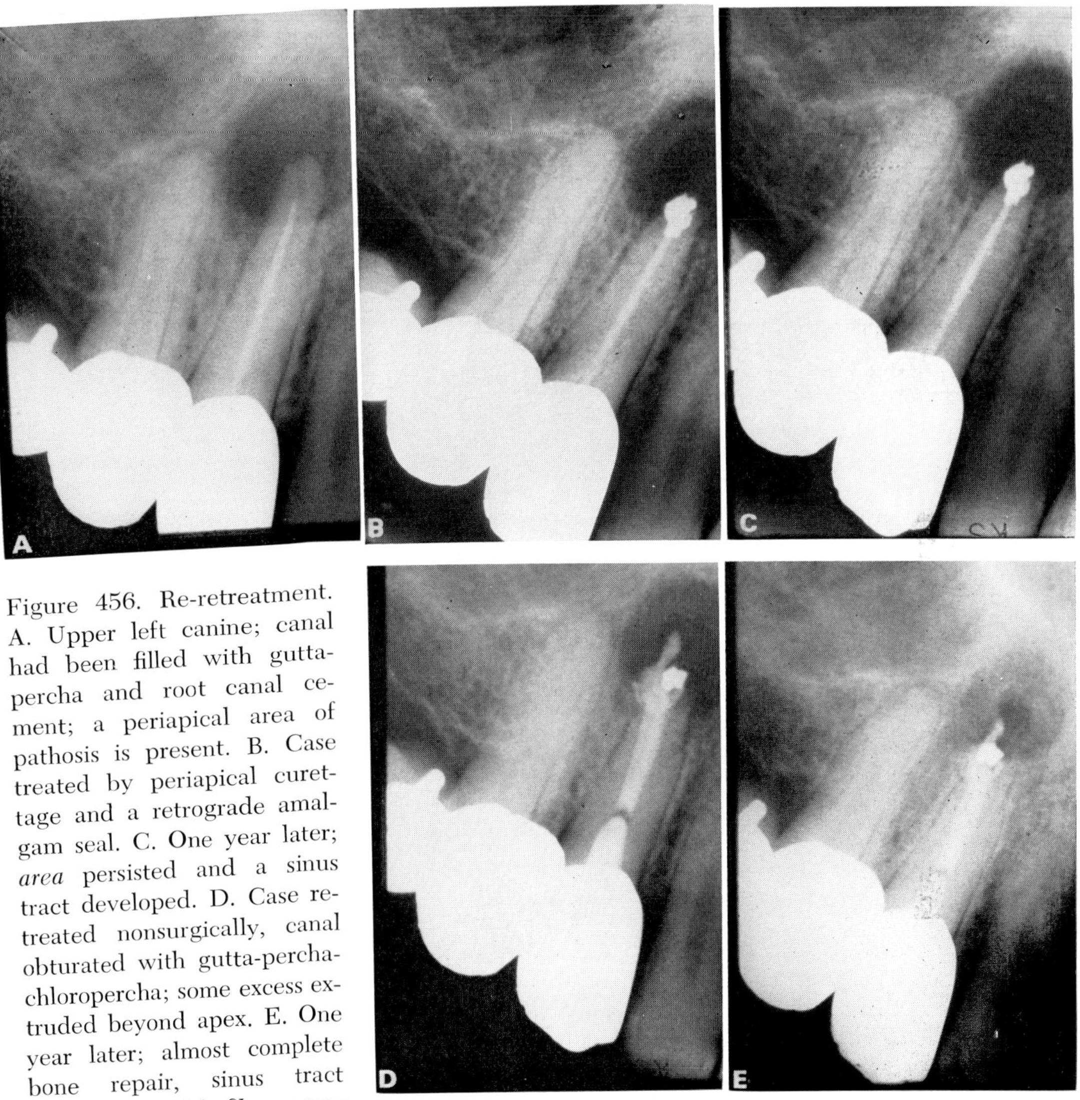

Figure 456. Re-retreatment. A. Upper left canine; canal had been filled with gutta-percha and root canal cement; a periapical area of pathosis is present. B. Case treated by periapical curettage and a retrograde amalgam seal. C. One year later; *area* persisted and a sinus tract developed. D. Case retreated nonsurgically, canal obturated with gutta-percha-chloropercha; some excess extruded beyond apex. E. One year later; almost complete bone repair, sinus tract healed, a possible fibrous scar is present (black area in center of periapical region). From D. R. Morse, "The Management of Endodontic Problem Cases," *JDA South Africa*, 27:387, 1972.)

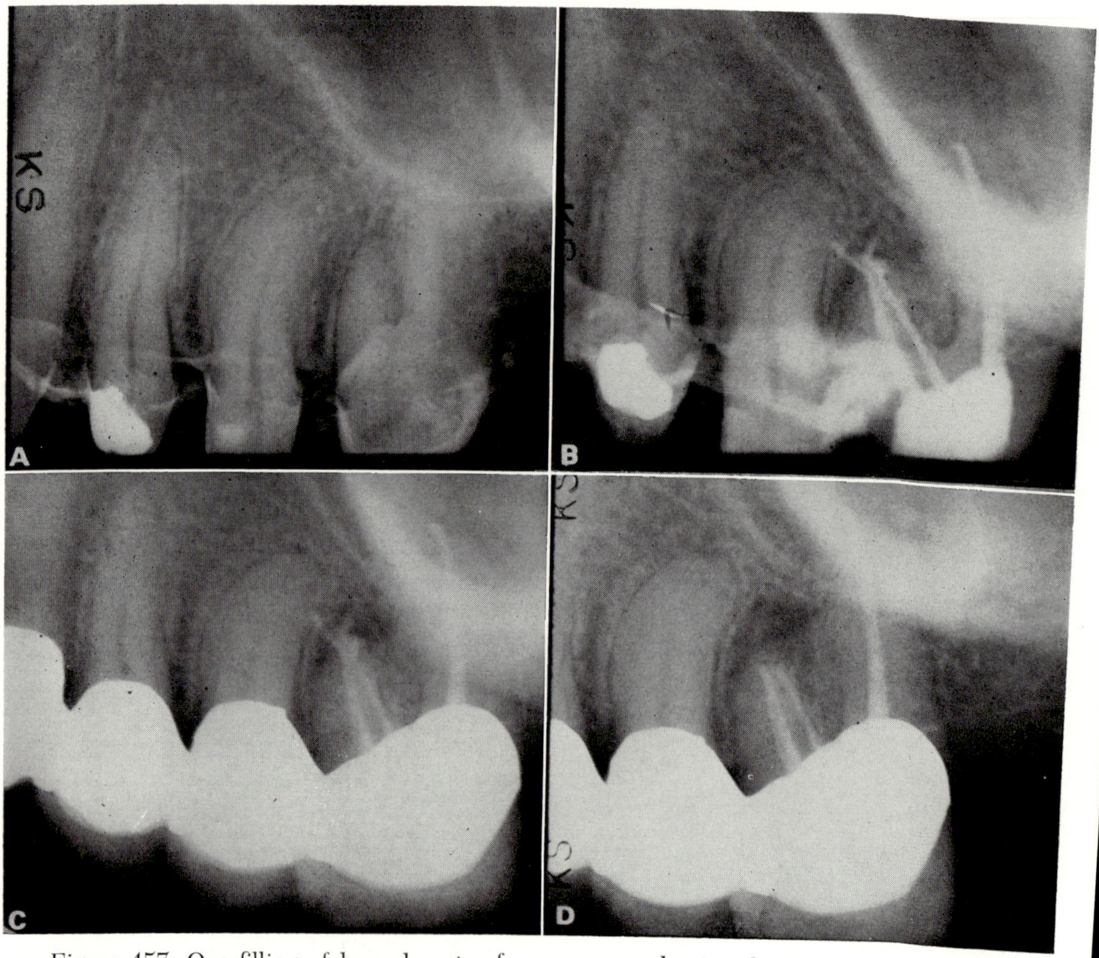

Figure 457. Overfilling of buccal roots of an upper molar in which fenestrations were present and pain developed; treatment was apicoectomy. A. Upper molar required endodontic therapy. B. Canals obturated with gutta-percha-chloropercha; excess went beyond the apex; extreme care must be used in instrumenting and obturating in upper molars; because of the superimposition of the maxillary sinus and zygoma it may be difficult to obtain accurate root canal measurements. C. A few months later, patient had a fixed bridge in position, and still had pain and sensitivity to apical palpation on the buccal roots. D. Apicoectomies were performed on the buccal roots; there were fenestrations present and the excess gutta-percha had been expressed into the alveolar mucosa rather than into the bone; this was apparently the cause of the pain as after the removal of the excess, the pain disappeared.

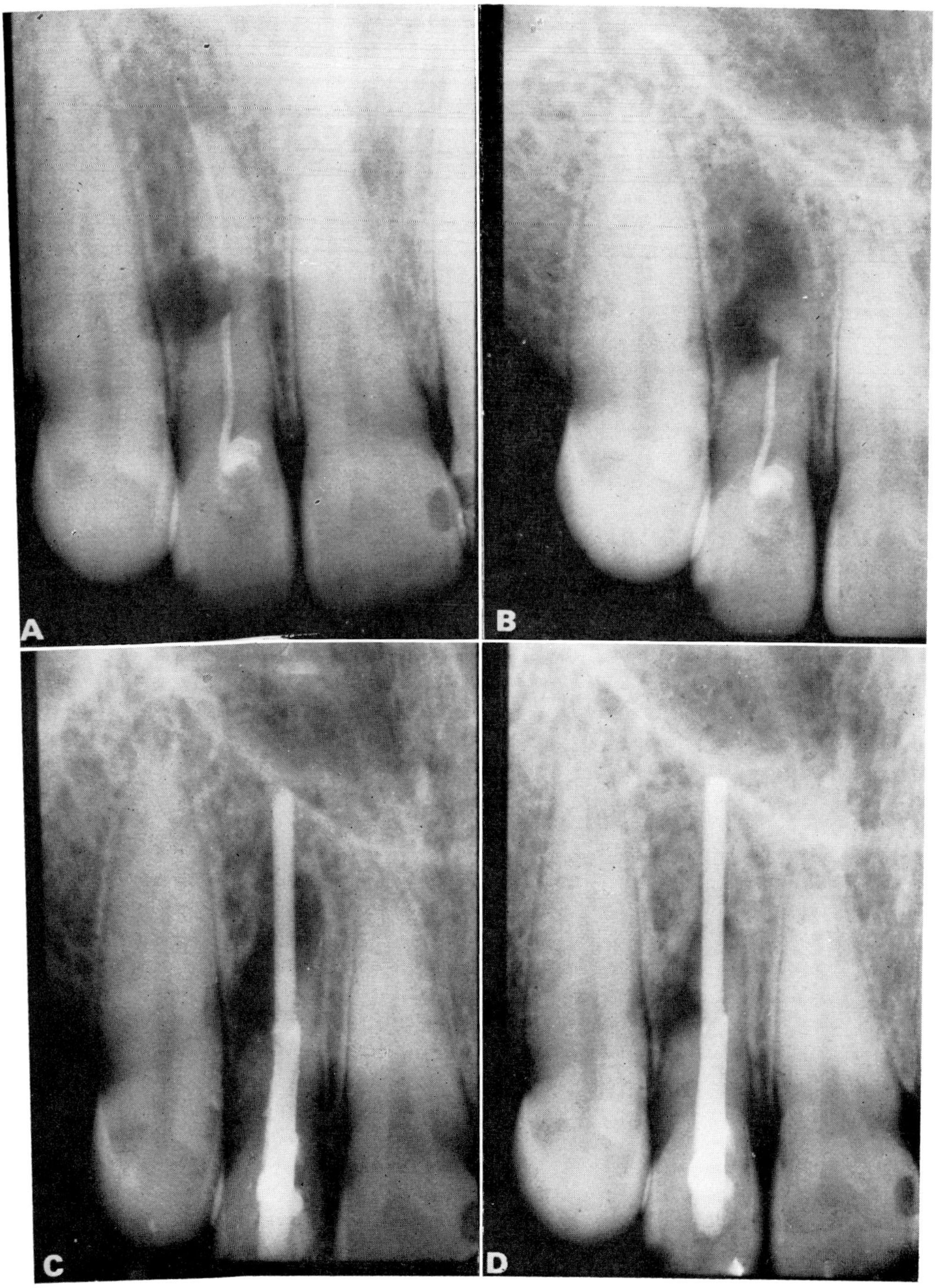

Figure 458. Retreatment with the use of an endodontic implant. A. Upper left lateral incisor; canal had been *filled* with a single gutta-percha cone, and an *apicoectomy* had been performed midway through the root. B. Apical region removed preserving the palatal aspect of the root. C. Endodontic implant cemented in place. D. Over six months later, tooth is firm; there is evidence of periapical repair. (From D. R. Morse, "The Management of Endodontic Problem Cases," *JDA South Africa,* 27:387, 1972.)

Cases of Dens Invaginatus (Dens in Dente)

Almost invariably these cases require periapical surgery and retroseals, because of the difficulty to instrument the canals from the lingual approach (Fig. 221).

Hypercementosis

In cases of hypercementosis, it is very difficult to see where the apex is located on the radiograph. The canal should be obturated as far as it goes without using excessive force, as quite often the canal ends short of the root apex (Fig. 395).

Management of Cases with Full Coverage

In order to drill through full crowns, the practitioner should use a new No. 35 inverted cone bur in an ultra-high speed contra-angle until dentin is reached. Then he (or she) should switch to a No. 701 bur. There are times when it is not possible to detect the long axis of the root(s) in crowned teeth with the rubber dam in position. This can occur when the crown is not in the same relationship to the root as the natural crown was. In these instances, it may be necessary not to use the rubber dam as the access preparation is made, in order to observe the root (to determine the long axis). See Figure 459A and B. Also in cases where it is difficult to locate the orifices, an examination of the cervical root contour gives an indication of where to look for the canal orifices (Fig. 459C). A good means of determining the contour of the natural

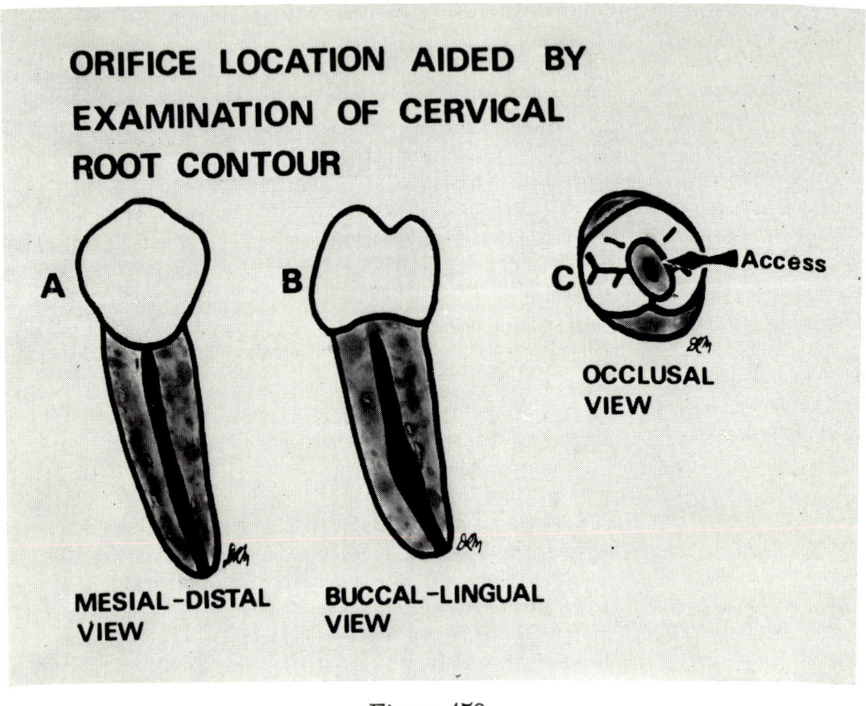

Figure 459

crown is to have available a model of the tooth before the crown (or bridge) was made. If these other methods fail, it may be necessary to remove the crown or bridge in order to be able to gain access into the canals. Some methods to aid in bridge removal are (1) have the patient bite on a tongue blade placed over the bridge; this may help loosen it; (2) use a crown remover at the interproximal surfaces and crown margins (if there is a catch present); and (3) place orthodontic 050 wire through the interproximal surfaces, twist it with a hemostat, and then elevate at each joint.

TREATMENT AIDS

Air in the Root Canal

Never blow air into a root canal. An air embolism can result. In this connection, if using alternating hydrogen peroxide and sodium hypochlorite as root canal irrigants, never use hydrogen peroxide as the last rinse. Oxygen can be released which also could conceivably result in an air embolism.

Treatment Acute Apical Periodontitis

For the patient who develops an acute apical periodontitis (acute pericementitis) during endodontic treatment, the following regimen is used. No local anesthesia is given but nitrous oxide-oxygen relative analgesia is used. This decreases the pain, but not to the extent that the patient cannot tell whether the condition is improving or not. The rubber dam is placed on the appropriate tooth. The temporary restoration is removed. Any fluid or gases that are present are evacuated or allowed to escape. The tooth is left open for five to ten minutes and is taken completely out of occlusion. A small pellet with either eugenol or Cresatin is then placed in the chamber, and the tooth is sealed with ZOE or Cavit. A corticosteroid paste can also be used if there are no systemic contraindications. Usually before the tooth is sealed, the pain has greatly diminished or stopped completely.

Separate or Joined Canals?

In order to determine whether two canals are separate or join each other, the following procedure is done. A file is placed into the first canal and the measurement is recorded. The file is removed and then placed into the second canal and the measurement is also recorded. If the two measurements are identical, this is a clue that there is only one apex. However, it is not unusual for two canals in the same tooth to have identical measurements. The next step is to take another file and place it into the first canal (with the original file remaining in the second canal). The file from the first canal is then removed and measured. If there is just one apex the measurement should be less than the first measurement in that canal (when no instrument was in the second canal; (Fig. 460). A final verification is to take two radiographs from different mesial-distal angulations. This would show in both X-rays that the two canals join each other. This procedure is especially helpful for lower anteriors and premolars where different mesio-distal angulations can help determine whether one or two canals are present.

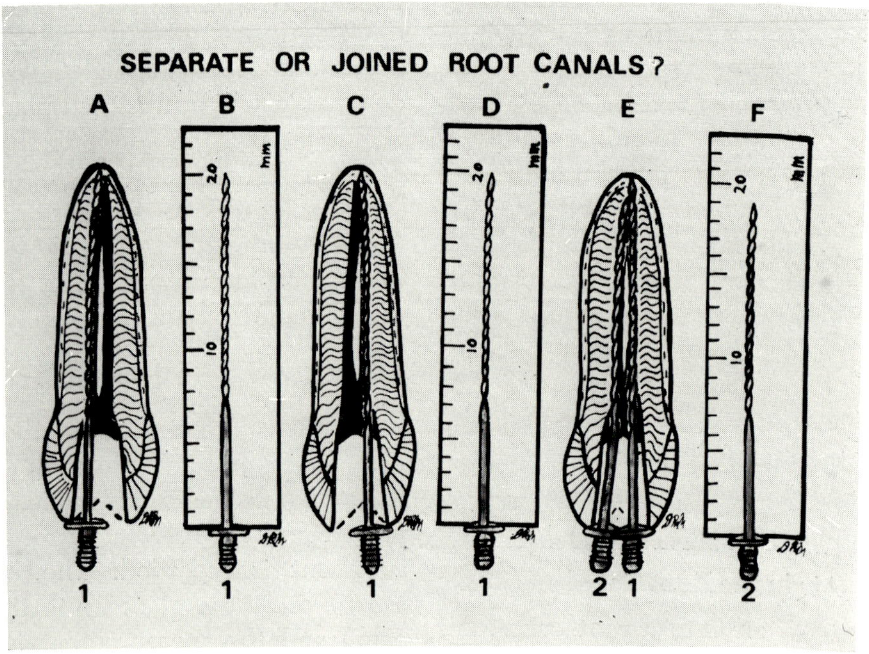

Figure 460

Nonhealing Sinus Tract or Fistula

Sinus tracts or fistulas almost always heal after nonsurgical endodontic therapy is successfully performed. In the rare case when the tract is lined by epithelium, then cauterization of the tract may be necessary. On an endodontic explorer, trichloroacetic acid is placed. A two by two gauze is held beneath the explorer as it is brought carefully towards the tract. The explorer is then inserted through the tract and immediately a white reaction is seen. This is repeated a couple of times, with care taken not to drop any of the highly caustic acid on the gingiva. Within a week the tract should heal. If it does not, then something is wrong with the endodontic therapy. There may be a defective apical seal, a patent lateral canal, or a root fracture may be present.

Treatment of Vertical Root Fractures

Generally speaking when vertical fractures occur, the tooth must be extracted. However, it is worth the probability of failure to try the following treatment for those patients who desperately want to try and retain their teeth. A full flap is made, and the root is exposed. Usually there is no bone over the labial surface. The fractured portion of the root is removed. With a No. 35 inverted cone bur, a trough is cut in the exposed root canal for the entire length of the canal. Undercuts are made in the most incisal and apical portions (Fig. 275M). Amalgam is condensed into the prepared trough and the flap is sutured. I have tried this procedure in four vertical root fracture cases, and have had a limited success. In

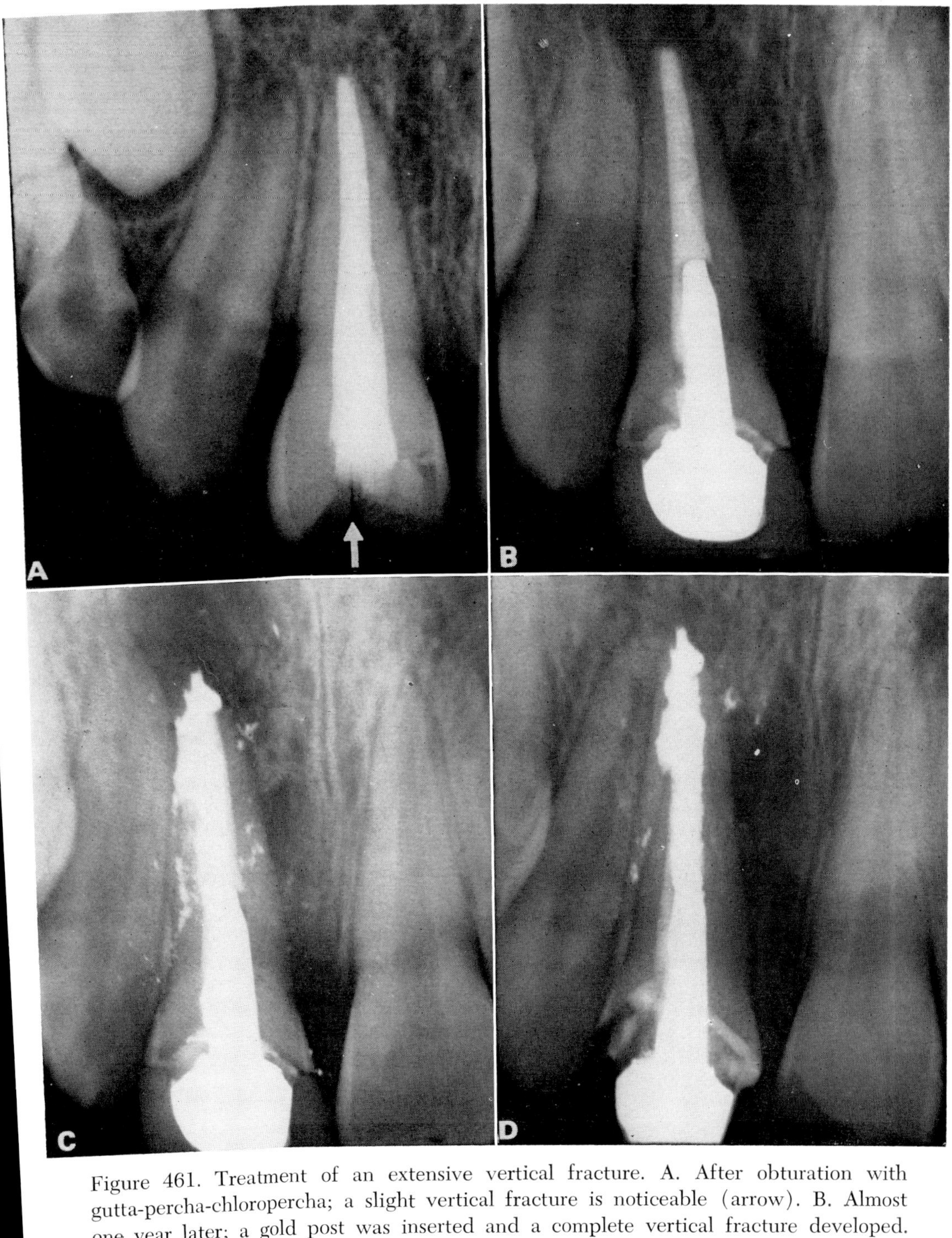

Figure 461. Treatment of an extensive vertical fracture. A. After obturation with gutta-percha-chloropercha; a slight vertical fracture is noticeable (arrow). B. Almost one year later; a gold post was inserted and a complete vertical fracture developed. C. The entire labial fractured surface was removed; a trough was prepared and amalgam was condensed into it. D. Four years later, the tooth was firm and symptomless; however, it refractured soon afterward and had to be extracted. Also notice that interproximal bone loss had occurred on the mesial.

one case, the tooth lasted for five years but then it refractured and had to be extracted (Fig. 461). In a second case in which the fracture was not as extensive, the tooth apparently is completely successful (Fig. 337). In the other two cases, failure occurred within two months. Hence, this is only a last chance procedure with 50 percent or less probability of success.

Orifice Location

The use of a drop of iodine tincture (or other disclosing solution) in the chamber is helpful. A dark spot indicates where the orifice is most likely located. Transillumination with fiber optics aids in orifice location (Fig. 129). At times it may be necessary to remove an entire cusp (decuspation) in order to gain access to the orifice. In rare cases, especially when crowns are in position and there is no indication of the presence of a pulp chamber, it may be necessary to remove the entire crown in order to find the root canal orifices.

Orifice Widening

The use of an orifice widener is helpful in facilitating subsequent instrumentation and obturation (Fig. 462B). A gates glidden drill can also be used for orifice widening (Fig. 462C), as

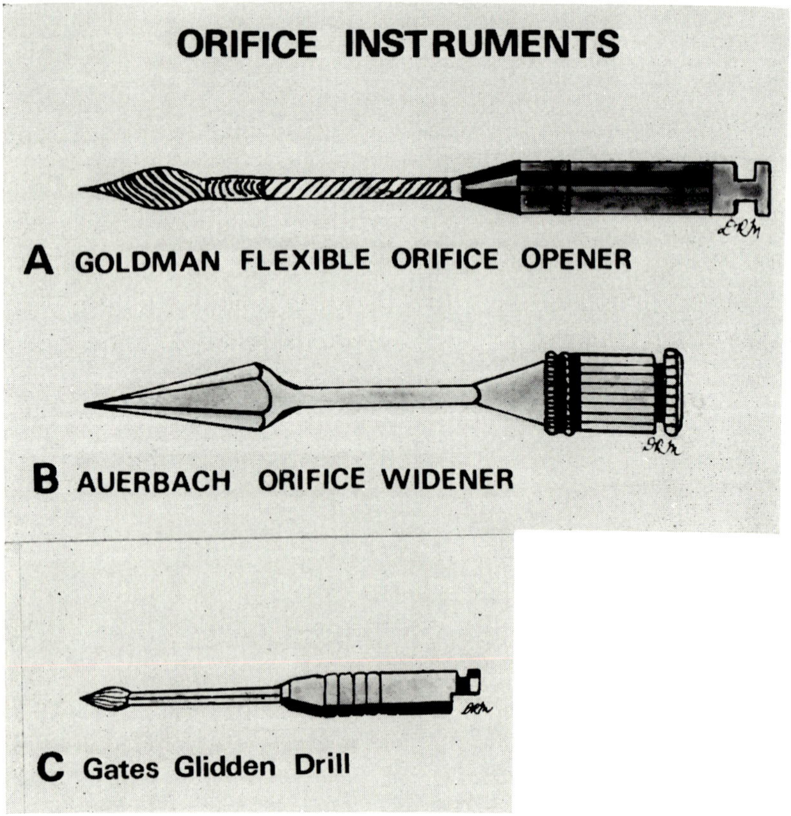

Figure 462

well as a Goldman orifice opener® (Medidenta®; Fig. 462A).

Apex Location

The best method of apex location is the use of an instrument in a root canal, followed by a periapical radiograph. However, there are times when the taking of a radiograph presents a problem (e.g. difficulty to take an x-ray with rubber dam in position because of small mouth, difficulty of opening, or gagging patient) (Figs. 453, 457). In these cases, there are other possible methods of apex determination. Three methods rely on going past the apex and are therefore not favored because of the detrimental effects of post-apical penetration. The first is to rely on the patient's subjective symptoms of pain. This is not reliable because there can be vital tissue remaining in the canal and the patient can be responding to that. Also, patients vary in their response, with some patients feeling no pain whatsoever when the apex is penetrated. A second method is the feel of the apical constriction by the operator. Some practitioners develop an uncanny perception with their fingertips and can detect when they reach the apex in a large majority of cases. However, this method is too subjective and cannot be routinely employed. A third method is the detection of bleeding on a paper point placed within the canal. This can be fairly accurate but it also has drawbacks. One is, if the pulp has not been completely removed, then bleeding can occur from pulpal blood vessels. A second problem results from capillary action. The absorbent point must not remain in the canal too long or the bleeding will go up the point for a short distance and the apex cannot be accurately estimated. A third deficiency in this method is that in pulpless teeth with periapical lesions, there may be capillaries present in the lesion at a distance from the apex. Therefore, the bleeding that is found on the absorbent point would not represent the apex.

Another method is based on estimation of average measurements of the roots involved as compared to the pretreatment radiograph. This method has two drawbacks. One is that average measurements might not be reliable for the particular case at hand. The second problem is that unless the radiograph is an exact replication of the true root measurement, or can be accurately estimated (see Chapter 1, section on treatment periapical radiographs) then considerable error in length is possible.

Recently, two new methods of apex location have come into vogue; these are the use of electronic measurements (Endometer®; Dent-O-Tronics®) and sonic measurements (Sono-Explorer; Electrodent). The Endometer is an electronic instrument that has a dial that is marked from 0 to 50 (Fig. 463). It is calibrated to respond to the electro-potential of the periodontal ligament. According to the manufacturer, as the file or reamer is placed within the root canal, the instrument reading increases until the periodontal ligament is reached. When that point occurs, the reading registers 40. Penetration past the apex results in a reading over 40. It is not clear what occurs in a pulpless tooth with periapical pathosis in which

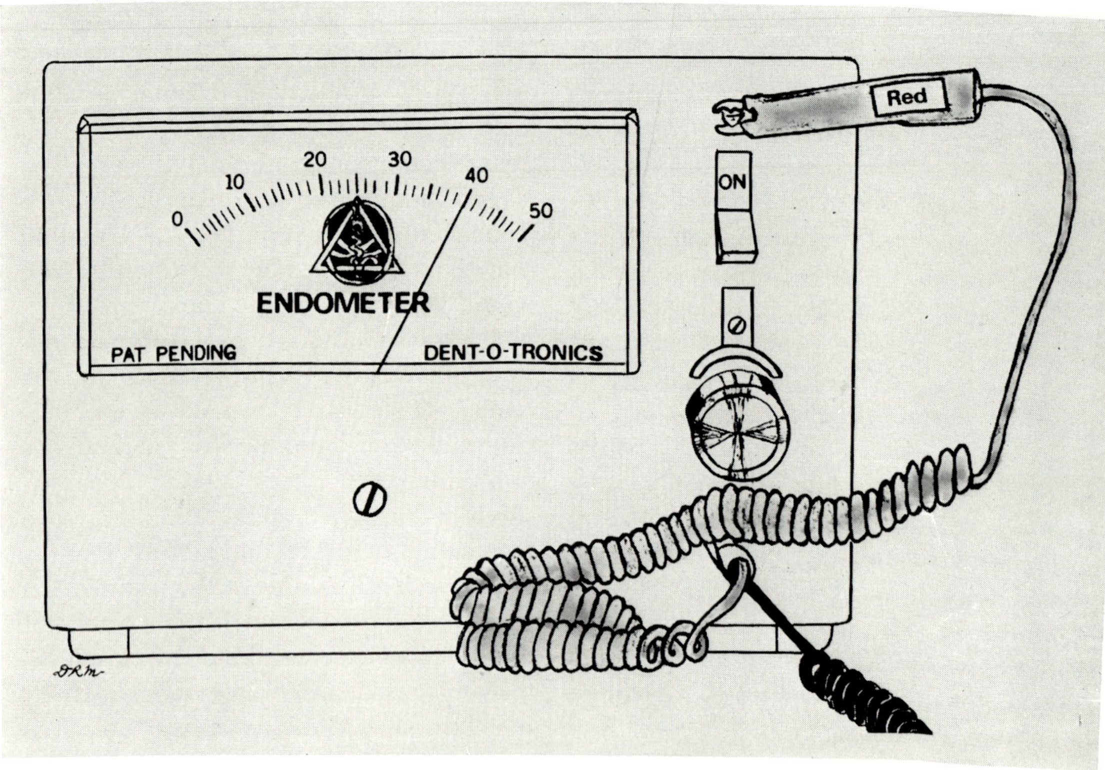

Figure 463. Endometer (Dent-O-Tronics).

Figure 464. Sono-Explorer (Electrodent).

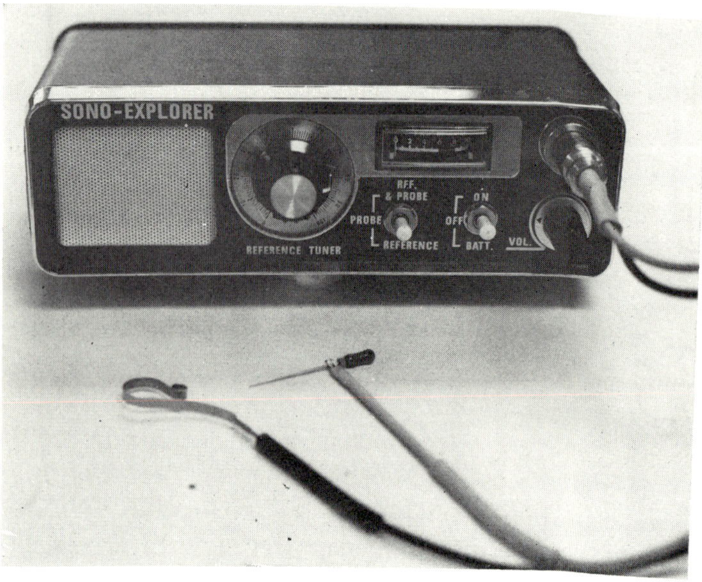

there is no intact apical periodontal ligament.

The Sono-Explorer works on sound measurements (Fig. 464). There are two separate sounds that are heard as the root canal is penetrated. Once the apex is reached, the two sounds are supposed to synchronize into one. Also, in this instrument, it is not definite how pulpless teeth with periapical areas respond. Currently, both of these instruments are undergoing clinical research (Sono-Explorer is being tested at Temple University School of Dentistry), and they may prove to be important adjuncts to clinical endodontic practice.

Marsupialization Procedure for Reduction of a Large Cyst*

Polyvinyl tubing of 0.184 inch diameter (available from medical supply houses) is autoclaved and cut into sections of approximately 20 mm. Local anesthesia is used. A small incision is made below the muco-buccal fold, and the mucoperiosteum is retracted (Fig. 324A). A small opening is made through the bone to accommodate the tubing (Fig. 324B). The fluid from the area is aspirated and then irrigation is done with sterile normal saline (Fig. 324C). The precut tube is inserted into the opening until it just touches the base of the periapical lesion. The portion of the tube that protrudes out of the opening is cut off so that it is about 2 mm beyond the alveolar mucosa (Fig. 324D, E). The exposed margins should not be left irregular or else gingival irritation will occur. The patient is given a plastic irrigation syringe and told to irrigate through the opening with saline solution several times a day (Fig. 324F). After one week, the patient returns and the tube is checked for patency and to see that the margins are not irritating to the soft tissues. The patient is shown how to reinsert the tube in case it comes out. At intervals of two to four weeks, the tube is reduced as the lesion resolves (Fig. 324G). Once drainage no longer is apparent, the tube is removed and nonsurgical endodontic therapy is performed (Fig. 324H).

* This discussion is based on a recent technique described by Dr. J. B. Freedland, of Charlotte, North Carolina.

Warm Anesthetic Cartridges

A method to warm anesthetic cartridges before injection (and make them less irritating to tissues) is to place

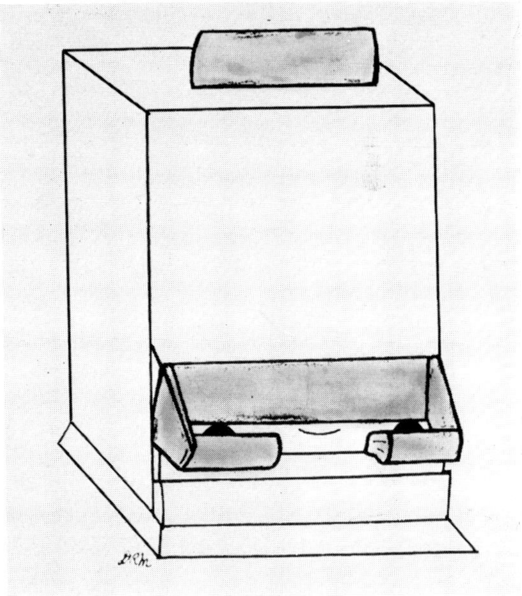

Figure 465. Premier carpule warmer and dispenser.

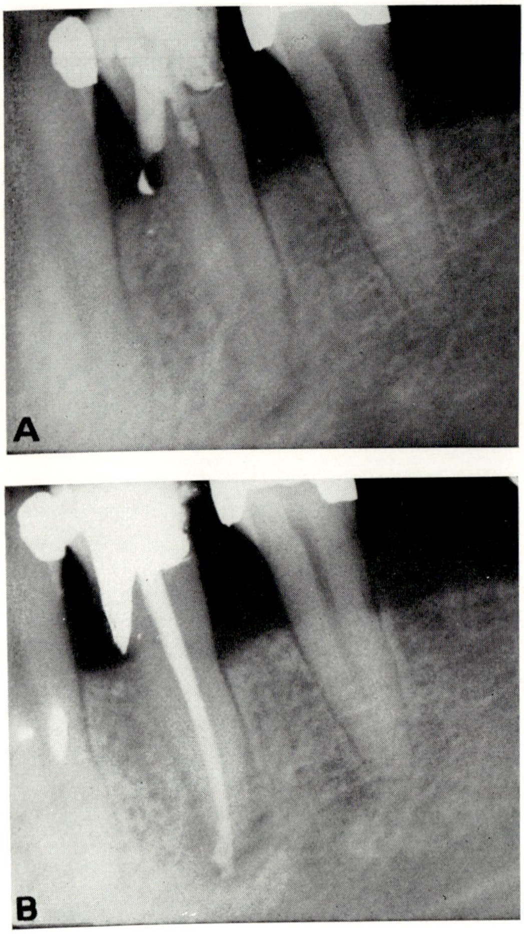

Figure 466. Nonsurgical treatment of a perforation in the occlusal third. A. Perforation occurred as a result of improper access. B. Perforation sealed with amalgam from within the chamber aided by the use of a band and a wedge placed interproximally.

them in an incubator set for 37°C for about ten minutes. Therefore, don't throw out that incubator yet; it still may have a use in endodontics. Also a carpule warmer can be used (Fig. 465). Epinephrine breaks down with excessive heat; so maintain the time and temperature as indicated above.

Treating Perforations and Internal Resorption Cases

These cases should first be treated by nonsurgical endodontic therapy. If that treatment is not successful, then surgical endodontic therapy should be attempted. The diagnosis of a perforation is made by these means. First there is evidence of considerable bleeding from the chamber after the removal of an explorer, bur, or a root canal instrument. Secondly, when a file or reamer is placed in the opening, it does not feel snug within *the canal* but it appears loose. If it were a true canal, depending upon the size of the canal and the size of the instrument used, it should feel relatively tight. Obvious evidence of a perforation is bleeding from the pulp chamber in a pulpless tooth. To confirm a perforation, a file or reamer is placed in the apparent canal and a radiograph is taken. If the x-ray image shows the instrument coming off at an angle rather than going into a canal, then it is definite that a perforation has occurred.

When a perforation is evident, the treatment is largely governed by the location of the perforation. A perforation in the occlusal third can often be sealed by amalgam inserted through the access opening (Fig. 466). If the perforation is in the apical third of the tooth, it is often possible to seal both the perforation and the apex by the use of the gutta-percha-chloropercha technique (see apical blockage section in this chapter). Typical cases are shown in Figure 467. If the perforation cannot be sealed by this method, then a

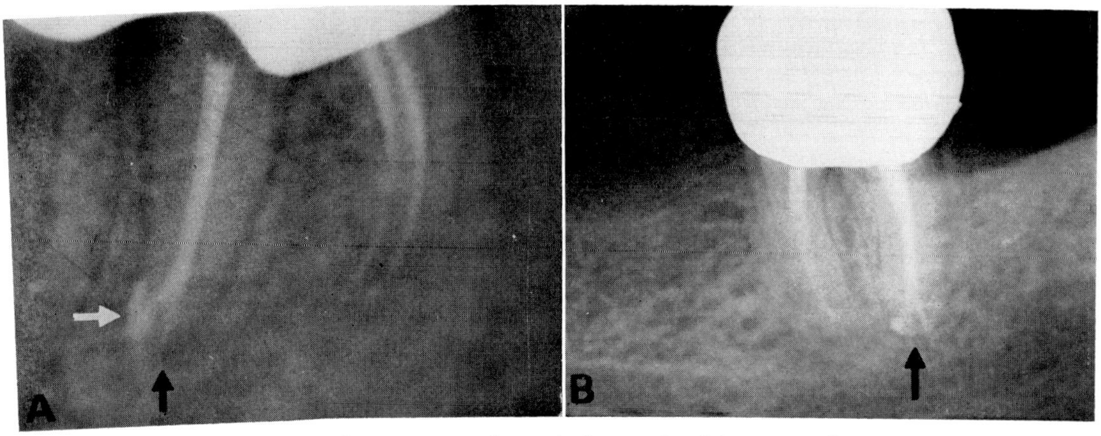

Figure 467. Sealing perforations in the apical one-third by a condensation technique using gutta-percha-chloropercha. A. White arrow indicates main canal sealed; black arrow indicates probable performation apparently sealed with gutta-percha. B. One of these branches (arrow) may be a perforation that is apparently sealed with gutta-percha. (From D. R. Morse, "The Management of Endodontic Problem Cases," *JDA South Africa,* 27:387, 1972.)

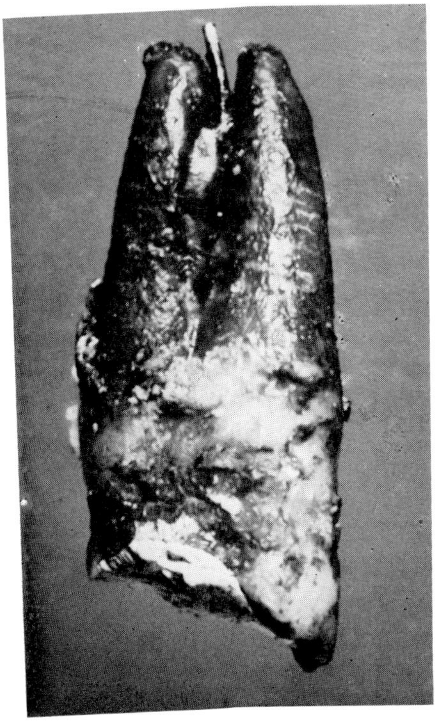

Figure 468. Extraction of an upper premolar because of perforation into the furca area by a silver cone which could not be removed; an x-ray of this tooth from a normal M-D angulation would show that the silver cone was apparently in a root canal, but the clinical feel (looseness) and bleeding should have verified that it was a perforation. (Courtesy of Dr. A. Schlossberg, Philadelphia, Pa.)

retrograde surgical approach should be used (Fig. 332). If the perforation occurs anywhere else on the root, nonsurgical endodontic therapy with gutta-percha-chloropercha is tried first. If it cannot be sealed by this method, then a surgical approach and a retrograde seal is used (Fig. 217). However, if the perforation is on the lingual (palatal) or proximal aspect of the root, then a surgical seal is not possible. In those cases intentional replantation with amalgam seal of the defect or extraction may have to be done, as the usual sequela is pocket formation up to the defect (Fig. 468). It may be possible to perform a gingivectomy and ostectomy

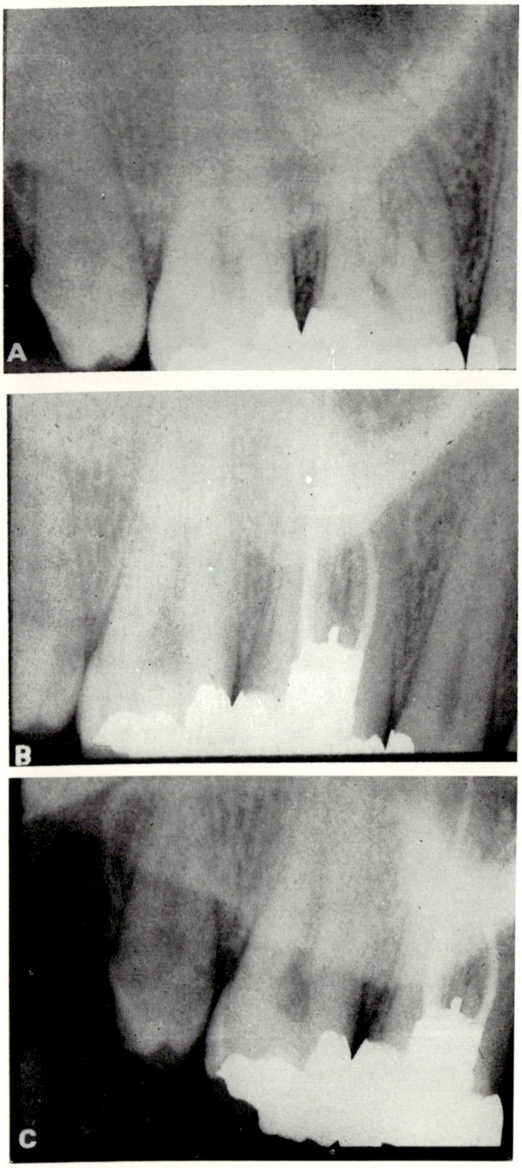

Figure 469. Sealing a small perforation in the furca area of an upper molar. A. Upper left first molar with pulpal involvement. B. Perforation developed in floor of chamber; canals obturated with gutta-percha-chloropercha; perforation sealed with amalgam. C. Over one year later; no pathological changes evident. (From D. R. Morse, "The Management of Endodontic Problem Cases," *JDA South Africa*, 27:387, 1972.)

up to the level of the perforation, if it is on the lingual (palatal) surface. This would then be followed by an amalgam seal. A small perforation in the floor of the chamber is treated by sealing it with amalgam from within the pulp chamber. This should be sealed at the time the defect is discovered (it should be before the root canal(s) is obturated). First the bleeding is stopped with a sterile saline-moistened cotton pellet or if this is not effective, a small amount of formocresol on a cotton pellet is usually sufficient. Then the defect is sealed with amalgam. If the root canal(s) has not yet been filled, care must be taken not to get amalgam into the canal(s). A good method is to place files, reamers, or silver cones into the canals before the amalgam is placed into the defect.

A perforation in a multirooted tooth into the furcation area is treated slightly differently. First, the bleeding is stopped as described previously. Gold foil, tin foil, or platinum foil is then placed over the defect. A thick mix of zinc polycarboxylate cement is placed over the foil or amalgam can be used (Fig. 469). Pressure is not applied during the placement or else irritation in the furcation area would cause the development of a furcation involvement (Fig. 470). If there is already a furca involvement present a wedge or a Stimudent® should be placed in the furca, prior to the placement of the foil and filling. This is to prevent further irritation.

Perforations can also occur after incorrect placement of posts. Treatment depends upon whether the perforation

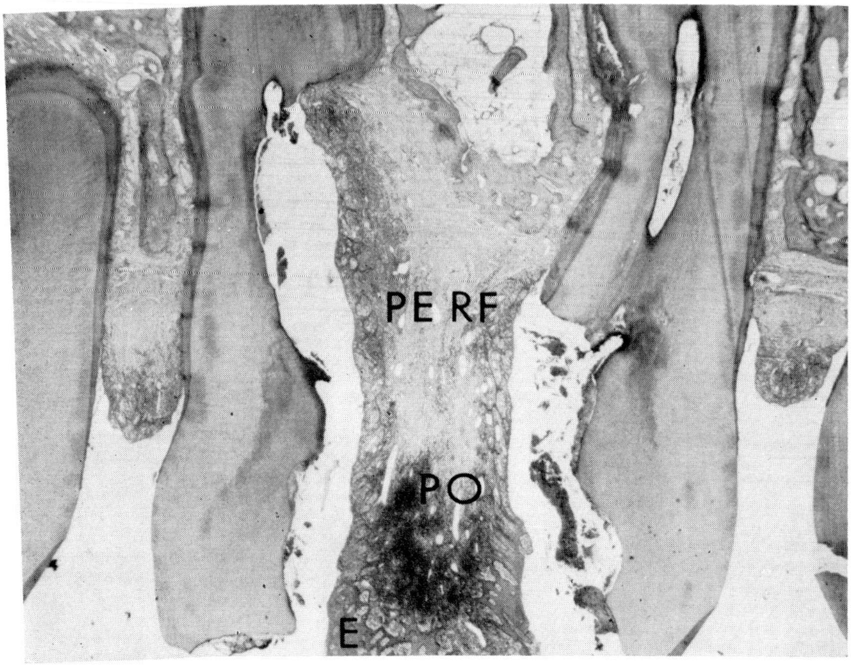

Figure 470. Periodontal pocket formation in the bifurcation region of a lower molar resulting from root perforation; histologic section. PERF = perforation, PO = pocket, E = proliferating epithelium (×10). (From S. Seltzer, *Endodontology,* McGraw-Hill, Inc., 1971. Used with permission of McGraw-Hill Book Company.)

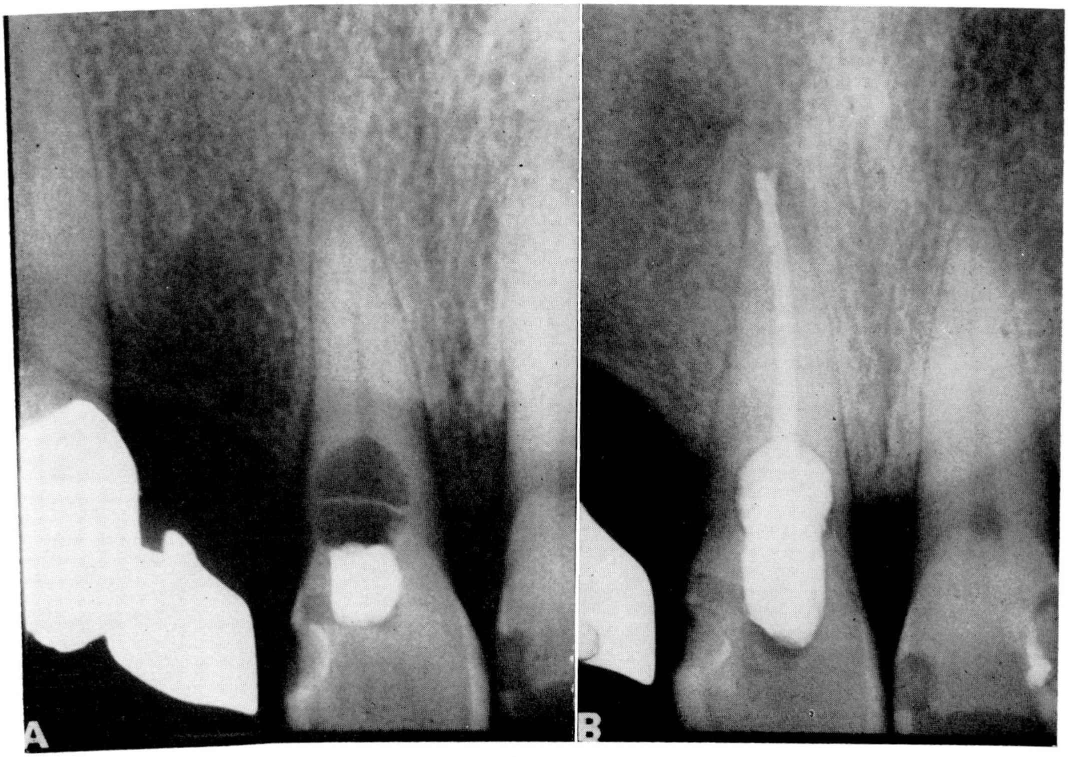

Figure 471. Internal resorption case sealed by nonsurgical endodontic therapy with gutta-percha-chloropercha. A. Upper left central incisor with internal resorption. B. Canal and resorption defect sealed. (From D. R. Morse, "The Management of Endodontic Problem Cases," *JDA South Africa,* 27:387, 1972.)

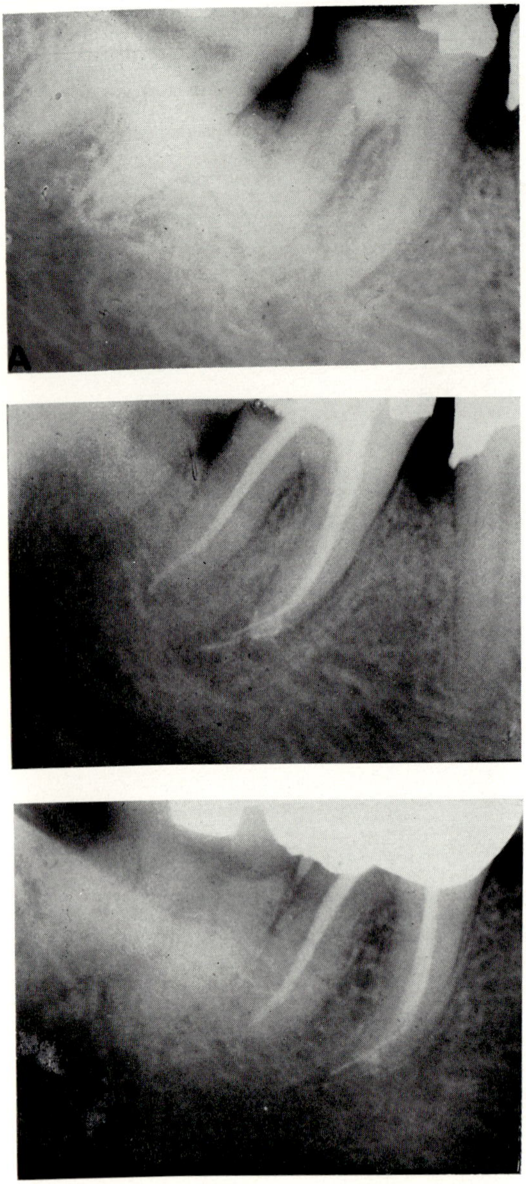

Figure 472. Bypassing a broken instrument. A. Lower left first molar with a pulpal involvement. B. File broken in mesio-buccal canal; it was dislodged beyond the apex during obturation with gutta-percha-chloropercha. C. Seven years later; no evidence of periapical pathosis. (From D. R. Morse, "The Management of Endodontic Problem Cases," *JDA South Africa*, 27:387, 1972.)

is in an area accessible to surgery. If the protruding post can be seen, the excessive portion is cut off and with a No. 35 bur, a preparation is made into the post. A restoration is placed into the preparation, and it is contoured even with the root surface (Fig. 445). Internal resorption cases are also first treated by nonsurgical endodontic therapy with gutta-percha and chloropercha. After the canal is obturated, condensation is completed until the defect is sealed (Figs. 144, 471). If the resorption defect cannot be sealed adequately by this method, then the case is treated surgically and the defect is sealed if it is on an accessible surface (Fig. 333). If complete perforation occurs, the apical portion is removed and an endodontic implant is inserted (Fig. 334).

Method of Bypassing "Calcified Canals," Root Canal Ledges, Denticles (Pulp Stones), Broken Instruments, Dentin Debris, and Silver Cones

If a canal is obstructed, an attempt should be made to bypass the obstruction before resorting to periapical surgery with a retrograde amalgam seal. RC-Prep is placed in the chamber and is passed up through the canal with a No. 20 or 25 file. A slight curve is first placed on the end of the instrument and it is gently rotated as apical penetration is attempted. It may take several applications and even several visits for the penetration to be effective. Once the obstruction is bypassed, the canal is widened with files and obturated with gutta-percha-choropercha by the previously described method (Fig. 472).

Method of Removing Gutta-percha Fillings

Chloroform is deposited with a syringe into the chamber. As the mass is softened, it is withdrawn by the use of an endodontic explorer and a No. 20 or 25 file. In upper molars, because of gravity, the chamber must be continuously replenished with the solution. Extreme care must be exercised to prevent getting the highly caustic solution on the patient's tissues or clothes. Once the filling is removed, retreatment can be performed (see this chapter, section on retreatments). In the removal of the gutta-percha, invariably some gutta-percha goes beyond the apex, but this is rarely a problem (Figs. 455, 456). The patient may have some pain for a brief moment from the irrritating effect of the chloroform. This soon dissipates as the liquid evaporates.

Methods of Removing Silver Cones, Posts or Broken Instruments

If the silver cones or instruments have been cut or broken off at the level of the orifice or within the canals, it is

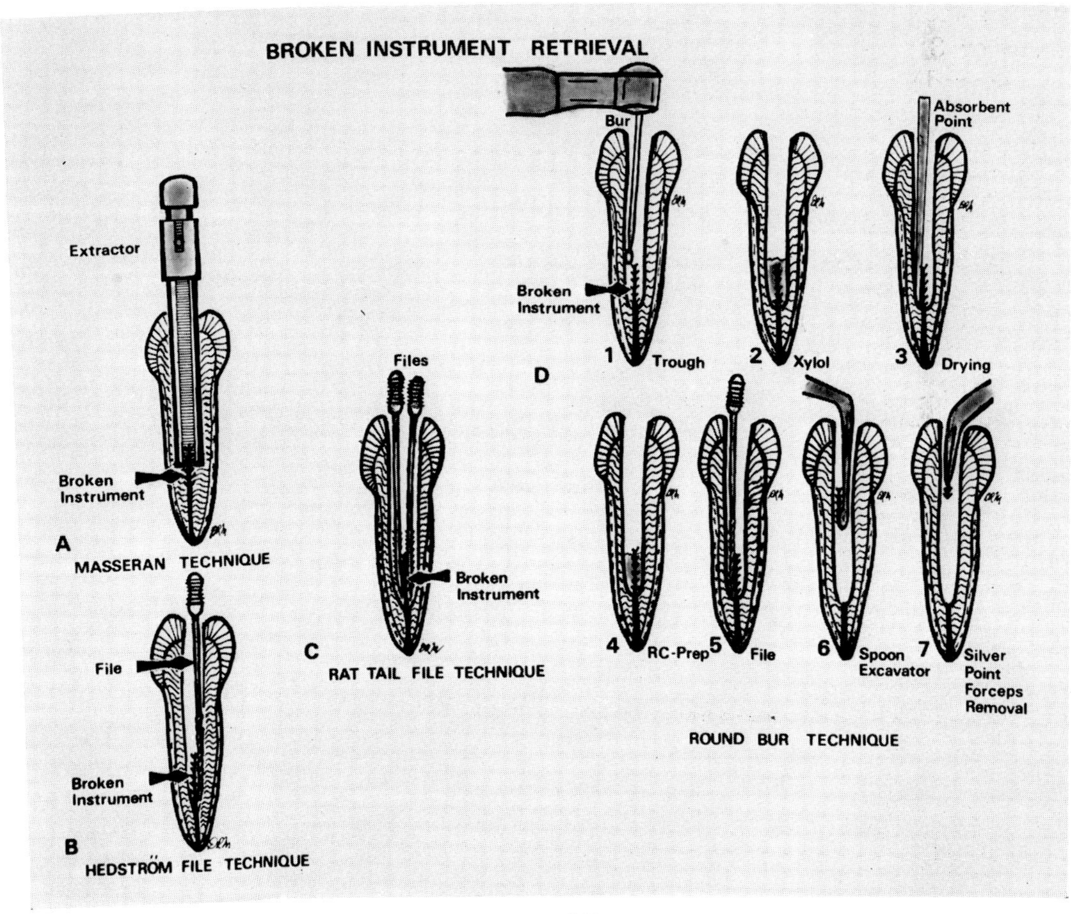

Figure 473

almost impossible to remove them. Techniques that may be attempted are (1) the use of magnets (usually ineffective); (2) the Masserann technique (Medidenta®), this is purported to be effective but entails the preparation of a large root channel, and it can only be used for straight roots (Fig. 473A); (3) the use of a Hedström file along the instrument (also very difficult to accomplish for fine canals; Fig. 473B); and (4) the use of two simultaneously placed rat-tail files (or small Hedström files) adjacent to the instrument (occasionally effective; Fig. 473C). A method that is sometimes effective is to rotate a No. 2 or 3 surgical length round bur (slow speed) adjacent to the instrument (or cone) in order to make a trough, with care taken not to nick the metal (Fig. 473D-1). Then, xylol is dropped into the trough and left there for several minutes to dissolve the cement (Fig. 473D-2). The canal is dried with absorbent points (Fig. 473D-3), and then RC-Prep is dropped into the canal for several minutes (Fig. 473D-4). A file (No. 20 or 25) is worked adjacent to the instrument, trying to pry it free (Fig. 473D-5). If the instrument is loosened, a long-shanked spoon excavator is worked between the instrument and dentin wall to move the instrument occlusally (Fig. 473D-6). Then a silver cone forceps (Fig. 473D-7) is used to take the instrument out of the canal. If the instrument cannot be removed then the RC-Prep is used to help bypass the instrument (as described previously). With all of the above-mentioned techniques, extreme care must be used to prevent a root perforation. This is because of the extensive widening of the canal that occurs in trying to dislodge the instrument. Generally, posts cannot be removed unless they are loose. In trying to remove a tight fitting post, it is possible to extract the tooth. Retroseal is the treatment of choice (see Chapter 10).

Giromatic® Technique*

The Giromatic contra-angle is an instrument that is designed to rotate special broaches, files, and reamers one-quarter turn in alternate directions (Medidenta, Fig. 474). It has been introduced into this country from Europe during the last few years, and has been widely promoted to general practitioners. The Giromatic technique has been advocated as a method that can perform instrumentation twenty times as fast as hand instrumentation. The manufacturer also states that instruments cannot be aspirated or swallowed, because they are attached to the contra-angle. Other claims are that instruments do not break, even with bending, ledges are not created, and perforations do not occur. The Giromatic is especially promoted for use in posterior teeth, and it is claimed by the proponents that hand instrumentation is not necessary.

Disadvantages are that there is a loss of tactile sense, which is so important to the effective practice of endodontics. Contrary to claims, complete instrumentation cannnot be satisfactorily performed with this instrument alone. The rubber dam is a far better means of

* The section on precautions is based on a discussion by Dr. A. Frank of Los Angeles, California.

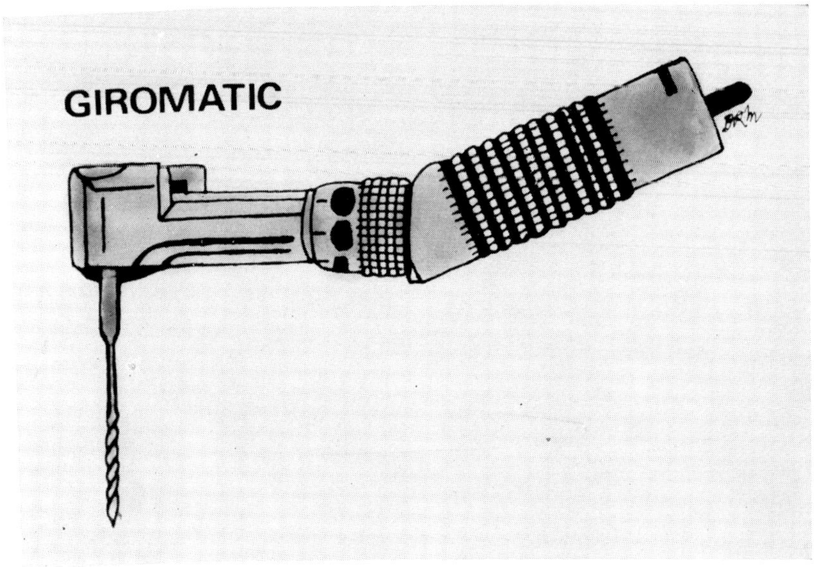

Figure 474. (Medidenta).

preventing aspiration and swallowing of instruments (and it also serves many other purposes) and although it is not usual to have ledging, perforation, or instrument breakage with the Giromatic, it is still possible for these mal-effects to occur.

Although, I do not advocate the routine use of engine-driven instrumentation for endodontic therapy, there may be a use for the Giromatic contra-angle as an adjunct in the instrumentation of fine and curved canals. We are currently investigating the use of this instrument at Temple University. As discussed in a recent publication the following precautions should be taken with the Giromatic:

(1) The initial penetration should be with a No. 10 reamer or file and a measurement should be taken and recorded.

(2) The initial Giromatic instrument to be used is an XXXX-fine broach.

(3) The broaches should be used only once; although the newest technique employs reamers and these are probably safer than broaches.

(4) The Giromatic should not be used in an attempt to bypass instruments, as breakage can occur.

(5) Slow speeds should be used, with an in and out motion, as apical penetration progresses; the instrument should not feel tight in the canal.

(6) The canal should be moistened with a lubricant such as RC-Prep during instrumentation.

Treating Patients in Their Homes

On occasion, a dentist may be asked to perform endodontic therapy for a bed-ridden patient. If the patient is

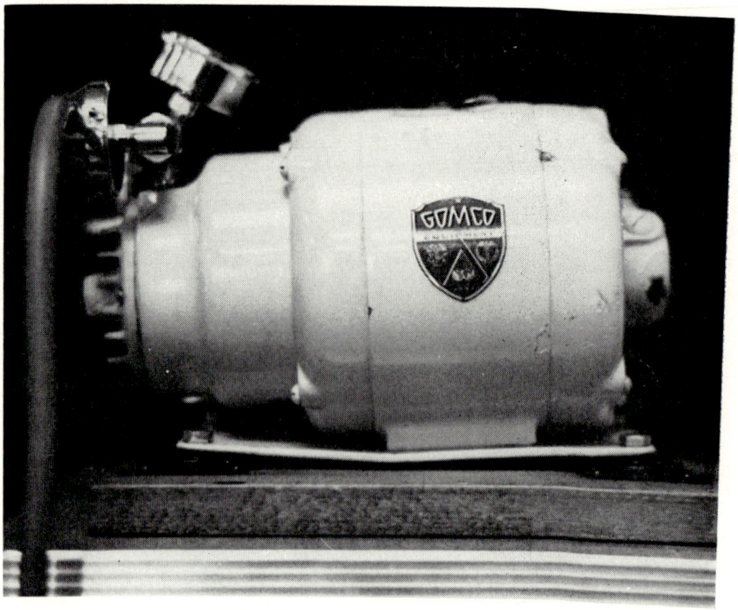

Figure 475. Gomco® portable suction apparatus.

temporarily incapacitated (for example as the result of a broken leg), then palliative treatment should be performed. However, if the patient would be bed-ridden for at least several months, then the dentist should attempt to do complete endodontic therapy. There are now available portable dental engines (high speed and low speed), transistorized pulp testers, as well as kits that contain a complete setup for endodontic therapy. The patient should be propped up with pillows and a bright bedroom lamp can be used for visibility. A portable suction apparatus is available for aspiration (Fig. 475).

Treating Patients in the Operating Room

There are patients who because of physical, medical, or psychological reasons cannot have endodontic therapy performed in the dental office. The dentist should be thoroughly familiar with operating room procedures before working on a patient under general anesthesia. There are certain considerations for endodontics under general anesthesia: (1) working on the operating table is different than working in the dental chair; the patient is supine, and direct vision is used; (2) as the patient cannot respond, the dentist should try not to over-instrument, spill caustic materials (such as sodium hypochlorite or chloroform), or overfill; (3) usually radiographs are not taken during the treatment, so the dentist has to try to use other methods of obtaining canal measurements (as described previously in this chapter); (4) because the patient is unconscious, it is possible to work more efficiently and complete the case in a faster time; and (5) as the patient has to recover from the general anesthesia (he (or she) usually stays overnight at the hospital or for at least an hour in the recovery room of an oral surgery office), the dentist should be certain that he (or she) sees the patient before the latter leaves the office or hospital.

Treating Lower Premolars

Treating lower premolars is often a problem. Pain occurs many times and there is a fairly high incidence of one canal bifurcating deep in the root into two branches (Fig. 291). It has been stated that there is poor circulation in this area, which is a possible reason for the pain. In treating lower premolars, one should try to complete the cases as rapidly as possible, and if necessary perform a trephination. It is also important to take a periapical radiograph with an instrument in position in order to ascertain that the trephination does not go into the region of the mental foramen. In cases of bifurcated roots, sometimes if the bifurcation is very far down, it is only possible to instrument and fill one canal. If the case fails, usually an apicoectomy is dangerous because of the mental nerve. An intentional replant can be attempted (Fig. 436). Sometimes it is possible to negotiate both canals. In order not to be blocked out, a silver cone should be temporarily placed in one canal, while the other canal is instrumented and obturated. Then when that canal is completed, the silver cone is removed and the second canal is instrumented and obturated. A case is shown in Figure 291 in which the silver cone was not removed and the second canal was sealed with gutta-percha and root canal cement.

RECALL PROCEDURES

Following the endodontic therapy, a recall is usually made at six months and then in one year. If possible, it is a good idea to see the patient or at least have a periapical radiograph available from the dentist currently treating the patient at yearly intervals for at least five years. It is not unusual to have *success* change to *failure* many years after completion of treatment. This can be related to periodontal disease with concomitant exposure of lateral canals, incomplete seal of canal with patient's local resistance decreasing and microbial virulence or numbers increasing, systemic disease such as diabetes lowering the patient's resistance, trauma causing a fracture or loosening of the restoration, caries destroying the support of the tooth, a post insertion causing a perforation and the presence of a cyst in which initial healing of the granulomatous tissue surrounding the cyst occurred, and then the cyst expanded at a later time. In determining the success or failure of endodontic therapy, the dentist should consider the effects of the treatment upon the patient's original complaints as well as the results of various testing methods (Table VIII).

Systemic

Considering the effect of the treatment upon the patient's systemic health, the dentist should determine if any systemic condition has improved or been

TABLE VIII

CRITERIA FOR SUCCESS

1. No spontaneous pain (pain could indicate an unfilled or poorly filled canal, a root fracture, or periapical inflammation).
2. No sensitivity to percussion or periapical palpation (positive responses could indicate periapical inflammation).
3. No sensitivity to hot, cold, sweet, or sour (sensitivity could indicate an accessory or unfilled canal).
4. No mobility (if mobility was caused by endodontic disease; mobility could indicate periapical inflammation).
5. No swelling (swelling could result from pulpal or periapical infection).
6. No sinus tract (could result from periapical inflammation or root fracture).
7. Root is not fractured (could result from instrumentation, obturation, or post insertion).
8. No development of a periapical area of pathosis as determined radiographically.
9. If a periapical, lateral or furcation area of pathosis was present before it should have resolved or noticeably decreased as judged by radiographic interpretation. Radiographs should be taken at 6 months, one year, and two years. In some cases it may take two years or longer for a periapical area of pathosis to resolve and sometimes "areas" decrease in size and then increase at a later date.
10. Even without clinical manifestations or radiographic changes, the quality of the root canal obturation must be satisfactory. Incomplete instrumentation and obturation are unacceptable. Teeth with poorly instrumented and obturated canals may fail years later.
11. The tooth must be restorable and salvageable. Endodontics should not be performed for nonrestorable teeth or severely periodontally involved teeth.

prevented. An example would be the improvement of an iritis as the result of successful endodontic therapy. As stated previously, focal infection per se may not occur, but the possibility of some auto-immune type response to oral microbes and tissue break-down products cannot be discounted (currently being investigated at Temple University School of Dentistry). As far as prevention of systemic complications, an example would be the prevention of subacute bacterial endocarditis in a rheumatic fever patient by a correct antibiotic regimen and a nonirritating method of treatment.

Psychologic

The dentist should consider the effect of endodontic therapy on the patient's psychologic health. A long-lasting toothache can make an individual depressed, irritable, excitable, unfriendly, among other possibilities. Alleviation of the pain can change his (or her) personality. A simple procedure such as restoring the natural appearance to a discolored tooth, can change a person's outlook on life. To many individuals, the loss of a tooth is equivalent to aging and the saving of that tooth can have tremendous psychologic advantages. The functional aspect is related to the psychologic. If the tooth previously was mobile and mastication of many foods was difficult, then the result of having a firm tooth (possibly by the use of an endodontic implant) allows the patient to eat previously untouchable foods. This may allow the patient to enjoy his meals more, resulting in a happier personality. Finally, those patients with non-endodontic complaints like atypical facial neuralgia may be relieved of their pain, temporarily, by the endodontic procedure. In the latter instances, it is possibly the psychologic role that the dentist assumes allows for the result. However, treatment in those cases is always a risky procedure and it is rarely indicated. One possible indication is when the dentist is not certain from the result of clinical tests and medical or other dental consultations as to whether the pain is of endodontic, or psychological origin. If it is of endodontic origin, then relief should occur, and as previously mentioned if it is of psychological origin, relief may occur for a time.

Local

The patient should be asked if he (or she) had any local symptoms or signs since completion of the endodontic therapy. If the patient had either pain, swelling, drainage, or lymphadenopathy related to the treated tooth, and the condition persisted after completion of therapy, then retreatment should be performed (if possible).

The dentist should palpate the apical region and percuss the tooth. If either or both of these procedures cause pain, this is an indication that there may possibly be a failure. However, sensitivity may be related to a high restoration, traumatic occlusion or the patient's biting or tongue-thrust habits. The dentist should correlate these test results with the radiologic evidence and the other clinical evidence. If the only manifestation of failure is percussion and/or palpation sensitivity, the tooth should be taken out of occlusal contact and checked periodically. If at a later date, there is radiologic evidence of periapical breakdown, then retreatment should be attempted.

The tooth should be inspected for fractures, caries, erosion, abrasion, or discoloration. The gingiva and alveolar mucosa should be examined and probed for possible pocket formation or evidence of a sinus tract. The patient should be notified if any of these conditions are present, so that remedial measures towards saving the tooth can be undertaken. If a sinus tract is present and it is related to the root apex or a lateral canal, then retreatment should be tried.

The most important evidence is radiographic. The periapical radiograph should be taken under the same conditions (angulation, density, etc.) as the previous one (if at all possible). If a periapical *area* was previously present, and it has enlarged, or an *area* has developed around the root apex of a tooth that had no *area,* then retreatment should be done (if possible). If the *area* remained the same size and the patient currently has signs or symptoms, then retreatment should be attempted. If the *area* became smaller, but has not yet disappeared, and the patient has no clinical manifestations, then the patient should be rechecked at six month intervals, until the *area* has disappeared. If the *area* does not disappear and the patient has no symptoms or signs, then the tooth should be kept under periodic observation. If the *area* enlarges or the patient develops clinical manifestations related to the tooth, then retreatment should be attempted.

CASE PRESENTATION*

Discussing the Case

There are various methods of explaining the advantages of endodontic therapy to the prospective patient:

(1) Informational handouts; the

* Preparation of this section was aided by Dr. Harold Nazimoff, Clinical Assistant Professor, Department of Endodontology, Temple University School of Dentistry, Philadelphia, Pa.

ADA has an excellent pamphlet on endodontics that the patient can read in the reception room. Another excellent pamphlet with a humorous tone is "Am I Losing My Nerve?" (Burns, R. C.).

(2) Audio-visual aids; there are several companies that produce endodontic film-strips that are synchronized with tape cassettes. These can be shown in the private office by the dental assistant approximately fifteen minutes before the scheduled appointment.

(3) Various chairside methods such as verbal communication, radiographs, study models, tooth sections, charts, diagrams, tables (e.g. tooth formation and eruption), demonstrations on extracted teeth, and use of the phase microscope to show oral and root canal microbes.

Some of the information that can be conveyed to the patient includes the following:

(1) The advantages of a natural tooth over nonreplacement, a partial denture, or a fixed bridge. Some advantages are: prevent migration of opposing and adjacent teeth, easier to clean, less costly than a *bridge,* and maintains the *feel* of a natural tooth.

(2) The advantages of a primary molar over nonreplacement or a space maintainer. Some advantages are to prevent malocclusion, and natural tooth is better than a space maintainer as often space maintainers loosen and are difficult to clean.

(3) The possibility of saving a crown or a bridge by the use of endodontic therapy.

(4) The use of endodontics to salvage roots to have a more stable denture.

(5) The advantage of endodontics as compared to extraction in preventing bacteremias.

(6) The probability that neither endodontic therapy nor exodontia will cure *focal* disease.

(7) The reasonable assurance that pulpal or periapical pain can be abolished after endodontic therapy.

(8) The relative painlessness of endodontic therapy during treatment and the fact that there are available excellent analgesics to control inter-visit and post-treatment pain.

(9) The reasonable assurance that endodontic therapy can relieve the patient's swelling and/or cause regression of the *gum boil* or discharging sinus tract.

(10) The probability that the tooth will *tighten up* after the therapy is completed (if the mobility was caused by a pulpal-periapical condition or if an endodontic implant was used).

(11) The probability that the *bony abscess* will heal.

(12) The reassurance that the lesion is not *cancer* (certain patients have a *cancerphobia*).

(13) Finally, that endodontic therapy is usually clinically success-

ful, probably over 90 per cent of the time; however, treatment can never be guaranteed.

Before treatment is begun, the patient should be told certain details: (1) cost; (2) the necessity of a post-treatment coronal restoration; (3) the possibility of alternate modes of treatment; (a) surgical vis-a-vis non-surgical, especially for cases with calcified or unnegotiable canals, perforations, porcelain jackets (the possibility of fracture should be discussed), precision attachments, and recurrent flare-ups; (b) pulpotomy vis-a-vis nonsurgical endodontic therapy, especially for financial reasons; (c) periapical surgery, intentional replantation, or extraction; and (d) gutta-percha technique as opposed to a paste filling technique, again with an explanation about the difference in cost and in prognosis; (4) the importance of recall check-ups.

If during treatment some irregularity occurs, the patient should always be informed. These irregularities include broken needles, broken root canal instruments, fractured roots, burns, lacerations, misplaced injections, and swallowed or aspirated instruments (with proper precautions, the latter should never occur). If the dentist is not competent to handle the incident, the patient should be referred to some practitioner who can treat the condition.

During treatment, the patient can be educated to other factors about endodontic therapy:

(1) It is the pulp and not the *nerve*.
(2) A tooth without a pulp can function normally.
(3) All three (or four) canals are interconnected and therapy must be performed on all canals even though only one is apparently inflamed.

When to Advise Extraction After Therapy Has Begun

There are times when the best treatment advice for the patient is "get an extraction." This could be for the following cases:

(1) The patient is unmanageable. If patient cooperation cannot be assured, then treatment should not be continued.
(2) Untreatable periodontal disease is detected after treatment has been begun.
(3) Vertical root fracture occurs that leaves no bony support.
(4) Root canals are unnegotiable; periapical surgery cannot be performed (e.g. inferior alveolar canal near root apexes); and intention replantation cannot be done (roots are severely curved).
(5) Tooth becomes nonrestorable because of nontreatable extensive caries, perforation, or fracture.
(6) Patient has uncontrollable pain.
(7) Patient has a superficial or deep cellulitis in which it is not possible to get adequate drainage without removing the tooth.
(8) Patient just does not want to continue treatment, because of pain, fear, swelling or any other reason.

USE OF AUXILIARIES

Aside from her regular office duties, the receptionist should have these specific duties relative to endodontic practice:

(1) Give the patient an information booklet and a history form.

(2) Show the patient audio-visual material on endodontics.

(3) Alleviate the patient's fears about the procedure.

The dental assistant should perform these duties:

(1) Take the pre-treatment radiograph (if qualified).

(2) Transfer the patient information and history to the dental chart.

(3) Underline with red on the chart any important medical information such as allergic to penicillin, diabetes, rheumatic fever, cardiovascular disease, hyperthyroidism and drug intake.

(4) Have ready for the doctor when he (or she) enters the treatment room: the patient's chart, the mounted radiograph, the patient draped in correct position in the chair, and a tray set-up for diagnosis.

Some dentists prefer taking radiographs and the history themselves, but a well trained assistant can perform these functions admirably. This saves the dentist time so that he (or she) can see more patients. Even with the history recorded on the chart, the dentist should ask the patient for details about any important medical conditions, drug intake, or oral manifestations.

At recall time, the trained assistant can take the periapical x-ray and the history. When the dentist enters the room with the radiograph mounted and the history indicated, relatively little time is needed to examine the tooth and surrounding tissues for any possible deviation from normal.

As most patients have some inherent fear of endodontics, during the treatment procedures, it is advisable for dentist and assistant to work from tray setups that are behind the patient (Fig. 476). The assistant should be thor-

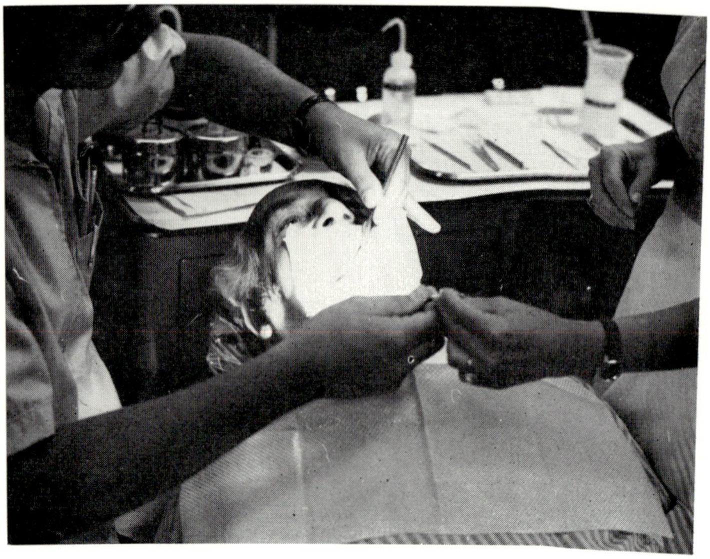

Figure 476. Four handed endodontics; tray set-up behind the patient.

oughly trained on how to use nitrous-oxide-oxygen analgesia including, any possible mal-effects (such as nausea, vomiting, approach of excitement stage). She can put the mask on and remove it. The patient should never be left alone while the analgesia is being used. Also after administration of a local anesthetic, if the doctor must leave the room, the assistant must remain with the patient. Any practitioner who uses intra-venous sedation, should have a well trained assistant who knows about administration and possible side effects. All members of the staff should be aware of where emergency equipment is, how to use it, and standard procedures to follow in case of medical emergencies (see Chapter 16).

DENTIST-ENDODONTIST INTERRELATIONSHIPS

The general practitioners and specialist must have a good working relationship with each other. If any doubts exist about a particular treatment, consultation is essential. It is the endodontist's responsibility to both the patient and the referring dentist, to inform the general practitioner about any deviations from normal that are found.

(1) Teeth adjacent to the one that was referred for treatment that have either caries, periodontal disease, traumatic occlusion, periapical *areas*, or an orthodontic problem.
(2) Poor fitting fixed bridges or partial dentures.
(3) Oral lesions.
(4) Pain and/or swelling of non-endodontic etiology.

The specialist should inform the general practitioner about his (or her) method of treatment and philosophy of treatment. For example: filling short, flush filling, button-type filling, overfilling. The endodontist should also tell the referring dentist before discussing it with the patient, if he (or she) believes that a post, core, crown or fixed bridge is essential, after the endodontic treatment is completed. If the endodontist wants to use a new or different method of treatment such as an endodontic implant, allogeneic transplant, or an intentional replant, he (or she) should inform the referring dentist. It is a good practice for an endodontist to send the referring dentist before and after radiographs. This is important in cases of clinically calcified canals, dilacerated roots, and complications that may have occurred prior to the time that the specialist first saw the patient. These complications include fractured roots, perforations, broken instruments, and root caries. The endodontist should inform the general practitioner about these conditions, prior to beginning therapy. There are times when the endodontist is asked by the patient to perform services that are not within his (or her) realm. Such services include placement of permanent restorations, adjusting clasps, balancing occlusion, performing extensive periodontal therapy, and recementing crowns. Although the specialist may be able to perform these services, he (or she) does not have the time or facilities to handle any complications that might result from such treatments. Therefore, the endodontist should politely inform the patient that as a specialist he (or she) cannot perform such services, but the patient's own dentist will be informed about the particular need.

The endodontist should inform the referring dentist about treatment complications such as broken instruments, fractured roots, perforations, and a nonmanageable patient.

It is also the endodontist's responsibility to inform the general practitioner if he (or she) feels the latter has not performed properly. The specialist should tell the referring dentist his (or her) beliefs, even if this means losing a referral as a result, because it is the patient's welfare that is of paramount interest. Some particular items that could be discussed are failure of general practitioner to take radiographs, to use the rubber dam, to take a good history, or to consider endodontics rather than exodontics.

The discussions between a general practitioner and an endodontist are not along a one-way path. There certainly are times when it is the duty of the generalist to inform the specialist when the specialist's work or methods are not up to par. If the general practitioner feels that a particular method of treatment is not satisfactory (e.g. use of silver cones), he (or she) should so inform the endodontist. If the dentist feels that the patient was poorly handled, this also should be discussed. Too many specialists only consider the technical aspects of the treatment. Only by mutual respect and understanding between the practitioners involved can endodontics become available to more people.

BIBLIOGRAPHY

Cash, P. W.: Electronics and root canals. *J Acad Gen Dent, 21(2)*:20, 1973.

Frank, A. L.: An evaluation of the giromatic endodontic handpiece. *Oral Surg, 24*:419, 1967.

Freedland, J. B.: Conservative reduction of large periapical lesions. *Oral Surg, 29*:455, 1970.

Grossman, L. I.: *Endodontic Practice*, 7th ed. Philadelphia, Lea & Febiger, 1970.

Ingle, J. I.: *Endodontics*. Philadelphia, Lea & Febiger, 1965.

Linaburg, R. G., and Marshall, F. J.: The diagnosis and treatment of vertical root fractures: report of case. *JADA, 86*:679, 1973.

Moon, D.: Helpful hints: warm cartridges. *Dent Surv, 49(1)*:49, 1973.

Parker, W. A., and Hutchins, D. W.: Periapical localization using fiber optics. *J Oral Med, 26*:17, 1971.

Sommer, R. F., Ostrander, F. D., and Crowley, M. C.: *Clinical Endodontics: A Manual of Scientific Endodontics*, 3rd ed. Philadelphia, Saunders, 1966.

Weine, F. S.: *Endodontic Therapy*. St. Louis, Mosby, 1972.

CHAPTER 16

MEDICAL EMERGENCIES

IN THIS CHAPTER, consideration is given to severe life-threatening medical emergencies, as well as less serious complications that can occur in endodontic practice. Topics covered include syncope; shock; toxic reactions to a local anesthetic; allergic reactions; cardiac emergencies; cerebrovascular accidents; obstruction of the respiratory passages; diabetes; epilepsy; adrenal crisis; thyroid crisis; vomiting; drug overdosage (narcotics); aspirated or swallowed root canal instruments; broken injection needles; hemorrhagic emergencies; surgical emphysema; injection of local anesthetic into region of eye, ear, buccal fat pad, skin, lip or tongue; burns by heat or drugs, of lips, skin or oral mucosa; dislocated mandible; accident in dental chair; swallowing of intracanal medicament or irrigant; and spilling of intracanal medicament or irrigant on patient's clothes. Ingredients of an emergency tray are shown in Figure 477.

SYNCOPE (FAINTING)

Syncope is usually psychogenic in origin and is directly caused by cerebral hypoxia. Signs and symptoms are moist skin; cold sweat; vertigo; pallor of skin, lips, mucosa, and nails; rapid pulse that becomes slow and weak; nausea; and fall in blood pressure. Treatment entails placing the patient so that the head is lower than the feet (shock position, Fig. 478), breaking ammonia pearl inhalant (aromatic spirits of ammonia)

INGREDIENTS OF AN EMERGENCY TRAY

aromatic spirits of ammonia	→ cns stimulant
amyl nitrate	→ coronary vasodilator
nitroglycerine	→ coronary vasodilator
epinephrine 1:1000	→ vasopressor
isoproterenol	→ bronchial dilator
secobarbital	→ sedative
diazepam	→ epilepsy treatment
hydrocortisone	→ corticosteriod
diphenhydramine	→ antihistamine
morphine	→ for severe pain
nalorphine	→ narcotic antagonist
instant glucose	→ hypoglycemia treatment
scalpel	→ for tracheostomy
syringe	→ for emergency injections
stethoscope	→ heart sounds
sphygmomanometer	→ blood pressure

Figure 477

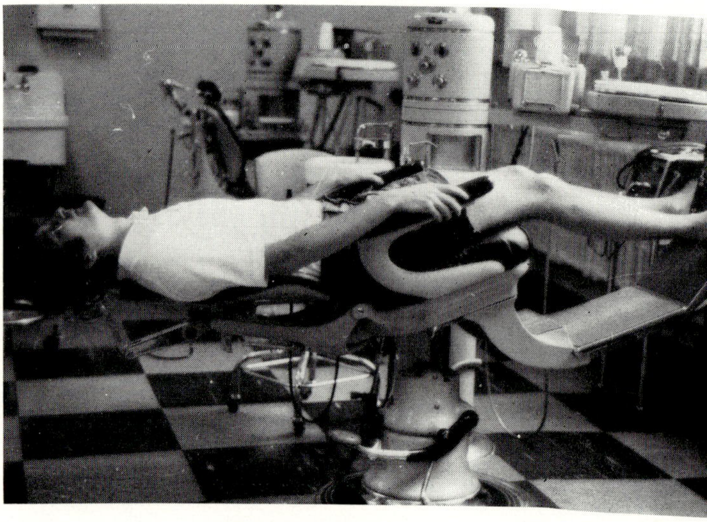

Figure 478. Shock position; head lower than the feet.

under the patient's nose, placing a cold compress on the patient's forehead, giving oxygen under positive pressure (Fig. 479), terminating any further dental treatment that visit, and giving a col[d] drink or coffee to the patient when h[e] recovers.

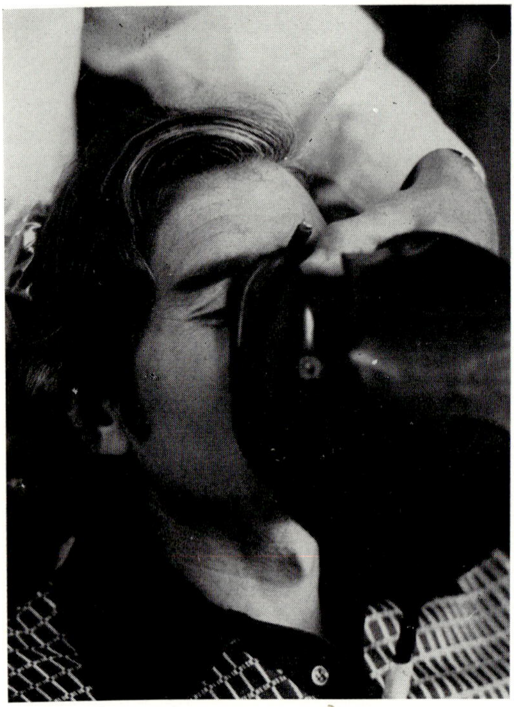

Figure 479. Oxygen given under positive pressure.

SHOCK (CIRCULATORY COLLAPSE)

Shock can be a component of many conditions including anaphylaxis, myocardial infarction, pulmonary emboli, severe hemorrhage, extensive burns, dehydration, severe liver and/or kidney disease, adrenal insufficiency, overwhelming infection, alcohol ingestion, and rarely as a complication of syncope. The clinical picture shows rapid, thready pulse; pallor; sweating; nausea; tachycardia; restlessness; confusion; apathy; decreased blood pressure; unconsciousness; dyspnea, leading to apnea; and increased cyanosis. Management includes several steps: (1) place the patient in the shock position; (2) give oxygen under positive pressure; (3) give a potent vasopressor such as mephentermine sulfate (Wyamine® Sulfate) in a dose of 30 to 45 mg IV or IM; or methoxamine (Vasoxyl®) 15 mg IM; (4) if cardiac arrest occurs, external massage must be used (see section on cardiac arrest); and (5) medical assistance should be obtained as soon as possible.

TOXIC REACTIONS TO A LOCAL ANESTHETIC

This results from an intravascular injection of a local anesthetic. Procaine and other ester-type derivatives produce central nervous system stimulation followed by depression, while amide-type derivatives (Xylocaine, Carbocaine, Citanest) only produce depression. Manifestations of the excitement stage are apprehension, nervousness and tremors, blurred vision, disorientation and dizziness, elevated blood pressure, rapid pulse, and fast breathing. Treatment of this stage includes placing the patient in the shock position, administration of oxygen under positive pressure, and secobarbital sodium (Seconal) or pentobarbital sodium (Nembutal), 100 to 200 mg (50 mg/cc) given by slow IV or IM administration.

Characteristics of the depressive stage are drowsiness leading to unconsciousness, convulsions, fall in blood pressure, weak, rapid pulse, decrease in rate and frequency of respiration, and cyanosis.

The convulsions can be controlled with the Seconal or Nembutal, but the patient must be carefully monitored to see that no further depression occurs. IV injection of succinycholine, 30 mg will also control convulsions, but it may be necessary to support respiration with positive pressure as a result of the respiratory depression action of this drug. To increase the force of myocardial contraction, and increase the blood pressure, mephentermine sulfate (Wyamine Sulfate) should be used. The dose is 30 to 45 mg by IV or IM administration. Oxygen administration must be continued during this phase.

Toxic reaction from the epinephrine in the local anesthetic solution may cause the manifestations of tachycardia, and central nervous system stimulation. Treatment is oxygen administration, and gentle reassurance. This is a transitory condition and the dental treatment can be continued in a few minutes.

On rare occasions, an epinephrine-reversal reaction may occur to the administered local anesthetic solution. It results from a reflex vasodilation. Signs and symptoms are tachycardia, fall in blood pressure, malaise, and unconsciousness. This is usually a transient reaction. Treatment is oxygen administration, after the patient has been placed in the shock position.

Allergic reactions can occur to any of the components of the local anesthetic solution. Diagnosis and treatment of these reactions are discussed in the following section.

ALLERGIC REACTIONS

These reactions include urticaria, rashes, other dermatitises, angioneurotic edema, nasal obstruction, sneezing, rhinorrhea, mucous membrane edema, swollen eyelids, asthma, and anaphylactic shock.

Generalized Reactions Aside from Asthma and Anaphylactic Shock

Antihistamines are of value in controlling the clinical manifestations of these reactions. A typical treatment is the use of oral diphenhydramine hydrochloride (Benadryl) 50 mg every four hours. In more severe cases, the same dose is given intravenously.

Asthma

This usually results from an allergy that causes bronchial spasm. Clinical manifestations are prolonged noisy expirations (wheezing), gasping for breath, productive cough, and cyanosis. Management of the attack involves bringing the patient to an upright position, administering oxygen under positive pressure and giving 0.2 to 0.5 ml of 1:1000 epinephrine IM, subcutaneously, or IV (if very severe dyspnea). An alternative drug is aminophylline 250 to 500 mg, diluted in 100 to 200 ml of 5% dextrose in water. It is given by slow IV administration (10-20 minutes). If the asthmatic attack fails to respond, a physician should be called and hydrocortisonc succinate (Solu-Cortef®, Mix-O-Vial®) should be administered (100 mg IV or IM).

Anaphylactic Shock

Symptoms and signs are rapidly appearing dyspnea which may lead to apnea; cyanosis; marked fall in blood pressure; weak pulse; angioedema of the glottis or laryngospasm may occur; shock may follow rapidly, leading to respiratory and circulatory collapse; and finally cardiac and respiratory arrest can occur. Treatment must be immediate and includes the following:

(1) The patient is placed in the shock position.

(2) Oxygen under positive pressure is given; if laryngospasm or glottis occlusion occurs, then an

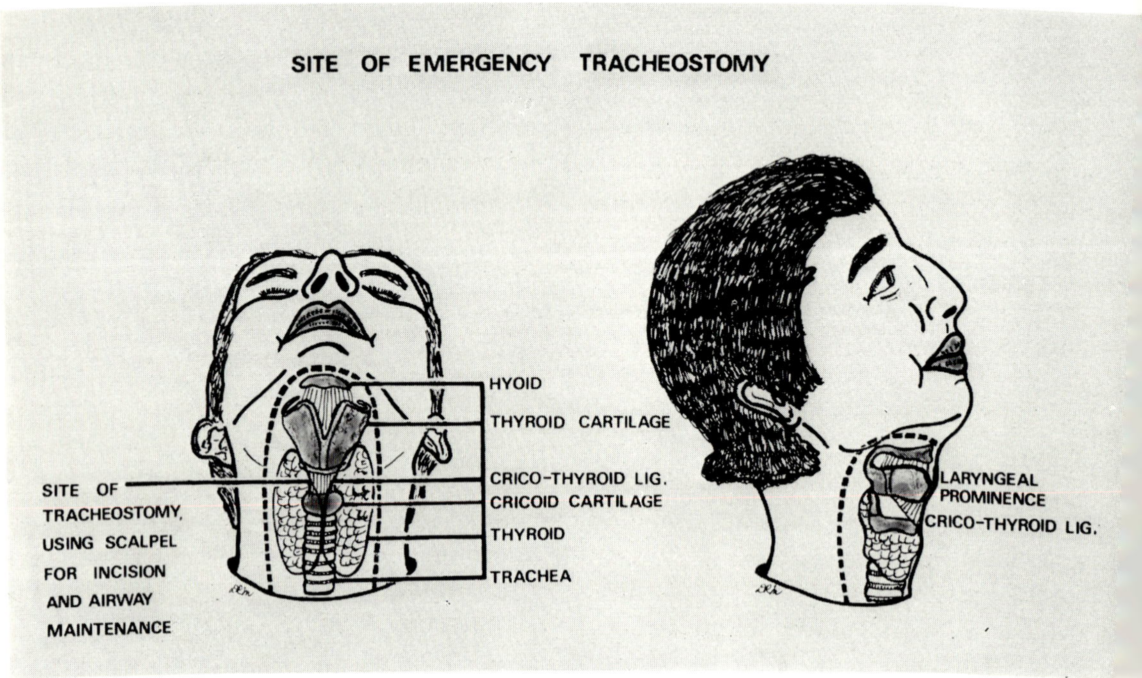

Figure 480

emergency tracheostomy must be done (Fig. 480).

(3) 0.5 ml of 1:1000 epinephrine is given IV or sublingually; if the mouth is clenched or veins are collapsed, one ml should be given IM.

(4) If the anaphylactic shock persists, then Solu-Cortef should be given by IV, or if not possible IM, in dosages of 200 to 400 mg.

(5) Once blood pressure is stabilized, then Benadryl, 50 mg by slow IV administration is used for supportive antihistamine therapy.

(6) As soon as possible, medical assistance should be obtained.

CARDIAC EMERGENCIES

These include angina pectoris, coronary occlusion, acute myocardial infarction, cardiac arrest, congestive heart failure, and cerebrovascular accident.

Angina Pectoris

Angina is caused by a decreased blood supply to the cardiac musculature. It is manifested by pre-cordial (sub-sternal) pain of short duration that radiates across the chest and possibly to the left arm, neck and on occasion to the mandible; strong pulse; and blood pressure rise. The patient is given a nitroglycerine (Glyceral Trinitrate) 0.4 mg tablet, to be placed under the tongue. The treatment can be repeated several times at ten minute intervals, but overdose can cause hypotension; amyl nitrite inhalant (pearls) can be used as an alternative treatment. Oxygen under positive pressure is administered. The patient's physician should be called, and no further treatment should be performed until a medical clearance is obtained.

Coronary Occlusion and Acute Myocardial Infarction (Heart Attack)

Coronary occlusion is caused by an obstruction to the blood flow of the myocardium (coronary vessels), usually resulting from a thrombus. The infarction results from the death of the myocardium. If a patient has a heart attack in the dental office, some diagnostic signs and symptoms that might occur are severe, prolonged precordial (substernal) pain radiating across the chest to the left arm; pallor; cyanosis; weak, rapid pulse (often irregular); clammy hands; drop in blood pressure; gastrointestinal upset; shortness of breath; occasionally pain referred to the mandible that can simulate a toothache; shock leading to circulatory and respiratory collapse; and cardiac arrest. The dentist should tilt the chair so that the patient is supine, administer oxygen under positive pressure, call a physician or ambulance and control pain by the administration of 10 to 15 mg morphine sulfate (intramuscularly or subcutaneously) or meperidine (Demerol), 75-100 mg (IM). If shock occurs, treat as discussed in the section on shock. Cardiac arrest treatment is discussed in the next section.

Cardiac Arrest

Cardiac arrest is the result of complete circulatory and respiratory failure. The signs and symptoms are obvious and include no detectable heart beat or pulse rate, rapidly dilating pupils that are nonresponsive, and apnea, which may be preceded by agonizing gasps. Treatment must be immediate and entails placing the patient supine on the floor; beginning artificial respiration by mouth to mouth resuscitation (Fig. 481); using equipment (if available) for positive pressure ventilation (oxygen mask, tank, endotracheal tube) (Fig. 29); performing closed chest cardiac massage (Fig. 482); and enlisting aid as soon as possible (physician and ambulance). For each fifteen chest compressions, two lung ventilations are given (if only one person is doing the treatment). If two people are available, then mouth to mouth resuscitation should be given at a rate of twelve to fourteen times per minute by one individual. The second person performs the cardiac compression at a rate of one per second. These treatments should be continued until spontaneous breathing and pulse recurs and/or a physician arrives.

Congestive Heart Failure

This results from an improper emptying of the ventricle because of myocardial fatigue. Manifestations are pain or discomfort in the chest, dyspnea, cough, edema, distention of cervical veins, and cyanosis. Treatment is (1) give oxygen under positive pressure;

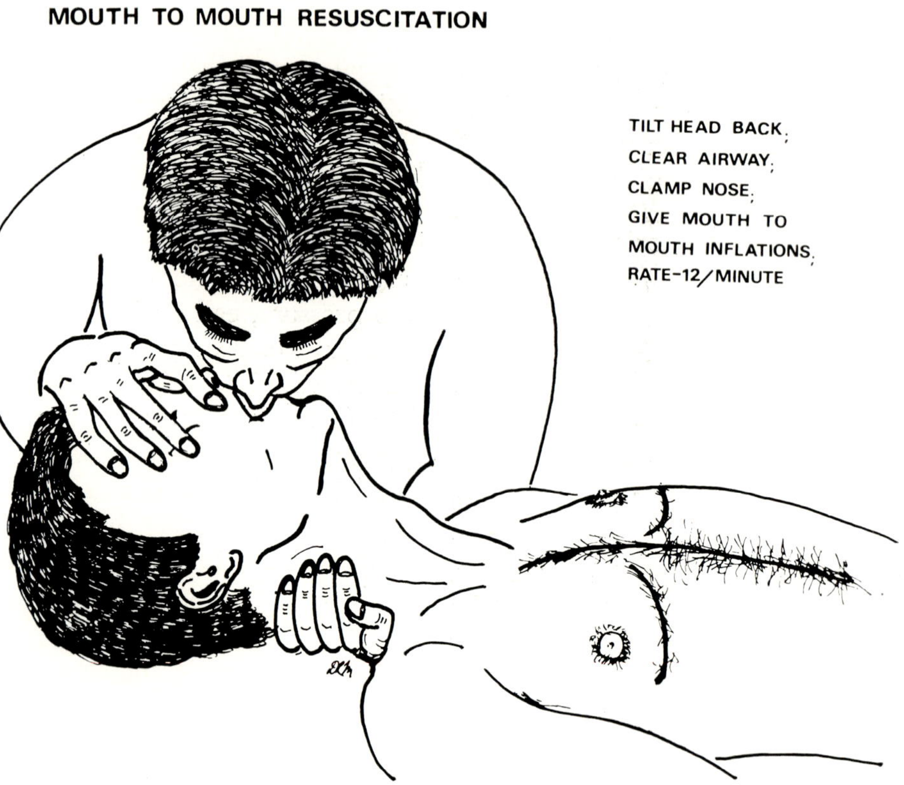

Figure 481

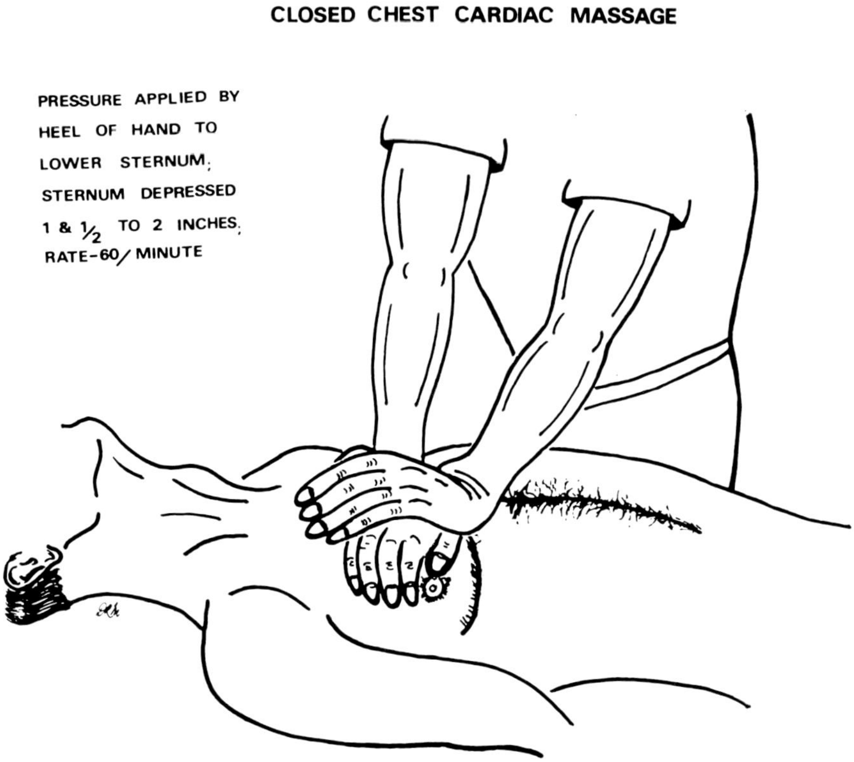

Figure 482

(2) give morphine sulfate 10-15 mg IM for pain; (3) give the patient a digitalis pill (digitoxin 0.6 mg); and (4) call the physician.

Cerebrovascular Accident (CVA)

Possible causes are hemorrhage, thrombosis, embolism, rupture, or spasm of a cerebral blood vessel. Clinical manifestations are vertigo rapidly leading to unconsciousness or convulsions, aphasia (speech impairment), headache, nausea and vomiting, and possible drop in blood pressure and slowing of pulse. Treatment is (1) keep patient quiet and do not move him (or her), (2) give oxygen, and (3) call physician.

OBSTRUCTION OF THE RESPIRATORY PASSAGES (PARTIAL OR COMPLETE)

This can result from aspiration of foreign objects (teeth, bridges, gauze, clamps, vomitus, etc.), laryngospasm, and laryngeal edema. Manifestations are choking, severe cough and wheezing, violent gasping for breath, and cyanosis of lips, mucosa and nail beds. Management includes the following: (1) bend patient forward and hit him (or her) sharply between the shoulders (to try and dislodge the object); if this is not effective, then (2) invert the chair so that the chin, thyroid cartilage and the suprasternal notch are in a horizontal

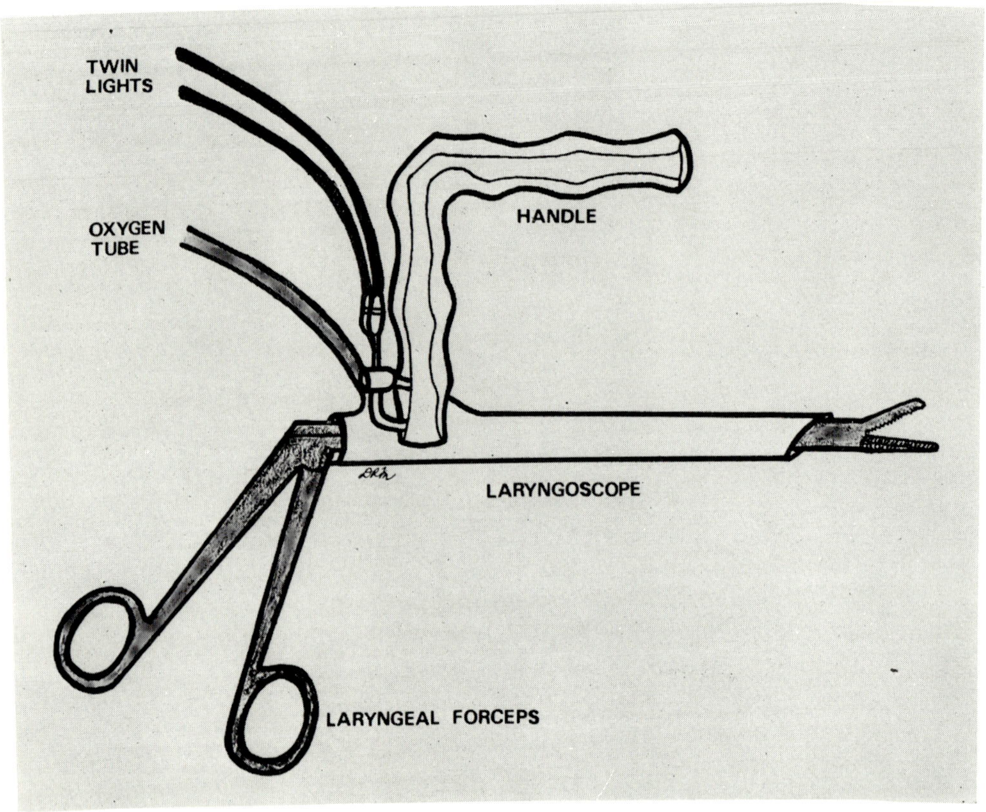

Figure 483

plane; (3) use suction to aspirate the airway; (4) if available, and the practitioner is facile in their use a laryngoscope, a laryngeal foreign body forceps, and/or a laryngeal suctioning cannula should be used for observation and attempted removal of the foreign body (Fig. 483); (5) give oxygen, if the obstruction is partially or completely removed; if it is still not possible to remove the obstruction, then (6) an emergency tracheostomy (Fig. 480) must be performed.

DIABETES

At times, it is difficult to differentiate diabetic coma from insulin shock. Diabetic coma is the rarer of the two reactions and results from insulin lack. It can occur in a controlled diabetic who forgets to take his (or her) insulin. It can also occur in an unknown diabetic. The clinical manifestations are drowsiness leading to unconsciousness, dry skin and mucous membranes, flushed (or very pale face), sunken eyes, breath with *fruity* acetone odor, headache, nausea and vomiting, malaise, epigastric pain, rapid, feeble pulse, and fall in blood pressure. Treatment is detailed and beyond the scope of the dental practitioner, as it is necessary to definitely determine the cause of the reactions, prior to treatment. The best treatment is to recognize the signs and symptoms and get medical help. If in doubt about differentiation between diabetic coma and insulin shock, a lump of sugar, a candy bar, or a glass of orange juice should be given to the patient. If the symptoms subside, then the condition was insulin shock. Insulin shock results from a hypoglycemia caused by too much insulin or skipping of a meal. It can be precipitated by a stressful situation. Symptoms and signs are nervous stomach, intense hunger, profuse sweating, pallor, rapid pulse, transient loss of memory, weakness, disorientation, dizziness, delusions, ataxia, aphasia, unconsciousness, convulsions, and coma. Treatment is sugar administration as mentioned above. If the patient will not swallow, 20 to 40 ml of 50 per cent glucose should be given IV.

EPILEPSY

Before an attack of grand mal (the more dangerous form of epilepsy), the patient usually has an aura which may be visual, olfactory, gustatory, tactile, or an irritable or depressive feeling. This is often followed by swinging movements of the head and arms, convulsions and then unconsciousness. The treatment is the following: (1) the patient is removed from the chair (if he (or she) is being treated at the time); (2) sharp objects are withdrawn from the vicinity; (3) clothing is loosened; (4) a mouth prop or tongue depressor is placed between the teeth, to prevent cheek or tongue biting; (5) the patient is observed carefully, and if respiratory obstruction occurs, the tongue must be pulled forward and oxygen administered; and (7) if the seizure is prolonged, the use of intravenous diazepam (Valium) by a slow administration of 5 to 30 mg helps in controlling the seizure.

ACUTE ADRENAL CORTICAL INSUFFICIENCY (ADRENAL CRISIS)

This can result from an acute exacerbation of Addison's disease, or in a patient who is on prolonged cortisone therapy, where there is a diminished or absent function of the pituitary-adrenal cortical system. Under the stress of a surgical procedure, the normal dosage of maintenance steroid therapy may be insufficient in such a patient and a condition of relative adrenal insufficiency can occur. Clinical manifestations are nausea and vomiting, anorexia, diarrhea, abdominal pain, dehydration, headache, restlessness, weakness, hypotension, and eventually coma and vascular collapse (shock). Immediate medical help is imperative. Emergency treatment would be the measures discussed under shock. It is important to give Solu-Cortef® in dose of 100 mg IV (if possible) or IM.

THYROID CRISIS (STORM)

Infections, anxiety, and an epinephrine containing local anesthetic injection can precipitate a thyroid crisis in a hyperthyroid patient. Fortunately, this complication is rare. Signs and symptoms are high fever, extreme tachycardia, persistent vomiting and diarrhea, profuse sweating, palpitation, and tremor. As these manifestations take time to occur, serious reactions usually do not develop in the dental office. However if reactions occur, the dentist should get medical help immediately, meanwhile keeping the patient calm and reassured.

VOMITING

If patient is receiving nitrous oxide analgesia, turn off the *nitrous* while maintaining the oxygen, and guide the patient's head to the cuspidor. If a rubber dam is in position, pull it to one side, and suction the vomitus with a large bore aspirating tip. Make sure that the patient does not occlude the glottis with the vomitus. If this occurs, follow instructions in the section on respiratory obstruction. Clean the patient's face and clothes and discontinue the treatment for that visit. Try to ascertain the cause of vomiting. If it is due to prior eating, advise the patient to eat a light meal at least one hour before the next appointment.

DRUG OVERDOSAGE—NARCOTICS

It is rare for the dentist to see a case of drug overdosage in the dental office, unless the patient is accidently given a toxic dose of a drug. However, it is possible for the patient to have taken an overdose just prior to the visit and then manifestations could occur in the office. Considering the fact that analgesics are probably the most widely prescribed drugs by dentists, the diagnosis and treatment of the analgesic overdosage is now to be discussed.

Manifestation of drug overdosage induced by any of the narcotic analgesics (codeine, Synalgos D-C, Percodan, Demerol, Dilaudid, Leritine, Dolophine, morphine), Darvon and its derivatives, and Talwin, is respiratory depression, leading to central paralysis of the respiratory centers. Treatment entails: (1) call a physician, (2) use a specific antagonist, (3) maintain a patent airway (described previously), and (4) administer oxygen (if necessary, initiate artificial respiration). The specific antagonists include (1) Nalorphine hydrochloride (Nalline®) for morphine, the other aforementioned narcotics, and Darvon. The initial dose is five to ten mg IV; to be repeated in ten to fifteen minutes; with the maximum being three doses. (2) Levallorphan tartrate (Lorfan®). This is also used for the same indications as Nalline, but it is much more potent and should be used when the precise extent of the overdose is known. The initial dose is one mg IV followed by another 0.5 mg three minutes later (if improvement in respiration is noted). Three administrations should be sufficient. (3) Naloxone hydrochloride (Narcan®). This is used specifically for Talwin overdosage. The initial dose is 0.4 mg IV. This can be repeated twice at three minute intervals.

ASPIRATED OR SWALLOWED ROOT CANAL INSTRUMENTS

With proper endodontic techniques (use of rubber dam, Endodontic Safety Chain) this complication should never occur. However, if the problem arises, certain measures should be taken:

(1) All methods should be undertaken to retrieve the instrument before it goes down the throat, such as use of aspiration, and in-

version of patient with slap between the back.

(2) If the glottis is occluded, follow the methods described in the section on respiratory passage obstruction.

(3) If the instrument is swallowed, give the patient water to drink to help prevent the instrument from being occluded in the wall of the intestinal tract.

(4) If the instrument has apparently been inhaled, then the patient should be referred to a physician for necessary radiographs.

(5) In both cases (aspiration or swallowing) medical referral is essential, and the patient must be informed of what has occurred.

BROKEN INJECTION NEEDLES

With the use of new, sterile, disposable needles, this complication is practically unknown. Nevertheless, if a needle breaks in the tissues, there should be an attempt to remove it with a hemostat. If this fails, the patient

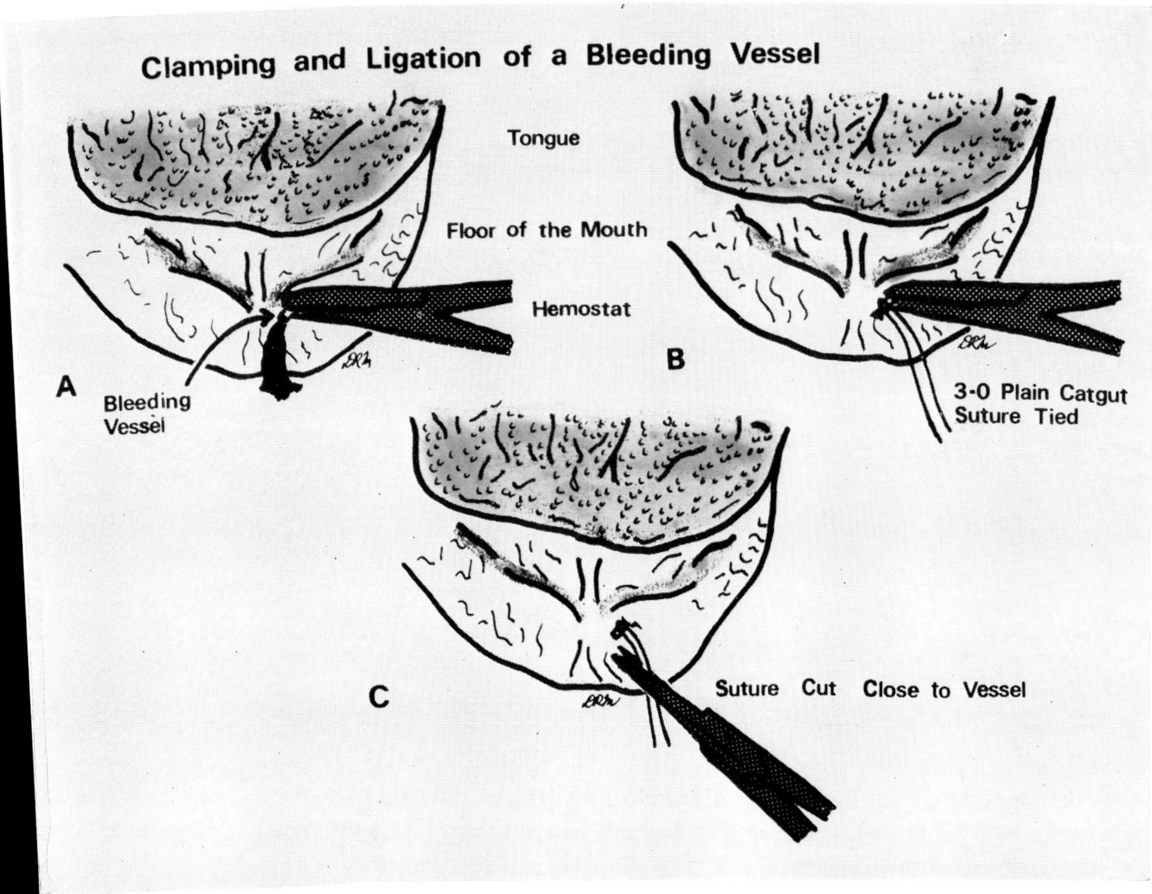

Figure 484

should be referred to an oral surgeon for attempted removal. Again, the patient should be immediately informed.

HEMORRHAGIC EMERGENCIES

Minor post-surgical hemorrhage is discussed in Chapter 10. In endodontic practice, hemorrhagic emergencies can result from bur or instrument laceration of blood vessels, post-surgically, or in patients with hemorrhagic diseases or tendencies. A thorough medical history should help prevent the latter etiology of hemorrhagic emergencies. Treatment is the following:

(1) The gross hemorrhage should be removed by aspiration in order to visualize the bleeding vessels.

(2) If the bleeding vessels are in soft tissue they should be clamped with a hemostat and tied off (Fig. 484); if they are in bone, the bone over the bleeding area should be crushed by forceful pressure of an instrument; alternatively, bone wax can be forced into the bleeding vessels.

(3) If bleeding cannot be controlled, medical assistance should be obtained and the patient should be kept calm.

SURGICAL EMPHYSEMA

Air in the tissues can cause sudden swelling that if it occurs in the neck region can interfere with respiration and this then constitutes a true emergency. The air mass can be infected and treatment should include the following:

(1) Prescription for penicillin or erythromycin (if allergy to penicillin is present) is given.

(2) The patient should be sent to a radiologist for a chest x-ray to see if mediastinal emphysema is present.

(3) A panograph or lateral jaw radiograph should be taken to see if radiolucent air masses are present in the jaw.

(4) Only if the condition gets worse should surgical intervention be done (usually the swelling resolves in a few days).

(5) If respiration is interfered with, the procedures described in section on management of respiratory obstruction should be done.

INJECTION OF LOCAL ANESTHETIC INTO REGION OF EYE, EAR, BUCCAL FAT PAD, SKIN, LIP, OR TONGUE

None of these reactions are serious. They can all be prevented with careful injection techniques. An injection in the region of the eye can cause a temporary diplopia (double vision) or blurring of vision (usually subsides in several minutes). If the ear is involved by an injection, a ringing or earache may occur that should subside within a couple of hours. An injection in the buccal fat pad can cause a swelling that may take several days to subside. For a skin, lip, or tongue injection, the bleeding should be stopped with gauze and an antiseptic such as tincture of metaphen should be placed. Another possible result is the formation of a hematoma. No treatment is necessary, as the extravasated blood is absorbed over a period of days to weeks. The patient should be informed about each of these conditions and of the probable outcome.

BURNS BY HEAT OR DRUGS OF LIPS, SKIN, OR ORAL MUCOSA

An anesthetic dressing (e.g. Xylocaine ointment) is placed on the wound. The patient should be informed that a scab will probably occur, but healing should take place. Unless it is a large burn, a scar usually does not result.

DISLOCATED MANDIBLE

This can occur if the patient keeps his (or her) mouth open too long. Also certain individuals are prone to this occurrence. The management entails:

(1) Try to relax the patient.
(2) The doctor positions himself in front of the patient.
(3) He places the thumbs in the inner aspect of the rami of the mandible with the four fingers of each hand wrapped around the outside of the mandible (Fig. 485).
(4) Pressure is exerted downward and then upward to get the condyle to snap into the glenoid fossa; this should be done as soon as possible, so that the masticatory muscles do not become spastic.
(5) If spasm occurs and the jaws cannot be positioned, it is necessary to inject a local anesthetic into the region of each condyle.
(6) It then may be possible to reposition the jaws.

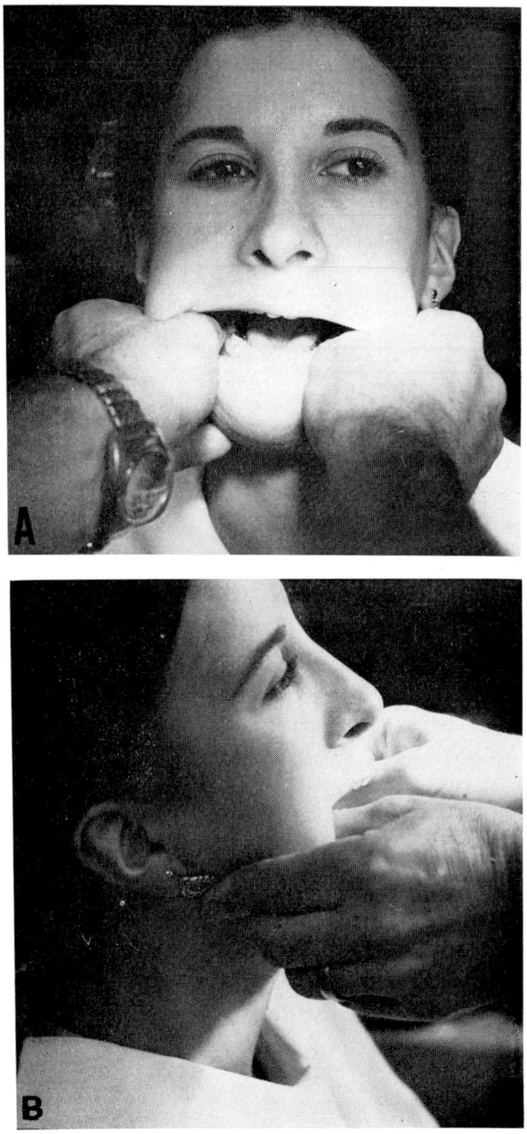

Figure 485. Repositioning a dislocated mandible (see text for description). A. Front view. B. Side view.

(7) If this still cannot be done, then the patient must be admitted to the operating room and the jaws are repositioned under general anesthesia.

ACCIDENT IN DENTAL CHAIR

The patient should be kept calm and if the accident is serious, medical assistance should be obtained immediately. The patient should not be moved, if there is possibility of damage to any internal organs.

SWALLOWING OF INTRACANAL MEDICAMENT OR IRRIGANT

With the use of a well fitted rubber dam, this complication should not occur. However, if the patient does swallow some medication, he (or she) should be informed that the small quantity will probably not cause any problem.

SPILLING OF INTRACANAL MEDICAMENT OR IRRIGANT ON PATIENT'S CLOTHES

Use of a drape would prevent this. If a caustic is used and damage occurs, it is up to the dentist to inform the p tient and remedy the situation.

BIBLIOGRAPHY

American Dental Association: Accepted De tal Therapeutics 1973/1974, 35th ed. C cago, American Dental Association, 1973.

Ballenger, J. J.: *Diseases of the Nose, Thro and Ear,* 11th ed. Philadelphia, Lea & Fe iger, 1969.

Beeson, P. B., and McDermott, W.: *Cec Loeb Textbook of Medicine,* 13th ed. Ph adelphia, Saunders, 1971.

Mann, D. E., Jr.: *Temple University Formu lary and Dental Therapeutics.* Baltimor Williams and Wilkins, In Preparation.

Mitchell, D. F., Standish, S. M., and Fas T. B.: *Oral Diagnosis/Oral Medicine,* 2n ed. Philadelphia, Lea & Febiger, 1971.

Roberts, M. W., and Morrill, G. S.: Medica emergencies and a standardized emergenc kit for the dental office. *J Acad Gen Dent* 20:36, 1972.

Selden, H. S.: Bone wax as an effective hemostat in periapical surgery. *Oral Surg, 29:* 262, 1970.

Welch, J. T.: Emergency drugs in dental practice. *Dent Clin North Am, 14:*821, 1970.

DIVISION FOUR

PREVENTION

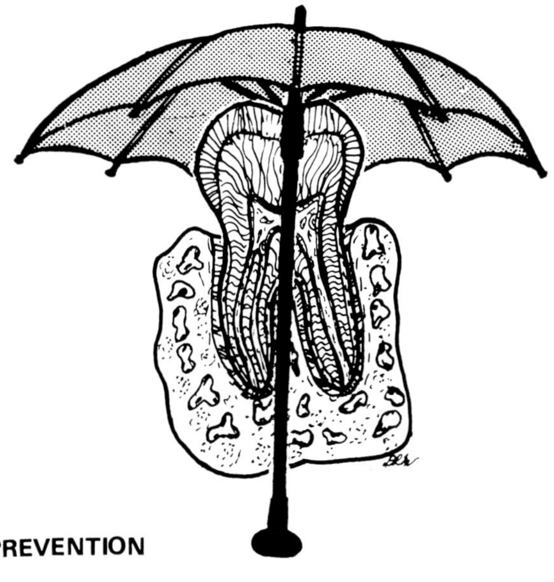

PREVENTION

CHAPTER 17

PREVENTION

THERE ARE SEVERAL aspects of prevention in endodontics. Most of these ave been alluded to in previous secons of this book. In this chapter, these reventative measures are categorized nd discussed briefly. The subjects covred include prevention of endodontic lisease, caries control methods, prevenion of extraction, prevention of treatment complications, prevention of retreatments, and prevention of serious medical complications by pulpal diagnosis.

TECHNIQUES AND METHODS TO PREVENT ENDODONTIC DISEASES

In the discussion of past and present oral history (Chapter 1) it was seen that

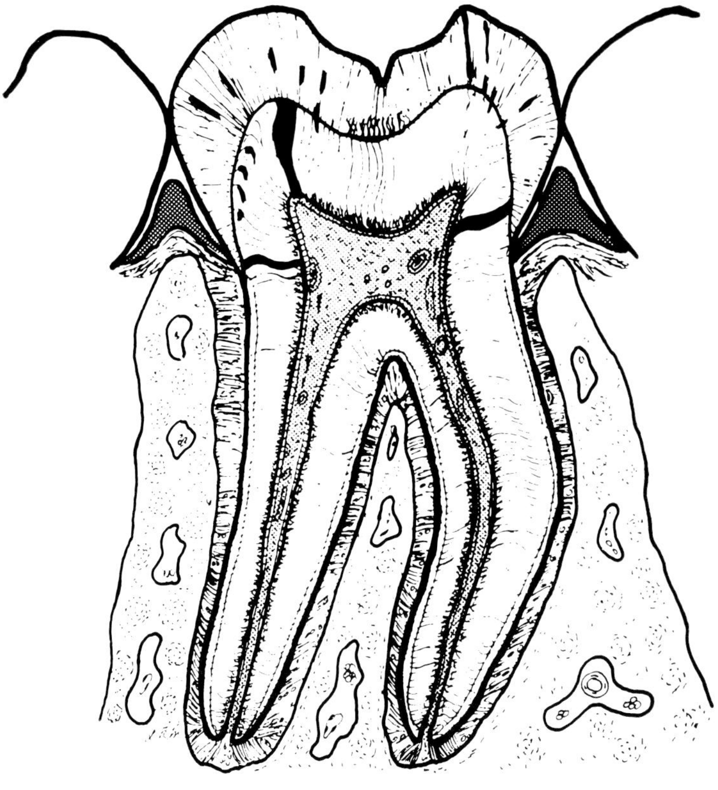

Figure 486. The normal pulp—goal of preventative endodontology.

there are many possible pulpal and periapical irritants. If the dentist follows these steps he will be able to prevent the development of most endodontic diseases (Fig. 486).

(1) Use adequate coolant during rotary instrumentation. Do not use speeds of 3,000 to 30,000 RPM. Ultra-high speed using small burs (larger burs and stones are more deleterious) with copious water spray at the actual site of cutting is the preferred method (Fig. 487). Cavity preparations should be as shallow as possible.

(2) Do not use compressed air blasts in deep unlined cavities.

(3) Do not dessicate cavities with alcohol, chloroform, or any other drying agent.

(4) Line deep cavities with a calcium hydroxide liner covered by a varnish.

(5) Do not polish restorations unless an adequate coolant is provided.

(6) Do not remove that last bit of leathery decay and cause an exposure; it is preferable to do indirect pulp capping.

(7) Do not place silver nitrate, phenol, or any other caustic drug on floor of cavity preparations, on surfaces of crown preparations, or on hypersensitive dentin or cementum, as these drugs can penetrate into

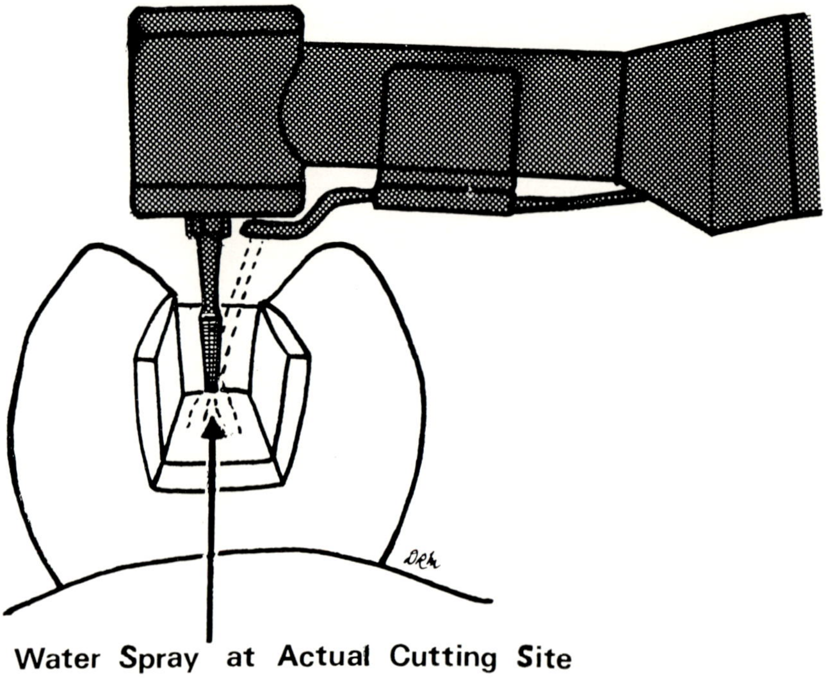

Figure 487

the pulp or cause pulpal damage.

(8) Do not repeatedly take hot compound copper band impressions on the same tooth as there is a double irritation to the pulp (heat and pressure) that is compounded with each impression. Use a well-fitting temporary crown or bridge, cemented in with zinc-oxide eugenol, in between visits to help allay the inflammation. These temporary restorations should not be fabricated in the mouth as the setting acrylics generate damaging heat.

(9) Do not perform tooth reduction and copper band impressions at the same visit. This is also to prevent compounding of pulpal irritation. Deep cutting of teeth to prepare parallel abutments is often dangerous. A possible alternative is the use of telescope crowns.

(10) If zinc phosphate cement is used as an insulation or for cementation, it is preferable to incorporate as much powder as possible into the mix to decrease the potential damaging effect of the acid. It is advisable to use a less irritating cement for insertion of restorations, such as a zinc polycarboxylate cement (Duralon, Poly-C) or a reinforced ZOE cement (EBA®, Final®). A calcium hydroxide base covered by a cavity varnish, placed beneath the zinc phosphate cement, should prevent the deleterious effects of the acid from reaching the pulp.

(11) Do not perform excessive malleting during gold foil insertion.

(12) Do not place silicates or acrylic resins in unlined cavities; use cavity sealers or varnish, as well as calcium hydroxide prior to the insertion of the synthetic restoration.

(13) Place a cavity varnish around the margins of amalgam restorations to help prevent seepage. Fluoride incorporation in amalgams may help prevent recurrent caries.

(14) Try not to use separation devices during operative dentistry. If they are used, separation should be very slow and not more than one mm.

(15) Be extremely careful in order to avoid pulp horn penetration when preparing and placing pins.

(16) When pulp testing a tooth, avoid excessive use of heat, cold, and electricity.

(17) Perform periodontal procedures judiciously so that there will not be pulpal injury or exposure of lateral canals. Microbial irritants may penetrate the pulp via lateral canals. Try not to remove excessive cementum, as this also can cause pulpal injury, resulting from exposure of lateral canals and dentinal tubules.

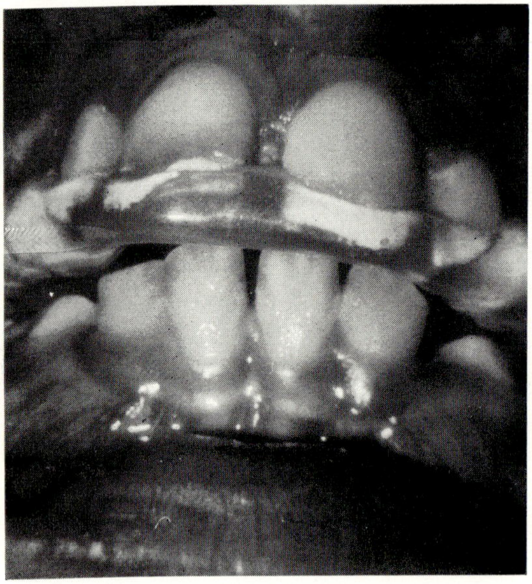

Figure 488. Processed acrylic mouth guard. (Courtesy of Dr. K. Bomze, Cherry Hill, N. J.)

(18) Use a rubber dam for cases of suspected pulp exposure during crown or cavity preparation, in order to prevent microbial contamination.

(19) Use a mouth guard for individuals engaged in conta sports (Fig. 488).

(20) Use a night guard for cases bruxism (Fig. 489).

(21) Explain to the patient the in portance of avoiding faci trauma in automobiles by th use of seat and shoulder belts.

(22) During orthodontic therapy, d not use excessive force or to rapid movement.

(23) Correct occlusal imbalances, o improper tooth contacts by th use of equilibration or properl contoured new restorations.

(24) Either remove developmenta grooves (prophylactic odontotomy) or use fissure sealants tc try to inhibit caries.

(25) During oral surgical procedures, be careful not to injure adjacent teeth.

(26) Advise other practitioners to try and avoid damage to teeth during nasal, sinus, and eye opera-

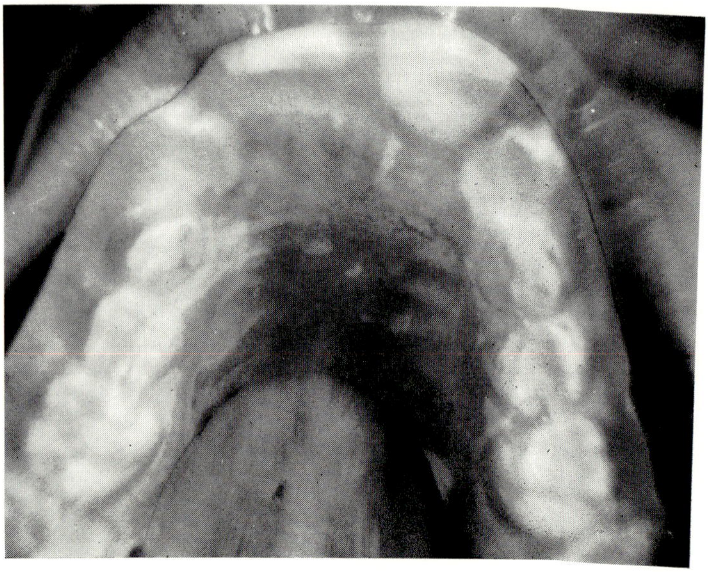

Figure 489. Processed acrylic night guard. (Courtesy of Dr. K. Bomze, Cherry Hill, N. J.)

tions, and during intubation procedures.

(27) Do bite-wing examinations every six months for caries detection. For any suspicious teeth or conditions, take periapical radiographs. Full mouth radiographs should be taken at least every three years.

(28) During examination for caries, pay particular attention to margins of orthodontic bands, beneath clasp attachments, and in cervical areas (possible root caries).

(29) Examine for abrasion, attrition and erosion (as well as caries).

(30) Recognize patient habits that have deleterious effects on teeth such as thumbsucking, biting on hard objects, and pushing the tongue against the lingual surfaces of anterior teeth. Try to correct these habits by explaining to the patients the results of their actions.

(31) Explain to the patient (or patient's parents) the importance of immediate replacement back into the socket of an avulsed tooth. The patient should be told that the tooth should be replaced by themselves (or their parents) if they cannot get to the dentist within one-half hour from the time the tooth was knocked out.

(32) Do not use electrocautery as a

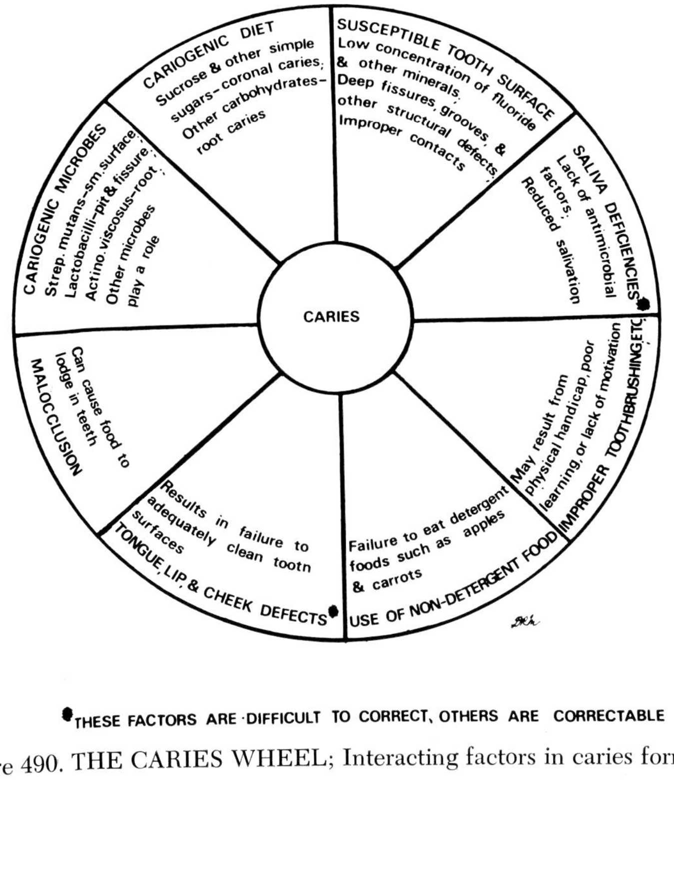

Figure 490. THE CARIES WHEEL; Interacting factors in caries formation.

treatment for hypersensitive dentin or cementum as the heat may cause pulpal damage.

CARIES CONTROL METHODS

As the predominant cause of endodontic disease is carious pulpal exposure, it is incumbent upon the dentist to instruct patients in methods of preventing or controlling dental caries. This would include methods of control of the interacting factors in the causation of dental caries: microbes, diet, tooth surfaces, etc. (Fig. 490). A brief summary of these methods is now given.

Plaque Control

Explain to the patient proper methods of plaque control to prevent dental caries. These include use of toothbrush, dental floss, irrigating devices, interdental stimulators and plaque disclosing agents.

Correct Use of Toothbrush

This is to remove food debris, stain, and plaque, and to prevent development of abrasion. In cases of surgery, the toothbrush should not be used for at least three days post-operatively in the vicinity of the surgical procedure. After the sutures are removed, brushing should be gentle for the following week.

Correct Use of Dental Floss

This is to remove plaque, the primary etiologic agent in caries and periodontal disease.

Correct Use of Irrigating Devices

This is to remove interproximal food debris and soft plaque from all tooth surfaces. This should not be used when there is an abscess present (to prevent spread of infection) or for at least one week after surgery (to prevent damage to the healing tissues). When it is then used, it should be at low pressure in the area where the surgery was performed, for another week, after which regular use can be reinstated.

Correct Use of Interdental Stimulators

These are used to stimulate the gingival tissues and aid in removing food debris from the interproximal areas.

Use of Plaque Disclosing Agents

These show the patient the effectiveness of his (or her) toothbrushing techniques.

Diet and Dental Caries

Explain to the patient the relationship of diet to dental caries. Subjects to be discussed are sucrose and other carbohydrates, proteins, detergent foods, abrasion, erosion, mineral supplements, mouthwashes, and toothpastes.

Sucrose and Other Carbohydrates

The patient should be informed of the deleterious effect of sucrose especially in the form of sticky-type candy. Sucrose in the form of sodas is not as detrimental as it does not remain on the tooth surface for a long enough period to aid in plaque formation. It is also a good idea to inform patients about the possible relationship of sucrose to heart disease, as well as dental caries. There is also recent evidence to show that other carbohydrates can act as substrata for the microorganism Actinomyces viscosus, which has been implicated

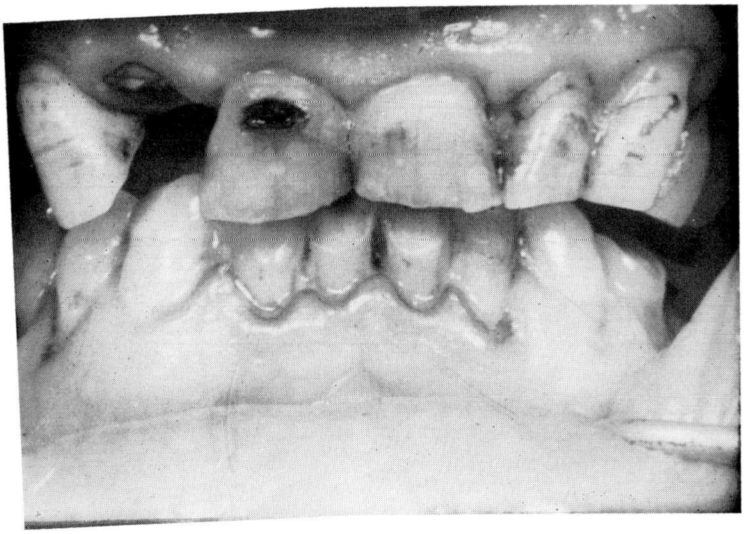

Figure 491. Excessive abrasion caused by overuse of abrasive foods. (Courtesy of Dr. T. Simpson, Philadelphia, Pa.)

in the etiology of root caries. Therefore, this reemphasizes the necessity of removing carbohydrates from root surfaces by mechanical means.

Proteins

A recent study with rats has shown that protein deficiency during gestation and lactation causes a markedly increased caries susceptibility. If this finding could be transferred to humans, it would show the importance of having adequate protein in the diet as a caries preventive measure.

Detergent Foods Such as Apples and Carrots

The patient should be informed that these type foods are preferable to sucrose snacks and they also have the bonus of helping in keeping teeth clean.

Abrasion

Explain to the patient the detrimental effects of eating excessively tough foods and/or of grinding the teeth (Fig. 491).

Erosion

Explain to the patient the corrosive effects of excessive intake of acidic fruit juices or excessive vomiting (Fig. 492).

Mineral Supplements

Explain to the patient, the advantage of mineral supplements. These supplements (fluorides and phosphates) are used to alter the tooth surface to make it less permeable to microbes and their products. The patient should be told about the use of the following:

FLUORIDATED WATER. In a concentration of one part per million in drinking water, most studies have shown a reduction of dental caries of approximately 60 per cent.

FLUORIDATED TOOTHPASTE. The effects appear to be additive to those achieved from drinking fluoridated water.

FLUORIDE TABLETS OR PHOSPHO-FLUORIDE TABLETS (OR DROPS). These must be prescribed by the dentist and are use-

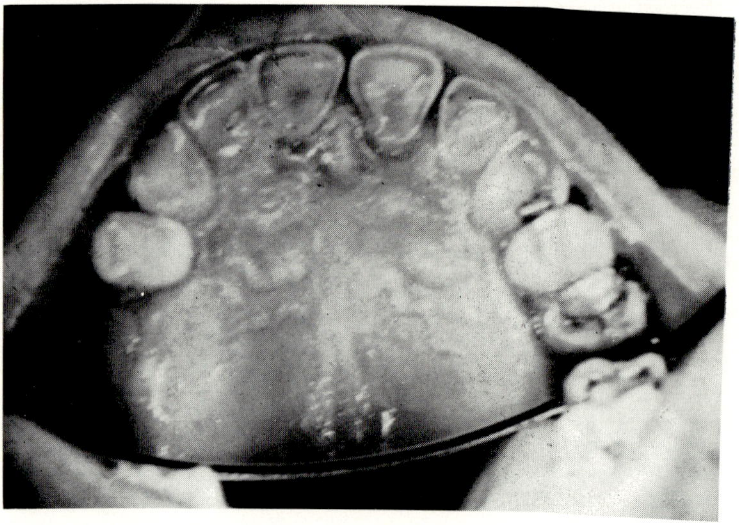

Figure 492. Erosion caused by acidic content of vomitus in a patient who had excessive vomiting. (Courtesy of Dr. T. Simpson, Philadelphia, Pa.)

ful for children in nonfluoridated areas.

FLUORIDE APPLICATIONS. Sodium fluoride or stannous fluoride can be used. Sodium fluoride must be applied in multiple sittings, while stannous fluoride appears to be just as effective in one sitting. Many dentists use solutions with acidulated phosphate (Luride® drops) which appear to give the best results. The fluoride should be applied at the completion of a prophylaxis and should be performed every six months. It is used for children and young adults. Recent findings show that a self application of an acidulated phosphate fluoride paste and gel is effective in reducing caries.

Microbial Reduction

Explain to the patient about methods of decreasing microbial populations. Use of mouthwashes have only a temporary effect but they do have a function in breath freshening. However, recent studies have shown that stannous fluoride mouth-rinses may be effective in reducing caries. Use of anti-microbial toothpastes such as those incorporating penicillin have had promising results in animal and clinical tests, but, this method has not yet been approved.

PREVENTION OF EXTRACTION

Prevention of extraction can be done by convincing dentists, physicians, and patients about the relative effectiveness and painlessness of endodontic therapy. It is still important to convince people that endodontically-treated teeth are not a menace to health, are not dead teeth, probably do not cause focal infection, and do not cause unbearable pain during or after treatment. These facts should be divulged by means of lectures, articles (in lay and professional journals), ordinary conversation, distribution of pamphlets, and use of audio-visual materials. It is also important to perform endodontic therapy in such a manner that the patient will no longer fear to have root canal therapy performed in the future. If enough patients have endodontic therapy performed in a satisfactory way, then fear of having root canal therapy will no longer prevent people from having this service.

Prevention of extraction by various surgical and nonsurgical endodontic procedures is what clinical endodontic practice is primarily concerned with. All the various treatment procedures discussed in division three are important because they either prevent or delay the loss of teeth. Tooth loss often leads to drifting and tilting of adjacent and opposing teeth, with the concomitant development of marginal periodontitis on those teeth. Performing endodontics rather than extraction prevents possible complications that can occur from extractions. These include *dry socket,* jaw fracture, broken root tip, and post-surgical pain and swelling.

PREVENTION OF TREATMENT COMPLICATIONS AND EMERGENCIES

This would be accomplished if the diagnostic and treatment procedures described in the previous chapters were followed carefully. A brief summary of complications followed by preventative methods is given in this section.

Tooth Discoloration

(1) Do complete access.
(2) Remove all pulp tissue or necrotic debris from pulp horns.
(3) Do prophylactic bleaching of anterior teeth.
(4) Do not use intracanal medicaments or cements that can stain dentinal tubules.
(5) Use an oxidizing irrigant (e.g. sodium hypochlorite, hydrogen peroxide, etc.).

Pain and Swelling

(1) Do not overinstrument vital cases.
(2) Do not irrigate beyond the apex with an irritating drug.
(3) Do not use irritating intracanal medicaments.
(4) Do not place medicaments on absorbent points.
(5) Do not leave restorations in supraocclusion.
(6) Do not leave pulpal remnants in the canal.
(7) Do not perforate root canals.
(8) Do not close root canals when there is active drainage present.

Broken Instruments

(1) Do not use old instruments.
(2) Do not use *worn out* instruments (stretched, open flutes).
(3) Do not use a broach as the first instrument in a root canal.
(4) Do not put too severe a bend on instruments (right angle or greater).
(5) Do not press directly apically with an instrument.
(6) Always use adequate irrigation while instrumenting.

Perforation and Ledges

(1) Curve each subsequent instrument with the same curvature as the previous one had.
(2) Return to the previous instrument after using a higher numbered instrument.

(3) Use adequate irrigation while instrumenting.
(4) Do not overuse calcium chelating agents (e.g. RC-Prep).
(5) Do not use fissure burs in the floor of the chamber.
(6) Be certain of the alignment of the long axis of the root during access preparation.

Burns, Eye Injuries, Swallowing of Medicaments, Staining of Clothes

(1) Drape the patient.
(2) Place eyeglasses on the patient.
(3) Use rubber dam.
(4) Be extremely careful with caustic chemicals such as formocresol, chloroform, paraformaldehyde pastes, chlorinated soda, 30% hydrogen peroxide (Superoxol).

Aspiration or Swallowing of Instruments

(1) Use rubber dam regularly.
(2) In those rare cases when that is not possible, use an Endodontic Safety Chain.

Broken Injection Needles

(1) Inject slowly.
(2) Do not force the needle into the tissues.
(3) Use new sterile disposable needles for each patient.

Bleeding Problems

(1) Take an adequate health history.
(2) Get blood tests or medical consultation when necessary.
(3) Be certain patient has whatever drugs or supplements they need.
(4) Do not traumatize the tissues.
(5) Clean the area well.
(6) Use firm pressure and adequate sutures.
(7) Give the patient appropriate post-operative instructions.

Oral-antral Fistula

(1) Try to avoid the sinus during periapical surgery.
(2) If this cannot be done, keep the opening into it as small as possible.
(3) Use enough sutures in order to get good closure of the incision.
(4) Do not use a semilunar incision when performing palatal surgery as this increases the possibility of creating an oral-antral fistula.
(5) Advise patient to try not to blow the nose or sneeze for the few day following sinus perforation.
(6) Prescribe a nasal decongestant.

Paresthesia

(1) Do not overinstrument or irrigate beyond the apex.
(2) Do not use irritating intracanal medicaments; especially do not use them on absorbent points.
(3) Do not overfill root canals of lower posterior teeth.
(4) When doing periapical surgery on lower posterior teeth, make the access from above.

Mobility

(1) Do not overinstrument.
(2) Do not traumatize the tooth during access and obturation.

Ecchymosis

(1) Do not traumatize tissues during periapical surgery.

Trismus

(1) Be certain inferior alveolar injections are correctly placed.
(2) Do not inject into muscles.
(3) Do not traumatize tissues.

Jaw Subluxation or Dislocation

(1) Do not have patient keep the mouth open too long (more than 45 minutes).
(2) Every few minutes allow the patient to partially close his (or her) mouth.

Syncope (Fainting)

(1) Have a gentle reassuring manner.
(2) Use nitrous oxide-oxygen relative analgesia regularly.
(3) Be especially careful with patients who have a previous history of syncope at the dental office.
(4) Patients who have a morning dental appointment should have a good breakfast, as some patients have a more pronounced tendency to faint if they have not eaten. However if the patient will be having nitrous oxide analgesia, he (or she) should not eat a heavy breakfast and should have the appointment delayed for at least an hour after eating.
(5) Patients who will have general anesthesia must not eat anything for several hours prior to the appointment.
(6) In patients taking anti-hypertensive drugs, sudden changes in position must be avoided, to prevent syncope.

Allergic Reactions

(1) Get a good medical history.
(2) Have skin tests taken if necessary.
(3) Get a medical consult if there is any doubt.
(4) Do not prescribe drugs to which the patient may be allergic.
(5) Use nitrous oxide with high oxygen concentration (80% or higher) for asthma patients. This insures that they will have a high alveolar oxygen content and will help prevent an asthma attack.

Serious Toxic Reactions

(1) Do not give drugs to patients for whom these drugs are contraindicated.
(2) Consider drug interactions when prescribing drugs.
(3) Be certain that a drug overdose is avoided; if necessary consult with the family pharmacist.
(4) Be certain that a good medical history is obtained.
(5) Use an aspirating syringe and aspirate before each injection, to prevent toxic systemic reaction resulting from blood vessel injection. When a local anesthetic has been given, and the dentist has to leave the room he should be certain that the assist-

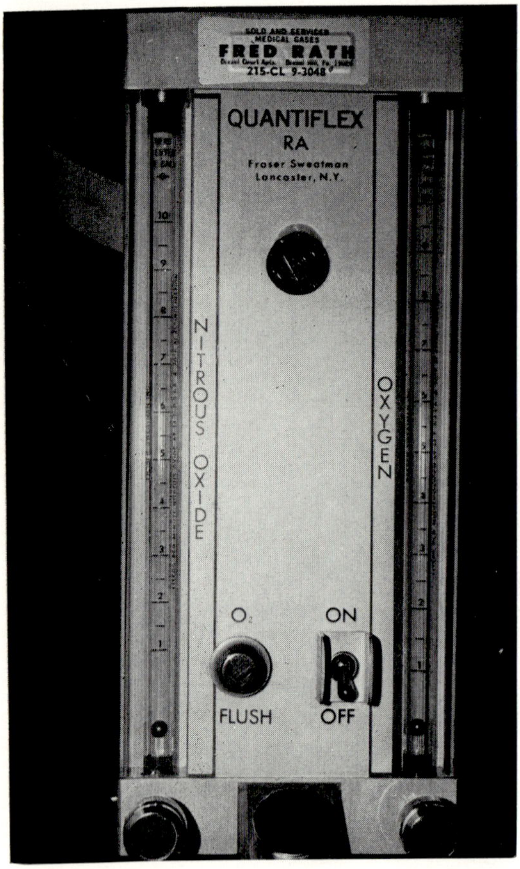

Figure 493. A constant flow-fail safe nitrous oxide-oxygen relative analgesia machine (Quantiflex RA-Fraser Sweatman).

ant stays in the room with the patient. This does two things: (a) it reassures the patient that he (or she) is not being deserted; and (b) it allows the assistant to monitor any untoward reactions, so they can be treated immediately.

(6) When using nitrous oxide-oxygen analgesia, only use a fail-safe machine (Fig. 493).

(7) Do not use *nitrous* for patients with colds, or bronchial, and lung diseases, to prevent dissemination of microbes.

(8) Have emergency drugs available; have the knowledge of how to use them; and have an office protocol for emergency treatment, including a list of whom to call for help.

(9) Prevent bacteremia results (subacute bacterial endocarditis and other systemic infectious diseases) by giving correct antibiotics for indicated patients, and by performing endodontics rather than extraction. Studies have shown a much higher incidence of bacteremia following extractions as compared to post-endodontic therapy.

(10) Prevent serious reactions in cardiac, diabetic, and other patients with severe systemic conditions by the proper use of sedatives, analgesics, other necsary drugs, and a reassuring manner.

(11) Prevent early death in leukemic patients by performing endodontic therapy rather than extractions.

(12) Prevent osteoradionecrosis by the use of nonsurgical endodontic therapy rather than extractions.

(13) Prevent transmission of hepatitis and other systemic diseases by only using sterile instruments and supplies and by wearing sterile gloves.

(14) Prevent interference with pacemaker action, by not using an electric pulp tester for patients having pacemakers.

Hematoma

(1) Do not inject into blood vessels.
(2) Do not injure major blood vessels during surgery.

Buccal Fat Pad Swelling

(1) Do not inject into the region of the buccal fat pad.

Air Embolism or Surgical Emphysema

(1) Do not blow air into root canals or into periapical *areas* during surgery.

Diplopia (Double Vision)

(1) Do not inject in region of orbit while giving an infraorbital or posterior superior alveolar injection.

Ringing in the Ears

(1) Do not inject in the region of the auriculo-temporal nerve while giving an inferior alveolar nerve injection.

Tooth Fracture

(1) Do not use excessive pressure during instrumentation or obturation.

Fracture of Jacket Crown

(1) To gain access into these crowns, use a new diamond stone or a No. 35 inverted cone bur in an ultra-high speed contra-angle with water spray.

Vomiting

(1) Do not use nitrous oxide analgesia immediately after the patient has eaten.
(2) Have the patient hold the x-ray film firmly, especially while the rubber dam is in position. This is especially true for patients who are prone to vomiting, such as those taking digitalis.

Accidents

(1) Have the patient remove their glasses after access preparation; they can get in the operator's way during treatment or can be accidently broken.
(2) If nitrous-oxide oxygen-analgesia or chemanalgesia has been used during treatment, carefully guide the patient to the cuspidor when they have to rinse. If not, a patient can hit their head against the cuspidor, as he (or she) may be dizzy. Also, at the conclusion of the visit, the patient should be helped out of the chair to prevent his (or her) falling and injuring himself (or herself).
(3) Be certain that a patient who has taken a drug such as phenobarbital, meperidine or Percodan, had chemanalgesia during treatment, or had taken any other drug that would impair the senses, has someone along to

drive him (or her) home. If not, a vehicular accident can occur.

Possible Damage to a Fetus

(1) Do not prescribe drugs to a pregnant woman during the first trimester.

(2) Use a lead apron, a properly shielded x-ray machine, and as few radiographs as possible when treating a pregnant woman.

PREVENTION OF RETREATMENTS

If correct endodontic therapy is performed in a healthy individual, then retreatment should not be necessary, unless systemic conditions change (e.g. development of diabetes, a hormonal deficiency or protein deprivation) periodontal disease occurs, or caries or trauma supervenes. Some of the factors included in correct endodontic therapy which would tend to prevent retreatments or loss of teeth following completion of therapy are correct diagnosis, complete access, complete instrumentation, control of infectious diseases (decrease of microbial population, increase of host resistance), and as complete obturation as possible. It is also essential to inform the patient about the necessity of coronal restoration, including the use of posts and pins when indicated (see Chapter 14). If periodontal disease is present, it must be treated; if it is not present, it must be prevented. The occlusion must be balanced and the patient must be made aware of the fact the decay can still occur in endodontically-treated teeth. In addition, trauma must be avoided to the treated tooth.

PREVENTION OF SERIOUS MEDICAL COMPLICATIONS BY PULPAL DIAGNOSIS

There is a new aspect of diagnosis of medical conditions that is performed by an examination of the dental pulp. The patients do not have to have any symptoms related to pulpal disease. The pulp is removed because it is an easily accessible connective tissue that can be sectioned, stained, and examined histologically. It has been possible to diagnose metachromatic leukodystrophy in this manner. This myelin degeneration disease shows the presence of sulfatide granules in the nerve fibers of the den-

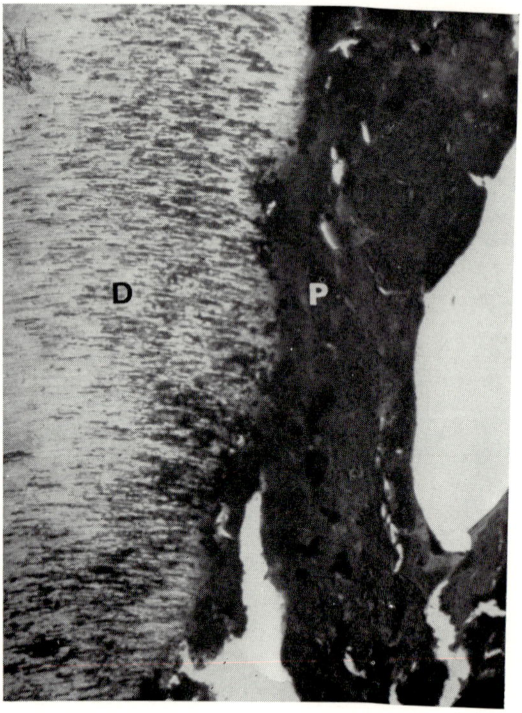

Figure 494. Mycobacteria leprae in the dentinal tubules and invading the pulp in a case of leprosy. (Courtesy of Dr. T. Simpson, Philadelphia, Pa.)

pulp. In primary hyperoxaluria and losis, biopsy of the dental pulp has ealed the presence of diagnostic oxa- crystals (in the soft tissue and ontoblasts). Although not specific to pulp, mycobacterium leprae have en found invading the pulp from dentin in cases of leprosy (Fig. 4). It is possible that in the future lpal diagnosis of systemic diseases ll allow for early diagnosis and pre- ntion of serious medical complica- ons.

BIBLIOGRAPHY

nerican Dental Association: Protein deficit appears to boost caries danger. *ADA News, 4(19)*:6, Sept. 10, 1973.

uonocore, M.: Sealants. *J Am Soc Prev Dent, 3*:Jan-Feb, 1973.

heraskin, E., Ringsdorf, W. M., and Clark, J. W.: *Diet and Disease*. Emmaus, Pennsylvania, Rodale Books, 1968.

ilass, R. T.: Oral manifestations in primary hyperoxaluria and oxalosis: report of a case. *Oral Surg, 35*:502, 1973.

Iazen, S. P., Chilton, N. W., and Mumma, R. D., Jr.: The problem of root caries. 1. Literature review and clinical description. *JADA, 86*:137, 1973.

Hoerman, K. C., Keene, H. J., Shklair, I. L., and Burmerster, J. A.: The association of streptococcus mutans with early carious lesions in human teeth. *JADA, 85*:1349, 1972.

Kopel, H. M., and Grenoble, D. E.: The pit and fissure sealants: a critical review. *JSCDA, 41*:103, 1973.

Morse, D. R.: Sucrose: A common enemy for medicine and dentistry. *J Am Soc Prev. Dent, 2(5)*:27, 1972.

Newbrun, E.: *Fluorides and Dental Caries*. Springfield, Thomas, 1972.

Nizel, A. E.: *Nutrition in Preventive Dentistry: Science and Practice*. Philadelphia, Saunders, 1972.

Ralcike, A. W., Gish, C. W., Peterson, J. K., King, J. D., and Segreto, V. A.: Clinical evaluation of stannous fluoride as an anticaries mouthrinse. *JADA, 86*:404, 1973.

Scherp, H. W.: Dental caries: prospects for prevention. *Science, 173*:1199, 1971.

Seltzer, S., and Bender, I. B.: *The Dental Pulp: Biologic Considerations in Dental Procedures*. Philadelphia, Lippincott, 1965.

Stanley, H. R.: The effects of systemic diseases on the human pulp. *Oral Surg, 33*:606, 1972.

Trubman, A., and Caellin, J. A.: Effect on dental caries of self-application of acidulated phosphate fluoride paste and gel. *JADA, 86*:153, 1973.

APPENDIX 1

SYSTEMIC DIAGNOSTIC TESTS

Test	*Normal Range*	*Disease or Condition and Range*
A. Blood Tests		
1. Acetone	0.3-2.0 mg%	Increased in diabetes (ketosis stage)
2. Amino acid nitrogen	4-6 mg%	Increased with extensive liver damage
3. Amylase	60-150 Somogyi units/100 ml	Increased in acute pancreatitis, cystic fibrosis, mumps, and in some cases of sialolithiasis
4. Ascorbic acid	0.6-1.6 mg% (plasma)	Low in scurvy and vitamin C deficiency; decreases during stress
5. Bilirubin		These are increased with most cases of jaundice
a. Direct	Up to 0.4 mg%	
b. Indirect	0.4-0.8 mg%	
c. Total	0.5-1.4 mg%	
6. Bromsulphalein (BSP)	Less than 5% dye retention at 45 minutes	Abnormal degrees of retention occur in various liver diseases
7. Calcium	9-10.6 mg% (4.5-5.3 mEq/liter)	Increased in: hyperparathyroidism; malignant bone lesions; hypervitaminosis D; sarcoidosis. Decreased in: hypoparathyroidism; advanced rickets; renal rickets; advanced osteomalacia; steatorrhea (as is found in some cases of cystic fibrosis)
8. Carbon Dioxide		
a. Content	24-30 mM/liter (Adults)	Increased in respiratory acidosis or metabolic alkalosis; decreased in metabolic acidosis or respiratory alkalosis
b. Pressure (PCO_2)	35-45 mm Hg	
9. Cells		
a. RBC		
(1) Number	4,500,000-5,500,000 per cu/mm (women); 4,000,000-5,000,000 per cu/mm (men)	Anemias show a relative decrease; polycythemia shows a marked increase
(2) Morphology and staining properties	Biconcave disc; saturated red color	Iron deficiency anemia; hypochromic microcytic Pernicious anemia; hyperchromic macrocytic Sickle cell anemia; moon or sickle shaped cells Cooley's anemia; "target cells"
(3) Sedimentation rate	Wintrobe test 0-9 mm/hr (men) 0-20 mm/hr (women)	Decreased in sickle cell anemia Increased in many diseases; indicator of course of rheumatic fever

Test	*Normal Range*	*Disease or Condition and Range*
(4) Indices		
(a) MCV	82-92 cu u	Increased in pernicious anemia; decreased in iron deficiency anemia
(b) MCH	27-31 u u	Increased in pernicious anemia; decreased in iron deficiency anemia
(c) MCHC	32-36%	Decreased in iron deficiency anemia
(5) Fragility test, osmotic	In % of NaCl; hemolysis begins 0.45-0.39; complete 0.33-0.30	More rapid destruction in certain hemolytic anemias
(6) Hematocrit	40-54 volumes % (men) 37-47 volumes % (women)	Decreased in anemias; increased in polycythemia vera
(7) Hemoglobin	14-18 gm% (men) 12-16 gm% (women)	Decreased in anemias; increased in polycythemia vera
b. WBC		
(1) Number	4,000-11,000 per cu/mm	
(2) Differential		Neutrophilic leucocytosis in: acute infections; after severe hemorrhage; chronic myelocytic leukemia; intestinal obstruction
(a) Myelocytes	0 (0%)	
(b) Meta-myelocytes	0-100 (1%)	
(c) Band	0-500 (0-5%)	Lymphocytosis in: chronic lymphatic leukemia; infectious mononucleosis; chronic infections
(d) Adult neutrophiles	2,500-6,000 (40-60%)	
(e) Lymphocytes	1,000-4,000 (20-40%)	Monocytosis in: monocytic leukemia; subacute bacterial endocarditis; tuberculosis
(f) Monocytes	200-800 (4-8%)	
(g) Eosinophiles	50-300 (1-3%)	Eosinophilia in: allergic diseases; parasitic infections
(h) Basophiles	0-100 (0-1%)	Leukopenia in: mumps; measles; typhoid fever; influenza; pernicious anemia; aplastic anemia; radiation therapy; aleukemic leukemia
		Agranulocytosis after ingestion of high doses of: sulfonamides; tetracyclines; streptomycin; chloramphenicol; and thorazine
		Shift to the left (immature forms) in: leukemias; infectious mononucleosis (some cases)
		Shift to the right (mature forms) in pernicious anemia
c. Platelets	200,000-500,000 per cu/mm	Decreased in the thrombocytopenias and the defibrination syndromes; *abnormal platelets with the qualitative platelet deficiencies*
10. Cephalin-Cholesterol Flocculation	Negative or 1+ after 24 hrs; 2+ or less after 48 hrs	Positive in many cases of hepatitis and cirrhosis
11. Chloride	95-103 mEq/liter	Increased in kidney disease; decreased with diarrhea and vomiting; important in the regulation of acid-base balance

12. Cholesterol (total)	150-250 mg%	Elevated in: cardiac diseases; hypothyroidism; diabetes; liver diseases (some types); decreased in other types of liver diseases
13. CPK	0-36 international units	Elevated in myocardial infarction and muscular dystrcphy
14. Glucose	Fasting level: 65-100 mg%	High in diabetes
15. Glucose tolerance	Fasting level: 70-110 mg%; 1 hr—20-50 mg above; 2 hrs—5-15 mg above; 3 hrs—fasting level or below	In diabetes: 1 hr-180 mg% or greater
16. Hemorrhage disorders evaluation tests		
a. ADP-induced platelet aggregation	Compared to a standard curve	Deficient in platelet disorders
b. Bleeding time (Duke)	1-6 minutes	Prolonged in platelet deficiencies, vascular defects, and Von Willebrand's disease
c. Clotting time (Lee & White)	6-10 minutes (glass tubes)	Prolonged in coagulation defects
d. Clot reaction time	In a normal individual, the clot decreases to one-half the original amount within 1 hr after clotting begins (3-4+)	Prolonged in platelet deficiencies; with disseminated intravascular coagulation, there is a small retracted clot that appears to lyse
e. Euglobulin lysis time	2-4 hrs for lysis	Rapid lysis is indicative of fibrinolysis defect
f. Fibrinogen	0.2-0.4 gm%	Decreased in liver damage and fibrinogen deficiency diseases
g. Fibrin split products	Less than 10 μg	Found with disseminated intravascular coagulation and fibrinolysis
h. Partial thromboplastin time (PTT)	60-70 seconds	Prolonged in coagulation deficiencies
i. Platelet adhesiveness	Greater than 15% adhesiveness in glass beads	Impaired with certain platelet disorders, including Von Willebrand's disease
j. Prothrombin time (Quick; PT)	12-14 seconds	Prolonged in prothrombin deficiency, Factors V, VII, and X deficiencies, disseminated intravascular coagulation, and with liver damage
k. Thrombin time (TT)	Less than 6 seconds	Prolonged with fibrinogen deficiencies
l. Thromboplastin generation	Conform to normal range of PTT	Impaired with classical hemophilia
m. Tourniquet test (Rumpel-Leede)	Less than 5 petechiae in a 1½ inch diameter on the volar surface of the arm	Increased in the platelet deficiencies, including Von Willebrand's disease, and in vitamin C deficiency
17. Hydrogen ion concentration (pH)	7.35-7.45	Varies with type of acidosis or alkalosis (respiratory or metabolic)
18. Iodine		
a. Protein bound	4-8 μg/100 ml	High in hyperthyroidism; low in hypothyroidism
b. Butanol extractable	3.5-6.5 μg/100 ml	High in hyperthyroidism; low in hypothyroidism

Test	*Normal Range*	*Disease or Condition and Range*
19. Iron	50-150 μg/100 ml	Low in iron deficiency anemia
20. LDH	80-120 Wacker units	Elevated in myocardial infarction
21. Lipase	0-1.5 Cherry Crandall units	Increased in pancreatic diseases
22. Non-protein nitrogen (NPN)	20-35 mg%	Increased in kidney disease
23. Microbes	None	Present with bacteremias and septicemias
24. Phosphatase (Acid)	0-1.1 Bodansky units; 1-4 King-Armstrong units	Increased in metastatic carcinoma of the prostate and Gaucher's disease
25. Phosphatase (Alkaline)	1.5-4.5 Bodansky units; 4-13 King-Armstrong units	Increased in: hyperparathyroidism; Paget's disease; rickets; osteomalacia; osteosarcoma; bony metastases; and liver diseases; decreased in hypophosphatasia
26. Phosphorus	3-4.5 mg%; 1.8-2.6 mEq/liter	Increased in: hypoparathyroidism; hypervitaminosis D; renal insufficiency Decreased in: hyperparathyroidism; rickets; osteomalacia; and vitamin D-resistant rickets
27. Potassium	4.0-4.8 mEq/liter	Increased in: renal failure; adrenal cortical insufficiency Decreased in: diarrhea; diabetic acidosis; chronic renal diseases; important in acid-base balance
28. Proteins		
a. Total b. Albumin	6.0-7.8 gm% 3.2-4.5 gm%	Low total protein and albumin is seen in: liver diseases (e.g. cirrhosis); intestinal diseases (e.g. sprue); starvation; and kidney diseases (e.g. nephrosis) High albumin levels are seen in dehydration and shock
c. Globulins (alpha, beta, gamma)	2.3-3.5 gm%	High alpha globulins are found with: acute febrile diseases; and wasting diseases such as malignancies and tuberculosis High beta globulins are found in: hepatitis; cirrhosis; and atherosclerosis High gamma globulins are found in: allergic responses and diseases; auto-immune type diseases (eg. rheumatoid arthritis; lupus erythematosus, Hashimoto's thyroiditis); multiple myeloma; hepatitis; cirrhosis; and macroglobulinemia No gamma *globulins are seen in patients with agammaglobulinemia*
d. C-reactive protein (ceruloplasmin)	23-50 mg/100 ml	Present in cases of inflammatory reactions and infectious diseases; is found in some cases of periodontal disease; may be present in periapical serum in cases of cysts and granulomas (see Figs. 126, 127)

e. A/G ratio	1.5:1-3:1	Reversal of ratio in patients with chronic or advanced liver disease, such as cirrhosis
29. Sodium	136-142 mEq/liter	High in dehydration and hypercortinism; low in kidney disease, Addison's disease
30. Thyroxine tests		Altered in thyroid diseases
a. Thyroxine serum (Murphy-Patee)	2.9-6.4 μg/100 ml	
b. T4 by column	3.4-6.4 μg/100 ml	
c. TBG	10-26 μg/100 ml	
31. Transaminases		
a. GOT	Up to 9-25 Karmen units	Increased in myocardial infarction, muscular dystrophy, and liver diseases
b. GPT	Up to 4-30 Karmen units	Increased in liver diseases
32. Urea Nitrogen (BUN)	8-20 mg%	Increased in advanced kidney disease Decreased in extensive liver disease
33. Uric Acid	2.1-7.8 mg% (men) 2.0-6.4 mg% (women)	Increased in gout
B. Urine Tests		
1. Acetone	0	Found in diabetes (ketosis stage)
2. Albumin	10-100 mg/24 hrs	Increased in kidney disease
3. Ammonia	20-70 mEq/liter	Increased in acidosis; decreased in alkalosis
4. Bence-Jones protein	0	Found in many cases of multiple myeloma
5. Bilirubin	0	Found in liver diseases
6. Blood cells	0	Found in kidney diseases
7. Calcium	Av. diet; 100-250 mg/24 hrs Low ca. diet; <150 mg/24 hrs High ca. diet; 250-350 mg/24 hrs	Increased excretion in: hyperparathyroidism; hyperthyroidism; osteoporosis (especially after immobilization); and hypervitaminosis D Decreased excretion in: hypoparathyroidism; steatorrhea; and vitamin D deficiency
8. Casts	0	Found in kidney diseases
9. Color	Clear yellow	Red in porphyrias and bleeding (kidney diseases); yellowish-brown or greenish-brown in gall bladder diseases
10. Epithelial cells	0-few	If occurs in large numbers, indicates bladder or urethra inflammation
11. Glucose	0	Found in diabetes
12. Hemoglobin	0	Found in kidney diseases
13. Hydrogen ion concentration (pH)	4.6-8	Varies with type of acidosis or alkalosis (respiratory or metabolic)

Test	*Normal Range*	*Disease or Condition and Range*
14. Microbes	0	Found in kidney infections
15. Odors	None	Found in kidney infections
16. Phosphorus	0.9-1.3 gm/24 hrs (varies with intake)	Increased excretion in hyperparathyroidism
17. Proteins (aside from albumin)	10-150 mg/24 hrs	Increased in kidney diseases
18. "Pus" (Polymorph leucocytes)	0	Found in kidney infections
19. Specific gravity	1.016-1.022 (24 hr period)	Increased in: dehydration; shock; diabetes mellitus: nephritis (some cases) Decreased in diabetes insipidus
20. Steroids (17 ketosteroids)	8-15 mg/24 hrs (men) 6-11.5 mg/24 hrs (women)	Increased in Cushing's disease Absent in Addison's disease
21. Urobilinogen	0.05-2.5 mg/24 hrs	Increased in liver diseases and hemolytic anemia
22. Volume (total)	600-1600 ml/24 hrs	Increased in: diabetes; (chronic) glomerulonephritis; and hyperparathyroidism Decreased in: acute glomerulonephritis; dehydration; and shock

APPENDIX 2

CALCIFICATION AND ERUPTION PATTERNS OF PERMANENT TEETH

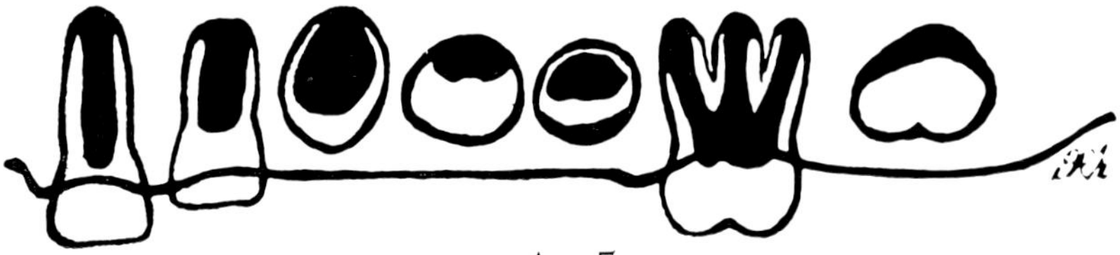

Age 7

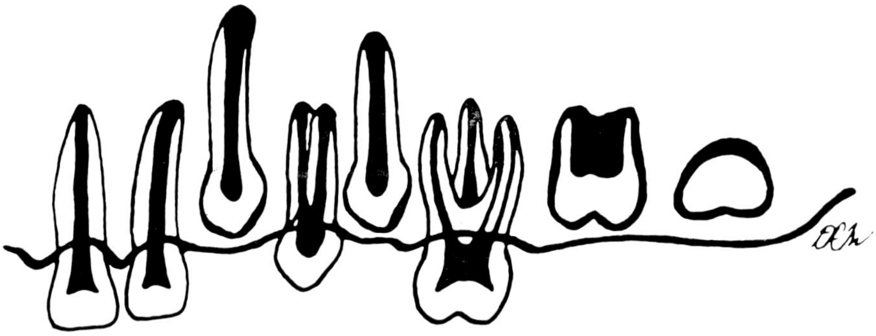

Age 10

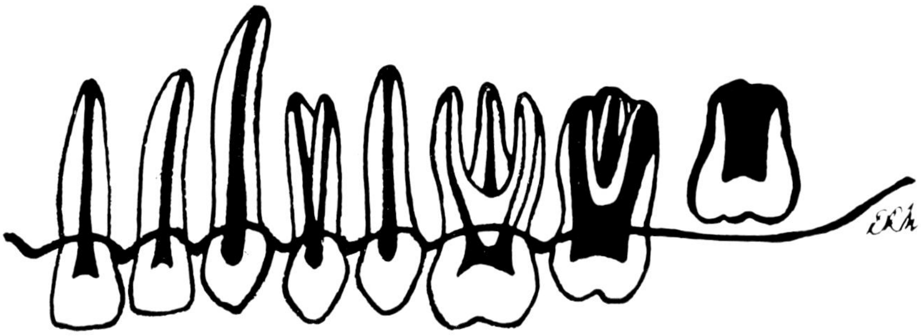

Age 13

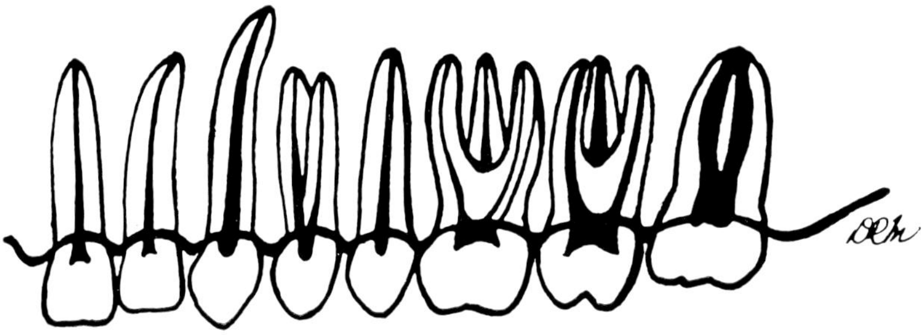

Age 18

APPENDIX 3

DRUG INTERACTIONS

This table is based on material derived from several sources (listed in the bibliography). The actions that may result from the various combinations have been reported in the literature but they do not always occur. They are listed here for informational use.

Drug Patient Is Taking	*Use*	*Drug Dentist Prescribes*	*Actions That Result From the Combination*
Acidifying agents: Ammonium chloride and nitrate; ascorbic acid (Vit. C); calcium chloride; cranberry juice; fowl and fish; lysine hydrochloride; methenamine hippurate and mandelate; methionine; orange juice; sodium acid phosphate; etc.	Foods and various uses; acidifiers tend to inhibit bases (increase excretion) and potentiate weak acids (decrease excretion)	Antihistamines	Acidifiers inhibit antihistamines
		Aspirin	Acidifiers potentiate aspirin
		Atropine	Acidifiers inhibit atropine
		Barbiturates	Acidifiers potentiate barbiturates
		Benzodiazepines (Librium, Valium, Serax)	Acidifiers inhibit benzodiazepines
		Erythromycin	Acidifiers inhibit erythromycin
		Levarterenol (Levophed)	Acidifiers inhibit levarterenol
		Mefenamic acid (Ponstel)	Acidifiers potentiate mefenamic acid
		Meperidine (Demerol) and other narcotic analgesics	Acidifiers inhibit meperidine and other narcotic analgesics
		Procaine (Novocain)	Acidifiers inhibit procaine
		Sulfonamides	Acidifiers potentiate sulfonamides
		Tetracyclines	Acidifiers potentiate tetracyclines
Adrenergic blocking agents: Alpha blockers; (*see* Anti-hypertensives) Beta blockers; propranolol (Inderal)	Heart disease treatment, especially for angina pectoris	Antihistamines	Propranolol antagonizes antihistamines
		Aspirin	Propranolol inhibits aspirin
		Barbiturates	Propranolol potentiates barbiturates
		Corticosteroids	Propranolol inhibits corticosteroids
		Morphine and narcotic agents	Propranolol potentiates narcotic agents; can be severe reaction
Alcohol	Beverage	Analgesics	Alcohol potentiates analgesics; alcohol plus morphine can be lethal; alcohol plus aspirin increases possibility of gastric hemorrhage; if patients are also taking thiazide diuretics, there is an increased chance of precipitating acute gout
		Anti-anxiety agents and	Alcohol potentiates sedative action; meprobamate (Equa-

		tranquilizers	nil, Miltown) plus alcohol can be lethal
		Antihistamines	Alcohol potentiates sedative action
		Atropine and similar agents	Alcohol plus atropine-like agents can cause prolonged mydriasis
		Barbiturates and other sedatives	Alcohol potentiates sedative action; can be lethal combination
		Sulfonamides	Sulfonamides potentiate the psychotoxic effects of alcohol
		Tetracyclines	Alcohol potentiates the tetracylines
Alkalinizing agents: Acetazolamide (Diamox); coffee, milk and milk products etc.; potassium citrate; sodium bicarbonate, citrate, and lactate	Foods and various uses; alkalinizers tend to inhibit weak acids (increase excretion) and potentiate weak bases (decrease excretion)	Antihistamines	Alkalinizers potentiate antihistamines
		Aspirin	Alkalinizers inhibit aspirin
		Atropine	Alkalinizers potentiate atropine
		Barbiturates	Alkalinizers inhibit barbiturates
		Benzodiazepines	Alkalinizers potentiate benzodiazepines (probably)
		Erythromycin	Alkalinizers potentiate erythromycin
		Levarterenol	Alkalinizers potentiate levarterenol
		Mefenamic acid	Alkalinizers inhibit mefenamic acid (probably)
		Narcotic analgesics	Alkalinizers potentiate narcotic analgesics
		Procaine	Alkalinizers potentiate procaine
		Sulfonamides	Alkalinizers inhibit sulfonamides
		Tetracyclines	Alkalinizers inhibit tetracyclines
Analgesics—weak: Acetaminophen (Tylenol, Tempra, Nebs); aspirin; dipyrone (Dipralone; it is rarely used); indomethacin (Indocin); phenacetin (acetophenetidin) Pyrazilone derivatives; aminopyrine (Pyramidon); antipyrine; oxyphenbutazone (Tandearil); phenylbutazone (Butazolidin); sulfinpyrazone (Anturane)	Pain relief; anti-inflammatory, anti-pyresis; treatment of arthritis	Antihistamines	Pyrazilone deriviatives and antihistamines inhibit each other
		Ascorbic acid (vitamin C)	Vitamin C potentiates analgesics; aspirin inhibits vitamin C
		Aspirin	Aspirin antagonizes the anti-inflammatory action of indomethacin and both together cause enhanced ulcerogenic effect in the gastrointestinal tract lining (can be severe); indomethacin and phenylbutazone enhance aspirin's action
		Barbiturates	Analgesics tend to potentiate sedative action; barbiturates inhibit analgesia produced by aspirin and dipyrone and increase breakdown of acetaminophen into its metabolites (tendency to form methemoglobin); pyrazilone derivatives and barbiturates inhibit each other
		Corticosteroids	Aspirin and indomethacin plus corticosteroids cause increased danger of ulceration of gastrointestinal tract lining, as well as an increased anti-inflammatory response; pyrazilone derivatives potentiate corticosteroids at first, later they antagonize the corticosteroids (enzyme action)

Drug Patient Is Taking	*Use*	*Drug Dentist Prescribes*	*Actions That Result From the Combination*
		Narcotic analgesics	Aspirin plus narcotic analgesics potentiate analgesia and CNS depression
		Penicillin	Aspirin and the pyrazilone derivatives potentiate penicillin
		Sulfonamides	Aspirin and the pyrazilone derivatives potentiate sulfonamides
		Tranquilizers and nonbarbiturate sedatives	These CNS depressants are potentiated by analgesics; glutethimide (Doriden) inhibits dipyrone
Analgesics—strong, including narcotics: Alphaprodine HCl (Nisentil); anileridine (Leritine); dihydrocodeine bitartrate (Drocode; in Synalgos-DC); dihydromorphinone HCl (Dilaudid); fentanyl citrate (Sublimaze); levorphanol tartrate (Levo-Dromoran); meperidine HCl (Demerol); methadone HCI (Adanon, Amidone, Dolophine); morphine HCl and sulfate; nalorphine HCl (Naline); opium alkaloids; oxycodone HCl (in Percodan); oxymorphone HCl (in Numorphan); pimnidine ethanesulfonate (Alvodine); pentazocine (Talwin)	Moderate to severe pain relief	Atropine	Meperidine plus atropine is a hazardous combination in patients with glaucoma; narcotics potentiate atropine
		CNS depressants	All CNS depressants are potentiated by the narcotic analgesics
		Corticosteroids	Meperidine plus corticosteroids is also dangerous in glaucoma patients
		Pentazocine (Talwin)	The interaction of the opiate narcotics with pentazocine can precipitate withdrawal symptoms
Androgens (male hormones): Androsten (Androtex); androsterone; fluoxymesterone (Halotestin; Ora-Testryl, Ultandren);	Increase muscle tone; treat certain tumors	Antihistamines	Antihistamines inhibit some androgens and vice versa
		Barbiturates	Barbiturates inhibit androgens and vice versa

methyltesterone (Metandren, Neo-Hombreol-M, Oreton-M); norethandrolone (Nilevar); stanozolol (Winstrol); testosterone; etc.			
Anesthetics, local: Lidocaine (Xylocaine); mepivicaine (Carbocaine); prilocaine (Citanest); procaine (Novocain)	Local analgesia	CNS depressants	Depressant effects may be enhanced
		Epinephrine	Contraindicated in hyperthyroid patients and patients receiving thyroid drugs; also contraindicated in patients receiving many antihypertensives (e.g. guanethidine, reserpine) and anti-depressants, especially the MAO inhibitors
		Local anesthetics	Enhanced toxicity may occur with certain combinations of local anesthetics
		Sulfonamides	Local anesthetics with PABA nucleus (e.g. procaine) inhibit sulfonamides
Antacids: Aluminum hydroxide; calcium carbonate; magnesium carbonate; magnesium hydroxide; magnesium trisilicate; sodium bicarbonate	Treat gastric hyperacidity Treat gastric hypersecretions	Antibiotics	Antacids decrease the absorption of antibiotics such as penicillin G and tetracyclines from the gastrointestinal tract
		Aspirin	Antacids decrease the absorption of aspirin from the gastrointestinal tract
		Barbiturates	Antacids decrease the absorption of barbiturates from the gastrointestinal tract
		Sulfonamides	Antacids decrease the absorption of sulfonamides from the gastrointestinal tract
Anti-alcoholism agents: Disulfiram (Antabuse)	To control alcoholism	Sedatives	Antabuse potentiates sedative action
Anti-arrhythmia agents: Procainamide (Pronestyl); quinidine; quinidex; quinine; quinora	Treatment of heart rhythm irregularities Quinines also used for treatment of malaria	Gentamycin	Anti-arrhythmia agents plus gentamycin causes enhanced neuromuscular blocking; leads to apnea and muscle weakness; reaction with quinidine can be serious
		Lidocaine (Xylocaine)	Lidocaine plus procainamide may cause restlessness, a noisy patient, and visual hallucinations
		Procaine (Novocain)	Procaine potentiates the action of procainamide, and there is a cross allergy between them
Antibiotics: Bacitracin; carbenicillin;	Treat infectious diseases	Analgesics	Aspirin potentiates penicillin; chloramphenicol potentiates codeine

Drug Patient Is Taking	*Use*	*Drug Dentist Prescribes*	*Actions That Result From the Combination*
cephalosporins; (cephaloridine [Loridine] cephalothin [Keflin] cephalexin [Keflex]) chloramphenicol (Chloromycetin); clindamycin (Cleocin); erythromycin (Erythrocin, Ilosone); griseofulvin (Fulvicin, Grifulvin, Grisactin); lincomycin (Lincocin); novobiocin (Albamycin); oleandomycin (TAO); paromomycin (Humatin); penicillins (V-cillin K, Pen-V-Oral, Pentids 400, Staphcillin, Ampicillin, etc.); polymyxin B; streptomycin and related compounds (kanamycin, neomycin, gentamycin, di-hydro-streptomycin, etc.); tetracyclines (Aureomycin, Achromycin, Terramycin, Declomycin, etc.) Viomycin		Antihistamines and other sedatives	Griseofulvin enhances CNS depression
		Barbiturates	The interaction of kanamycin and some barbiturates may produce apnea and muscle weakness; chloramphenicol potentiates barbiturates; barbiturates inhibit griseofulvin; griseofulvin enhances CNS depression
		Chymotrypsin	Chymotrypsin potentiates tetracyclines
		Miscellaneous antibiotics	Bactericidal antibiotics (cephalosporins, penicillin) generally antagonize bacteriostatic antibiotics (erythromycin, tetracyclines, etc.); ampicillin (Alpen, polycillin) inhibits carbenicillin; chloramphenicol inhibits penicillin; neomycin inhibits penicillin; oleandomycin inhibits penicillin; paromomycin inhibits penicillin; tetracyclines inhibit novobiocin and penicillin; the neuromuscular blocking antibiotics (streptomycin, kanamycin, gentamycin, etc.) can cause a serious apnea and muscle weakness when they interact with each other; there is cross allergenicity between the cephalosporins and penicillin
		Promethazine (Phenergan)	Bacitracin, dihydro-streptomycin, gentamycin, kanamycin, neomycin, polymyxin B and streptomycin may produce a dangerous reaction with promethazine
Anticholinergic agents: Atropine; chlorphenoxamine (Phenoxene); scopolamine (Hyoscine); trihexphenidyl (Artane)	Dry secretions; decrease gastrointestinal mobility and secretions; anti-ulcer; anti-diarrhea	Antihistamines	*Hazardous combination in glaucoma; additive effect;* very dry mouth can occur
		Ascorbic acid (vitamin C)	Atropine inhibits vitamin C and vice versa
		Barbiturates	Chlorphenoxamine potentiates sedation by barbiturates
		CNS depressants	Scopolamine potentiates CNS depressants

		Corticosteroids	Hazardous combination in glaucoma
		Narcotic analgesics (meperidine [Demerol], alphaprodine [Nisentil])	Hazardous combination in glaucoma; narcotics potentiate atropine
		Sympatheticomimetics (epinephrine, norepinephrine, etc.)	Hazardous combination in glaucoma (narrow angle)
		Tranquilizers (benzodiazepines, phenothiazines)	Anticholinergics potentiate sedative effect of tranquilizers; tranquilizers potentiate anticholinergic effects
Anticoagulants (oral): Bishydroxycoumarin (Dicumarol); Danilone ethyl biscoumacetate (Tromexan); Indon; Miradon; phenindione (Dindevan, Hedulin) sodium warfarin (Merevan, Coumadin, Panwarfin)	Prevent clots in cardiac patients	Analgesics, aspirin, acetaminophen (Tylenol), mefenamic acid (Ponstel), narcotics	Analgesics increase the anticoagulant response; with aspirin and mefenamic acid, in combination with an anticoagulant, may get severe hemorrhage
		Antibiotics and sulfonamides	Antimicrobials inhibit vitamin K and thereby increase action of anticoagulants
		Antihistamines	Antihistamines vary in their response with anticoagulants
		Anti-inflammatory enzymes; bromelins (Ananase), chymotrypsin, papase, trypsin, Varidase	Anti-inflammatory enzymes may increase the anticoagulant effect
		Barbiturates	Barbiturates inhibit anticoagulants; combination may be serious
		Benzodiazepines (Librium, Valium, Serax)	Benzodiazepines vary in their response with anticoagulants
		Chloral hydrate (Noctec)	This action varies; some authorities stating chloral hydrate potentiates action of anticoagulants and others stating the reverse; can have severe hemorrhage through gastric lesion
		Corticosteroids	Corticosteroids tend to inhibit anticoagulants
		Ethchlorvynol (Placidyl), glutethimide (Doriden) and paraldehyde	These sedatives decrease the anticoagulant response
		Meprobamate (Equanil, Miltown)	Meprobamate decreases the anticoagulant response
		Methaqualone (Quaalude, Soper)	Methaqualone may potentiate the anticoagulant response
		Vitamin B complex	Vitamin B complex potentiates the anticoagulant response by increasing the prothrombin time

Drug Patient Is Taking	*Use*	*Drug Dentist Prescribes*	*Actions That Result From the Combination*
		Vitamin C	Vitamin C decreases the anticoagulant response by decreasing the prothrombin time
Anticonvulsants: Includes barbiturates and the sedatives diphenylhydantoin (Dilantin); ethosuximide; glutethimide (Doriden); phenacemide; primidone (Mysoline)	Treatment and prevention of epilepsy	Antihistamines, barbiturates, chloral hydrate, and glutethimide (Doriden)	These sedatives, which may also act as anticonvulsants, inhibit the other anticonvulsants; Dilantin and Mysoline may potentiate the sedative action of the barbiturates; the interaction of Dilantin and the barbiturates may also decrease the action of the barbiturates
		Aspirin	Aspirin (large doses) may potentiate Dilantin
		Corticosteroids	Dilantin inhibits the corticosteroids
		Diazepam (Valium)	Valium potentiates the anticonvulsants
		Narcotic analgesics	Narcotics potentiate the anticonvulsants; may be serious reaction
		Sulfonamides	Sulfonamides potentiate Dilantin; may cause serious reaction
Antidepressants: Tricyclic; amitriptyline (Elavil, Tryptizol); carbamazepine (Tegretol); desipramine (Norpramin, Pertofrane); doxepin (Sinequan); imipramine (Tofranil); nortriptyline (Aventyl); protriptyline (Vivactil, Concordin) *MAO inhibitors;* Furazolidone (Furoxone); iproniazid (Marsilid); isocarboxazid (Marplan); mebanazine (Actomol); nialamide (Niamid); pargyline (Eutonyl); phenelzine (Nardil); pivalolyl hydrazine, procarbazine (Matulane),	For depressed patients, neuroses, psychoses	Aspirin	Aspirin plus tricyclic antidepressants can be a serious reaction, especially if large doses of aspirin are taken
		Barbiturates and other sedatives	Anti-depressants potentiate sedation, may get severe hypotension (especially with MAOI's)
		Benzodiazepines, meprobamate and other tranquilizers	Antidepressants potentiate sedation, may get severe hypotension (especially with MAOI's); chlordiazepoxide (Librium) plus amitriptyline (Elavil) is potentially lethal
		CNS depressants such as: antihistamines; meperidine and other narcotics; glutethimide (Doriden)	These CNS depressants, when reacting with the tricyclic anti-depressants, produce a dangerous reaction for patients with glaucoma; can get severe dry mouth and potentiation of the CNS depression (potentially lethal) when any of the anti-depressants react with these CNS depressants; the interaction of an MAOI and meperidine may result in the inhibition of the MAOI
		Corticosteroids	Corticosteroids plus tricyclic depressants is a hazardous

			combination in glaucoma
tranylcypromine (Parnate)		Lidocaine (Xylocaine)	Patients receiving an MAOI (e.g. pargyline) may be refractory to local anesthetic effects of lidocaine
		Procaine (Novocain)	MAOI's may augment procaine effects
		Sympatheticomimetics (epinephrine, norepinephrine etc.)	Enhanced adrenergic effect from interaction of sympatheticomimetic with tricyclines; sympatheticomimetic plus MAOI's can cause acute hypertensive crisis (cranial hemorrhage, convulsions, coma, death)
Anti-diabetic agents: Insulin; sulfonureas; acetahexamide (Dymelor); chlorpropramide (Diabinese); tolazamide (Tolinase); tolbutamide (Orinase)	Hypoglycemic agents; used to treat diabetes	Aspirin	Aspirin potentiates action of antidiabetic agents
		Barbiturates and other sedatives	Antidiabetics may potentiate the depressive action of the sedatives
		Corticosteroids	Corticosteroids antagonize the anti-diabetic agents
		Epinephrine	Epinephrine antagonizes the anti-diabetic agents
		Sulfonamides	Sulfonamides potentiate the anti-diabetic agents
Anti-diarrheal medication: Attapulgite; diphenoxylate (in Lomotil); kaolin pectin (Kaopectate)	Prevent or treat diarrhea; anti-spasmotic	Antibiotics, especially lincomycin (Lincocin)	Kaopectate interferes with the adsorption and absorption of antibiotics, especially lincomycin
		Barbiturates	Lomotil may potentiate barbiturate sedation
Anti-diuretic hormones: Felypressin vasopressin (ADH, Pitressin)	Retain fluids	Acetaminophen (Nebs, Tempra, Tylenol)	Acetaminophen potentiates vasopressin
		Barbiturates	The interaction of barbiturates and antidiuretic hormones can cause cardiovascular collapse
Anti-emetics: Cyclizine (Marezine); dimenhydrinate (Dramamine); diphenidol (Vontrol)	Prevent vomiting (anti-nauseant)	Mepivicaine (Carbocaine)	In children and the aged, the combination of anti-emetics (high dose) and mepivicaine may cause CNS depression and extrapyramidal effects
Antihistamines: Antazoline (Antistine); brompheniramine maleate (Dimetane); carbinoxamine maleate (Clistin); chlorcyclizine HCl (Perazil); chlorpheniramine (Chlor-trimeton); clemizole (Allecur, Reactrol®);	Anti-allergy Anti-nauseant; sedative; tranquilizer (some); anti-cholinergic (some)	Analgesics	Interaction of antihistamines and analgesics potentiates CNS depression, especially in the beginning; some analgesics antagonize antihistamines; phenothiazines and meperidine is a dangerous combination
		Antihistamines	Use of more than one drug such as a phenothiazine and another antihistaminic potentiates the CNS depression
		Atropine	Atropine plus a phenothiazine potentiates the phenothiazine and the combination may precipitate glaucoma; atropine plus an antihistamine is dangerous in glaucoma.

Drug Patient Is Taking	Use	Drug Dentist Prescribes	Actions That Result From the Combination
cyproheptadiene HCl (Periactin); dimethindene maleate (Forhistal); dextro-brompheniramine maleate (Disomer); dextro-chlorpheniramine maleate (Polaramine); diphenhydramine HCl (Benadryl); diphenylpyraline HCl (Diafen, Hispril); methapyrilene (Histadyl, Thenylene); methdilazine HCl (Tacaryl); pheniramine maleate (Trimeton); phenothiazine and related drugs; chlorpromazine (Thorazine), mesoridazine (Serentil), pipazethate (Theratuss®), prochlorperazine (Compazine), promethazine HCl (Phenergan), pyrrobutamine phosphate (Pyronil), thioridazine (Mellaril), thonzylamine HCl (Anahist), trimeprazine tartrate (Temaril®), tripelennamine HCl (Pyribenzamine); triprolidine HCl (Actidil®); pyrilamine		Barbiturates and other sedatives	Interaction of sedative and antihistamine potentiates CNS depression, especially in the beginning; barbiturates inhibit antihistaminic action
		Benzodiazepines and other tranquilizers	Interaction of tranquilizer and antihistamine potentiates CNS depression, especially in the beginning; some tranquilizers inhibit antihistaminic action
		Corticosteroids	Antihistamines decrease effects of corticosteroids; combination is dangerous in glaucoma
		Gentamycin	Promethazine (Phenergan) plus gentamycin may cause enhanced neuro-muscular blocking with resultant apnea and muscle weakness
		Sympatheticomimetics (epinephrine, norepinephrine, phenylephrine)	Epinephrine plus a phenothiazine may cause paradoxical hypotension; with most antihistamines and sympatheticomimetic combinations, an enhanced adrenergic effect occurs

Antihypertensives: Alpha adrenergic blockers; phenoxybenzamine HCl (Dibenzyline), phentolamine HCl (Regitine), pronethalol, tolazoline HCl (Priscoline®), ganglionic blocking agents; chlorisondamine chloride (Ecolid), hexamethonium chloride, mecamylamine HCl (Inversive,) pentolinium tartrate (Ansolysen, Pempidine), tetra-ethylammonium chloride and bromide, trimethapan camyslate (Arfonad), trimethidinium, methosulfate (Ostensin) Norepinephrine depleters; guanethidine (Ismelin), methyldopa (Aldomet); Rauwolfia alkaloids; alseroxylon, rau (plus a suffix)— a whole host of drugs, rescinnamine, reserpine (Serpasil) Vasodilators including nitrates and nitrites; amyl nitrite, cyclandelate (Cyclospasmol); dioxyline phosphate (Paveril), erithrityl tetranitrate (Cardilate), glyceryl trinitrate,	Lower blood pressure for cardiacs, potential cardiacs, kidney disease, etc.	Acetaminophen (Tylenol)	Acetaminophen potentiates some antihypertensives
		Antihistamines	Tripelennamine and pyrilamine (antihistamines) partially inhibit the action of guanethidine (Ismelin); reserpine plus an antihistamine causes an increased CNS depression; nitrates and nitrites may potentiate anticholinergic effects of antihistamines
		Atropine	Atropine inhibits some veratrum alkaloids
		CNS depressants	Reserpine inhibits analgesic effect of morphine, meperidine (Demerol) and aspirin; combination of anti-hypertensives and CNS depressants (barbiturates, tranquilizers, sedatives, analgesics antihistamines, etc.) can cause increased CNS depression and orthostatic (postural) hypotension
		Corticosteroids	Chlorthalidone (Hygroton®) plus corticosteroids can cause the occurrence of excessive potassium depletion
		Diazepam (Valium)	Diazepam potentiates the antihypertensives
		Norepinephrine	Antihypertensives (guanethidine, methyl dopa) potentiate norepinephrine; phenylamine (Segontin) potentiates epinephrine

Drug Patient Is Taking	*Use*	*Drug Dentist Prescribes*	*Actions That Result From the Combination*
isosorbide dinitrate (Isordil); isoxsuprine (Vasodilan); mannitol hexanitrate (Nitranitol); nitroglycerin, pentaerythritol tetranitrate (Peritrate); phenylamine (Segontin) peutsery thrital tetranitrate, sodium nitrate, trolnitrate phosphate (Metamine, Nitrematin)			
Veratrum alkaloids; alkavervir (Veriloid); chlorthalidone (Hygroton); cryptenamine (Unitensen), hydralazine HCl (Apresoline), mebutamate (Capla); protoveratrines A and B			
Anti-inflammatory enzymes and flufenamic acid (an anti-inflammatory agent): Ananase; Buclamase; chymotrypsin (Chymar), flufenamic acid (Arlef), streptokinase, streptodornase (Varidase), trypsin	Resolve swellings; decrease swellings and other inflammatory responses	Aspirin	Aspirin inhibits flufenamic acid
		Penicillin, tetracyclines	Chymotrypsin plus either of these antibiotics results in an increased antibiotic action
		Sedatives	Many sedatives may inhibit the anti-inflammatory enzymes
Anti-microbials (*other than antibiotics*):	To prevent and treat infectious diseases	Ascorbic acid (vitamin C)	Sulfonamides inhibit vitamin C; vitamin C potentiates sulfonamides
Furazolidone (Furoxone; also see MAOI drugs); methenamine;		Aspirin	Aspirin potentiates sulfonamides
		Barbiturates and chloral hydrate	Some barbiturates inhibit nitrofurantoin and sulfonamides; furazolidone plus barbiturates or chloral hydrate

			results in potentiation of the sedative action
nitrofurantoin (Furadantin); sulfonamides		Local anesthetics of PABA type (e.g. procaine)	Local anesthetics inhibit sulfonamides
		Meperidine (Demerol)	The result of the interaction of furazolidone and meperidine is an enhanced CNS depression and an inhibition of furazolidone
		Paraldehyde	The sedative paraldehyde inhibits sulfonamides
		Penicillin	These are varying reactions with penicillin and sulfonamides, but sulfonamides usually potentiate penicillin
		Promethazine (Phenergan)	Phenergan potentiates sulfonamides
Anti-neoplastic and alkylating agents: Alkyl sulfonates; busulfan (Myleran) Ethlenimines; TEM, Thio-Tepa® Nitrogen mustards; chlorambucil (Leukeran), cyclophosphamide (Cytoxan, Endoxan),	Anti-neoplastic; treat nephrosis, collagen diseases; immunosupressives (for transplants)	Analgesics	Aspirin potentiates 5-fluorouracil, mercapto-purine, Imuran, methotrexate and thiotepa; methotrexate plus aspirin can lead to pancytopenia; interaction of narcotics with methotrexate may also increase the toxicity of the methotrexate
mechlorethamine HCl (Mustargen), melphalan (Alkeran), uracil mustard,		Barbiturates and tranquilizers	Barbiturates potentiate cyclophosphamide; barbiturates and tranquilizers potentiate 5-fluorouracil, mercaptopurine, Imuran, methotrexate and Thio-Tepa; urethan inhibits some barbiturates
anti-metabolites; azothioprine (Imuran), D-actinomycin (Actinomycin D), 5-fluorouracil etc.		Corticosteroids	Negative nitrogen balance and muscle wasting occurs from reaction between Imuran and corticosteroids; prednisone plus mercapto-purine can cause hyperuricemia; prednisone may inhibit cyclophosphamide
6-mercapto-purine (Purimethol, Purinethol)		Penicillin	Actinomycin inhibits penicillin
Methotrexate Urethan (Urethane)		Sulfonamides	Sulfonamides potentiate 5-fluorouracil, mercaptopurine, Imuran, methotrexate and Thio-Tepa; methotrexate plus sulfonamides can lead to pancytopenia
Anti-parkisonism drugs: Benztropine mesylate (Cogentin);		Antihistamines	Anti-parkinsonism drugs plus antihistamines can lead to a dry mouth and constipation
biperiden (Akineton);		Barbiturates	Orphenadrine antagonizes some barbiturates
chlorphenoxamine HCl (Phenoxene);		Propoxyphene (Darvon)	The interaction of propoxyphene and orphenadrine can cause mental confusion, tremors and anxiety

Drug Patient Is Taking	Use	Drug Dentist Prescribes	Actions That Result From the Combination
cycrimine HCl (Pagitane HCl); ethopropazine HCl (Parsidol); L-dopa Orphenadrine HCl (Disipal, Norflex); Procyclidine (Kemadrin); trihexyphenidyl (Artane)		Vitamin B-6 (Pyridoxine)	Interaction of L-dopa and vitamin B-6 reduces the effect of L-dopa
Anti-thyroid drugs	Treat hyperthyroidism	Benzodiazepine and tranquilizers (Librium, Valium)	Increased anti-thyroid effect; probably only of importance with prolonged use of tranquilizers
Anti-tuberculosis drugs (e.g. isoniazid)	Treat tuberculosis	Atropine	Hazardous combination for patients with glaucoma
		Barbiturates and other sedatives	Isoniazid potentiates the sedative action
		Narcotic analgesics	Isoniazid potentiates the narcotics; meperidine and isoniazid is a hazardous combination for glaucoma patients
		Sulfonamides	Isoniazid plus sulfonamides may cause acute hemolytic anemia
Anti-viral eye preparations (e.g. Stoxil)	Treat eye infections	Corticosteroids	This combination can cause the spread of infection
Barbiturates: Amobarbital (Amytal); cabrital; pentobarbital (Nembutal); phenobarbital (Luminal); secobarbital (Seconal)	Sedative and hypnotic	Analgesics	CNS depression is enhanced; barbiturates inhibit meperidine (Demerol) and aspirin
		Antihistamines	Interaction of barbiturates and antihistamines especially in the beginning results in enhancement of CNS depression; barbiturates inhibit antihistaminic action
		Anti-inflammatory enzymes	Barbiturates inhibit anti-inflammatory enzymes
		Ascorbic acid (vitamin C)	Vitamin C potentiates barbiturates; barbiturates inhibit vitamin C
		Benzodiazepines (Valium, Librium)	Barbiturates potentiate Benzodiazepines
		Corticosteroids	Barbiturates inhibit corticosteroids; corticosteroids potentiate barbiturates
		Felypressin (a vasoconstrictor found in some local anesthetics such as Citanest [non U.S.	Barbiturates plus felypressin can cause cardiovascular collapse

		preparations])	
		Meprobamate (Equanil, Miltown) and other tranquilizers	Interaction of barbiturates and tranquilizers results in augmentation of CNS depression; later interference occurs between the groups
		Sedatives	Interaction of barbiturates and sedatives results in increase of CNS depression in the beginning; later interference occurs between the groups
		Sulfonamides	Barbiturates inhibit sulfonamides
Calcium salts: Calcium carbonate; calcium chloride; calcium gluconate; calcium lactate	Antacids; nutritional supplement; treat hypoparathyroidism; for use in electrolyte balancing	Cephalosporins (Keflex, etc.)	Cephalosporins are incompatible with calcium
		Narcotic analgesics	Calcium may inhibit the narcotics
		Tetracyclines	Calcium inhibits tetracyclines
Cathartics: e.g. mineral oil	Laxative	Tetracyclines	Cathartics inhibit tetracyclines
Cholinergics: Indirect type; (anticholinesterases), ambenonium (Mytelase), demecarium bromide (Humorsol), echothiophate iodide (Phospholine), isofluorophate (Floropryl), neostigmine (Prostigmin), physostigmine, pyridostigmine (Mestinon), direct type; acetylcholine, bethanechol, carbachol, methacholine, pilocarpine	Treat glaucoma	Antihistamines	Antihistamines antagonize cholinergics; anticholinesterases potentiate sedation of antihistamines
		Atropine	Atropine inhibits the cholinergics
		Barbiturates	Anticholinesterases potentiate sedation of barbiturates
		Corticosteroids	Corticosteroids antagonize cholinergic effect
		Morphine and other narcotics	Morphine potentiates cholinergic effect; neostigmine potentiates action of morphine, meperidine, and methadone
		Procaine (Novocain)	Physostigmine antagonizes the action of procaine at the neuro-muscular junction
		Sympatheticomimetics (epinephrine, norepinephrine, etc.)	Sympatheticomimetics antagonize the cholinergics

Drug Patient Is Taking	Use	Drug Dentist Prescribes	Actions That Result From the Combination
Cocaine	Formerly a local anesthetic; a CNS stimulant; drug abuse; limited use in some nasal preparations as a topical anesthetic	Sympatheticomimetics (epinephrine, norepinephrine)	If the patient receives this combination systemically, serious results may follow such as cardiac arrhythmias, convulsions, and vasomotor collapse.
Corticosteroids: Cortisone (Cortone); dexamethasone (Decadron); desoxycorticosterone (Percoten); hydrocortisone (Cortiphate, Cortisol, Cortril); neo-Cortef; prednisolone (Meticortelone, Paracortrol, Delta-Cortef, Hydeltra); prednisone (Meticorten, Paracort, Deltasone, Deltra) Triamcinolone (Aristacort)	Anti-inflammatory; treat collagen diseases	Antihistamines	Antihistamines antagonize corticosteroids; combination is dangerous in glaucoma
		Aspirin	Aspirin plus corticosteroids causes increased danger of ulceration of gastrointestinal tract lining; also an increased anti-inflammatory response and analgesic effect
		Barbiturates and other sedatives	Barbiturates and other sedatives inhibit corticosteroids; corticosteroids potentiate barbiturates and other sedatives
		Meperidine (Demerol)	Meperidine plus corticosteroids is a dangerous combination in glaucoma patients
		Sympatheticomimetics (epinephrine, norepinephrine, etc.)	Corticosteroids plus sympatheticomimetics is also hazardous in glaucoma and dangerous in asthma
Digitalis and digitalis glycosides: Acetyldigitoxin (Acylanid); deslanoside (Cedilanid-D); digitoxin (Crystodigin, Digitalline nativelle, Myodigin, Purodigin); digoxin (Davoxin, Lanoxin, Saroxin); gitalin (Gitaligin); lanatoside C (Cedilanid)	Treat congestive heart failure	Corticosteroids	This combination can lead to hypokalemia, which would lead to enhanced digitalis toxicity
		Sympatheticomimetics (epinephrine, etc.)	Sympatheticomimetics plus digitalis can lead to cardiac arrhythmias
		Tetracyclines and lincomycin	Use of tetracyclines and lincomycin can cause diarrhea, which results in potassium loss; the effect increases the toxicity of digitalis
Diuretics: Amisometradine (Rolicton); chlorthalidone; ethacrynic acid; furosemide	To lose fluid; treat edema (especially in cardiacs)	Aspirin	Thiazide diuretics plus aspirin can increase the chance of acute gout occurring in predisposed individuals; the tendency is enhanced if alcohol is added to the combination

(Frusemide, Lasix); guinethazone (Hydromox); spironolactone triamterene (Dyrenium); mercurial diuretics; chlormerodrin (Neohydrin), meralluride (Mercuhydrin), mercaptomerin (Thiomerin), mercurophylline (Mercupurine), merethoxylline (Dicurin), thiazide diuretics; bendroflumethiazide (Naturetin), benzthiazide (Aquatag, Exna), chlorothiazide (Diuril), cyclothiazide (Anhydron), hydrochlorthiazide (HydroDIURIL), hydroflumethiazide (Saluron); polythiazide (Renese); trichlormethiazide (Metahydrin, Naqua)		Barbiturates	Barbiturates plus thiazide diuretics [illegible] static hypotension
		Corticosteroids	Corticosteroids plus diuretics can cause excessive potassium loss
		Narcotic analgesics	Narcotics may inhibit mercurial diuretics; the combination of diuretics plus the narcotics can potentiate orthostatic hypotension
Ergot alkaloids: ergonovine (Ergotrate); ergotamine tartrate (Cafergot, Gynergen, Medihaler-Ergotamine); methylergonovine tartrate (Methergine)	To treat vasodilating pain and migraine headaches; induce labor	Sympatheticomimetics (epinephrine, etc.)	This interaction may cause extreme elevation of blood pressure
Estrogens e.g. estradiol	Menopausal therapy; to treat some male tumors	Barbiturates	Barbiturates may inhibit estrogens
		Meprobamate (Equanil, Miltown)	Meprobamate may inhibit estrogens
Foods, drink and dietary supplements: Blue cheese; iron salts; ferrous bromide, ferrous fumarate,	Food; dietary supplement; to treat iron-deficiency anemia	Ascorbic acid (vitamin C)	High vitamin C enhances iron absorption
		Penicillin	Blue cheese inhibits penicillin
		Tetracyclines	Iron salts inhibit tetracylines

Drug Patient Is Taking	*Use*	*Drug Dentist Prescribes*	*Actions That Result From the Combination*
ferrous carbonate, ferrous gluconate, ferrous iodide, ferrous lactate, ferrous sulfate etc.,			
1-glutavite (monosodium 1-glutamate and vitamins);	Dietary supplement	Meprobamate (Equanil, Miltown)	1-glutavite potentiates meprobamate's action
milk and milk products;	Drink	Tetracyclines	Milk and milk products inhibit tetracyclines
Pressor containing foods; broad bean pods (contain dopa), fruits such as bananas, pineapples, plums (contain serotonin), some alcoholic beverages (contain histamine)			
Tyramine-rich foods; beer, brie, beef liver, chicken, cheddar cheeses such as camembert, Stilton and other ripe types, Chianti-wine, chocolate, fermented foods, figs, kippered herring, meat extracts (Bovril), pickled herring;	Food	Morphine	Tyramine antagonizes analgesic effect
Vitamins; ascorbic acid (vitamin C),	Aid in healing	Aspirin	Vitamin C potentiates aspirin; aspirin inhibits vitamin C
		Atropine	Vitamin C inhibits atropine; atropine inhibits vitamin C
		Barbiturates	Vitamin C potentiates barbiturates; barbiturates inhibit vitamin C
		Sulfonamides	Vitamin C potentiates sulfonamides; sulfonamides inhibit vitamin C
riboflavin,		Tetracylines	Riboflavin inhibits tetracyclines
vitamin K (menadiol sodium diphosphate [Kappadione, Synkayvite], menadione [vitamin K_3], menadione sodium bisulfite [Hykinone], phytomenad-		Antibiotics	Antibiotics inhibit intestinal vitamin K; hence a decreased action would occur from a vitamin K supplement

ione, phytonadione [Aqua MEPHYTON, Konakion, Mephyton, Mono-Kay], Vitamin Kl);			
Xanthines—in drinks; caffeine (in coffee, cocoa, kola-nut, cola, maté and tea); theobromine (in cocoa); theophylline (in tea); Xanthines—not in drinks; aminophylline, choledyl, glucophylline, neothylline, tulfyllin	Stimulating beverage, CNS stimulants, diuretics	Propoxyphene (Darvon)	Excessive caffeine plus propoxyphene can be a dangerous combination
		Sedatives	Patients who have consumed several cups of beverages containing xanthines would require a higher dose of a sedative
Hallucinogenic agents: Lysergic acid-diethyl amide (LSD); mescaline; psilocybin	Drug abuse	Sedatives and tranquilizers	Normal dose of sedative or tranquilizer may not be effective
Histamine producers: Betahistine HCl; Betazole (Histalog)	To treat Meniere's syndrome (middle ear disease); action is vasodilation	Antihistamines	Antihistamines antagonize histamine producers
Muscle relaxants: Central acting; carisoprodol (Rela, Soma), chlorzoxazone (Paraflex),	Muscle relaxation	Antihistamines, barbiturates and other sedatives	Antihistamines, barbiturates and other sedatives may inhibit muscle relaxants
		Diazepam (Valium)	Valium plus curariform muscle relaxants can induce neuromuscular blockage with apnea and muscle weakness
mephenesin (Myanesin, Tolseram, Tolserol), methocarbamol (Robaxin),		Epinephrine	Epinephrine inhibits curariform agents
		Gentamycin (Garomycin)	Gentamycin plus peripheral acting muscle relaxants potentiate neuromuscular blockage; can cause apnea and muscle weakness
styramate (Sinaxar), zoxazolamine (Flexin) Peripheral acting (neuromuscular blocking agents); curariform; dimethyl tubocurarine iodide (Metubine, Mesotrin), d-tubocurarine, gallamine triethiodide (Flaxedil), depolarizing;		Local anesthetics	Local anesthetics plus succinylcholine can prolong apnea
		Meprobamate (Equanil, Miltown)	Carisoprodol and meprobamate show cross allergenicity; carisoprodol inhibits meprobamate
		Other CNS depressants	Muscle relaxants enhance CNS depressants

Drug Patient Is Taking	*Use*	*Drug Dentist Prescribes*	*Actions That Result From the Combination*
benzoquinonium (Mytolon), decamethonium (Syncurine), succinylcholine chloride (Anectine)			
Oral contraceptives: Demulen; Enovid; Norlestrin; Norinyl; Ortho-novum; Ovulen; progesterone (in oral contraceptives)	Prevent pregnancy	Antihistamines; barbiturates, meprobamate, and other tranquilizers	These CNS depressants tend to inhibit oral contraceptives and progesterone
		Meperidine (Demerol)	Oral contraceptives potentiate meperidine
Oxytocics: Oxytocin (Pitocin, Synctocinon)	Induce labor	Sympatheticomimetics (epinephrine, norepinephine)	The result of this interaction can cause a severe persistent hypertension
Parathormone Parathyroid hormone	To treat hypoparathyroid patients	Corticosteroids	Corticosteroids inhibit parathormone
PABA (para amino benzoic acid)	Can be used to treat "collagen diseases"	Aspirin	PABA potentiates aspirin
		Penicillin	PABA potentiates penicillin
		Sulfonamides	PABA inhibits sulfonamides
Pollutants, Air: Polluted air may contain; carbon monoxide, halogenated insecticides (Aldrin, chlordane, DDT); hydrocarbons, nitrogen, phosphorus compounds, sulfur	Insecticides, indirectly causes air pollution	Barbiturates	Halogenated insecticides are enzyme inducers and can decrease the action of barbiturates
		Pentazocine (Talwin)	Air pollutants can interfere with the action of pentazocine
Sedatives (other than barbiturates): Chloral hydrate (Noctec); ethchlorvynol (Placidyl); glutethimide (Doriden); methaqualone (Quaalude, Soper); paraldehyde	Sedation and hypnosis	Barbiturates, sedatives and other CNS depressants	Interaction of these drugs potentiates CNS depression; glutethimide inhibits antihistamines and meprobamate
		Corticosteroids	Chloral hydrate and glutethimide decrease corticosteroid action
		Sulfonamides	Paraldehyde inhibits sulfonamides

Smoking: Charcoal broiled foods (contain benzpyrene); tobacco smoke (contains benzyprene, nicotine)	Satisfaction, habit	Barbiturates and benzodiazepines (Librium, Valium)	Smoking inhibits barbiturates and benzodiazepines (by enzyme induction)
		Corticosteroids	Smoking increases endogenous corticosteroids; hence action of corticosteroids is potentiated
		Pentazocine (Talwin)	Smoking inhibits pentazocine
Sympatheticomimetics: Amphetamines; amphetamine (Benzedrine, Raphetamine), dextro-amphetamine (Dexedrine, d-Amfetasul), metamphetamine (Desoxyn, Amphedroxyn, Desyphed, Desoxephedrine, Doxyfed, Dexoval, Norordin, Efroxine, Semoxydrine, Syndrox), Anorexiants; benzphetamine, diethylpropion, phendimetrazine, phenmetrazine, phentermine, Catecholamines; dopamine, epinephrine (Adrenaline), ephedrine, isoproterenol (Isuprel), isoxysuprine, metaproterenol, metaraminol, mephentermine, nordefrin, norepinephrine (Levarterenol, Levophed, Noradrenaline), nylidrin, phenylephrine (Neo-Synephrine), protokylol, tyramine Local vasconstrictors; cyclopentamine, hylometazoline, naphazoline, oxymetazoline, phenylpropanolamine, propylhexedrine, tetrahydrozoline, tuaminoheptane	Treat asthma; nasal decongestion; weight loss; keep alert (CNS stimulants); emergency treatment of depression	Antihistamines	Antihistamines counteract the effects of amphetamines; antihistamines may potentiate the pressor effects of the other sympatheticomimetics
		Corticosteroids	Corticosteroids plus sympatheticomimetics can be a hazardous combination in asthma and glaucoma
		Epinephrine	Epinephrine with one of the other sympatheticomimetics can be a hazardous combination in asthma; methylphenidate plus epinephrine can precipitate a hypertensive crisis, and is a hazardous combination in asthma
		Narcotic analgesics	Dopamine and tyramine antagonize morphine; amphetamines enhance meperidine
		Propoxyphene (Darvon)	Interaction of Darvon (excessive amounts) and amphetamine is a potentially lethal interaction

Drug Patient Is Taking	*Use*	*Drug Dentist Prescribes*	*Actions That Result From the Combination*
Methylphenidate (Ritalin)	Psychomotor stimulant		
Thyroid preparations: Cytomel; dextrothyroxine (Choloxin); Euthroid; 1-thyroxine (Synthroid); Letter; Levoid; levothyroxine; liothyronine; liotrix; Proloid; thyroid gland; thyrolar; triodothyronine (Cytomel)	To treat hypothyroid condition, for weight reduction	Barbiturates	Because of increased metabolism produced by the thyroid hormone, may need increased barbiturate dosage to get effective sedation; however, interaction of Synthroid and a barbiturate leads to a decreased rate of metabolism
		Meperidine (Demerol)	Cholexin potentiates meperidine
		Sympatheticomimetics (epinephrine, norepinephrine)	Interaction may precipitate cardiac insufficiency
Tranquilizers and anti-anxiety agents: Acetophenazine maleate (Tindal); azacyclonol HCl (Frenquel); buclizine (Softran); butaperazine maleate (Repoise); captodiame HCl (Suvren); chlordiazepoxide HCl (Librium); chlormezanone (Trancopal); chlorpromazine (Thorazine); diazepam (Valium); droperidol (Inapsine); fluphenazine (Prolixin); haloperidol (Haldol); hydroxyphenamate (Listica); hydroxyzine (Atarax, Vistaril); meprobamate (Equanil, Miltown); mesoridazine besylate (Serentil); oxanamide (Quiactin); oxazepam (Serax);	Tranquilization; treat neuroses; relax patients	Atropine	Atropine is potentiated by the thioxanthenes
		Barbiturates	This interaction results in pronounced CNS depression; later inhibition occurs as a result of enzyme induction
		CNS depressants: e.g. antihistamines, narcotics, and tranquilizers	This interaction results in potentiation of CNS depression; interaction of tranquilizers and meperidine can lead to severe depression; interaction of Librium and codeine can lead to coma
		Epinephrine	The thioxanthenes (Clopenthixol, chlorprothixene and triothixene) inteaction with epinephrine causes epinephrine reversal and severe hypotension

perphenazine (Trilafon); phenaglycodol (Ultran); prochlorperazine (Compazine); piperactazine (Quide); promazine HCl (Sparine); thiopropazate HCl (Dartal); thioridazine HCl (Mellaril); thiothixene (Navane); thioxanthenes; clopenthixol (Sordinol), chlorprothixene (Taractan), triothixene; trifluoperazine (Stelazine); triflupromazine HCl (Vesprin); tybamate (Solacen)			
Uricosuric agents: Allopurinol (Zyloprim); probenecid (Benemid)	To treat gout	Aspirin	Aspirin inhibits the action of the uricosuric agents
		Erythromycin	Probencid inhibits erythromycin
		Penicillin	Probencid potentiates penicillin
		Sulfonamides	Probencid potentiates sulfonamides

BIBLIOGRAPHY

Medical Tests

American Dental Association: *Accepted Dental Therapeutics 1973/1974,* 35th ed. Chicago, American Dental Association, 1973.

Davidsohn, I., and Henry, J. B.: *Todd-Sanford Clinical Diagnosis by Laboratory Methods,* 14th ed. Philadelphia, Saunders, 1969.

Mitchell, D. F., Standish, S. M., and Fast, T. B.: *Oral Diagnosis/Oral Medicine,* 2nd ed. Philadelphia, Lea & Febiger, 1971.

Eruption and Calcification Table

Mitchell, D. F., Standish, S. M., and Fast, T. B.: *Oral Diagnosis/Oral Medicine,* 2nd ed. Philadelphia, Lea & Febiger, 1971.

Seltzer, S.: *Endodontology: Biologic Considerations in Endodontic Procedures.* New York, McGraw, 1971.

Drug Interactions

American Dental Association: *Accepted Dental Therapeutics 1973/1974,* 35th ed. Chicago, American Dental Association, 1973.

Arthur, J.: A dental viewpoint of drug interactions. *J Indiana Dent Assoc, 52*:52, 1973.

Cadwallader, D. E.: *Biopharmaceutics and Drug Interactions.* Nutley, Roche Laboratories, 1971.

Goldman, V., Astrom, A., and Evers, H.: A study of the interaction between a tricyclic antidepressant and some local anaesthetic solutions containing vasoconstrictors. *J Hosp Dent Prac, 5*:176, 1971.

Hussar, D. A.: Interactions involving drugs used in dental practice. *JADA, 87*:349, 1973.

Martin, E. W.: *Hazards of Medication: A Manual on Drug Interactions, Incompatibilities, Contraindications, and Adverse Effects.* Philadelphia, Lippincott, 1971.

Wynn, R. L.: Interactions of drugs used in dentistry-clinical implications and methods of prevention. *J Baltimore Coll Dent Surg, 26*:20, 1971.

INDEX

B

D

I

J

K

L

O